Preface

Congratulations! You are about to read the most factual book on menopause in existence today. This textbook, *Menopause Practice: A Clinician's Guide*, 3rd edition, has been developed by the NAMS Professional Education Committee to meet the need for updated provider education. This textbook is published solely by The North American Menopause Society (NAMS) and is approved by the NAMS Board of Trustees. The book thus represents a collaborative input of dozens of experts in all modes of medical expertise. In its pages are practical recommendations to assist clinicians in every aspect of menopause management.

The need for menopause education has never been greater. The numbers of aging women are increasing worldwide to a record level. Every day in just North America alone, over 6,000 women reach menopause. Menopause presents an ideal opportunity to change and improve health practices and enhance quality of life for women.

In the research arena, new findings continue to add to our knowledge. Conflicting findings, however, may add to the challenges to inform our patients and impact their health decisions through menopause and beyond. That's where NAMS plays an important role. As the preeminent scientific organization addressing menopause, NAMS is committed to quality educational offerings.

Knowledge about and the need to manage menopause are increasing at a phenomenal pace. This book is state of the science. But, to maintain your expertise, I truly encourage you to join NAMS. The Society has multiple offerings that will keep you up to date and on the front lines.

Special thanks are owed to the experts who wrote the sections, as well as the NAMS Professional Education Committee, the NAMS Board of Trustees, and the editorial staff who all contributed so much of their knowledge, time, and energy. The Society is grateful to Novo Nordisk, Inc., for its generous grant that supported the textbook's development; please note that the grantor exercised absolutely no control over its contents.

Best wishes in your efforts. We know that menopause practitioners and their patients will benefit from *Menopause Practice*.

Wulf H. Utian

Wulf H. Utian, MD, PhD, FRCOG, FACOG, FICS
Executive Director
Chair, CME Committee
The North American Menopause Society

Table of Contents

CME Activity

Menopause Practice: A Clinician's Guide has been developed by The North American Menopause Society (NAMS) to meet the healthcare provider's need for updated menopause education. NAMS has designated this textbook a continuing medical education (CME) activity.

Release date. October 31, 2007.

Expiration date. October 31, 2009.

Goal. To demonstrate an increase in, or affirmation of, knowledge regarding the clinical management of menopause-associated symptoms and diseases later in life that are associated with diminished hormone levels and aging.

Learning objectives. After reading this textbook, participants should be able to:

- Utilize correct terminology for menopause-related conditions and treatments.
- Distinguish normal physical, hormonal, and emotional changes at menopause from the pathophysiologic conditions and effects related to aging.
- Identify women's risk factors for development of common diseases at midlife and beyond, such as osteoporosis, cardiovascular disease, diabetes, and cancer.
- Describe appropriate health evaluation, risk assessment, and screening methods for women in peri- and postmenopause.
- Integrate the clinical findings and develop lifestyle and pharmacologic risk reduction and treatment strategies in collaboration with each woman for menopause symptoms and disease.
- Summarize current research regarding the use of complementary and alternative medicine (CAM) treatments for menopause-related conditions.
- Prepare appropriate counseling strategies that lead to positive lifestyle changes for women at menopause and beyond.

Target audience. This educational activity has been developed to meet the educational needs of multidisciplinary healthcare professionals who provide care to peri- and postmenopausal women.

Accreditation. NAMS is accredited by the Accreditation Council for Continuing Medical Education (ACCME) to provide continuing medical education for physicians. NAMS designates this educational activity for a maximum of 25 *AMA PRA Category I Credits*™. Physicians should only claim credit commensurate with the extent of their participation in the activity.

Instructions. Program participants should complete the CME self-assessment examination provided on page **to come** of this textbook. No administrative fee is required.

Commercial support. The CME activity is supported by an unrestricted educational grant from Novo Nordisk, Inc.

Contributors

NAMS appreciates the efforts of all contributors to the content of this textbook. Authors, editors, and reviewers are listed on the following pages. The textbook was approved by the NAMS 2006-2007 Professional Education Committee (*), then approved by the NAMS 2006-2007 Board of Trustees (†).

Gloria A. Bachmann, MD*
Associate Dean for Women's Health
Professor of Obstetrics and Gynecology and Medicine
University of Medicine and Dentistry of New Jersey
Director of Women's Health Institute
Chief of OB/GYN Service
Robert Wood Johnson University Hospital
New Brunswick, NJ

Glenn D. Braunstein, MD
Chairman
Department of Medicine
Cedars-Sinai Medical Center
Professor of Medicine
The David Geffen School of Medicine at UCLA
Los Angeles, CA

Thomas B. Clarkson, DVM†*
Professor of Comparative Medicine
Comparative Medicine Clinical Research Center
Wake Forest University School of Medicine
Winston-Salem, NC

Elizabeth Contestabile, RNC, BScN
Nurse Educator
Shirley E. Greenberg Women's Health Centre
The Ottawa Hospital
Ottawa, ON, Canada

Odelia Cooper, MD
Fellow
Division of Endocrinology, Diabetes, and Metabolism
Department of Medicine
Cedars-Sinai Medical Center
The David Geffen School of Medicine at UCLA
Los Angeles, CA

Esther Eisenberg, MD, MPH*
Professor of Obstetrics and Gynecology
Vanderbilt University School of Medicine
Nashville, TN

Robert R. Freedman, PhD†
Professor
Departments of Psychiatry and Obstetrics and Gynecology
Wayne State University School of Medicine
Detroit, MI

J. Chris Gallagher, MD†
Professor of Medicine
Creighton University
Division of Endocrinology
Section of Bone Metabolism
Omaha, NE

Steven R. Goldstein, MD†*
Professor of Obstetrics and Gynecology
New York University School of Medicine
New York, NY

George I. Gorodeski, MD, PhD†
Professor of Reproductive Biology, Oncology,
  and Physiology and Biophysics
Case Western Reserve University School of Medicine
Case Medical Center
Department of Obstetrics and Gynecology
Cleveland, OH

Keri L. Greenseid, MD
Fellow
Division of Reproductive Endocrinology
Department of Obstetrics and Gynecology
Albert Einstein College of Medicine
Bronx, NY

Robert P. Heaney, MD
John A. Creighton University Professor and
  Professor of Medicine
Department of Internal Medicine
Creighton University
Omaha, NE

Victor W. Henderson, MD, MS†
Professor
Departments of Health Research & Policy and of
  Neurology & Neurological Sciences
Stanford School of Medicine
Stanford, CA

Andrew G. Herzog, MD, MSc
Professor of Neurology
Harvard Medical School
Director, Neuroendocrine Unit
Beth Israel Deaconess Medical Center
Boston, MA

Susan R. Johnson, MD, MS
Associate Provost for Faculty
University of Iowa
Iowa City, IA

Catherine Juve, PhD, MSPH, MN, CNP, RN*
Senior Teaching Specialist
School of Nursing
University of Minnesota Twin Cities
Minneapolis, MN

Risa Kagan, MD†*
Clinical Professor
Department of Obstetrics, Gynecology, and
  Reproductive Sciences
University of California, San Francisco
San Francisco, CA

Andrew M. Kaunitz, MD
Professor and Assistant Chairman
Department of Obstetrics and Gynecology
University of Florida College of Medicine
Jacksonville, FL

Julie Lew, MD
Clinical Fellow
National Eye Institute
National Institutes of Health
Bethesda, MD

Tieraona Low Dog, MD
Director of Education
Program in Integrative Medicine
Clinical Assistant Professor
Department of Medicine
University of Arizona Health Sciences
Tucson, AZ

Mark G. Martens, MD
Professor of Obstetrics and Gynecology
University of Oklahoma
Tulsa, OK

Michael R. McClung, MD, FACP
Founding Director
Oregon Osteoporosis Center
Assistant Director
Department of Medical Education
Providence Portland Medical Center
Portland, OR

Margaret F. Moloney, RN, PhD, ANP
Associate Professor
Byrdine F. Lewis School of Nursing
Georgia State University
Atlanta, GA

Katherine M. Newton, PhD
Associate Director for External Research
Group Health Center for Health Studies
Affiliate Associate Professor
Department of Epidemiology and School of Nursing
University of Washington
Seattle, WA

Joan Otomo-Corgel, DDS, MPH, FACD
Adjunct Assistant Professor
UCLA School of Dentistry
Department of Periodontics
Faculty and Chair, Postgraduate Research
Greater Los Angeles VA Health Care Center
Los Angeles, CA

JoAnn V. Pinkerton, MD†
Professor
Department of Obstetrics and Gynecology
Medical Director, The Women's Place, Midlife Health Center
University of Virginia Health Sciences Center
Charlottesville, VA

Natalie Rasgon, MD, PhD
Professor of Psychiatry and Obstetrics and Gynecology
Stanford School of Medicine
Director, Stanford Center for Neuroscience in Women's Health
Stanford, CA

Veronica A. Ravnikar, MD
Associate Clinical Professor
Harvard Medical School
Boston, MA
Chair of Obstetrics and Gynecology
South Shore Hospital
South Weymouth, MA

Nancy K. Reame, MSN, PhD, FAAN†
Mary Dickey Lindsay Professor of Nursing
Director, DNSc Program
Columbia University School of Nursing
New York, NY

Marcie K. Richardson, MD
Co-Director
Harvard Vanguard Menopause Consultation Service
Boston, MA

Marilyn L. Rothert, PhD, RN, FAAN
Professor Emerita and Dean Emerita
College of Nursing
Michigan State University
East Lansing, MI

Nanette Santoro, MD
Director, Division of Reproductive Endocrinology
Department of Obstetrics, Gynecology and Women's Health
Albert Einstein College of Medicine
Bronx, NY

Isaac Schiff, MD†
Joe Vincent Meigs Professor of Gynecology
Harvard Medical School
Chief, Vincent Memorial Obstetrics and Gynecology Service
Massachusetts General Hospital
Boston, MA

Peter E. Schwartz, MD
John Slate Ely Professor of Obstetrics and Gynecology
Vice Chair, Gynecology
Department of Obstetrics, Gynecology and the
 Reproductive Sciences
Yale University School of Medicine
New Haven, CT

Joan L. Shaver, PhD, RN, FAAN
Professor and Dean
College of Nursing
University of Illinois at Chicago
Chicago, IL

Jan L. Shifren, MD
Associate Professor of Obstetrics, Gynecology and
 Reproductive Biology
Harvard Medical School
Director, Vincent Menopause Program
Vincent Memorial Obstetrics and Gynecology Service
Massachusetts General Hospital
Boston, MA

Janine A. Smith, MD
Deputy Clinical Director
National Eye Institute
National Institutes of Health
Bethesda, MD

Steven Sorin, MD
Assistant Professor of Medicine
Case Western Reserve University School of Medicine
Cleveland, OH

Leon Speroff, MD†
Professor of Obstetrics and Gynecology
Oregon Health and Science University
Portland, OR

Martha G. Stassinos, PharmD
Clinical Pharmacist Specialist
Berkeley, CA

Cynthia A. Stuenkel, MD†
Clinical Professor of Medicine
University of California, San Diego
La Jolla, CA

Holly L. Thacker, MD, FACP*
Director, Women's Health Center
Cleveland Clinic
Associate Professor, Cleveland Clinic Lerner
 College of Medicine
Case Western Reserve University
Cleveland, OH

James A. Underberg, MD, MS, FACPM, FACP
Clinical Assistant Professor
Department of Medicine
New York University Medical School
New York, NY

Wulf H. Utian, MD, PhD†
Arthur H. Bill Professor Emeritus of Reproductive Biology
Case Western Reserve University School of Medicine
Chairman, Advisory Board
Rapid Medical Research
Consultant in Women's Health
Cleveland Clinic
Executive Director
The North American Menopause Society
Cleveland, OH

John J. Vogel, DO
Private Practitioner
Atlanta, GA

L. Elaine Waetjen, MD
Assistant Professor
Department of Obstetrics and Gynecology
University of California Davis Medical Center
Sacramento, CA

Michelle P. Warren, MD*
Professor of Medicine and Obstetrics and Gynecology
Medical Director
Center for Menopause, Hormone Disorders, and
 Women's Health
Wyeth-Ayerst Professor of Women's Health
Columbia University
New York, NY

Robert A. Wild, MD, PhD, MPH*
Professor of Reproductive Endocrinology
Adjunct Professor of Biostatistics and Epidemiology
Adjunct Professor of Medicine (Cardiology)
Oklahoma University Health Sciences Center
Oklahoma City, OK

Tonita Wroolie, PhD
Clinical Instructor
Stanford Center for Neuroscience in Women's Health
Department of Psychiatry & Behavioral Sciences
Stanford School of Medicine
Stanford, CA

The Society wishes to extend a very special thank you to the two editors who volunteered much of their time to this major project: Risa Kagan, MD, and Steven R. Goldstein, MD—both members of the 2006-2007 Professional Education Committee and the 2006-2007 NAMS Board of Trustees. NAMS is also grateful to Elizabeth Contestabile, RNC, BScN, a member of the 2006-2007 Consumer Education Committee, for Canadian-specific content of the entire textbook.

NAMS also acknowledges the contributions of Pamela P. Boggs, MBA, NAMS Director of Education and Development; Kathryn J. Wisch, NAMS Managing Editor; Angela M. Bilancini, NAMS Assistant Medical Editor; and the assistance of editors Eva-Lynne Greene, Nancy Ortman, Anne Rossi, and Stephanie L. Skernivitz.

NAMS is grateful to Novo Nordisk, Inc., for the unrestricted educational grant that helped defray development costs for this textbook. Note that this company did not exercise any control over its contents.

Disclosures

NAMS is committed to ensuring balance, independence, and objectivity in all its educational offerings. All contributors are expected to disclose any significant financial interest or other relationship with the manufacturer of any commercial product and/or provider of commercial services discussed in the educational activity and with any commercial supporters of the activity. This information is found in the chart below. (See Key on page 8.)

Contributor	Research support	Consultant	Speaker's bureau	Advisory board	Major stockholder	Other
Bachmann	8, 19, 25, 27, 42, 43, 52	8, 19, 25, 27, 42, 43, 52	8, 25, 43, 52	•	•	•
Braunstein	•	•	•	•	•	•
Clarkson	•	•	•	•	•	•
Contestabile	•	•	•	•	•	•
Cooper	•	•	•	•	•	•
Eisenberg	•	39	•	•	•	•
Freedman	25, 34, 40	2, 19, 25, 36, 40, 42, 50, 52	•	•	•	•
Gallagher	40, 42, 52	40, 42, 52	•	•	•	•
Goldstein	•	12, 41	•	10, 20, 25, 31, 32, 39, 42	•	49
Gorodeski	•	•	•	15	•	•
Greenseid	•	•	•	•	•	•
Heaney	•	•	•	•	•	•
Henderson	•	•	•	•	•	•
Herzog	•	•	•	•	•	•
Johnson	•	•	•	•	•	•
Juve	•	•	•	•	•	•
Kagan	9, 10, 36, 43, 52	25, 32, 45	7, 8, 20, 22, 25, 32, 38, 45	•	•	•
Kaunitz	6, 8, 30, 40, 51	3, 6, 8, 27, 40, 51	3, 32, 40, 51	•	6, 27, 37, 43, 45, 46	•
Lew	•	•	•	•	•	•
Low Dog	•	•	•	•	•	•
Martens	•	•	•	•	•	•
McClung	20, 32, 36, 43, 45, 46	20, 32, 36, 43, 46	•	•	•	•
Moloney	•	•	•	21	*	•
Newton	42	•	•	•	•	•
Otomo-Corgel	•	•	•	•	•	•
Pinkerton	48, 52	9, 13, 19, 32	32	•	•	35
Rasgon	1, 23, 25, 52	25, 52	1, 11, 23, 25, 42	•	•	•
Ravnikar	•	19	19	•	•	•
Reame	39, 43	14, 43	•	•	•	•
Richardson	•	•	•	•	•	•
Rothert	•	•	•	•	•	•
Santoro	•	42, 44	•	52	•	•
Schiff	•	•	•	3	•	•
Schwartz	•	•	•	•	•	•
Shaver	•	•	•	•	•	•
Shifren	43	43	•	43, 52	•	43
Smith	•	•	•	•	•	•
Sorin	•	•	•	•	•	•
Speroff	6, 8, 40, 52	51	•	•	•	•
Stassinos	•	•	•	•	•	•
Stuenkel	•	•	•	•	•	•
Thacker	•	•	•	•	•	•
Underberg	5, 7, 32, 36	28, 42	1, 5, 16, 18, 28, 33, 36, 42, 47	•	•	•
Utian	•	6, 8, 10, 17, 19, 24, 26, 29, 39, 40, 42	•	20, 25, 32, 45	•	•
Vogel	•	•	•	•	•	•
Waetjen	•	•	•	•	•	•
Warren	4, 25, 36, 48, 52	4, 7, 10, 52	7, 52	7, 52	•	•
Wild	•	•	•	•	•	•
Wroolie	•	•	•	•	•	•

• = Nothing to disclose.

For additional contributors, Ms. Bilancini, Ms. Boggs, Ms. Greene, Ms. Ortman, Ms. Rossi, Ms. Skernivitz, and Ms. Wisch have nothing to disclose.

Key to contributor disclosure statements

1 Abbott Laboratories
2 Alexza Pharmaceuticals
3 American College of Obstetricians and Gynecologists
4 Amylin
5 AstraZeneca
6 Barr Laboratories
7 Bayer Corporation
8 Berlex Laboratories, Inc.
9 Boehringer-Ingelheim
10 Bradley Pharmaceuticals
11 Bristol-Myers Squibb
12 Cook Medical
13 Council on Hormone Education
14 Cypress Bioscience
15 CytoCore, Inc.
16 Daiichi Sankyo
17 Depomed
18 diaDexus
19 Duramed Pharmaceuticals, Inc.
20 Eli Lilly and Company
21 Endocrine Pharmaceuticals, Inc.
22 Esprit Pharma, Inc.
23 Forest Laboratories, Inc.
24 Gerson Lehrman Group
25 GlaxoSmithKline
26 Goldman Sachs
27 Johnson & Johnson
28 Liposcience
29 McKinsey & Company
30 Medical Diagnostic Laboratories, LLC
31 Meditrina Pharmaceuticals, Inc.
32 Merck & Co., Inc
33 Merck Schering-Plough
34 National Institutes of Health
35 National Women's Health Resource Center
36 Novartis Pharmaceuticals
37 Noven Pharmaceuticals, Inc.
38 Novogyne Pharmaceuticals, Inc.
39 Novo Nordisk, Inc.
40 Organon Inc.
41 Phillips Medical Systems
42 Pfizer Inc.
43 Procter & Gamble Pharmaceuticals
44 Quatrx Pharmaceuticals
45 Roche Laboratories
46 sanofi-aventis
47 Schering-Plough
48 Solvay Pharmaceuticals, Inc.
49 Sonosite, Inc.
50 Vela Pharmaceuticals, Inc.
51 Warner Chilcott
52 Wyeth

Menopause is a normal, natural event—defined as the final menstrual period (FMP). It represents the permanent cessation of menses resulting from loss of ovarian follicular function usually due to aging. Menopause can occur naturally (spontaneously)—occurring on average around age 51—or be induced through a medical intervention (surgery, chemotherapy, or pelvic radiation therapy).

Aging is the natural progression of changes in structure and function that occur with the passage of time in the absence of known disease. Aging of the female reproductive system begins at birth and proceeds as a continuum. It consists of a steady loss of oocytes from atresia or ovulation, and does not necessarily occur at a constant rate. Because of the relatively wide age range (40-58 y) for natural menopause, chronologic age is a poor indicator of the beginning or the end of the menopause transition.

Menopause affects every woman. And, as the large baby-boom generation reaches midlife and beyond, an unprecedented number of women are now postmeno-pausal. An estimated 6,000 US women reach menopause every day (over 2 million per year). In addition, more women are living beyond age 65. A woman's life expectancy in the Western world is estimated at 79.7 years. Today, a woman who reaches age 54 can expect to reach age 84.3. About two thirds of the total US population is expected to survive to age 85 or longer.

During the transition from the reproductive years through menopause and beyond, a woman experiences many physical changes, most of which are normal consequences of both menopause and aging. Some of the physical changes observed around menopause may be signs of illness that develop during midlife, such as diabetes. Sometimes, health problems arise when changing hormone levels and the physical effects of aging are coupled with an individual's genetic makeup, certain unhealthy lifestyles, and/or other stresses of midlife.

Survey research does not verify the concept of a "midlife crisis" as universal or even widely present in the general population. However, women in midlife may fear aging for a variety of reasons, some of which are universal, some peculiar to their culture, and the rest reflecting their personal and family circumstances. Women at midlife may be reacting to a multitude of changes that are common at this time of life, such as financial, relationship, and caregiving burdens, that can elicit fear and anxiety.

All women experience menopause, but each one does so in a unique way. How a woman responds to the physical changes of menopause may be similar to the way her mother responded, although the evidence to support this notion is limited.

Lifestyle, demographic factors, and attitudes all influence a woman's perception of menopause. The menopause experience is often perceived as merely the cessation of menses. A woman may view the end of fertility as liberation from the possibility of pregnancy, or she may grieve for the children she never had. For women who have had an unexpected early menopause, either natural or induced, their experience may be more negative. The level of menopause-related symptoms will also have an influence. Some women will have troublesome symptoms, whereas others may navigate the transition with few or even no symptoms at all.

Diverse social and cultural differences can also affect a woman's experience of menopause and her view of menopause treatments as well as her overall health and well-being. Risk factors, patterns of disease and mortality, access to health care, economic status, existing medical therapies, and societal norms related to femininity and aging all differ across groups of women. There is very little research on how these differences affect the experience of menopause. To date, menopause research has focused mostly on middle-class white women. Although different populations are now being studied, considerable information is needed before many aspects of menopause are better understood.

In one study, 80% of women experiencing menopause reported no decrease in quality of life (QOL), and 75% of the women denied experiencing any loss in their attractiveness. Most women (62%) reported positive attitudes toward menopause itself. In another study, most women viewed menopause as inconsequential, and suggested that other events of midlife were more important or stressful. A cohort of well-educated, midlife women described the menopause transition as a normal developmental event. Only about 10% of peri- and postmenopausal women participating in community-based studies reported feelings of despair, irritability, or fatigue during the menopause transition.

The QOL and health status of a generally low-income and poorly educated population of menopause-aged women were examined in a cross-sectional study. Women who were employed, had attained higher levels of education, or had higher levels of income reported better overall health and fewer menopausal symptoms. There were no significant differences between ethnic groups with respect to either menopausal QOL or health status. The surgical intervention of hysterectomy (with bilateral oophorectomy) did not appear to be a factor in decreasing QOL. Compared with women with an intact uterus, women who underwent hysterectomy expressed more improvement, especially in the areas of sexual relationships, spouse or partner relationships, personal fulfillment, and physical health. This improvement did not appear to be the result of menopausal hormone therapy (HT).

Most US postmenopausal women (51%) surveyed in a 1998 NAMS-sponsored Gallup Poll reported being happiest and most fulfilled between ages 50 and 65 compared with when they were in their 20s (10%), 30s (17%), or 40s (16%). Many women reported improvement in various areas of their lives since menopause. They reported a sense of personal fulfillment, an ability to focus on hobbies or other interests, and improved relationships with their spouse or partner and with friends. A majority (51%) said their sexual relationships had remained unchanged. Lifestyle behavioral changes were often initiated during this midlife period.

Fortunately, menopause is now better understood and more openly discussed than ever before. Menopause can be viewed as a sentinel event that presents a unique opportunity for women, working with their healthcare providers, to evaluate personal health and improve health practices. Collaboration between the woman and her provider, characterized by mutual respect and trust, is the goal of menopause counseling. Menopause counseling can facilitate informed decision making and validate the woman's confidence in her decisions, and in her ability to carry them out or modify them over time. Individualized screening and management approaches are essential components of this collaboration.

Accurate information about physiologic changes, management of menopause symptoms, and reducing disease risk is essential. Although menopause is perhaps the most obvious physical event, general knowledge about the aging process is also needed. Additionally, psychological support may be required for the many psychosocial issues women encounter in midlife.

By considering a woman's preferences, values, and concerns, the menopause practitioner will enhance the woman's sense of well-being, not only around menopause but for the rest of her life.

Terminology

Clinicians and researchers in the field of menopause have long recognized the need for universally accepted menopause terminology as well as a staging system useful in categorizing the last 10 to 15 years of reproductive aging. In 2001, the Stages of Reproductive Aging Workshop (STRAW), sponsored by The North American Menopause Society (NAMS), the National Institutes of Health, the American Society for Reproductive Medicine, and the National Institute of Child Health and Human Development, addressed nomenclature and a staging system. Previously, the Council of Affiliated Menopause Societies (CAMS), an international policy organ of the International Menopause Society, had developed standardized definitions for menopause-related events. Although STRAW redefined some terms, other CAMS terms remain in use.

The reproductive aging continuum created by STRAW is divided into seven stages: five precede and two follow the FMP (see Fig. 1). STRAW points out, however, that not all healthy women will follow this pattern; some will seesaw between stages or skip a stage altogether.

Menopause. As defined by STRAW, *menopause* (ie, "spontaneous" or "natural" menopause) is recognized to have occurred after 12 months of amenorrhea with no obvious pathologic cause. It reflects a near-complete but natural diminution of ovarian hormone secretion. There is no adequate independent biological marker for menopause.

Menopause is one point in time. The phrases "in menopause" and "going through menopause" are

---

Figure 1. Stages/nomenclature of normal reproductive aging in women

Final Menstrual Period (FMP) ▼ 0

Stages:	-5	-4	-3	-2	-1	0	+1	+2
Terminology:	Reproductive			Menopausal Transition			Postmenopause	
	Early	Peak	Late	Early	Late*		Early*	Late*
				Perimenopause				
Duration of Stage:	variable			variable		ⓐ 1 yr	ⓑ 4 yrs	until demise
Menstrual Cycles:	variable to regular	regular		variable cycle length (*>7 days different from normal*)	≥2 skipped cycles and an interval of amenorrhea (≥60 days)	Amen. x 12 mos	none	
Endocrine:	normal FSH		↑ FSH	↑ FSH			↑ FSH	

*Stages most likely to be characterized by vasomotor symptoms.

Source: Stages of Reproductive Aging Workshop (STRAW), *Menopause* 2001.

misnomers sometimes used to describe perimenopause or the menopause transition. It is appropriate to say that one "reaches" menopause.

Menopause transition. According to STRAW, the term *menopause transition* (or *menopausal transition*) refers to the span of time when menstrual cycle and endocrine changes occur, and is divided into stage –2 (early) through stage –1 (late). The menopause transition begins with variation in the length of the menstrual cycle caused by a rise in levels of monotropic follicle-stimulating hormone (FSH) and ends with the FMP (which is recognized only after 12 consecutive months of amenorrhea). Women experiencing induced menopause (see below) do not experience this menopause transition.

Perimenopause. The term *perimenopause* is somewhat confusing. According to STRAW, perimenopause is defined as about or around menopause, beginning with stage –2 (early transition) and ending 12 months *after* the FMP (not *with* the FMP). NAMS prefers to use the term interchangeably with *menopause transition*, although there is a difference in the STRAW system. STRAW suggests that the term be used only with patients or in the lay press; NAMS uses the term for all audiences.

Premenopause. The term *premenopause* is used ambiguously. The literal meaning of the word implies the whole time preceding menopause, that is, the time before the FMP. CAMS recommends that this term encompass the entire *reproductive* period up to the FMP. STRAW does not use this term, but prefers classifying the reproductive stage as early, peak, and late (with "late" being the time when levels of FSH increase). In recent years, NAMS has used the term "premenopause" to refer to the time from menarche to the beginning of perimenopause. However, it is not appropriate to consider a young teenager "premenopausal." To obviate confusion, NAMS concurs with the recommendation of CAMS to abandon the term "premenopause." NAMS prefers the term recommended by STRAW—*menopause transition*.

Postmenopause. The term *postmenopause* refers to any span of time dating from the FMP, regardless of whether menopause was natural or induced. It is defined by STRAW as extending from stage +1 (early menopause) through stage +2 (late menopause).

Stage +1 is defined as the time span within 5 years after the FMP. During stage +1, ovarian hormone function is further dampened, resulting in a permanently low level. Stage +1 is also the time of accelerated bone loss. STRAW further divides stage +1 into segments *a* (the first 12 mo after the FMP) and *b* (the next 4 y). Stage +2 has a definite beginning (5 y after the FMP), but its duration is variable as it ends with death. STRAW concluded that further divisions may be warranted as more information is accumulated about the physiology of menopause.

Induced menopause. According to CAMS, the term *induced menopause* is defined as the cessation of menstruation that follows either surgical removal of both ovaries (bilateral oophorectomy, with or without hysterectomy) or iatrogenic ablation of ovarian function (eg, by chemotherapy or pelvic radiation therapy). Bilateral oophorectomy is the most common cause of induced menopause.

Fertility ends abruptly for women who experience surgically induced menopause (*surgical menopause*). With other types of induced menopause, fertility may end immediately or over several months. Depending upon the age of the woman, chemotherapy-induced ovarian failure may only be transient.

Premature menopause. According to CAMS, *premature menopause* should be defined as natural menopause that occurs at an age less than 2 SD below the mean estimated age for the reference population. In practice, CAMS states, the age of 40 years is frequently used as an arbitrary cutoff point below which menopause is said to be premature.

NAMS uses the term *premature menopause* to describe menopause reached at or under age 40, whether menopause is natural or induced.

Early menopause. NAMS uses this term to describe natural or induced menopause that occurs well before the average age of natural menopause (age 51 y)—at or under age 45. Early menopause encompasses premature menopause.

Premature ovarian failure. The term *premature ovarian failure* (POF) is used to describe ovarian insufficiency leading to amenorrhea that occurs in women younger than age 40. POF may be transient when caused by autoimmune disease or chemotherapy, but permanent loss of ovarian function is the usual outcome. Genetic abnormalities of the X chromosome are another important cause. POF reflects primary failure of the ovary with resultant high levels of luteinizing hormone (LH) and FSH. POF should not be confused with hypothalamic amenorrhea (HA). Overexercising, eating disorders, or high levels of stress can induce a reduction in ovarian hormone production, but as opposed to POF, the lack of ovarian function in HA reflects central suppression of the hypothalamic-pituitary-ovarian axis resulting in low levels of LH and FSH. Resumption of a normal lifestyle by women with HA is usually followed by resumption of normal menstrual cyclicity.

Temporary menopause. The term *temporary menopause* is used to describe a span of time when normal ovarian function is interrupted and temporary amenorrhea results. Since menopause is by definition the very last menses, NAMS does not use the term "temporary menopause" and recommends that the term be abandoned.

Climacteric. STRAW suggests that the term *climacteric* be used interchangeably with "perimenopause." However,

CAMS defines climacteric as the age-related transition in women from the reproductive to the nonreproductive state. It is a process rather than a specific point in time. According to CAMS, the climacteric for women is sometimes, but not necessarily always, associated with symptomatology. When symptoms occur, they may be termed the "climacteric syndrome."

STRAW has suggested that the term "climacteric" not be used in scientific papers. Global consensus on this terminology has not been achieved. NAMS does not use the term, but it is still widely used outside North America.

Demographics

Exact figures on the number of postmenopausal women and the number reaching menopause each year are not known. To provide estimates, NAMS has extrapolated data from several sources to determine the number of postmenopausal women by age, by surgically induced menopause, and by premature menopause, and has presented them in Table 1.

Table 1. Estimates of numbers of postmenopausal US women in 2000

Total number (prevalence)	(in millions)
Age 51 and older*	39.944
Age 40 to 50 (natural menopause)	3.123
Surgical menopause**	2.000
Premature natural menopause†	0.504
Total	45.571

Total reaching menopause during 2000	
Age 51 and older	1.796
Surgical menopause†	0.228
Premature natural menopause	NA
Total	2.024

Total/day reaching menopause during 2000	5,640

* Includes women who may have experienced menopause earlier in life (induced or premature natural menopause).
** From the National Hospital Discharge Survey, 2004; includes only women younger than age 50.
† Includes only women younger than age 40.

Source: US Census Bureau *Census 2000.*

United States. In 2000, there were an estimated 45.6 million postmenopausal women in the United States. About 39.9 million of them were older than age 51, the average age of natural menopause in the Western world. By the year 2020, the number of US women older than age 51 is expected to be more than 50 million.

NAMS estimated the number of postmenopausal women (see Table 1), extrapolating data from the 2000 US Census

and other resources. Details regarding the calculation of these estimates follow.

Postmenopause by age. Nearly 40 million US women are past the average age of natural menopause (51 y). Although the US Census Bureau year 2000 report does not provide the exact number of women over 51, it does report numbers for women aged 55 and older, who can all be assumed to be postmenopausal. An estimated 75% of women in the 50- to 55-year-old age category are assumed to be postmenopausal. These estimates include women who may have had induced or premature natural menopause earlier in life.

Among women aged 40 to 45 years, an estimated 5% have experienced natural menopause, based primarily on data from the Study of Women's Health Across the Nation (SWAN). For naturally postmenopausal women in the next oldest category (45 to 55 years), a rough estimate is 25%.

For a 1-year estimate of the number of women experiencing natural menopause during 2002, the number of women aged 50 to 55 years was divided by 5 (approximately one fifth of the 50- to-55-year-old age group turned 51 in 2000).

Surgical menopause. The US hysterectomy surveillance (1994-1999) from the Centers for Disease Control provides estimated overall rates for hysterectomies by age plus percentages for those hysterectomies that included bilateral oophorectomy. Applying those rates to US Census Bureau data for premenopausal-aged women provides an estimate of the number of women who had undergone a hysterectomy with bilateral oophorectomy before age 50. No overall numbers are published for bilateral oophorectomies without hysterectomy. Given that bilateral oophorectomy without hysterectomy is relatively rare, a conservative estimate was added to round the number up to 2 million.

Data are inconclusive regarding the association of hysterectomy with ovarian failure occurring earlier than normal. Thus, numbers for that group are not included.

Annual numbers for surgical menopause come from the 2004 National Hospital Discharge Survey. Oophorectomy data for women aged 15 to 44 years plus 25% of women aged 45 to 64 years were combined to provide an estimate. The survey also provides data on hysterectomies, but it is not known whether those hysterectomies were with or without bilateral oophorectomy.

Premature natural menopause. Several studies, including SWAN, indicate that the percentage of US women experiencing premature natural menopause is approximately 1%. Applying this estimate to the number of women aged 15 to 40 years in the 2000 US census gave an estimate of the number of US women who experienced premature natural menopause. This is based on the total number of US cases; the annual figure is not known.

Induced menopause from chemotherapy or pelvic radiation therapy. There are no hard data from which to calculate estimates, so these women are not included.

Canada. Canadian statistics also demonstrate an increase in life expectancy for midlife women. In 1922, a 50-year-old woman lived until age 75 on average. Today, a woman the same age can expect to live until her mid-80s. Thus, Canadian women are living at least one third of their lives after menopause. By 2026, it is estimated that almost one quarter (22%) of the Canadian population will be comprised of women over the age of 50.

Worldwide. In 1998, there were more than 477 million postmenopausal women in the world and approximately 9% were expected to live to age 80. By 2025, the number of postmenopausal women is expected to rise to 1.1 billion. Life expectancy for women worldwide was 65 years in 1998 (79 y in more developed countries). This is expected to rise to 72 years worldwide by 2025 (82 y in developed countries).

How to evaluate the medical literature

As new studies are published, the evidence base increases for understanding the risks and benefits of treatment options. A basic understanding of the types of studies and the meaning of the analyses helps healthcare providers evaluate the evidence and implications for clinical practice. Readers in search of more sophisticated discussions are urged to consult current clinical epidemiology texts.

Types of studies. Two major types of studies are *experimental* and *observational*. In experimental studies, interventions and conditions are strictly defined and controlled by the investigators. In observational studies, investigators observe outcomes in relation to variables of interest. They do not assign participants to an exposure of interest. The most common types of studies are listed here, ordered by the strength of evidence they provide.

Experimental studies. Types of experimental studies are randomized controlled trials (RCTs), crossover trials, and quasi-experimental studies.

- *Randomized controlled trials* are considered the strongest for therapeutic interventions. In RCTs, a group of participants with similar characteristics is identified (eg, low bone density). Each participant is then "randomly assigned" (neither the participants nor the investigator chooses) to an intervention group (or groups) or to a control group. Participants typically have an equal and unbiased (ie, random) chance of being assigned to each treatment under study. RCTs have the best chance of avoiding selection bias if the randomization is adequate. This is because known and unknown characteristics should be the same in each group. The baseline characteristics of the two groups should be presented and statistically compared in an

RCT's final report. The Women's Health Initiative is an example of an RCT.

RCTs are best suited to situations in which exposure to treatment is modifiable, a legitimate uncertainty exists regarding benefit and/or harm of treatment, and outcomes are reasonably common. However, inclusion and exclusion criteria may limit the extrapolation of the results to other groups (ie, whether the results can be generalized).

The "power" of a trial is the likelihood that it will determine the effect of the intervention. The number of participants is determined when the trial is designed based on the likelihood of the measured outcome events and the anticipated magnitude of the intervention's effect. If events do not occur as often as predicted, the trial may not have adequate power to determine the effect of the intervention. The Methods section of the published trial results will describe how the investigator calculated the number of participants required and will quantify the range of effect the study can detect (eg, the study was powered to detect more than a 20% reduction in heart attacks). Publication bias favors small trials with positive outcomes. An international registry of clinical trials requires submission of the planned trial so that a full accounting of the status of trials that are not completed or are completed regardless of their outcomes can be assessed.

Depending on the intervention, participants and investigators may be purposefully blinded or masked (ie, they do not know which treatment a participant is receiving). This helps reduce some forms of bias and the effects of the participant's or investigator's expectations of intervention benefit.

Classically, RCTs are used to assess for *efficacy* of the treatment in an ideal controlled setting. More often now, an RCT will assess *effectiveness* (not efficacy) by studying the intervention under more usual circumstances. This is because a study for efficacy may not reflect its actual effectiveness in a real-world, clinical practice setting. Both these types of RCTs often use a relatively narrowly defined patient population. Even though an RCT is quite "internally valid" (ie, the study was done well), it may not be accurate to extrapolate (generalize) the results from one RCT to another patient population that was not studied in the trial.

Other important issues when evaluating the results of an RCT include checking to see whether all participants who started the trial were accounted for at trial conclusion and whether the groups were treated equally aside from the experimental intervention.

- *Crossover trials* allow participants to serve as their own controls. Participants are randomly assigned to one treatment arm and later switched to the other treatment arm. This "crossover" study methodology has often been used in trials to assess the efficacy of medications. The design is difficult to do well because of its potential for residual effects between interventions. Often there will be a washout period (time during which no intervention is given) between interventions.

- *Quasi-experimental studies* are of two general varieties. In one, two interventions are simultaneously compared in two groups of participants, but interventions are not randomized for any given participant (eg, two hospitals comparing two types of wound closure for the same type of surgery).

  Another common quasi-experimental study is when participants serve as their own controls and the investigator controls the intervention. The intervention is neither randomized nor is there a control population to which the response can be compared. After baseline evaluation, the intervention is given and the participants are reevaluated to observe any changes in characteristics because of the intervention.

Observational studies. Types of observational studies include purely *analytic* (or *descriptive*) studies. Analytic studies (including cohort studies, case-control studies, and cross-sectional studies) have a nonrandomized control group (eg, women who did not use HT for any number of reasons would be compared with women who elected to use HT). What is sampled first—risk factor, outcome, or both risk factor and outcome simultaneously—determines which analytic study design is being used. Case reports and case series are not analytic because they do not have control comparisons.

- *Cohort studies* (or *longitudinal studies*) begin with a defined group of participants (eg, individuals of a certain age or those who work in a certain industry) called the "cohort." These studies sample individuals from the general population and determine if they have risk factors of interest (eg, HT users vs nonusers). This cohort of individuals is then followed over time to study a variety of outcomes. Data are collected in a similar manner on all participants from the beginning of the study (the baseline) and frequently at set intervals during follow-up. The Nurses' Health Study is one of the best-known cohort studies.

  These studies provide a clearer temporal sequence of exposures and/or outcomes, are well suited for common exposures, and can study multiple exposures and/or outcomes. However, they can be time-consuming and expensive, they have the potential for many forms of bias, and participants may be lost during follow-up. When too many patients are lost, the validity of the study is compromised.

Cohort studies may follow relevant events as they occur over time (prospective), but they may also be performed in an historical or a concurrent (cross-sectional) manner. Evidence from prospective cohort studies is considered stronger than the other forms of analytic studies because data on exposures are collected before the outcomes occur.

The term *retrospective* is sometimes used when referring to an historical cohort study, and it can be confusing. If the data are easily accessible, the researcher can retrospectively evaluate a cohort that was followed in time, but the time was in the past moving forward (historical cohort), not progressing from current time onwards (concurrent cohort). In the Nurses' Health Study and the Framingham Study, information was gleaned in a concurrent and retrospective fashion (where a historical cohort was evaluated). All participants in each of these circumstances were followed longitudinally forward in some time frame.

- *Case-control studies* begin with an outcome or disease of interest (eg, myocardial infarction [MI], breast cancer) and then compare the characteristics or risk factors of individuals with the outcome (cases) to controls who do not have the outcome or disease of interest. Case-control studies are prone to many more forms of bias. A frequent one is "recall bias" (ie, participants cannot remember accurately).

  Matching participants for specific characteristics and defining strict eligibility criteria lessens, but cannot eliminate, the possibility that the results are "confounded." For example, women who use HT are known to smoke less and lead generally healthier lifestyles. HT users have less cardiovascular disease primarily because of better lifestyle habits rather than any beneficial effect from HT use. Smoking or other lifestyle patterns can confound the results when observational studies analyze HT use and health outcomes. Matching cases and controls for smoking status helps reduce this confounding.

  Despite these limitations, case-control studies have many advantages. Because they begin with an outcome of interest, they can be performed efficiently and at less cost than cohort studies. They are important in situations in which it would be unethical to assign individuals to an exposure (eg, chemotherapy) or when an outcome is rare (eg, X-chromosome abnormalities associated with POF).

- *Cross-sectional studies* are snapshots in time. Here, cases and controls are evaluated at the same time for both risk factors or characteristics and outcomes of interest. Cross-sectional studies are very useful for determining prevalence, for planning for healthcare needs, and for generating hypotheses.

- *Case reports* and *case series* describe the experience of a single patient or series of patients. Such reports are useful in bringing new diseases or phenomena to the attention of the clinical and scientific community and for generating new hypotheses. However, lacking a control group, case reports or series without further study are only suggestive.

Many of these basic designs can be modified or combined, and many hybrid studies exist. An example is a case-control study within a cohort; this is a very useful study design and can provide many advantages, including cost.

Analyses. The bottom line in evaluating a study is, "What are the results?" The results of cohort studies and clinical trials are most frequently presented as a relative risk (RR)—the likely level of greater risk (eg, for HT users compared to nonusers). The RR can be determined because these study designs follow participants longitudinally and risk (which is time-dependent) can be determined in each comparison group. Definitions of key terms used in analyzing study results are as follows:

Rate/risk. The term *rate* is the number of events per number of individuals per time interval (eg, 44 per 10,000 per year). Knowing the exact number of events over time is very useful, as this determines the *risk*.

The Council for International Organizations of Medical Sciences Task Force has provided the following nomenclature to guide the interpretation of risks:

- Rare = less than or equal to 10/10,000 per year
- Very rare = less than or equal to 1/10,000 per year

Rare outcomes would not be of such great concern to an individual woman making a decision about treatment. However, it is important to recognize that common exposures that produce rare outcomes can still have profound public health impact.

Relative risk (RR). RR is a ratio—the rate of disease or the outcome of interest in a group exposed to a potential risk factor or treatment, or having a characteristic of interest, divided by the rate of disease or interest in an unexposed group (ie, those without the risk factor, treatment, or characteristic of interest). The RR should be used only for prospective studies.

Rate is used as above in both the numerator and the denominator. These are the numbers of events, per numbers of individuals, per time interval (eg, 50/100,000/year). For example, if the annual rate of MI in women who smoke is 220 per 100,000, and the annual rate in women who do not smoke is 110 per 100,000, the RR associated with smoking is:

$$RR = \frac{220}{100,000/year} \div \frac{110}{100,000/year} = 2.00$$

This means that compared with nonsmoking women, the risk of MI for a smoking woman is twice that of a nonsmoking woman in the study.

An RR *less than 1.0* suggests lower risk. For example, an RR of 0.50 means there is a 50% less chance (or risk) of the outcome studied in those with versus those without the risk factor of interest. An RR of 0.3 means a 70% less relative risk.

An RR *greater than 1.0* suggests that the factor increases risk. For example, an RR of 1.2 means there is a 20% increase in risk in the group with the factor versus the group without the risk factor. An RR of 2.0 means double the risk.

Odds ratio (OR). The OR is an estimate used in any of the analytic studies. It best approximates the RR when the outcome is rare.

Confidence interval (CI). The CI, usually cited with the RR or the OR, indicates with a certain degree of assurance the range within which lies the true magnitude of the measured effect. The CI has two components—the point estimate and a range (eg, RR, 1.20; 95% CI, 1.09-1.32). The point estimate (the RR or OR number) is the best mathematical estimate from the data. Understanding the upper and lower limits of the range is often clinically useful. If the CI is "wide," the reader's confidence in the validity of the RR would be less than if the CI is "narrow" (ie, closer to the value of the RR).

Often, a 95% CI is used. A 95% CI gives the range of values that have a 95% probability of containing the true RR or OR. When a 95% CI does not contain the number 1.0 (eg, 0.40-0.80 or 1.12-1.37), the measured RR or OR is significant by at least $P < 0.05$. The CI is more clinically useful than the P value (see below) because the CI helps the reader to understand the best estimate of the effect and it also provides the mathematical estimated limits, which are useful in determining the best-case and worse-case scenarios.

P value. This term is the probability of obtaining the observed RR or OR by chance alone. A P value of .01 means that there is a 1% mathematical probability that the observed difference between two groups occurred by chance. By convention, P is generally deemed significant if below .05. This means that if 20 outcomes are evaluated in a single study, one of these outcomes is likely to show a positive result just due to chance alone ($P = .05$, or 1/20). By the time $P = .001$, the likelihood is only 1/1,000 that the results occurred by chance—in other words, the finding is more likely to be real.

It is important to remember that a study can be *statistically* significant and not *clinically* significant. However, if it is not statistically significant, it cannot reach clinical significance and the result could be "clinically nonsignificant" or "inconclusive." An example is when the study is underpowered.

Attributable risk/absolute risk (AR). The impact of RR on both a population and an individual basis depends on "incidence" (ie, the number of new cases). This can be quantified by the AR, which is the difference between the incidence rates in the exposed and unexposed groups—in other words, the "risk difference." The AR quantifies the effect of exposure, providing a measure of its public health impact. For example, for the calculation presented earlier about the risk of MI in smoking women, the AR is:

$$AR = \frac{220}{100,000/year} - \frac{110}{100,000/year} = \frac{110}{100,000/year}$$

This means that for every 100,000 women who smoke, there would be 110 additional cases of MIs per year.

Often, AR is more clinically useful than RR in explaining risk to patients.

Number needed to treat (NNT). To communicate this risk difference to patients, the NNT can be useful. The NNT is merely the reciprocal of the AR (ie, 1 divided by the AR). For example, in a 1-year study, if the rate of an outcome was 20 per 1,000 in an untreated group, and 10 per 1,000 in a treated group, the NNT is:

$$NNT = \frac{1}{(20/1,000) - (10/1,000)} = \frac{1}{(10/1,000)} = \frac{1}{0.01} = 100$$

This means that for every 100 people treated, there would be 1 less negative outcome over the year.

Meta-analysis. This term describes an analytic technique used to pool the results of clinical trials. Often, a meta-analysis is performed on a group of studies that are too small to have statistical significance by themselves but that may show significance when pooled. Specific criteria (eg, eligibility criteria of participants, data completeness) are established to determine which studies will be included in the analysis. Since any biases present in the contributing studies will be present in the meta-analysis, the outcome of a meta-analysis is only as good as the studies included.

In general, meta-analyses are difficult to perform. They are best performed based on the original data obtained from each investigator from each individual study. International guidelines provide checklists to understand the quality of a meta-analysis of clinical trials (CONSORT guidelines) and observational studies (MOOSE guidelines).

Suggested reading

Administration on Aging. *A Profile of Older Americans: 2000.* Washington, DC: U.S. Department of Health and Human Services, Administration on Aging, 2000.

Avis NE, Stellato R, Crawford S, et al. Is there a menopausal syndrome? Menopausal status and symptoms across racial/ethnic groups. *Soc Sci Med* 2001;52:345-356.

Brzyski RG, Medrano MA, Hyatt-Santos JM, Ross JS. Quality of life in low-income menopausal women attending primary care clinics. *Fertil Steril* 2001;76:44-50.

Chalmers C, Lindsay M, Usher D, Warner P, Evans D, Ferguson M. Hysterectomy and ovarian function: levels of follicle stimulating hormone and incidence of menopausal symptoms are not affected by hysterectomy in women under age 45 years. *Climacteric* 2002;5:366-373.

Coulam CB, Adamson SC, Annegers JF. Incidence of premature ovarian failure. *Obstet Gynecol* 1986;67:604-606.

Council for International Organizations of Medical Sciences (CIOMS). Guidelines for Preparing Core Clinical-Safety Information on Drugs, 2nd ed. Geneva, Switzerland: CIOMS, 1998.

Cramer DW, Harlow BL, Xu H, et al. Cross-sectional and case-controlled analyses of the association between smoking and early menopause. *Maturitas* 1995;22:79-87.

Cramer DW, Xu H, Harlow BL. Family history as a predictor of early menopause. *Fertil Steril* 1995;64:740-745.

Ettinger B, Woods NF, Barrett-Connor E, Pressman A. The North American Menopause Society 1998 menopause survey: Part II. Counseling about hormone replacement therapy: association with socioeconomic status and access to care. *Menopause* 2000;7:143-148.

Gold EB, Bromberger J, Crawford S, et al. Factors associated with age at natural menopause in a multiethnic sample of midlife women. *Am J Epidemiol* 2001;153:865-874.

Gold EB, Sternfeld B, Kelsey JL, et al. Relation of demographic and lifestyle factors to symptoms in a multi-racial/ethnic population of women 40-55 years of age. *Am J Epidemiol* 2000;152:463-473.

Gracia CR, Sammel MD, Freeman EW, et al. Defining menopause status: creation of a new definition to identify the early changes of the menopausal transition. *Menopause* 2005;12:128-135.

Hardy R, Kuh D. Reproductive characteristics and the age at inception of the perimenopause in a British national cohort. *Am J Epidemiol* 1999;149:612-620.

Harlow SD, Cain K, Crawford S, et al. Evaluation of four proposed bleeding criteria for the onset of late menopausal transition. *J Clin Endocrinol Metab* 2006;91:3432-3438.

Harlow SD, Crawford S, Dennerstein L, Burger HG, Mitchell ES, Sowers MF, for the ReSTAGE Collaboration. Recommendations from a multi-study evaluation of proposed criteria for staging reproductive aging. *Climacteric* 2007;10:112-119.

Hersh AL, Stefanick ML, Stafford RS. National use of postmenopausal hormone therapy: annual trends and response to recent evidence. *JAMA* 2004;291:47-53.

Hing E, Brett K. Changes in U.S. prescribing patterns of menopausal hormone therapy, 2001-2003. *Obstet Gynecol* 2006;108:33-40.

Jacobs Institute of Women's Health, Expert Panel on Menopause Counseling. *Guidelines for Counseling Women on the Management of Menopause.* Washington, DC: Jacobs Institute of Women's Health, 2000.

Johnston JM, Colvin A, Johnson BD, et al. Comparison of SWAN and WISE menopausal status classification algorithms. *J Womens Health* 2006;15:1184-1194.

Kato I, Toniolo P, Akmedkhanov A, et al. Prospective study of factors influencing the onset of natural menopause. *J Clin Epidemiol* 1998;51:1271-1276.

Keshavarz H, Hillis SD, Kieke BA, Marchbanks PA. Hysterectomy surveillance—United States, 1994-1999. *MMWR CDC Surveill Summ* 2002;51:1-8.

Koepsell TD, Weiss NS. *Epidemiologic Methods: Studying the Occurrence of Illness.* New York, NY: Oxford University Press, 2003.

Kozak LJ, DeFrances CJ, Hall MJ. National hospital discharge survey: 2004 annual summary with detailed diagnosis and procedure data. *Vital Health Stat 13* 2006;162:1-209.

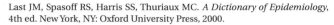

Last JM, Spasoff RS, Harris SS, Thuriaux MC. *A Dictionary of Epidemiology*, 4th ed. New York, NY: Oxford University Press, 2000.

Lawlor DA, Ebrahim S, Smith GD. The association of socio-economic position across the life course and age at menopause: the British Women's Heart and Health Study. *BJOG* 2003;110:1078-1087.

LeLorier J, Gregoire G, Benhaddad A, Lapierre J, Derderian F. Discrepancies between meta-analyses and subsequent large randomized, controlled trials. *N Engl J Med* 1997;337:536-542.

Lock M, Kaufert P. Menopause, local biologies, and cultures of aging. *Am J Hum Biol* 2001;3:494-504.

Luborsky JL, Meyer P, Sowers MF, Gold EB, Santoro N. Premature menopause in a multi-ethnic population study of the menopause transition. *Hum Reprod* 2003;18:199-206.

Mansfield PK, Carey M, Anderson A, et al. Staging the menopausal transition: data from the TREMIN Research Program on Women's Health. *Womens Health Issues* 2004;14:220-226.

McKinlay SM. Issues in design, measurement, and analysis for menopause research. *Exp Gerontol* 1994;29:479-493.

McKinlay SM, Brambilla J, Posner JG. The normal menopause transition. *Maturitas* 1992;14:103-115.

Miro F, Parker SW, Aspinall LJ, et al. Sequential classification of endocrine stages during reproductive aging in women: the FREEDOM study. *Menopause* 2005;12:281-290.

Mitchell ES, Woods NF, Mariella A. Three stages of the menopausal transition from the Seattle Midlife Women's Health Study: toward a more precise definition. *Menopause* 2000;7:334-349.

Moher D, Cook DJ, Eastwood S, Olkin I, Rennie D, Stroup DF. Improving the quality of reports of meta-analyses of randomised controlled trials: the QUOROM statement. Quality of reporting of meta-analyses. *Lancet* 1999;354:1896-1900.

Moher D, Schulz KF, Altman D, for the CONSORT Group (Consolidated Standards of Reporting Trials). The CONSORT statement: revised recommendations for improving the quality of reports of parallel-group randomized trials. *JAMA* 2001;285:1987-1991. Checklist available at: http://www.consort-statement.org/downloads/checklist.pdf. Accessed July 25, 2007.

The North American Menopause Society. Clinical challenges of perimenopause: consensus opinion of The North American Menopause Society. *Menopause* 2000;7:5-13.

The North American Menopause Society. Estrogen and progestogen use in peri- and postmenopausal women: March 2007 position statement of The North American Menopause Society *Menopause* 2007;14:168-182

Obermeyer CM. Menopause across cultures: a review of the evidence. *Menopause* 2000;7:184-192.

Palmer JR, Rosenberg L, Wise LA, Horton NJ, Adams-Campbell LL. Onset of natural menopause in African American women. *Am J Public Health* 2003;30:97-108.

Progetto Menopausa Italia Study Group. Premature ovarian failure, frequency and risk factors among women attending a network of menopause clinics in Italy. *BJOG* 2003;110:59-63.

Randolph JF Jr, Crawford S, Dennerstein L, et al. The value of follicle-stimulating hormone concentration and clinical findings as markers of the late menopausal transition. *J Clin Endocrinol Metab* 2006;91:3034-3040.

Richards M, Kuh D, Hardy R, Wadsworth M. Lifetime cognitive function and timing of the natural menopause. *Neurology* 1999;53:308-314.

Santoro N, Brockwell S, Johnston J, et al. Helping midlife women predict the onset of the final menses: SWAN, the Study of Women's Health Across the Nation. *Menopause* 2007;14:415-424.

Schneider HP, Schultz-Zehden B, Rosemeier H, Behre H. Assessing well-being in menopausal women. In: Studd J, ed. *The Management of the Menopause: The Millennium Review 2000*. Pearl River, NY: Parthenon Publishing Group, 2000:11-19.

Siddle N, Sarrel P, Whitehead M. The effect of hysterectomy on the age at ovarian failure: identification of a subgroup of women with premature loss of ovarian function and literature review. *Fertil Steril* 1987;47:94-100.

Smith T, Contestabile E. Executive summary: Canadian consensus on menopause and osteoporosis. *J SOGC* 2001;23:829-835.

Sommer B, Avis N, Meyer P, et al. Attitudes toward menopause and aging across ethnic/racial groups. *Psychosom Med* 1999;61:868-875.

Soules MR, Sherman S, Parrott E, et al. Executive summary: stages of reproductive aging workshop (STRAW) Park City, Utah, July 2001. *Menopause* 2001;8:402-407.

Statistics Canada. Population projections for 2001, 2006, 2011, 2016, 2021 and 2026. Based on 2000 population estimates. 2005. Available at: http://www40.statcan.ca. Accessed August 10, 2007.

Stroup DF, Berlin JA, Morton SC et al, for the Meta-analysis Of Observational Studies in Epidemiology (MOOSE) Group. *JAMA* 2000;283:2008-2012. Checklist available at: http://www.consort-statement.org/Initiatives/MOOSE/Moosecheck.pdf. Accessed June 29, 2007.

Torgerson DJ, Thomas RE, Reid DM. Mothers' and daughters' menopausal ages: is there a link? *Eur J Obstet Gynecol Reprod Biol* 1997;74:63-66.

US Census Bureau. Census 2000 PHC-T-9: Female population by age, race, and Hispanic or Latino origin for the United States: 2000. Available at: http://www.census.gov/population/cen2000/phc-t9/tab03.pdf. Accessed August 10, 2007.

US Census Bureau. Population survey: Female population by age, sex, and race and Hispanic origin: March 2002. Available at: http://www.census.gov/population/socdemo/race/api/ppl-163/tab01.pdf. Accessed August 10, 2007.

Utian WH, Boggs PP. The North American Menopause Society 1998 menopause survey. Part I: postmenopausal women's perceptions about menopause and midlife. *Menopause* 1999;6:122-128.

Weel AE, Uitterlinden AG, Westendorp IC. Estrogen receptor polymorphism predicts the onset of natural and surgical menopause. *J Clin Endocrinol Metab* 1999;84:3146-3150.

Winterich JA, Umberson D. How women experience menopause: the importance of social context. *J Women Aging* 1999;11:57-73.

Woods NF, Mitchell ES. Anticipating menopause: observations from the Seattle Midlife Women's Health Study. *Menopause* 1999;6:167-173.

World Health Organization Scientific Group on Research on the Menopause in the 1990s. Geneva, Switzerland: *WHO Technical Report Series* 866, 1996.

As each woman moves from the reproductive phase of life through the menopause transition into the postmenopausal years, a number of physical and psychological changes may occur. Clinicians may be challenged to differentiate changes related to menopause from those related to aging. Several hormonal systems manifest age-related changes that may or may not have their onset during the menopause transition. Furthermore, medical conditions such as obesity, diabetes, lipid disorders, thyroid disorders, and hypertension often develop or worsen during midlife.

Age at menopause

In the Western world, spontaneous menopause occurs at an average age of 51.4 years, with a Gaussian distribution ranging roughly from 40 to 60 years. Extremes in age at menopause are rare and are often associated with other medical conditions. Menopause in a woman younger than 40 years of age constitutes premature ovarian failure. No set age formally constitutes "delayed menopause," but a woman well past the usual age of menopause with irregular vaginal bleeding should be evaluated to rule out gynecologic and possible endocrine or hematologic disorders. (See Section D for more about premature menopause.)

Although women today enjoy an increase in life expectancy, the average age of natural menopause has not substantially changed during the past few centuries, even with improved nutrition and reduction of disease. Age at menopause is influenced by multiple genetic and environmental factors.

Earlier menopause can be induced by factors that accelerate ovarian follicular atresia (cell death and degeneration). Genetic variations, ovarian "toxins" such as smoking, metabolic disorders, autoimmune syndromes, HIV infection, and cancer therapies, as well as lifestyle variables, may contribute. The dose and duration of exposure are important. Aberrations in central neuroendocrine control of reproduction might also alter the timing of menopause. See Tables 1 and 2.

To predict the age of menopause, a model has been proposed that incorporates the number of full-term pregnancies, body mass index, history of breast surgery, and the presence of either of two specific single nucleotide polymorphisms of estrogen-metabolizing genes (CYP17 or CYP1B1-4).

Table 1. Genetic and environmental factors affecting age at menopause

Genetic variations

- Alterations in the X-chromosome and possibly in chromosome 9.
- Polymorphisms (common genetic variations in DNA) of estrogen receptor-α.
- Polymorphisms of estrogen-metabolizing genes.

Environmental exposure

- Current smoking accelerates age of menopause by approximately 1.5 years with a dose-response relationship between the number of cigarettes smoked, the duration of smoking, and age at menopause.
- Survivors of childhood cancers have an 8% incidence of premature menopause compared with 0.8% in siblings. Risk factors include ovarian exposure to increasing doses of radiation, number of alkylating agents and cumulative dose, and the diagnosis of Hodgkin's lymphoma.

Lifestyle and concurrent medical conditions

- Nulliparity may be associated with earlier menopause.
- In the Framingham Heart Study cohort, each 1% higher premenopausal Framingham risk score for cardiovascular risk was associated with a 1.8-year decrease in the age at menopause, suggesting that heart disease risk factors influence the age of menopause, rather than the converse. In the prospective evaluation of women during the menopause transition—the Study of Women's Health Across the Nation (SWAN)—a history of heart disease was independently associated with earlier menopause.
- In one report, women with type 1 diabetes mellitus (DM) experienced menopause approximately 8 years earlier than their female siblings without DM; those with type 2 DM did not experience an earlier menopause.
- Women with epilepsy have an increased risk for developing menopause earlier. Women who experienced menopause earlier were more likely to have had exacerbation of their seizures.
- In a study of Latin American women, women living at high altitudes had earlier menopause.
- In an Italian cohort, season of birth was associated with timing of menopause. The earliest age of menopause was in women born in March; the latest was among those born in October.
- Adverse socioeconomic conditions across the life span, measured in terms of economic hardship and low educational attainment, may be associated with an earlier perimenopause.
- Being separated, widowed, divorced, or unemployed was associated with earlier natural menopause in SWAN.
- Women with a lifetime history of major depression, particularly if accompanied by the use of anti-depressants, had nearly three times the risk of an earlier perimenopause.

Table 2. Factors affecting delayed menopause

- Menopause may be delayed in direct proportion to the number of full-term pregnancies.

- In SWAN, prior use of oral contraceptives was associated with later age at natural menopause.

- No association between total alcohol consumption and onset of perimenopause was reported in the Harvard Study of Moods and Cycles; there was some suggestion that red wine consumption delayed entry into perimenopause.

- Japanese race/ethnicity was associated with a later age of menopause in SWAN.

- Limited data support the association of a later menopause with increased body mass index.

- Experience of sexual or physical violence was associated with delayed onset of perimenopause.

Ovarian aging, hormone production, and regulation

The changes characteristic of ovarian aging are best examined from the perspective and clear understanding of the physiology of the normal menstrual cycle.

Chronologic age is an inaccurate predictor of reproductive age because individual women vary widely in timing of the menopause transition. To establish a more specific measurement, a standardized definition of the stages of reproductive aging has been proposed (see Fig. 1 in Section A, page 10). The major categories are reproductive interval, menopause transition, and postmenopause.

Reproductive interval. The normal menstrual cycle involves three phases: follicular (or proliferative), periovulatory, and luteal (or secretory) (see Fig. 1 below). Menses coincides with the beginning of the follicular phase. At the onset of the menstrual cycle, circulating levels of estrogen and progesterone are low, signaling the hypothalamus and pituitary through a negative feedback loop to increase follicle-stimulating hormone (FSH). FSH initiates the process of follicular maturation, and the follicle (the fluid-filled sac containing an ovum, or egg) increases estrogen production, which stimulates new endometrial growth. At the end of the follicular phase, the endometrium thickens threefold, and a primordial follicle matures in preparation for the release of an ovum.

During the periovulatory phase, increased estrogen from the mature follicle, through a positive feedback mechanism, triggers a sharp increase in luteinizing hormone (LH)—

Figure 1. The menstrual cycle

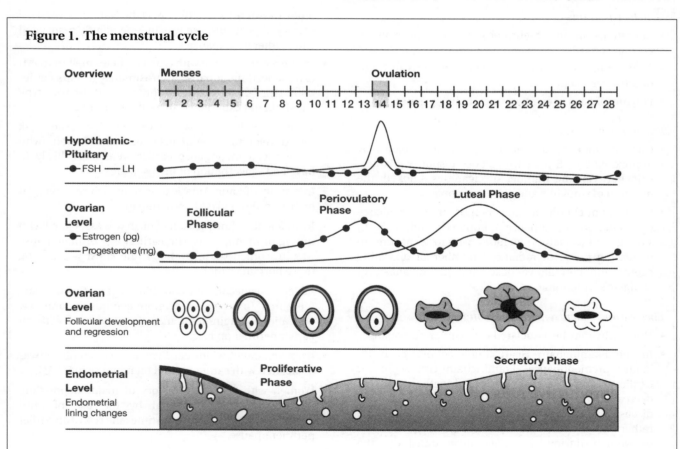

the LH surge—leading to release of the ovum. Pituitary LH continues to stimulate the residual ovarian follicle, transforming it into the corpus luteum.

The luteal phase is marked by estrogen and progesterone secretion from the corpus luteum. Increased progesterone supports and enriches the thickened endothelium in preparation for implantation and possible pregnancy. If fertilization of the ovum does not occur, the corpus luteum regresses, estrogen and progesterone levels decline, and as a result menses (ie, shedding of the endometrial lining and uterine bleeding) ensues.

The cyclical release of FSH and LH from the pituitary gland is tightly regulated and easily disturbed. When the pituitary gland does not release appropriate quantities of FSH or LH, ovulation may not occur, potentially disrupting the cycle.

Estradiol is the primary estrogen produced by the ovaries. In the normal ovarian cycle, circulating serum estradiol levels fluctuate from less than 10 to 100 pg/mL (37-370 pmol/L) in the early follicular phase, 200 to 800 pg/mL (730-2,930 pmol/L) at midcycle, and 200 to 340 pg/mL (730-1,250 pmol/L) during the luteal phase.

During the menstrual cycle, ovarian production of estradiol ranges from 36 µg/day in the follicular phase to 250 µg/day in the luteal phase. More than 95% of the circulatory estradiol comes from the dominant follicle and corpus luteum; most of the remaining amount is derived from peripheral conversion of estrone.

Estrone is the second most abundant estrogen in women. Estrone is derived primarily from the metabolism of estradiol and from peripheral aromatization of androstenedione to estrone in adipose tissue and muscle. Ovarian and adrenal secretion supplies a small amount. During the menstrual cycle, serum estrone levels vary from 30 to 180 pg/mL (110-660 pmol/L). In premenopausal women, the ratio of circulating estradiol to estrone is greater than 1.0.

The major gonadal peptides involved in the feedback loop are inhibin A and inhibin B. During the menstrual cycle, inhibin A levels are low for most of the follicular phase, then rise in midcycle, subsequently falling and then rising again to reach the highest levels during the luteal phase. Inhibin A secretion is in parallel with the secretion of estradiol and progesterone. Inhibin B levels rise and fall in the first half of the follicular phase, also show a midcycle peak, then subsequently fall to their lowest concentrations during the luteal phase. It is hypothesized that inhibin B and FSH form a closed-loop feedback system during the first half of the cycle, with the levels of inhibin B fine-tuning FSH regulation. Thus, both ovarian estradiol and the inhibins contribute to pituitary feedback.

In reproductive-age women, circulating androgens are produced in the ovaries, the adrenal glands, and through peripheral conversion of circulating androstenedione and dehydroepiandrosterone (DHEA) to testosterone. Five androgens are clinically important: testosterone, dihydrotestosterone (DHT), androstenedione, DHEA, and dehydroepiandrosterone sulfate (DHEAS).

Some androgens circulate in blood bound to proteins; others circulate in an unbound state. DHEAS binds strongly to albumin, resulting in a very low metabolic clearance rate. DHEA and androgen bind weakly to albumin, and their metabolic clearance rates are higher.

One quarter of circulating testosterone originates in the ovaries, one quarter in the adrenals, and one half from peripheral conversion of androstenedione. Testosterone levels range from 0.2 to 0.81 ng/mL (0.7 to 2.8 nmol/L). During the menstrual cycle, there is a slight but significant preovulatory rise in testosterone concentration.

Menopause transition. The menopause transition (or perimenopause) is characterized by erratic hormone secretion presenting as menstrual cycle irregularity, and finally complete cessation of menses. Changes in both central nervous system control and accelerated follicular atresia within the ovary likely contribute to the initiation and progression of the menopause transition.

During the late reproductive stage, elevation of FSH (>10 mIU/mL or IU/L) in the early follicular phase (between days 2 and 5) of the menstrual cycle is the sentinel mark of reproductive aging. The accelerated loss of follicles and resultant reduction of inhibin B contribute to further rapid elevation of FSH during the menopause transition. In the Melbourne Women's Midlife Health Study, an increase in FSH was apparent at least 2 years before the final menstrual period (FMP). A marked increase occurred in the year before the FMP with a plateau within 2 years after the FMP.

The ovary contains the maximal number of oocytes during a woman's fetal development; follicular loss begins in utero. Women are born with 1 to 2 million follicles. By menopause, only a few hundred to a few thousand remain. Most follicular loss results from atresia, not ovulation (<500 follicles over a lifetime). The number of follicles falls at a linear rate until approximately age 37, followed by a steeper decline until menopause. The rate of atresia, however, varies from woman to woman.

Anti-Müllerian hormone (AMH) is produced by the granulosa cells of primary, secondary, and antral follicles and has been identified as a potential marker of ovarian reserve. As opposed to other menstrually related hormones, AMH does not seem to fluctuate across the menstrual cycle. Longitudinal studies demonstrate an age-related decline; serial measurement of AMH might offer the potential of predicting the onset of menopause.

As ovarian follicle numbers decrease, levels of inhibin B fall, allowing FSH to rise and, for a time, sustain follicular development and ovulatory function. The higher levels of FSH recruit relatively more follicles per cycle, which may contribute to accelerated follicular atresia after age 37. Overproduction of estradiol by this enlarged cohort of recruited follicles may be responsible for common midlife symptoms such as bloating, irritability, mastalgia, menorrhagia, growth of uterine fibroids, and endometrial hyperplasia. Conversion of androgen to estrogen through aromatization increases with age and body weight. Normal (for reproductive-age women) to elevated estradiol levels might also be explained by this mechanism. Other symptoms characteristic of the late reproductive phase include vasomotor symptoms, insomnia, migraines, and premenstrual dysphoria. These symptoms may occur in the face of "regular" menstrual cycles.

According to the Stages of Reproductive Aging Workshop (STRAW) definition, the formal onset of the menopause transition is marked by a change in menstrual cycle length of at least 7 days. Later in the menopause transition, as the number of ovarian follicles decreases, the follicles remaining often respond poorly to FSH and LH. As a result, ovulation is erratic and cycle irregularity develops. Some cycles may be anovulatory (ie, no follicle released), whereas several follicles may be released during other cycles, perhaps accounting for the increased incidence of twins born to midlife women. In SWAN, three patterns of anovulatory cycles were described. One group of women had a normal increase in estradiol and midcycle LH surge but very low progesterone production; a second group had an estrogen increase but the LH surge was absent; a third group had a hormonal pattern similar to that of postmenopausal women characterized by elevated levels of LH and FSH and low levels of ovarian steroids.

In the late menopause transition, ovulation becomes more irregular. The rhythmic cyclical fluctuations in estrogen and progesterone levels are disrupted, and women experience irregular uterine bleeding and episodes of oligomenorrhea followed by eventual amenorrhea. In one study, during the year before menopause, women experienced cycles more than 40 days long for more than 75% of their cycles. Estradiol levels initially drop 2 years before the FMP, but the most dramatic drop is at the time of the FMP. Symptoms of genital atrophy and vaginal atrophy, often associated with painful sexual intercourse, may arise at this time.

Despite the resulting reduction in fertility, women should be aware that pregnancy is possible until menopause occurs, which is confirmed by either 12 consecutive months of amenorrhea or consistently elevated levels of FSH ($\geq$30 mIU/mL or IU/L).

In women of reproductive age, the ovary is the major source of estrogen. During the late menopause transition, a marked reduction in ovarian secretion of estrogen occurs. The greatest fall in estrogen secretion takes place during the first year postmenopause and is followed by a more gradual decline during the next few years.

In SWAN, women of different races and ethnic groups demonstrated similar patterns of hormonal changes with the menopause transition, but the levels of hormones differed. Both Chinese and Japanese women had lower estradiol concentrations compared than Caucasian, African-American, and Hispanic women. FSH concentrations were higher in African-American women than in women of other races. Ethnic differences in the pituitary-ovarian relation might explain these findings.

In the Melbourne Women's Midlife Health Study, the menopause transition was also associated with a drop in the levels of sex hormone-binding globulin (SHBG). During the 4 years before menopause to 2 years after menopause, SHBG levels decreased by approximately 40%, with the greatest change occurring 2 years before menopause concurrent with a dramatic decline in serum estradiol. Lower SHBG levels affect the free androgen index, calculated as the ratio of testosterone to SHBG. The index rises by nearly 80% during the menopause transition, with the maximal change occurring 2 years before the FMP. In a large Australian cross-sectional study, SHBG did not seem to vary from young adult to postmenopausal age. There was a minimal increase in the women aged 65 to 75 years.

Progesterone production depends on the integrity of the menstrual cycle. Early in the menopause transition, progesterone levels are usually normal. In anovulatory cycles, progesterone levels are low. During the menopause transition, progesterone is often lower than in normal-cycling women, even during ovulatory cycles.

Testosterone levels do not change during the menopause transition (from 4 y before menopause to 2 y after). Studies regarding testosterone concentrations are conflicting. In one small study, the midcycle rise in bioavailable testosterone and androstenedione, characteristic of younger regularly cycling women (19-37 y), was found to be consistently and significantly absent in older, regularly cycling women (43-47 y). Total testosterone levels did not differ significantly in any cycle stage between older and younger women. A prospective longitudinal study from Australia did not show a difference in total testosterone levels in the same women in the years before and after their FMP. A longitudinal study from Norway reported a 15% decrease in testosterone after menopause. Data from the Rancho Bernardo Study suggest that reductions in testosterone levels at menopause may be transient and followed by normalization of testosterone levels in older women. In a large cross-sectional Australian study, serum androgen levels were shown to decline with age from the early reproductive years without changing at the menopause transition. As in the Rancho Bernardo study, testosterone levels increased slightly during the seventh decade.

The concentration of DHT does not seem to be affected by aging or menopause. Metabolic clearance rates do not change significantly at menopause or with age. The pathways of metabolism are not altered at menopause, but aromatization of DHEA, androstenedione, and testosterone to estrone and estradiol all increase with age. Thus, androgen metabolism in general is affected more by gradual aging than by declining ovarian function.

Postmenopause stages. The hallmark for postmenopause is the FMP. The early postmenopause phase is defined as the 5 years after the FMP. This period encompasses a further dampening of ovarian hormones to a permanent low level. Late postmenopause begins 5 years after the FMP and continues until death.

The classic endocrine findings during postmenopause include elevated FSH and LH levels (10- to 15-fold) with FSH greater than LH, and marked reductions in serum concentrations of estradiol and estrone. Characteristically high gonadotropin levels after menopause progressively diminish with age. Postmenopausal estradiol levels are 10% or less of concentrations attained during reproductive life, and range from less than 10 to 37 pg/mL (37-140 pmol/L). Estrone levels range from 6 to 63 pg/mL (22-233 pmol/L). The ratio of estradiol to estrone reverses, and estrone becomes the predominant circulating estrogen. Estrone is derived primarily from peripheral conversion (ie, aromatization) of androstenedione. Estrogen levels, therefore, may be higher in obese women because aromatization increases as a function of the mass of adipose tissue.

Transient elevations of estradiol in postmenopausal women may reflect activity in a residual follicle, but such activity does not usually result in ovulation, though at least one case has been reported. Progesterone levels remain low after menopause. Because of the reduction in estradiol concentration after menopause, the ratio of estrogen to androgen is decreased.

The postmenopausal ovary continues to produce androstenedione and testosterone. Higher levels of androgens in some postmenopausal women might reflect ovarian stromal hyperplasia and luteinization. In the Rancho Bernardo Study, women aged 50 to 89 years with intact ovaries had total but not bioavailable (ie, free) testosterone levels that increased with age, reaching premenopausal levels by age 70, with relatively stable levels thereafter. In a report from the Cardiovascular Health Study, total testosterone levels declined with age until 80, whereas free testosterone levels did not vary by age. White race, greater education, lower body mass index, present use of estrogens, and oral corticosteroid use were each associated with lower total and free testosterone levels in women over age 65 years.

Surgical menopause results in lower testosterone levels. In the same Rancho Bernardo study, women who had undergone bilateral oophorectomy with hysterectomy had total

and bioavailable testosterone levels that did not vary with age, and were 40% to 50% lower than levels in women with intact uterus and ovaries. Levels of bioavailable estradiol, estrone, and SHBG were essentially the same regardless of oophorectomy status.

Hypothalamic-pituitary-ovarian axis

It is evident from the preceding material that a complex interplay through the hypothalamic-pituitary-ovarian axis controls the normal menstrual cycle and responds to ovarian aging. This section reemphasizes some of the key mechanisms.

Pulsatile hypothalamic release of gonadotropin-releasing hormone (GnRH) stimulates the pituitary gland to secrete FSH and LH. The gonadotropins then stimulate the ovary to secrete estrogen and progesterone. The pattern of pulsatile release of GnRH, pituitary hormones, and subsequent ovarian hormone secretion varies through the normal menstrual cycle (see Fig. 1).

As reproductive aging ensues, the hypothalamic-pituitary-ovarian axis changes in several ways. The first measurable sign is an increase in FSH. Ovarian inhibin production declines, resulting in a loss in negative feedback or "disinhibition" of pituitary FSH secretion. A rise in FSH can be detected as early as the late stage of the reproductive interval before any menstrual irregularity, although FSH is highly variable. Postmenopausal FSH levels continue to increase and then plateau within 1 year. Although FSH levels decrease somewhat after several years, they remain elevated above premenopausal concentrations even in elderly women.

Concurrent with or possibly preceding the decline in inhibin and resultant increase in FSH, the neuroendocrine control of GnRH secretion may also be altered. There is speculation based upon animal and some human studies that GnRH neurons change in their capacity to synthesize and release GnRH and to respond to neural inputs and steroid hormone sensitivity. Alterations of the GnRH pulse generator might contribute to the compromise or complete absence of the LH surge in perimenopausal women, thought to reflect a reduction in the sensitivity of the hypothalamic-pituitary-ovarian axis to positive feedback by estrogen.

During the menopause transition, LH levels usually remain in the normal range or increase slightly. After menopause, basal LH levels continue to rise and then plateau in about 1 year. The loss of gonadal steroid feedback after menopause alters the forms of LH and FSH secreted, resulting in slower clearance and prolonged half-life.

After menopause, the steady age-related decline in serum levels of LH and FSH provides clear evidence for additional hypothalamic-pituitary changes independent of those due to loss of ovarian hormonal feedback. The capacity of the hypothalamus to secrete GnRH is not diminished with age, although the dynamics of its control are altered. The amount of GnRH secreted is increased in postmenopausal women, although there is a decrease in GnRH pulse frequency. The decline of LH and FSH in the presence of increased GnRH secretion implies an age-related diminution of the ability of the pituitary to secrete gonadotropins. Gonadotropin secretion in postmenopausal women does not follow a circadian rhythm, although the circadian rhythmicity of the pituitary hormones adrenocorticotropic hormone (ACTH) and thyroid-stimulating hormone remains intact.

Low-level pituitary production of human chorionic gonadotropin (hCG) seems to be normal in postmenopausal women (levels <32 mIU/ml or IU/L). Pituitary hCG in postmenopausal women is the pregnancy-type hCG, and production parallels the increasing postmenopausal production of LH. The pituitary origin of hCG in a postmenopausal woman can be confirmed by suppression of hCG to less than 2 mIU/ml or IU/L after 2 weeks of menopausal hormone therapy (HT).

Adrenal physiology and menopause

The adrenal glands consist of two predominant regions—the cortex and the medulla. The adrenal medulla secretes epinephrine, norepinephrine, and dopamine in response to neural signals. The adrenal cortex is made up of three distinct zones, each of which secretes primarily one class of steroid hormone: glucocorticoids, androgens, or mineralocorticoids.

The zona fasciculata (the thick middle of the three layers of the adrenal cortex) secretes glucocorticoids, primarily cortisol, under control of the pituitary hormones ACTH and arginine vasopressin, as well as neural elements of the stress response. ACTH is regulated by hypothalamic corticotropin-releasing hormone (CRH) and by other central influences. Glucocorticoids provide feedback inhibition to both ACTH and CRH.

Adrenal glucocorticoid secretion follows a circadian pattern of secretion, with peak values in the morning and a nadir in the late afternoon. Cortisol and ACTH levels rise with increasing age, and serum concentrations at all ages are higher in women than in men. A blunting of the cortisol circadian rhythm is characteristic of aging in both sexes. Feedback inhibition of ACTH secretion by cortisol may be impaired in older persons, leading to prolonged glucocorticoid exposure.

In the Seattle Midlife Women's Health Study, during the 7 to 12 months after the onset of the late menopause transition stage (defined as skipped menstrual periods), cortisol levels were reported to rise significantly, coinciding with an increase in DHEAS, urinary metabolites of estrogen, and FSH. Women with an increase in cortisol were found to have significantly more severe hot flashes and vasomotor symptoms. Cortisol levels stabilized around the time of FMP.

Serum cortisol circulates bound to cortisol-binding globulin (CBG). In a cross-sectional study comparing postmenopausal women receiving oral estrogen therapy (ET), transdermal ET, or placebo, total serum cortisol concentrations were 67% higher in those receiving oral ET than in control subjects or women receiving transdermal ET. This was associated with a higher level of CBG in the women taking oral ET. Salivary cortisol concentration, a measure of free cortisol, was similar in all three groups. In another small study, transdermal ET administration for 3 months did not alter adrenal steroid levels or adrenal response to ACTH. Transdermal ET induced a significant reduction in ACTH response to CRH stimulation in women with a high waist-to-hip ratio and improved adrenal sensitivity in women with low waist-to-hip ratio. Estrogen effects on the hypothalamic-pituitary-adrenal axis may differ based upon a woman's weight and weight distribution. In another study of 11 women, 1 year of raloxifene therapy reduced circulating levels of adrenal steroids, sensitivity to ACTH, and estrogen levels, all hypothesized to be of benefit in both reducing exposure to endogenous glucocorticoids and reducing breast exposure to endogenous estrogens.

The zona reticularis (the innermost layer of the adrenal cortex) secretes adrenal androgens DHEA and androstenedione, also regulated by pituitary ACTH. Levels of adrenal androgens, particularly DHEA, fall with progressive age and are lower in women than in men. In older postmenopausal women, the disparity of lower DHEA and increased cortisol secretion is thought to be related to a defect in adrenal production of DHEA. The capacity of the adrenal glands to produce androstenedione does not seem compromised, and the age-related decrease in androstenedione likely reflects reduced production by the ovary. Smoking is associated with increased adrenal androgens; in the Rancho Bernardo study, the levels of DHEA and androstenedione increased concomitantly with cigarette smoking.

Reports about changes in DHEAS with the menopause transition have been mixed. A transient rise in DHEAS level was found in SWAN during the late menopause transition despite a preceding overall age-related decline. In the Melbourne Women's Midlife Health Project, DHEAS levels were unchanged during the menopause transition.

The zona glomerulosa (the thin outermost layer of the adrenal cortex) secretes mineralocorticoids, predominantly aldosterone. Secretion is primarily regulated by the renin-angiotensin system. Other regulators include sodium and potassium concentrations, ACTH, and neural components of the adrenergic and dopaminergic systems. Mineralocorticoid feedback at the level of the hippocampus might have important implications for regulation of glucocorticoid and adrenal androgen secretion, particularly with aging.

Receptor activity

Hormones such as estrogen are released from the cells in which they are produced and are carried in the bloodstream throughout the body to target cells in many different tissues where they trigger a response. Ovarian hormones diffuse freely into cells, but activity within a cell depends on the presence of specific hormone receptors or estrogen-binding proteins.

Two distinct estrogen receptors (ER) have been identified: ER-α and ER-β. Concentrations of the two receptors vary in different body tissues, with states of health, and possibly with age. In general, there are more ER-α receptors in the reproductive system (eg, uterus, breast) and liver whereas ER-β receptors are more prevalent in other tissues (eg, bone, blood vessels, and lungs). Both ER-α and ER-β are present in the ovary and the central nervous system.

The ER can bind to a variety of substances known as ligands. Different ligands have different affinities for ER-α and ER-β. For example, 17β-estradiol binds to both ER-α and ER-β, whereas phytoestrogens seem to have a higher affinity for ER-β.

A number of ER gene polymorphisms have been identified that may contribute to individual differences in menopause symptoms and development of osteoporosis, cardiovascular disease, cognitive dysfunction, diabetes, depression, and possibly breast cancer. Large population studies to date yield interesting though conflicting results. More research will determine how best to apply knowledge about ER polymorphisms in clinical practice.

Ligand binding to the ER initiates receptor activation. Depending on the ligand, the shape or conformation of the ER changes in a unique way specific to that ligand.

In the classic pathway of hormone action, estrogen binds to an ER in the cell nucleus. Depending on the tissue in which the particular ligand-receptor complex resides, tissue-specific cofactors interact with both the receptor and specific locations on the target gene, known as *estrogen response elements* (EREs). This usually involves the AP2 portion of the ERE. The DNA receptor-ligand complex will either turn on (activate) or turn off (repress) gene transcription depending on the ligand, the tissue, and the cofactors (coactivators or corepressors). A variety of proteins play a role in the interaction of ERs with EREs, a process that transpires over hours.

Alternatively, rapidly acting ERs located in close proximity to the cell membrane trigger release of intracellular messengers such as calcium, nitrous oxide, or activated kinases. Estrogen-binding portions of nonreceptor molecules in cell membranes seem to be responsible for rapid, nonclassic effects (no DNA binding of ERs required for action). The G-coupled membrane protein receptor, GPR30, has been identified as an estrogen-binding protein that is involved in rapid signaling of estrogen and may be clinically important in determining estrogen sensitivity of breast cancers.

Certain molecules such as growth factors and neurotransmitters are capable of activating the ER in the absence of estrogen (or other ligands), a process known as ligand-independent activation. Thus, the ERs/EREs modulate a potentially enormous number of different actions by different mechanisms in different tissues throughout the body.

Estrogen-related receptors (-α, -β, -γ) are orphan nuclear receptors that do not seem to require a classic ligand to facilitate interactions with coactivators and hormone response elements within target genes to stimulate transcription. Study of these estrogen-related receptors indicates an emerging role in modulating estrogen responsiveness, substituting for estrogen receptor activities, and serving as prognosticators in breast, ovarian, and colorectal cancers.

Our evolving understanding of ER action has broad clinical importance for the health of postmenopausal women, strategies for disease prevention, and development of cancer therapeutics.

Progesterone also acts via both genomic and nongenomic mechanisms. Two progesterone receptors (PRs), PR-α and PR-β, are coexpressed in most tissues, with PR-α dominating in the uterus and ovary and PR-β in the breast. Pure progesterone antagonists (eg, mifepristone, RU-486) bind to progesterone receptors and recruit corepressors to prevent progesterone action. Selective progesterone receptor modifiers (SPRMs, also known as J-compounds) have mixed agonist/antagonist activity depending on the structure of the ligand and the tissue where binding occurs. Current clinical applications of progesterone antagonists and SPRMs focus on labor induction and pregnancy termination. Potential uses under exploration include contraception, management of endometriosis and uterine fibroids, menopausal hormone therapy, and treatment of hormone-dependent tumors.

Suggested reading

Age at menopause

Allsworth JE, Zierler S, Lapane KL, Krieger N, Hogan JW, Harlow BL. Longitudinal study of the inception of perimenopause in relation to lifetime history of sexual or physical violence. *J Epidemiol Community Health* 2004;58:938-943.

Blumel JE, Chedraui P, Calie A, et al. Age at menopause in Latin America. *Menopause* 2006;13:706-712.

Cagnacci A, Pansini FS, Bacchi-Modena A, et al. Season of birth influences the timing of menopause. *Hum Reprod* 2005;20:2190-2193.

Dorman JS, Steenkiste AR, Foley TP, et al. Menopause in type 1 diabetic women: is it premature? *Diabetes* 2001;50:1857-1862.

Gold EB, Bromberger J, Crawford S, et al. Factors associated with age at natural menopause in a multiethnic sample of midlife women. *Am J Epidemiol* 2001;153:865-874.

Harden CL, Koppel BS, Herzog AG, Nikolov BG, Hauser WA. Seizure frequency is associated with age at menopause in women with epilepsy. *Neurology* 2003;61:451-455.

Harlow BL, Wise LA, Otto MW, Soares CN, Cohen LS. Depression and its influence on reproductive endocrine and menstrual cycle markers associated with perimenopause: the Harvard Study of Moods and Cycles. *Arch Gen Psychiatry* 2003;60:29-36.

Hefler LA, Grimm C, Bentz EK, Reinthaller A, Heinze G, Tempfer CB. A model for predicting age at menopause in white women. *Fertil Steril* 2006;85:451-454.

Hefler LA, Grimm C, Heinze G, et al. Estrogen-metabolizing gene polymorphisms and age at natural menopause in Caucasian women. *Hum Reprod* 2005;20:1422-1427.

Klein P, Serje A, Pezzullo JC. Premature ovarian failure in women with epilepsy. *Epilepsia* 2001;42:1584-1589.

Kok HS, van Asselt KM, van der Schouw YT, et al. Heart disease risk determines menopausal age rather than the reverse. *J Am Coll Cardiol* 2006;47:1976-1983.

Kok HS, van Asselt KM, van der Schouw YT, Peeters PH, Wijmenga C. Genetic studies to identify genes underlying menopausal age. *Hum Reprod Update* 2005;11:483-493.

Phillips GS, Wise LA, Harlow BL. A prospective analysis of alcohol consumption and onset of perimenopause. *Maturitas* 2007;56:263-272.

Parazzini F, Progetto Menopausa Italia Study Group. Determinants of age at menopause in women attending menopause clinics in Italy. *Maturitas* 2007;56:280-287.

Schoenbaum EE, Hartel D, Lo Y, et al. HIV infection, drug use, and onset of natural menopause. *Clin Infect Dis* 2005;41:1517-1524.

Sklar CA, Mertens AC, Mitby P, et al. Premature menopause in survivors of childhood cancer: a report from the Childhood Cancer Survivor Study. *J Natl Cancer Inst* 2006;98:890-896.

Sowers MR, Jannausch ML, McConnell DS, Kardia SR, Randolph JF Jr. Menstrual cycle markers of ovarian aging and sex steroid hormone genotypes. *Am J Med* 2006;119:531-543.

Wise LA, Kreiger N, Zierler S, Harlow BL. Lifetime socioeconomic position in relation to onset of perimenopause. *J Epidemiol Community Health* 2002;56:851-860.

Ovarian aging, hormone production, and regulation

Burger HG, Dudley EC, Cui J, Dennerstein L, Hopper JL. A prospective longitudinal study of serum testosterone, dehydroepiandrosterone sulfate, and sex hormone-binding globulin levels through the menopause transition. *J Clin Endocrinol Metab* 2000;85:2832-2838.

Berger HG, Dudley EC, Hopper JL, et al. Prospectively measured levels of serum follicle-stimulating hormone, estradiol, and the dimeric inhibins during the menopausal transition in a population-based cohort of women. *J Clin Endocrinol Metab* 1999;84:4025-4030.

Cappola AR, Ratcliffe SJ, Bhasin S, et al. Determinants of serum total and free testosterone levels in women over the age of 65 years. *J Clin Endocrinol Metab* 2007;92:509-516.

Davison SL, Bell R, Donath S, et al. Androgen levels in adult females: changes with age, menopause, and oophorectomy. *J Clin Endocrinol Metab* 2005;90:3847-3853.

Ferrell RJ, O'Connor KA, Rodriguez G, et al. Monitoring reproductive aging in a 5-year prospective study: aggregate and individual changes in steroid hormones and menstrual cycle lengths with age. *Menopause* 2005;12:567-577.

Ferrell RJ, Simon JA, Pincus SM, et al. The length of perimenopausal menstrual cycles increases later and to a greater degree than previously reported. *Fertil Steril* 2006;86:619-624.

Hehenkamp WJ, Looman CW, Themmen AP, et al. Anti-Müllerian hormone levels in the spontaneous menstrual cycle do not show substantial fluctuation. *J Clin Endocrinol Metab* 2006;91:3760-3762.

Klein NA, Battaglia DE, Miller PB, Branigan EF, Giudice LC, Soules MR. Ovarian follicular development and the follicular fluid hormones and growth factors in normal women of advanced reproductive age. *J Clin Endocrinol Metab* 1996;81:1946-1951.

La Marca A, Stabile G, Artensio AC, Volpe A. Serum anti-Mullerian hormone throughout the human menstrual cycle. *Hum Reprod* 2006;21:3103-3107.

Lasley BL, Santoro N, Randolf JF, et al. The relationship of circulating dehydroepiandrosterone, testosterone, and estradiol to stages of the menopausal transition and ethnicity. *J Clin Endocrinol Metab* 2002;87:3760-3767.

Laughlin GA, Barrett-Connor E. Sexual dimorphism in the influence of advanced aging on adrenal hormone levels: the Rancho Bernardo Study. *J Clin Endocrinol Metab* 2000;85:3561-3568.

Laughlin GA, Barrett-Connor E, Kritz-Silverstein D, von Muhlen D. Hysterectomy, oophorectomy, and endogenous sex hormone levels in older women: the Rancho Bernardo Study. *J Clin Endocrinol Metab* 2000; 85:645-651.

Mitchell ES, Woods NF, Marielle A. Three stages of the menopausal transition from the Seattle Midlife Women's Health Study: toward a more precise definition. *Menopause* 2000;7:334-349.

Mushayandebvu T, Castracane VD, Gimpel T, Adel T, Santoro N. Evidence for diminished midcycle ovarian androgen production in older reproductive aged women. *Fertil Steril* 1996;65:721-723.

Randolph JF, Sowers M, Bondarenko IV, et al. Change in estradiol and follicle-stimulating hormone across the early menopausal transition: effects of ethnicity and age. *J Clin Endocrinol Metab* 2003;89:1555-1561.

Santoro N. The menopausal transition. *Am J Med* 2005;118:85-135.

Santoro N, Brown JR, Adel T, Skurnick JH. Characterization of reproductive hormonal dynamics in the perimenopause. *J Clin Endocrinol Metab* 1996;81:1495-1501.

Santoro N, Lasley B, McConnell D, et al. Body size and ethnicity are associated with menstrual cycle alterations in women in the early menopausal transition: the Study of Women's Health Across the Nation (SWAN) daily hormone study. *J Clin Endocrinol Metab* 2004;89:2622-2631.

van Rooij IA, Broekmans FJ, te Velde ER, et al. Serum anti-Müllerian hormone levels: a novel measure of ovarian reserve. *Hum Reprod* 2002;17:3065-3071.

van Rooij IA, Tonkelaar I, Broekmans FJ, et al. Anti-müllerian hormone is a promising predictor of the occurrence of the menopausal transition. *Menopause* 2004;11:601-606.

Welt CK, Jimenez Y, Sluss PM, et al. Control of estradiol secretion in reproductive ageing. *Hum Reprod* 2006;22:2189-2193.

Hypothalamic-pituitary-ovarian axis

Cole LA, Sasaki Y, Muller CY. Normal production of human chorionic gonadotropin in menopause [letter to editor]. *N Engl J Med* 2007; 356:1184-1186.

Ferrell RJ, O'Connor KA, Holman DJ, et al. Monitoring reproductive aging in a 5-year prospective study: aggregate and individual changes in luteinizing hormone and follicle-stimulating hormone with age. *Menopause* 2007;14:29-37.

Hall JE. Neuroendocrine physiology of the early and late menopause. *Endocrinol Metab Clin North Am* 2004;33:637-659.

Lavoie BH, Marsh EE, Hall JE. Absence of apparent circadian rhythms of gonadotropins and free alpha-subunit in postmenopausal women: evidence for distinct regulation relative to other hormonal rhythms. *J Biol Rhythms* 2006;21:58-67.

Weiss G, Skurnick JH, Goldsmith LT, et al. Menopause and hypothalamic-pituitary sensitivity to estrogen. *JAMA* 2004;292:2991-2996.

Wise PM, Smith MJ, Dubai DB, et al. Neuroendocrine modulation and repercussions of female reproductive aging. *Recent Prog Horm Res* 2002; 57:235-256.

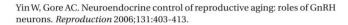

Yin W, Gore AC. Neuroendocrine control of reproductive aging: roles of GnRH neurons. *Reproduction* 2006;131:403-413.

Adrenal physiology and menopause

Cucinelli F, Soranna L, Barini A, et al. Estrogen treatment and body fat distribution are involved in corticotropin and cortisol response to corticotropin-releasing hormone in postmenopausal women. *Metabolism* 2002;51:137-143.

Genazzani AR, Lombardi I, Borgioli G, et al. Adrenal function under long-term raloxifene administration. *Gynecol Endocrinol* 2003;17:159-168.

Giordano R, Bo M, Pellegrino M, et al. Hypothalamus-pituitary-adrenal hyperactivity in human aging is partially refractory to stimulation by mineralocorticoid receptor blockade. *J Clin Endocrinol Metab* 2005;90:5656-5662.

Guthrie JR, Dennerstein L, Taffe JR, et al. The menopausal transition: a 9-year prospective population-based study. The Melbourne Women's Midlife Health Project. *Climacteric* 2004;7:375-389.

Khaw KT, Tazuke S, Barrett-Connor E. Cigarette smoking and levels of adrenal androgens in postmenopausal women. *N Engl J Med* 1988;318:1705-1709.

Lasley BL, Santoro N, Randolf JF, et al. The relationship of circulating dehydroepiandrosterone, testosterone, and estradiol to stages of the menopausal transition and ethnicity. *J Clin Endocrinol Metab* 2002;87:3760-3767.

Laughlin GA, Barrett-Connor E. Sexual dimorphism in the influence of advanced aging on adrenal hormone levels: the Rancho Bernardo Study. *J Clin Endocrinol Metab* 2000;85:3561-3568.

Liu CH, Laughlin GA, Fischer UG, Yen SS. Marked attenuation of ultradian and circadian rhythms of dehydroepiandrosterone in postmenopausal women: evidence for a reduced 17,20-desmolase enzymatic activity. *J Clin Endocrinol Metab* 1990;71:900-906.

Parker CR, Slayden SM, Azziz R, et al. Effects of aging on adrenal function in the human: responsiveness and sensitivity of adrenal androgens and cortisol to adrenocorticotropin in premenopausal and postmenopausal women. *J Clin Endocrinol Metab* 2000;85:48-54.

Qureshi AC, Bahri A, Breen LA, et al. The influence of the route of oestrogen administration on serum levels of cortisol-binding globulin and total cholesterol. *Clin Endocrinol (Oxf)* 2007;66:632-635.

Slayden SM, Crabbe L, Bae S, Potter HD, Azziz R, Parker CR Jr. The effect of 17 beta-estradiol on adrenocortical sensitivity, responsiveness, and steroidogenesis in postmenopausal women. *J Clin Endocrinol Metab* 1998;83:519-524.

Van Cauter E, Leproult R, Kupfer DJ. Effects of gender and age on the levels and circadian rhythmicity of plasma cortisol. *J Clin Endocrinol Metab* 1996;81:2468-2473.

Wilkinson CW, Petrie EC, Murray SR, et al. Human glucocorticoid feedback inhibition is reduced in older individuals: evening study. *J Clin Endocrinol Metab* 2001;86:545-550.

Woods NF, Carr MC, Tao EY, et al. Increased urinary cortisol levels during the menopausal transition. *Menopause* 2006;13:212-221.

Receptor activity

Ariazi EA, Jordan VC. Estrogen-related receptors as emerging targets in cancer and metabolic disorders. *Curr Top Med Chem* 2006;6:203-215.

Chabbert-Buffet N, Meduri G, Bouchard P, Spitz IM. Selective progesterone receptor modulators and progesterone antagonists: mechanisms of action and clinical applications. *Hum Reprod Update* 2005;11:293-307.

Cordera F, Jordan VC. Steroid receptors and their role in the biology and control of breast cancer growth. *Semin Oncol* 2006;33:631-641.

Deroo BJ, Korach KS. Estrogen receptors and human disease. *J Clin Invest* 2006;116:561-570.

Gaillard S, Dwyer MA, McDonnell DP. Definition of the molecular basis for estrogen receptor-related receptor-alpha-cofactor interactions. *Mol Endocrinol* 2007;21:62-76.

Jensen EV, Jordan VC. The estrogen receptor: a model for molecular medicine. *Clin Cancer Research* 2003;9:1980-1989.

Kjaergaard AD, Ellervik C, Tybjaerg-Hansen A, et al. Estrogen receptor alpha polymorphism and risk of cardiovascular disease, cancer, and hip fracture: cross-sectional, cohort, and case-control studies and a meta-analysis. *Circulation* 2007;115:861-871.

Kuiper GG, Carlsson B, Grandien K, et al. Comparison of the ligand binding specificity and transcript tissue distribution of estrogen receptors alpha and beta. *Endocrinology* 1997;138:863-870.

McDonnell DP. The molecular pharmacology of estrogen receptor modulators: implications for the treatment of breast cancer. *Clin Cancer Res* 2005;11(2 Pt 2):871S-877S.

Moriarty K, Kim KH, Bender JR. Minireview: estrogen receptor-mediated rapid signaling. *Endocrinology* 2006;147:5557-5563.

Prossnitz ER, Arterburn JB, Sklar LA. GPR30: a G protein-coupled receptor for estrogen. *Mol Cell Endocrinol* 2007;265-266:138-142.

Silvestri S, Thomsen AB, Gozzini A, et al. Estrogen receptor A and B polymorphisms: is there an association with bone mineral density, plasma lipids, and response to postmenopausal hormone therapy? *Menopause* 2006;13:451-461.

Sowers MF, Kardia SR, Johnson S, eds. Genetics and the sex steroid hormone pathway in women at midlife. *Am J Med* 2006;119(Suppl 1):S1-S112.

Woods NF, Mitchell ES, Tao Y, et al. Polymorphisms in the estrogen synthesis and metabolism pathways and symptoms during the menopausal transition: observations from the Seattle Midlife Women's Health Study. *Menopause* 2006;13:902-910.

As a woman moves through perimenopause and beyond, she may experience one or more of various menopause-related symptoms and other health effects. This section reviews the most common potential symptoms and effects. Risk factors for common diseases experienced by midlife women (such as osteoporosis, cardiovascular disease, and cancers), as well as strategies to lower risk and treat, are discussed in Section E, page 113.

Decline in fertility

Fertility declines significantly in women around age 35 to 38, or 10 to 15 years before menopause. In addition, advanced maternal age (age 35 and older) is associated with increased risks for spontaneous miscarriage (50% by age 45), chromosomal abnormalities in the fetus, and other pregnancy complications (eg, premature labor, fetal mortality, or need for cesarean section). Many women in industrialized countries are delaying childbearing and thus may face increased risk of fertility problems.

The functional activity of the ovary changes more with age than does almost any other organ in the human body. With aging, there is a subtle but real increase in follicle-stimulating hormone (FSH) and a decrease in inhibin A and B, which are responsible for the feedback regulation of FSH throughout the menstrual cycle. Declining secretion of inhibin B seems to contribute significantly to the rising FSH levels during the menopause transition and after menopause. The increase in FSH reflects the quality and quantity of aging follicles. Once the oocyte pool decreases to approximately 1,000 follicles, menopause is reached.

In addition to oocyte quality, the primary determinant of reproductive potential, age-related uterine changes may contribute to decreased fertility without creating any major change in the hormonal dynamics of the menstrual cycle.

Fertility-enhancing options. Research for assisted reproductive technologies has provided significant information regarding aging and fertility. It is now thought that functional ovarian reserve (as directly measured by a basal day 3 serum FSH and/or other markers) is the most important indicator of age-related infertility. Ovarian reserve describes a woman's reproductive potential as it relates to follicular depletion and oocyte quality. Although some intercycle variability exists, women with elevations of FSH in one cycle usually have elevations in subsequent cycles. Many other markers of ovarian function are currently being evaluated to optimize testing of ovarian reserve.

For women of advanced reproductive age who still desire to have children, fertility-enhancing technologies are an option. Alternatives include in vitro fertilization, intrauterine insemination, oocyte donation, and embryo transfer as well as surrogacy/gestational carriers. Hormonal therapies are also available to promote ovulation.

The success of the fertility-enhancing technology depends on the woman's age, general health, reasons for treatment, and the modality used. Many of these options are expensive, involve some risks, and are not always successful; the success rate decreases closer to menopause. Women of advanced reproductive age often have a number of health risks. In general, fertility-enhancing techniques are discouraged for women older than age 43 and are not recommended after age 51. If a woman is considering these alternatives, she should be fully apprised of the risks and benefits of each technique.

Birth control options during perimenopause. Despite a decline in fertility during perimenopause, unplanned pregnancy is still possible until menopause (ie, no menstrual periods for 12 consecutive months) or until levels of FSH are consistently elevated (>30 mIU/mL).

Perimenopausal women have a range of excellent nonhormonal contraception options.

Sterilization (tubal ligation and vasectomy) is safe and effective and has a very low failure rate (about 4-8 per 1,000). The primary disadvantages are the risks associated with anesthesia and the surgical procedure as well as difficulty reversing the process. Sterilization offers no protection from sexually transmitted infections (STIs). Sterilization is a good option for midlife women (or their male partners) if they are in a mutually monogamous, long-term relationship and desire permanent contraception.

Permanent female sterilization is available through hysterectomy, salpingectomy, tubal ligation, tubal fulguration, and application of clips. In addition, noninvasive irreversible sterilization is offered through the Essure Contraceptive Tubal Occlusion Device and Delivery System, available in several countries, including the United States and Canada. Using hysteroscopy in the outpatient setting without anesthesia, a drug-free nitrol-dacron device is inserted into the proximal section of each fallopian tube. When released from the delivery system, the outer coil expands in diameter to anchor the micro-insert in the varied diameters and shapes of the fallopian tube. This spring-like device is intended to provide the necessary anchoring forces for 3 months, during which time the device fibers elicit tissue growth into the coils, contributing to device retention and pregnancy prevention. During this 3-month period, the patient must use an alternate form of contraception. A hysterosalpingogram is performed to determine the proper location of the device and to document tubal occlusion. Studies have found the device to be 99.8% effective after 4 years of follow-up. Performed correctly (following manufacturer's training), the procedure is considered safe, with minimal post-procedure patient discomfort and sequelae and minimal adverse events. The majority of clinical data is based on 12 to 24 months of use; the risks of long-term implantation are not known.

Other nonhormonal methods of contraception include spermicides and barrier methods, including the male condom, female condom, diaphragm, cervical cap, and cervical sponge. These methods are highly effective if used correctly and consistently during every act of vaginal sex. The condom is the only proven effective protection against both pregnancy and STIs (during vaginal, oral, and anal sex). Barrier methods can be used in combination with other birth control methods. Disadvantages include potential allergic reaction to latex or spermicides, the need to be used during every act of sex, and (with condoms) the potential to break, leak, or spill when removed. Nonlatex diaphragms and male condoms as well as polyurethane female condoms are available. The diaphragm and cervical cap are available only from a healthcare provider.

Natural family planning (the rhythm method or periodic abstinence) and the withdrawal method are other options. These methods have the advantages of no cost, no need for surgery, and no need to take a drug or use a device. Disadvantages include a high failure rate compared with other methods and no protection against STIs. Natural family planning is not a reliable option during perimenopause, because ovulation occurs sporadically and is difficult to predict because of irregular menstrual periods. When using the withdrawal method, which is never a reliable method of birth control, enough sperm to cause pregnancy may seep from the penis prior to ejaculation.

Hormonal contraceptives and nonhormonal intrauterine devices are discussed in Section G.

It is important for women to know that fertility becomes significantly compromised long before overt clinical signs of perimenopause occur. Exact relations among the FSH rise, accelerated follicular atresia, shortened follicular phase, and oocyte quality remain to be determined. Research in assisted reproductive technologies continues to define these issues and offers improved options for women with decreased fertility.

Uterine bleeding changes

Changes in both menstrual flow and frequency are the hallmarks of perimenopause. There is no universal definition of irregular uterine bleeding patterns; rather, each woman will experience a pattern that is irregular for her.

Approximately 90% of women experience 4 to 8 years of menstrual cycle changes before natural menopause. Most report irregular menses that are attributed to decreased frequency of ovulation and erratic levels of ovarian-secreted hormones. Initial menstrual cycle changes as women approach menopause can be subtle, and a variety of menstrual patterns are possible (see Table 1).

The following are some terms used to describe menstrual periods and menstrual patterns:

- Amenorrhea: absence of menses
- Dysmenorrhea: painful menses
- Hypermenorrhea: increased uterine bleeding occurring at regular intervals
- Hypomenorrhea: decreased uterine bleeding occurring at regular intervals
- Menometrorrhagia: frequent bleeding that is excessive and irregular in amount and duration
- Menorrhagia: prolonged or excessive uterine bleeding occurring at the regular intervals of menstruation, a loss of 80 mL or more of blood each menstrual cycle, or bleeding that lasts longer than 7 days
- Metrorrhagia: bleeding that occurs between periods
- Oligomenorrhea: decreased frequency of menstrual periods
- Polymenorrhea: bleeding that occurs every 21 days or less

Table 1. Possible menstrual changes during perimenopause
- Lighter bleeding (avg blood loss, <20 mL)
- Heavier bleeding (avg blood loss, >40 mL)
- Bleeding lasting for <2 days or >4 days
- Cycle length <7 days or >28 days
- Skipped menstrual periods
- No changes

Bleeding irregularities reported in one population-based study of 380 perimenopausal women included the following changes: menstrual flow only (23%), both frequency and flow (28%), and frequency only (9%), as well as absence of menses for at least 3 months (13%). A chart review of 500 perimenopausal patients found that alterations in menstrual flow fit one of three patterns: oligomenorrhea and/or hypomenorrhea (70%); menorrhagia, metrorrhagia, and/or hypermenorrhea (18%); and sudden amenorrhea (12%).

Changes in menstrual patterns and flow are considered normal, natural phenomena of the menopause transition. Anovulatory uterine bleeding, which arises from anovulation or oligoovulation, is often seen during perimenopause.

The Stages of Reproductive Aging Workshop (STRAW) proposed a summary of a woman's reproductive life in seven stages (see Section A, page 10, for a diagram). Five stages occur before the final menstrual period (FMP) and two occur afterwards. Investigators from four cohort studies analyzing menstrual cycle changes in the transition around menopause formed a ReSTAGE collaboration to validate STRAW's guidelines. They concluded that 60 days of amenorrhea defines the onset of the late menopause transition. Follicular phase hormone levels of estradiol, FSH, inhibin B, and luteinizing hormone are associated with menstrual bleeding patterns and differentiate the earliest stages of the menopause transition. With future analysis of the cohort studies in peri- and postmenopausal women compartmentalized without the outline of the STRAW criteria, we will be able to further define menstrual cycle patterns and follicular hormone levels that may be able to predict the onset of the postmenopausal stage of life.

Irregular uterine bleeding has an array of consequences, such as heavy or prolonged flow, potential social embarrassment, avoidance of sexual activity, and diminished quality of life. In some cases, anemia may result, with associated fatigue, pica (unusual food cravings), and/or headaches.

Abnormal uterine bleeding. Terminology for uterine bleeding is inconsistent. NAMS distinguishes normal, irregular bleeding from abnormal uterine bleeding (AUB). In NAMS materials, the term *abnormal uterine bleeding* is used broadly to describe excessive and/or erratic bleeding (see Table 2).

Table 2. AUB patterns in perimenopausal women
• Heavy menstrual bleeding (avg blood loss, >80 mL), especially with clots
• Menstrual bleeding lasting >7 days or ≥2 days longer than usual
• Intervals <21 days from the onset of one menstrual period to the onset of the next period
• Any spotting or bleeding between periods
• Uterine bleeding after sexual intercourse

Anovulatory uterine bleeding is defined as menstrual bleeding arising from anovulation or oligoovulation. The normal, irregular bleeding characteristic of the perimenopause transition represents a type of anovulatory uterine bleeding.

Dysfunctional uterine bleeding describes AUB without known structural or endocrine cause.

The terms *uterine bleeding* and *vaginal bleeding* should not be used interchangeably.

Causes of uterine bleeding changes. Anovulatory and abnormal uterine bleeding may be related to a number of benign and malignant diseases of the reproductive tract and systemic diseases (see Table 3). The predominant cause of AUB in perimenopausal women is less predictable ovulation. If the woman is sexually active, pregnancy should also be considered. Endometrial hyperplasia and carcinoma also become more prevalent with age. Infection is another potential cause. Thyroid abnormalities, hyperprolactinemia, and polycystic ovarian syndrome may cause anovulation and bleeding irregularities. Systemic diseases other than endocrinopathies, such as leukemia, infrequently present with uterine bleeding as the only sign or symptom. AUB in perimenopausal women may also be caused by anatomic conditions, including endometrial polyps or uterine fibroids.

Table 3. Possible causes of anovulatory and abnormal uterine bleeding
Benign reproductive tract conditions
Anovulation
Pregnancy
Leiomyomata uteri
Endometrial or endocervical polyps
Adenomyosis
Endometritis
Endometriosis
Pelvic inflammatory disease
Vaginal/cervical infection
Endometrial neoplasia
Endometrial hyperplasia without atypia
Endometrial hyperplasia with atypia
Endometrial adenocarcinoma
Systemic causes
Coagulation disorders (thrombocytopenia, von Willebrand's disease, leukemia)
Hyperprolactinemia
Liver disease
Thyroid dysfunction
Obesity
Anorexia
Rapid fluctuations in weight
Chronic illness
Other causes
Corticosteroids
Exogenous progestogen withdrawal
Hormonal contraceptives
Contraceptive devices
Anticoagulants
Tamoxifen
Select herbs

Hormonal imbalance. The predominant cause of AUB in perimenopausal women is less predictable ovulation, reflecting hypothalamic-pituitary-ovarian dysfunction. Anovulatory uterine bleeding presents as noncyclic menstrual blood flow ranging from spotting to heavy. Timing of the bleeding episodes and the amount of blood loss are erratic. Without cyclic progesterone, the endometrium becomes proliferative and, in some women, can become hyperplastic. Either condition is prone to unpredictable localized bleeding. If estrogen exposure is continuous, an abnormal overgrowth of cells may develop within the endometrium (endometrial hyperplasia) that could lead to endometrial cancer.

Hormonal contraceptives. Hormonal contraceptive use may result in a variety of menstrual patterns. Missed oral contraceptive (OC) tablets may cause breakthrough bleeding. Long-cycle or continuous OCs are associated with breakthrough bleeding or spotting, which decreases over time. Progestin-only contraceptives often result in irregular bleeding or spotting, which diminishes over time. Progestin-secreting intrauterine devices (IUDs) reduce bleeding at menses; both unmedicated and copper devices may increase menstrual blood loss. Certain medications (most notably common anticonvulsants and the antibiotic rifampin) may interfere with absorption of hormonal contraceptives, resulting in spotting or bleeding (as well as a potential decrease in efficacy). (See Section G, page 201, for more about contraceptives.)

Menopausal hormone therapy. Women who use systemic menopausal estrogen-progestogen therapy (EPT) often have progestogen-induced uterine bleeding. If bleeding starts only after initiation of EPT, the bleeding may simply reflect the iatrogenic impact of hormones. Uterine bleeding is generally not associated with unopposed estrogen therapy (ET). (See Section E, page 146, for more about using progestogen to reduce endometrial cancer risk with ET.)

Pregnancy. Until menopause is reached, pregnancy can occur, causing amenorrhea or other aberrations in menstrual flow. Spontaneous and induced abortions as well as ectopic pregnancies can also cause AUB in reproductive-age women.

Thyroid and pituitary dysfunction. Hypothyroidism may result in menorrhagia. Both hypo- and hyperthyroidism as well as hyperprolactinemia are associated with amenorrhea. (See Section E, page 158, for more about thyroid disease.)

Fibroids. Benign uterine fibroid tumors are commonly associated with AUB. While most fibroids are asymptomatic, others produce dramatic changes in menstrual periods (eg, heavier and prolonged periods) as well as a range of other symptoms, such as excessive menstrual cramps, back pain, dyspareunia, and difficulties with bowel movements or urination.

Although the cause of fibroids is unknown, estrogen can stimulate their growth. Because fibroids are estrogen sensitive, they often shrink after menopause, when ovarian production of estrogen diminishes. Rarely, systemic estrogen therapy may cause fibroids to resume growth. Fibroids can undergo torsion, degenerate, or become necrotic. Postmenopausal women who have uterine fibroids and take tamoxifen may experience uterine bleeding.

Abnormalities of the endometrium. Endometrial hyperplasia, benign endometrial or endocervical polyps, and occasionally endometriosis can result in AUB.

Cancer. A small percentage of cases of AUB are caused by cancer of the uterus or cervix. (See Section E for more about these cancers, including evaluation.)

Other causes. Coagulopathies may result in heavy uterine bleeding. Women with renal or liver disease may experience AUB. Although bleeding usually originates in the uterus, it is possible for the vagina or the cervix to be the source. Vaginal or cervical infections or vaginal atrophy may result

in postcoital bleeding. In postmenopausal women with cervical stenosis, bleeding may be caused by hematometra or pyometra.

Evaluation of AUB. Evaluation of AUB will vary depending on a woman's age and stage of menopause. Although the most common cause of uterine bleeding in a postmenopausal woman is endometrial atrophy, if she is not using menopausal therapy with combined estrogen plus progestogen (EPT), *any* uterine bleeding should be considered abnormal and warrants further investigation; endometrial evaluation is mandatory (see Section F, page 146, for details regarding available methods).

For the perimenopausal woman not using any type of systemic hormone therapy who presents with AUB, the history should emphasize the clinical features of menstrual flow, intermenstrual uterine bleeding, contraceptive and other medication use, and systemic diseases. The impact of the bleeding on daily activities is also important.

Charting of uterine bleeding is helpful in assessing reported menstrual abnormalities. Information should include the days of the bleeding, the amount and color of the flow, the presence of clots, and any pain associated with the bleeding. These reports are limited by the subjective nature of each woman's assessment. Printed forms (eg, Menstrual Calendar offered as a NAMS MenoNote®) often help women keep more reliable records.

A pelvic examination is mandatory in all perimenopausal women with AUB. The following should be ordered selectively: pregnancy test, complete blood cell count (to determine if anemia is present), coagulation studies, and tests of thyroid-stimulating hormone and serum prolactin.

For women who start bleeding only after initiation of EPT (which may simply reflect the iatrogenic impact of EPT), the bleeding is not heavy and declines in amount over time, so no evaluation is needed. If these parameters are not met, or if there is concern regarding the cause of the bleeding, endometrial evaluation is warranted. Pathology should also be suspected in peri- or postmenopausal women using EPT if uterine bleeding persists longer than 6 months or longer than 1 week each month in the first 6 months of therapy.

The following strategies represent a prudent approach to endometrial evaluation of the perimenopausal woman presenting with AUB as well as the postmenopausal woman requiring endometrial evaluation for uterine bleeding.

- Begin with endometrial biopsy or enhanced transvaginal sonography. If the histology demonstrates benign endometrium, including hyperplasia without atypia, proceed with medical or expectant management. Likewise, if unenhanced transvaginal sonography is reassuring, proceed with medical management.

- If such management does not result in a satisfactory bleeding pattern or if endometrial measurements are

5 mm or greater or not adequately visualized (eg, in the case of axial uterus, coexisting fibroids, or obesity), proceed with sonohysteroscopy or hysteroscopy as early as possible.

Given the absence of large randomized controlled trials (RCTs) comparing different evaluation strategies in the evaluation of AUB in peri- and postmenopausal women, clinicians—guided by patient preference—should use the techniques with which they are most technically comfortable and which are most accessible and cost-effective in their practices.

Management of AUB. For the management of AUB in peri- and postmenopausal women, a number of effective options, both medical and surgical, are available. Prior to recommending these options, anatomic issues should first be identified and treated.

Hormonal treatments. There is no treatment government approved in the United States or Canada for treating AUB. However, for perimenopausal women with AUB, hormonal management options include combination estrogen-progestin OCs, as well as transdermal and vaginal ring contraceptives, continuous injectable or intrauterine progestin contraceptives, oral EPT, cyclic oral progestogen alone, and parenteral estrogen. Gonadotropic-releasing hormone (GnRH) agonists occasionally have a role, especially if the woman is very anemic.

- *Estrogen-containing contraceptives.* Use of a low-dose combination estrogen-progestin OC is considered to be the first-line treatment of AUB in otherwise healthy, nonsmoking, perimenopausal women, regardless of their contraceptive needs. OCs are the only combination hormonal products assessed in clinical trials for this use, but no OC is government approved in the United States or Canada for treating AUB. Perhaps other estrogen-containing contraceptives have similar effects.

In clinical trials, OCs have normalized irregular bleeding and decreased menstrual flow. However, the effectiveness of OCs in treating AUB for women with fibroids is variable. OCs also offer other benefits, including contraception (if needed) and relief of vasomotor symptoms (see Section G, page 201, for more about hormonal contraceptives).

Estrogen-containing contraception is not recommended for women with a history of deep vein thrombosis, those with other cardiovascular risk factors, or those over age 35 who smoke. Some clinicians are reluctant to use these agents in perimenopausal women.

Cycle control is an important issue for perimenopausal women experiencing AUB. The hormonal contraceptive formulation selected should result in minimal breakthrough bleeding or irregular bleeding. Different formulations have different effects on irregular bleeding depending on the estrogen dose and type of progestin. In comparative trials, less unscheduled bleeding was observed in women taking OCs with lower-dose (≤20 µg) ethinyl estradiol than higher dose (30-35 µg).

Perimenopausal women with menorrhagia may benefit from less frequent menses or even amenorrhea, which can be achieved with an extended estrogen-progestin OC regimen (eg, Seasonale, Lybrel). Seasonale provides 12 weeks of continuous hormonally active tablets followed by seven placebo tablets. The same outcome can often be achieved by using standard OC formulations off label in an extended regimen by skipping the placebo week. Some women can identify the frequency with which withdrawal-bleeding episodes (uterine bleeding after each cycle of progestogen is ended) are required to avoid unscheduled breakthrough bleeding. If the placebo weeks are spaced farther apart than the usual 3 weeks, this extended cycle can control bleeding while still providing contraception. Lybrel has no placebo and is packaged for 365 days of use.

Transdermal and vaginal ring contraceptive systems provide other options to treat AUB.

- *Continuous progestin-only contraceptives.* For a perimenopausal woman with AUB, depot medroxyprogesterone acetate (DMPA) injections gradually produce amenorrhea and provide contraception, if needed. Use of the levonorgestrel-releasing intrauterine system (Mirena IUS) also reduces bleeding over time, and is effective in the treatment of menorrhagia; contraception (if needed) is provided. An RCT in Finland found that use of the IUS for 1 year was a cost-effective alternative to hysterectomy in treating AUB, although after 5 years of follow-up, 42% of women assigned to the IUS group eventually underwent hysterectomy.

For perimenopausal women with AUB and vasomotor symptoms, menopausal doses of estrogen can be added to DMPA or an IUS. This combined approach also prevents vaginal atrophy and has a positive effect on bone density while minimizing uterine bleeding, endometrial hyperplasia, and uterine cancer. (See Section G, page 201, for more about contraceptives.)

- *High-dose progestin plus low-dose estrogen.* Many perimenopausal women with AUB are not candidates for combination OCs (see Section G, page 201, for contraindications). Cyclic progestin therapy may be an option, although women with vasomotor symptoms, low bone density, or hypoestrogenism associated with cigarette smoking may benefit from the addition of estrogen (in postmenopausal doses).

It is important to use contraceptive doses of progestins in perimenopausal women with AUB because the doses in some EPT regimens do not suppress ovulation and could consequently aggravate the bleeding problem. Continuous-combined regimens using high-dose progestin and low-dose estrogen may initially cause irregular uterine bleeding or spotting, with eventual amenorrhea.

- *Cyclic oral progestogen.* Traditionally, cyclic oral progestogen therapy (progestin or progesterone) has been the standard medical therapy for anovulatory AUB in perimenopausal women. Continuous progestogen therapy could result in breakthrough bleeding. Table 4 shows common oral progestogens and dosing recommendations.

Administering cyclic progestogen for 12 to 14 days each month should result in predictable bleeding episodes. It may be appropriate to add estrogen in postmenopausal doses if vasomotor symptoms occur.

Withdrawal bleeding may continue indefinitely in some perimenopausal women treated with cyclic progestogen-only therapy, particularly those who are overweight and have higher levels of endogenous estrogen. If this occurs, it is appropriate to continue progestogen therapy because of the increased risk of endometrial hyperplasia and neoplasia in these women.

For perimenopausal women with anovulatory AUB and women with postmenopausal bleeding, if endometrial proliferation or hyperplasia without atypia is found on endometrial biopsy, cyclic or continuous progestogen-based medical management is indicated with follow-up evaluation after 3 or 4 months. If progestogen therapy does not result in histologic regression, dilation and curettage (D&C) with hysteroscopy should be performed before surgical therapy due to the possibility of underlying endometrial malignancy. There is nearly a 30% chance that complex endometrial hyperplasia with atypia will progress to cancer if untreated; therefore, for some women, hysterectomy represents appropriate surgical management in this setting.

- *Parenteral estrogen.* In emergency situations, treatment with parenteral estrogen can be considered for severe AUB in perimenopausal women. In one controlled study, intravenous administration of conjugated estrogens (CE) stopped AUB in 71% of women compared with 38% who received placebo. Because high-dose intravenous estrogen can acutely increase thrombosis risk, measures to prevent thrombosis should be considered in this setting.

- *Gonadotropin-releasing hormone agonists.* GnRH agonists induce a reversible hypoestrogenic state that causes endometrial atrophy. GnRH agonists are effective in reducing menstrual blood loss in perimenopausal women, but they are limited by their expense and side effects, including hot flashes and reduction of bone

Table 4. Examples of cyclic progestogen-only regimens for the treatment of anovulatory AUB in perimenopausal women

	Available strengths	Recommended dose
Tablet		
medroxyprogesterone acetate	2.5, 5.0, 10.0 mg	5-10 mg/d, 12-14 d/mo
norethindrone acetate	5.0 mg	2.5-5.0 mg (1/2-1 tablet)/d
norethindrone	0.35 mg	7.0-1.05 mg (2-3 tablets)/d
progesterone (micronized)	100, 200 mg	100-400 mg/d, 12-14 d/mo
Intrauterine system		
levonorgestrel	52 mg (5 y)	After insertion, initial release is 20 µg/d; after a few weeks, 150-200 pg/mL; average concentration is <25% of 150 µg oral levonorgestrel

density. Examples include injectable leuprolide acetate (Lupron) and nafarelin acetate nasal spray (Synarel).

Nonhormonal treatments. The following are nonhormonal options for treatments of AUB.

- *Nonsteroidal anti-inflammatory drugs.* NSAIDs inhibit cyclooxygenase and reduce endometrial prostaglandin levels. In a review of RCTs, NSAIDs taken at menses decreased menstrual blood loss by 20% to 50% and improved dysmenorrhea in up to 70% of women. Therapy is usually started 24 to 48 hours before menses and then continued for 5 days or until cessation of menstruation.

- *Antibiotics.* If pyometra is encountered, antibiotic therapy followed by repeat endometrial sampling to ensure resolution and exclude underlying neoplasia is appropriate. For some women who experience recurrent bleeding due to pyometra or hematometra, repeated cervical dilation to assure drainage may be necessary.

- *Iron.* All women experiencing AUB should be evaluated for iron deficiency (anemia). In addition to the medical and surgical treatments described in this section, iron supplementation is appropriate for women with AUB who are found to have iron deficiency anemia. (See Section H, page 247, for more about iron.)

Surgical treatment. There are several surgical approaches for treating perimenopausal women with anovulatory AUB and women with postmenopausal bleeding.

- *Dilation and curettage.* D&C (sometimes called dilatation and curettage) is a surgical procedure now considered obsolete for the treatment of AUB. Because it is a blind procedure, localized disease, such as polyps, can be missed. Neither does D&C completely remove intracavity tissue. Another limiting factor is that D&C usually requires general anesthesia. However, D&C with hysteroscopy is still effective for diagnosis.

- *Endometrial ablation.* Surgical techniques for endometrial resection and ablation have emerged as effective, safe, and cost-effective alternatives to hysterectomy for the treatment of AUB. Postprocedure amenorrhea occurs in 20% to 50% of patients. Newer technologies for endometrial ablation include cryoablation, heated intrauterine fluid, and radio-frequency electrical energy. The various systems are ThermaChoice, Hydro ThermAblator, Her Option, NovaSure, and Microwave Endometrial Ablation System.

  Endometrial ablation should be performed only in women for whom endometrial evaluation excludes pathology and preservation of fertility is not desired.

  Some approaches to ablation (eg, thermal balloon ablation) do not involve visualization of the endometrial cavity and may not effectively treat AUB caused by endometrial polyps or submucous fibroids. Clinicians should evaluate the endometrial cavity with sonohysterography or diagnostic hysteroscopy before endometrial destructive therapy. Clinicians planning hysteroscopic endometrial ablation should be prepared to resect any polypoid lesions encountered intraoperatively.

  Endometrial ablation may not successfully treat AUB caused by anatomic lesions located in the uterine wall, either intramural fibroids or adenomyosis. Endometrial ablation and the scarring it produces may limit the ability to evaluate subsequent AUB with traditional methods.

  Endometrial ablation offers effective therapy for heavy uterine bleeding without the need for inpatient stay or time off work usually associated with hysterectomy. Nonetheless, serious complications and even death have resulted, underscoring the need for appropriate surgical training and meticulous patient selection.

- *Hysterectomy.* Before the development of newer techniques, hysterectomy was the only definitive cure for benign AUB that failed to respond to medical treatment. Although surgical mortality is low, postoperative complications occur in approximately 30% of patients. In many women with AUB, medical management can prevent the need for hysterectomy.

Vasomotor symptoms

Perimenopausal and early postmenopausal fluctuations in estrogen and progesterone levels are often accompanied by vasomotor symptoms (hot flashes)—recurrent, transient episodes of flushing, and a sensation ranging from warmth to intense heat on the upper body and face, sometimes followed by chills. Vasomotor symptoms while sleeping can produce intense perspiration (*night sweats*).

The terms *vasomotor symptoms*, *hot flash*, and *hot flush* are often used to describe the same phenomenon. NAMS defines vasomotor symptoms as a global term that encompasses both hot flashes and night sweats. NAMS prefers the term "hot flash" rather than "hot flush."

The cause of these vasomotor symptoms is still a matter of speculation, and the initiating stimulus is unknown. Few studies have estimated the effect of hot flashes on quality of life, even though the potential for hot flashes to disrupt daily activities and sleep quality is widely accepted. They can negatively affect a woman's quality of life by causing acute physical discomfort as well as sleep disturbances that may result in fatigue, irritability, and forgetfulness.

The hot flash is the second most frequently reported perimenopausal symptom (after irregular menses). As many as 75% of perimenopausal women in the United States have hot flashes. It is considered one of the hallmarks of perimenopause.

Hot flash frequency usually increases during perimenopause, reaching highest occurrence during the first 2 years of postmenopause, and then declining over time. Most women experience hot flashes for 6 months to 2 years, although some have them for 10 years or longer.

An individual hot flash generally lasts 1 to 5 minutes; about 7% are longer and about 17% are shorter. During a hot flash, skin temperatures rise as a result of peripheral vasodilation. This change is particularly marked in the fingers and toes, where skin temperature can increase 1°C to 7°C.

Most women experience a sudden wave of heat sensation that spreads over the body, particularly on the upper body and face. Sweating begins primarily on the upper body, and it corresponds closely in time with the increase in skin conductance.

Modest heart rate increases of about 7 to 15 beats per minute occur at approximately the same time as the peripheral vasodilation and sweating. Heart rate and skin blood flow usually peak within 3 minutes of the onset of a hot flash. Significant elevations in metabolic rate occur simultaneously with sweating and peripheral vasodilation.

Skin temperatures return to normal gradually, possibly taking 30 minutes or longer. Decreases in core body temperatures of 0.1°C to 0.9°C, occurring approximately

5 to 9 minutes after the hot flash begins, have been observed, probably due to heat loss through perspiration and increased peripheral vasodilation. If the heat loss is significant, chills may be experienced.

Hot flashes can occur infrequently (monthly, weekly) or frequently (hourly), although there is usually a consistent individual pattern. A circadian rhythm has been observed, with hot flash frequency peaking in the early evening hours (about 3 hours after the peak in core body temperature).

Prevalence. Hot flash prevalence rates vary widely, both within the United States and in other countries. Reasons for these differences are not known, but they may be influenced by a number of factors, including climate, diet, lifestyle, women's roles, and attitudes regarding the end of reproductive life and aging. In addition to demographic variables, methodologic differences of studies no doubt come into play.

A 2007 systematic review of 66 papers addressing prevalence of vasomotor symptoms around the world concluded that fewer premenopausal women reported having hot flashes than perimenopausal women, but still at clinically significant levels (21.5% and 41%, respectively). Prevalence of reporting hot flashes by postmenopausal women was 41.5%. Inconsistent definitions of menopause status, however, plagued some of the studies.

In the United States, hot flash prevalence also differs among racial and ethnic groups. According to the Study of Women's Health Across the Nation (SWAN)—a multiracial, multiethnic sample of 16,065 women aged 40-55 y)—African-American women reported vasomotor symptoms most frequently (45.6%), followed by Hispanic (35.4%), Caucasian (31.2%), Chinese (20.5%), and Japanese (17.6%) women. Differences in body mass index (BMI) may be a more important predictor of having hot flashes than ethnicity. Other studies suggest that African-American women may experience hot flashes more frequently than women in other ethnic groups, especially Caucasians.

Most hot flashes are mild to moderate in intensity. However, approximately 10% to 15% of women have severe and/or very frequent hot flashes. Hot flashes tend to be more frequent and severe after surgically induced menopause. In US women who undergo bilateral oophorectomy, hot flash rates of up to 90% have been reported. Over time, symptoms decline to a level similar to women who have reached menopause naturally.

Causes and associations. The precise cause of vasomotor symptoms is not known. The changing endogenous estrogen levels and/or progesterone levels associated with menopause may play a role; however, these levels alone are not predictive of hot flash frequency or severity.

Other conditions that can cause hot flashes include thyroid disease, epilepsy, infection, insulinoma, pheochromocytoma, carcinoid syndromes, leukemia, pancreatic tumors, autoimmune disorders, new onset hypertension, and mast-cell disorders. Some drugs, such as tamoxifen and raloxifene, can cause hot flashes. Night sweats can also be associated with more serious diseases, such as tuberculosis and lymphoma.

A history of premenstrual complaints is also significantly associated with hot flashes in perimenopausal women. Approximately 47% of perimenopausal women with a history of moderate to severe premenstrual complaints experienced hot flashes compared with 32% of women without such a history. Low socioeconomic status has been associated with more frequent reporting of hot flashes.

Vasomotor symptoms can occur when menopausal hormone therapy (HT) is discontinued. A large cross-sectional survey showed that in women aged 70 years and older, 11% experienced vasomotor symptoms after stopping HT.

Management of vasomotor symptoms. Nearly 25% of US women experience sufficient discomfort from vasomotor symptoms to seek help from their healthcare provider. Although the available treatments do not "cure" hot flashes, they offer symptomatic relief. Hot flashes typically stop without treatment, but there is no reliable method for determining when that will occur. In 2004, NAMS published a position statement on the management of vasomotor symptoms in peri- and postmenopausal women. The following presents some recommendations from that position statement.

The treatment of menopause-associated vasomotor symptoms is a common clinical challenge. Before treatment begins, a detailed patient history of hot flashes is needed, including frequency and severity as well as their effect on activities of daily living. No treatment is needed unless the hot flashes are bothersome to the woman.

As with all treatments, the decision to undertake treatment for vasomotor symptoms should be based on the severity of the symptoms, an assessment of treatment-related risks, and the woman's personal attitudes about menopause and medication. Some women seek only to reduce their symptoms slightly, whereas others request complete amelioration. The clinical goal is to tailor therapy to each individual woman's needs, using the various options.

When therapy is needed to treat vasomotor symptoms, various pharmacologic and nonpharmacologic options are available (see Table 5). With many of these treatment options, efficacy has not been determined in RCTs, yet the option is included on the list because of its low (or no) cost and/or its low potential for harm. Nonetheless, evidence of efficacy from sources other than RCTs must be viewed with caution, as RCTs have demonstrated a relatively high (up to 40%) placebo response with hot flashes.

> **Table 5. Suggested options for women to manage vasomotor symptoms**
>
> - Enhance relaxation with meditation, yoga, massage, or a leisurely lukewarm bath
> - Get regular exercise to promote better, more restorative sleep
> - Keep cool by dressing in layers, using a fan, and sleeping in a cool room
> - Maintain a healthy body weight
> - Don't smoke
> - When a hot flash starts, try using paced respiration (deep, slow, abdominal breathing)
> - Avoid perceived personal hot flash triggers (eg, hot drinks, caffeine, spicy foods, alcohol), although studies among large numbers of women do not support an association
> - Try nonprescription therapies (eg, soy foods/isoflavones, black cohosh, or vitamin E) for mild hot flashes, although evidence is mixed
> - For moderate to severe hot flashes, consider HT (the only government-approved treatment) or nonestrogen prescription drugs (eg, progestogens, transdermal clonidine, venlafaxine, gabapentin)

In women with breast cancer or other hormone-dependent neoplasias, no therapy has been approved by either the US or Canadian government for treating hot flashes. However, a variety of nonprescription and nonhormonal treatments have been used to relieve hot flashes in these populations. Caution is advised when recommending therapies to these women, as some therapies may have estrogenic activity or interact with estrogen or some chemopreventive treatments in women at high risk of hormone-dependent cancers or those with breast cancer. Data are inadequate to determine if the physiologic mechanisms for hot flashes in breast cancer survivors using tamoxifen are different from hot flashes in women experiencing natural menopause. At this time, it is reasonable to assume that the therapeutic results seen in women with hot flashes may be applicable to either population.

Lifestyle changes. For women requesting relief from mild, menopause-related hot flashes, NAMS recommends first considering lifestyle changes. Clinicians might recommend the following:

- Keep core body temperature as cool as possible. Warm ambient air temperatures increase a woman's core body temperature and make her more likely to reach the sweating threshold for triggering a hot flash. Conversely, cooler air temperatures are associated with a lower incidence of hot flashes.

- Maintain a healthy body weight. Previously, it was believed that hot flash risk was inversely related to body mass index (BMI), as estradiol is elevated as a result of aromatization in adipose tissue. However, several studies have found a higher BMI (≥ 27 kg/m^2) to be a predictor of hot flash frequency. It has been postulated that, at least in pre- and perimenopausal women, any increase in estradiol is offset by increased insulation from body fat, resulting in a higher core body temperature and more hot flashes.

- Refrain from smoking. Cigarette smoking (both past and current) increases the relative risk of hot flashes, perhaps because of its effect on estrogen metabolism. One study found that among current smokers, hot flash risk increased with greater amounts smoked. A 2006 case-control study showed higher odds of number and severity of hot flashes in current and ever-smokers. However, smoking was not associated with lower estradiol or estrone levels.

- Exercise regularly. Less physical activity increases the relative risk of hot flashes whereas daily exercise is associated with an overall decreased incidence. However, strenuous exercise has been shown to trigger hot flashes in symptomatic, unconditioned women. Physical activity may trigger hot flashes by raising core body temperature. A 2006 study found that a significant association between increasing physical activity and decreasing vasomotor symptoms was observed in women with a lifetime history of major depression, but no association was seen in women without this history.

- Practice relaxation techniques. Anxiety has been associated with an increased occurrence, as well as increased severity and frequency, of hot flashes.

Anecdotal reports from individual women have suggested a relationship between the frequency and/or severity of hot flashes and emotional stress or perceived personal hot flash triggers, including consumption of particular types of foods (eg, thermally hot or spicy food) or drinks (eg, caffeine, alcohol). Trial evidence among large groups of women, however, does not support such a relationship. The Melbourne Women's Midlife Health Project found no significant association between alcohol intake and hot flash rates.

Nonprescription remedies. When lifestyle changes are not adequate to achieve the desired level of relief from mild hot flashes, adding a nonprescription remedy may be considered. Trying soy foods or isoflavone supplements, black cohosh, or vitamin E may be an option, primarily because these remedies are not associated with serious side effects. Due to the inconclusive efficacy data, this is not a consensus recommendation. (See Section H, page 242, and Section I, page 259, for more about nonprescription remedies.)

For women with frequent hot flashes, clinicians may consider recommending soy foods or soy isoflavone supplements. Most hot flash studies used isoflavone amounts of 40 to 80 mg/day. Rather than isoflavone supplements or fortified foods, which can lead to isoflavone "overdose," whole foods are a better choice for achieving the suggested intake. Effects, if any, can take several weeks. It is not known whether women with breast cancer can safely consume isoflavone supplements.

Older and smaller trials from Germany showed some efficacy for hot flashes with black cohosh. The most-tested black cohosh supplement is Remifemin, a 27-deoxyactein standardized preparation. With a dosage of two 20-mg tablets/day, this product has few side effects, and use for less than 6 months is unlikely to cause harm and may provide some relief of mild hot flashes. The most recent trials of black cohosh have shown efficacy similar to placebo. A 2006 RCT (Herbal Alternatives for Menopause Trial) found no difference in hot flash frequency or intensity between women taking black cohosh, a multibotanical with black cohosh and nine other ingredients, a multibotanical plus dietary soy counseling, and placebo; this trial did not use the type of black cohosh found in Remifemin. (See Section I, page 259, for more about herbal remedies, including risks.)

Vitamin E, 400 to 800 IU/day, is another nonprescription option for hot flash relief. The clinical evidence is mixed. A statistically but not clinically significant decrease in hot flashes among breast cancer survivors was noted in one trial, although previous trials found no benefit of vitamin E over placebo. (See Section H, page 242, for more about vitamin E, including risks.)

Scientific data are lacking regarding both efficacy and safety of topical progesterone creams for relief of hot flashes. Contents and concentrations vary widely in different nonprescription brands. Additionally, the same safety concerns outlined in government-approved labeling (package inserts) for prescription systemic progestogen preparations (eg, potential breast cancer effect) also apply to topical progesterone preparations. Therefore, NAMS does not recommend use of progesterone creams for hot flash relief. (See Section G, page 223, for more about topical progesterone creams.)

Given the lack of efficacy data, NAMS also does not recommend dong quai, evening primrose oil, ginseng, licorice, Chinese herb mixtures, acupuncture, or magnet therapy for hot flash relief. (See Section I for more about CAM therapies.)

Prescription therapies: hormonal options. When lifestyle changes and nonprescription approaches do not provide the desired relief, prescription options are available.

- *Estrogen therapy/estrogen-progestogen therapy (ET/EPT).* Prescription systemic ET or, for women with a uterus, EPT, remains the therapeutic standard for treating moderate to severe menopause-related hot flashes in women without contraindications—and these therapies

are the only treatments government approved in the United States and Canada for this indication. Estrogen-containing contraceptives are an option to consider for use off label for healthy, nonsmoking perimenopausal women, especially those needing contraception. (See Section G, page 201, for more about contraceptives.)

NAMS considers treatment for moderate to severe menopause-related hot flashes to be a primary indication for systemic ET/EPT. Use of these therapies should be limited to the shortest duration consistent with treatment goals, benefits, and risks for the individual woman. Initiating ET/EPT during perimenopause is associated with lower risk compared to starting therapy several years after menopause. (See Section G for more.)

NAMS recommends considering lower-than-standard doses of ET (ie, daily doses of 0.3 mg CE tablet; 0.25-0.5 mg 17β-estradiol tablet; 0.025 mg 17β-estradiol patch; or the equivalent). Many studies have demonstrated that these doses provide vasomotor symptom relief similar to that of standard dosing. Lower ET/EPT doses are better tolerated, but may or may not have a more positive safety profile than standard doses. However, lower doses have not been tested for outcomes in long-term trials.

If the initial ET dose is not effective, it may be increased. If symptom relief is not obtained with once-daily dosing of oral ET (because of the possibility of more rapid metabolism of the hormone), a trial of twice-daily dosing with half doses or switching to transdermal ET may be advised. There is often no need to increase the total daily oral dose in women suspected of having rapid or irregular metabolism of exogenous estrogen. Maintaining a stable circulating estrogen level may be more important than attainment of an absolute level. Changing the route of administration may also be helpful. Transdermal ET may provide more stable levels of circulating estrogen than oral therapies. Another option is one of the vaginal estrogen rings, Femring; this product offers higher doses of systemic estrogen than local therapies and is approved by the US Food and Drug Administration (FDA) for treating hot flashes. It is not available in Canada.

If hot flashes persist after an adequate trial (ie, 2-3 mo) of ET, other conditions associated with hot flashes should be considered in the differential diagnosis.

When systemic ET/EPT is discontinued abruptly or by gradually decreasing the dose, hot flashes often return within several days or weeks, depending on the type and route of therapy. A large 2005 cross-sectional survey showed that in women age 70 or older, 11% experience vasomotor symptoms after stopping hormones. No specific protocols can be recommended for discontinuing therapy to avoid rebound hot flashes. Some clinicians lengthen the time between doses. There are no data to suggest that one method is superior to the other.

If hot flashes recur, HT may be reinstituted, and then discontinued at a later time.

- *Progestogen.* Prescription progestogen therapy alone has been used off label to treat hot flashes of varying severity. In clinical trials, DMPA, oral medroxyprogesterone acetate (MPA), and megestrol acetate have demonstrated efficacy. Short-term use of these drugs seems reasonable in women without contraindications who do not wish to try estrogen but who are not opposed to trying another hormone, although progestogens have been linked to increased breast cancer risk in some studies of HT.

Combined OCs. Perimenopausal women who require hot flash relief and contraception may achieve both goals with a low-dose combined estrogen-progestin OC. NAMS supports this use for healthy women who do not smoke or have no other contraindications. The potential side effects of nausea, mood swings, and headaches can usually be decreased or eliminated by altering the regimen or dose. Relief of hot flashes should be achieved within 4 weeks of starting therapy. If hot flashes occur during the placebo week, adding a low dose of supplemental estrogen or shortening or eliminating the placebo interval may provide relief. DMPA is another option for hot flash relief and contraception, although the adverse effect clinical profile is different from that for OCs.

Prescription therapies: nonhormonal options. When hormones are not an option, off-label use of nonhormonal prescription drugs is an alternative to consider. Some have demonstrated effectiveness in relieving hot flashes but none is as effective as systemic ET. However, there are no comparative trials in similar patient populations to guide clinicians in selecting a particular option.

- *Antidepressants.* If there are no contraindications, NAMS recommends the antidepressants fluoxetine (Prozac; 20 mg/d), paroxetine (Paxil; 12.5-25 mg/d), sertraline (Zoloft; 50 mg/d), or venlafaxine (Effexor; 37.5-75 mg/d) as options for women with hot flashes who are not candidates for HT, including those with a history of breast cancer. RCTs have demonstrated positive results for treatment of hot flashes using each of these antidepressants. However, there is no safety evidence for long-term use.

Venlaxafine is a serotonin-norepinephrine reuptake inhibitor (SNRI), and paroxetine, fluoxetine, and setraline are selective serotonin reuptake inhibitors (SSRIs). The additional antidepressant effect may benefit some women who suffer from mood disorders. A new SNRI, desvenlafaxine, is in development as a treatment for vasomotor symptoms. (See page 47 for more about depression, bone mass, and SSRIs.)

Hot flash relief, if any, is almost immediate with these therapies, whereas relief of depression may not be observed for 6 to 8 weeks. This rapid onset of action can be a powerful reinforcement for women who do not find hot flash relief with other, simpler methods. A brief trial of 1 week may determine whether these agents are going to be effective.

Side effects for both SSRIs and SNRIs, especially nausea and sexual dysfunction, should be monitored. Nausea is dose related and usually subsides within 2 weeks of starting treatment. Women who experience drowsiness should take the drug at night. Caution is advised for women using tamoxifen who decide to take SSRIs or SNRIs.

The SSRI paroxetine has been shown in studies to interfere with the enzyme that converts tamoxifen to its active metabolites and may therefore influence the therapeutic outcome from tamoxifen treatment. Paroxetine can cause weight gain and blurred vision, although this is rare. Fluoxetine is less likely to cause acute withdrawal side effects because of its longer half-life. Recent clinical studies have implicated SSRIs in both reduced bone mass and clinical fragility fractures.

The SNRI venlafaxine is the most likely in its class to promote weight loss (by causing anorexia), and may be preferred by overweight women.

To minimize adverse side effects, very low doses of these antidepressants should be used when starting therapy. If not effective, the dose can be increased after 1 week. Higher doses than those used in trials do not seem appropriate, given the lack of additional efficacy and the potential for increased toxicity. Taking the drugs with food may lessen nausea.

These antidepressant medications should not be stopped abruptly, as sudden withdrawal has been associated with headaches and anxiety. Women who have been using an antidepressant for at least 1 week should taper off the drug. Tapering may require up to 2 weeks, depending on the initial dosage.

- *Gabapentin.* The anticonvulsant drug gabapentin (Neurontin) is another nonhormonal option recommended by NAMS for treating hot flashes. An RCT that compared hot flash composite scores (severity and frequency) in women taking CE, gabapentin, or placebo, a statistically significant decrease in hot flash composite scores for both estrogen and gabapentin was found over placebo. Therapy can be initiated at a daily dose of 300 mg (although starting at 100 mg/d may be advisable in women >65 y). Bedtime administration is advised, given the initial side effect of dizziness and drowsiness. In women who continue to have hot flashes, the dose can be increased to 300 mg twice daily and then to three times daily at 3- to 4-day intervals. Increased efficacy may be seen at even higher doses, although this has not been well studied. Antacids may reduce the bioavailability of gabapentin; the drug should be taken at least 2 hours after antacid use. Gabapentin can cause weight gain. Tapering is advised when discontinuing gabapentin therapy.

- *Combination gabapentin and antidepressants.* A 2007 RCT evaluated women with inadequate hot flash control who were taking an antidepressant alone. The investigators compared the addition of gabapentin to the antidepressant versus weaning the antidepressant and starting gabapentin alone. Results showed comparable efficacy in both groups. Both treatments decreased hot flash frequencies and scores by approximately 50%.

- *Clonidine.* The antihypertensive agent clonidine (Catapres in the United States, Dixarit in Canada) is sometimes used to treat mild hot flashes, although it is less effective than the newer antidepressants or gabapentin. In addition, clonidine has a side effect profile that limits its use in many women. Clonidine lowers blood pressure, heart rate, and pulse rate; arrhythmias have been observed at high doses. Adverse effects include dry mouth, drowsiness, dizziness, constipation, and sedation. The initial oral dose for hot flash treatment is 0.05 mg twice daily, but women may require at least 0.1 mg twice daily. The clonidine patch (Catapres-TTS), delivering 0.1 mg/day, can also be considered. When discontinuing higher-dose therapy, the dose should be gradually tapered to avoid adverse side effects, including nervousness, headache, agitation, confusion, and a rapid rise in blood pressure.

- *Others.* Although sometimes prescribed for hot flash treatment, given the limited efficacy data and potential for adverse effects, NAMS does not recommend methyldopa (Aldomet) or the product combining phenobarbital, ergotamine tartrate, and belladonna alkaloids (Bellergal) as hot flash treatments for most women. The evidence supporting the use of acupuncture to treat hot flashes is scant and mixed; NAMS cannot support this approach until adequately powered RCTs provide more positive clinical data.

Ongoing treatment. Any hot flash treatment may need to be adjusted periodically because of gradually lower levels of ovarian hormones during the menopause transition and the possible appearance of medical conditions unrelated to menopause or menopause treatments. New research and changing ideas about treatments may have an impact on health decisions. Before switching from one therapy to another, a washout period may be required.

Regardless of the management option utilized, treatment should be periodically evaluated to determine if it is still necessary because, in almost all women, menopause-related vasomotor symptoms will abate over time.

Sleep disturbances

About 46% of US women aged 40 to 54 years and 48% aged 55 to 64 years report sleep problems, according to a 2007 National Sleep Foundation survey. The survey revealed that peri- and postmenopausal women sleep less, have more frequent insomnia symptoms, and are more than twice as likely to use prescription sleeping aids as premenopausal women. Most people do not voluntarily report sleep disturbances to their healthcare clinicians, nor do most clinicians ask about sleep disturbances.

In the SWAN community-based survey, a multiethnic sample of 12,603 US women aged 40 to 55 years, difficulty sleeping was reported by 38%. Age-adjusted rates were highest in the late perimenopausal (45.4%) and surgically postmenopausal (47.6%) groups. Among ethnic groups, rates ranged from 28% in Japanese women to 40% in Caucasian women. In the multivariate analysis, menopause status, ethnicity, vasomotor and psychological symptoms, self-perceived health and health behaviors, arthritis, and education were significantly associated with difficulty sleeping. Older age per se was not significantly associated with insomnia.

Sleep is considered adequate if one can function in an alert state during desired waking hours. Most adults require between 6 and 9 hours of sleep per night.

Poor sleep (ie, inadequate quantity or poor quality) is associated with somatic and mood/cognition symptoms as well as performance deficits, including muscle aches, dysphoria, tension, irritability, fatigue, lethargy, inability to concentrate, lack of motivation, and difficulty performing tasks. It has also been linked to risk of chronic illness, especially cardiac problems and mood disorders, such as depression. Increased automobile and work-related injuries are associated with excessive daytime (waking) sleepiness from multiple causes.

Insomnia can include lengthy times to fall asleep, inability to stay asleep through the night, or premature awakening without being able to resume sleep. It can be transient (lasting only a few days) or short term (lasting no more than 3 to 4 wk), usually accompanying acute emotional life situations or environmental changes. Chronic or persistent insomnia (defined as occurring at least three nights per week for a month or longer) may benefit from medical intervention.

Reports of insomnia increase as women make the transition through midlife. Perceived declines in sleep quality may be attributed to general aging effects (eg, nocturnal urination), the onset of sleep-related disorders (eg, apnea) or other illness-related disorders (eg, chronic pain conditions, depression), stress and social strain, negative mood, or ovarian hormone changes. Women in midlife are as likely to report sleep difficulties as they are to being troubled by weight gain.

Sleep efficiency rarely varies by menopause status. Most studies of menopause status and physiologic sleep revealed that disturbances emerging during transition to menopause occur mainly in women bothered by nighttime hot flashes, even though actual time awake is low. However, this has not been confirmed by laboratory studies. The Wisconsin Sleep Cohort Study of 589 pre-, peri-, and postmenopausal women found that postmenopausal women had the best physiologically recorded sleep and that this was somewhat worsened by HT. In studies conducted by Freedman et al, no evidence was found that hot flashes caused sleep disturbances in postmenopausal women. The authors suggested that previous work attributing sleep disturbances to hot flashes may be confounded by the inclusion of test subjects whose sleep disturbances actually arise from factors such as prescription drug use and sleep apnea. Primary sleep disorders (eg, sleep apnea, restless leg syndrome) are common in this population. But these investigators and others have noted that skin conductance recording can measure the frequency but not the severity or bothersomeness of hot flashes. To postmenopausal women, subjective sleep quality may be more important than objective sleep quality.

Additional studies by Freedman et al found that hot flashes triggered awakenings and arousals in the first, but not the second, half of the night. The investigators attributed the lack of arousals during the second half of the night to the predominance of rapid eye movement (REM) sleep, which occurs then and suppresses thermoregulation. Motor movements expend energy, which also elicits a thermoregulatory response. Awakenings increase norepinephrine, which also alters the thermoneutral zone in which body temperature changes occur without eliciting a thermoregulatory response. Thus, there appears to be an interaction between hot flashes, thermoregulation, and endocrine mechanisms (also including cortisol and growth hormone secretion).

Other studies have addressed the relationship of hot flashes to sleep in postmenopausal women with varying results. Studies do not universally support a causal relationship between hot flashes and sleep disturbances. Women and their healthcare providers frequently attribute sleep disturbances during perimenopause to vasomotor symptoms, when in fact they may be more etiologically linked to a primary sleep disorder or psychiatric symptomatology.

Stress and insomnia are closely linked. In addition to ovarian hormonal changes, many midlife women also experience significant life challenges (eg, job-related stress, loss of life partners through divorce or death, caregiving for young or old family members, or development of chronic illness).

Insomnia can also be associated with painful chronic illnesses, such as arthritis, fibromyalgia, and gastrointestinal disturbances, as well as CVD, respiratory disease, neurologic and psychiatric conditions, thyroid abnormalities, and allergies. Drugs that can disturb sleep include thyroid medication, theophylline, phenytoin, levodopa, SSRIs, and progestin (if estrogen deficient).

Sleep-disordered breathing. Characterized as the sleep apnea/hypopnea syndrome, sleep-disordered breathing (SDB) can emerge in midlife for women. Symptoms occur on a continuum from increased airway resistance (manifested as snoring or airflow reductions [hypopneas]) to periodic cessation of breathing effort or airflow (apneas). Severe or long-standing manifestations have been linked to cardiovascular disease. Episodes of SDB are associated with loud snoring, sleep arousals, and varying blood desaturated oxygen levels. These episodes lead to fragmented sleep, reports of waking from sleep unrefreshed, and excessive daytime sleepiness.

More postmenopausal women experience SDB episodes than premenopausal women, but comparisons of pre-, peri-, and postmenopausal women have shown no clear differences in apnea/hypopnea, sleep arousal, or arterial oxygen desaturation episodes among the groups. Heavy body weight and facial morphology with a crowded oropharynx (with or without obesity) have more importance than ovarian hormone factors in the SDB patterns of midlife women, but a functional breathing difference over and above anatomic factors has also been associated with menopause status. The occurrence of SDB has been linked to polycystic ovary syndrome and fibromyalgia.

Women seem similar to men in reporting snoring and daytime sleepiness, but they report less restless sleep or witnessed apneas. Women with SBD are more likely than men to report morning headaches, fatigue, and mood changes and to exhibit upper airway resistance than complete breathing pauses. Consequently, they may be less likely to be referred to sleep centers for evaluation. Various factors to explain risk of and gender differences in SDB are being pursued, including upper airway dynamics, pattern of fat distribution, effects of sex-related hormones, and obesity-hypoventilation syndrome.

Management of sleep disturbances. Healthcare providers are encouraged to assess sleep quality in all women during perimenopause and beyond. The decision to use behavioral and/or drug treatments for insomnia depends on the type of insomnia (acute or chronic, primary or secondary to other conditions), the context of the insomnia (high vasomotor symptoms or life strain), and the severity of daytime consequences. Primary sleep disorders, apnea, restless leg syndrome, anxiety, and depression need to be addressed. SDB is associated with increased risk of hypertension and sudden cardiac death, requiring prompt evaluation in a sleep center and appropriate management.

Behavioral therapies. For people with sustained sleep problems, behavioral therapies include avoiding behaviors that interfere with sleep and reinforcing those that promote sleep (eg, sleep hygiene measures), ritualizing environmental cues, regularizing the sleep/wake schedule, and relaxing to control tension. Behavioral therapies can be used alone or with adjunctive pharmacologic or botanical therapies.

Caffeine, alcohol, and nicotine should be avoided close to bedtime, if sleep induction is difficult. About 15 to 30 minutes are required for caffeine from a cup of coffee (80-115 mg) to affect the brain, and up to 7 hours are required to rid the system of caffeine; its stimulant effects have lasted up to 20 hours as it stacks up during the day. Besides being found in coffee, tea, "energy drinks," cola drinks, and chocolate, caffeine is also present in nonprescription pain relievers, premenstrual syndrome remedies, diuretics, alertness and allergy/cold medications, and weight-control aids.

Alcohol initially promotes drowsiness, thus assisting with falling asleep. However, it often results in rebound early awakening and fragmented sleep, leading to feeling unrefreshed upon awakening (ie, unrestorative sleep). Alcohol also affects breathing and tends to swell oral and nasal mucous membranes, which may worsen SDB. Nicotine is frequently overlooked as contributing to sleep disturbances, but it has been observed to prolong sleep onset and decrease sleep duration. Illicit drugs, such as marijuana, morphine, and heroin, also disrupt normal sleep patterns.

Although eating a large, heavy meal before bed can interfere with sleep, a snack with protein (to support central nervous system neurochemical production, especially serotonin) and carbohydrates (to promote blood/brain barrier entry) is recommended. Strenuous exercise close to a desired sleep time amplifies arousal, making it difficult to fall asleep; however, regular daily exercise is considered beneficial.

Nightly rituals and establishing a sleep-conducive environment (quiet, cool, dark, and safe) can "condition" better sleep. The bedroom should be reserved only for sleep, sex, and perhaps relaxation activities. If individuals are not asleep within 10 to 15 minutes, they should leave the bedroom to engage in relaxing activities elsewhere until drowsy, then return to bed again for sleep. This should be repeated as necessary. Resisting the temptation to check the clock will help avoid habitual awakenings.

A regular sleep schedule promotes sleep induction and stability. Choosing a consistent time to get up (regardless of time to bed and even on weekends) promotes synchrony with the light/dark cycle, which is important to a restorative sleep pattern.

Sleep-restriction therapy is a technique that can help reestablish a restorative sleep pattern for someone unable to get quality hours of sleep. The process is as follows:

- Determine current sleep duration (eg, 4 hours) and select a consistent time to arise (eg, 7:00 ʂṁ)

- Spend time in bed equal to perceived current sleep time (eg, go to bed at 3:00 ʂṁand arise at 7:00 ʂṁ)
- When able to sleep 95% of this duration for several nights, go to bed 30 minutes earlier (eg, 2:30 ʂṁ)
- When sleeping 95% of lengthened time for several nights, go to bed another 30 minutes earlier (eg, 2:00 ʂṁ)
- Repeat this procedure until bedtime-to-wake time equals desired duration of sleep.

Learning relaxation techniques can help individuals with insomnia. Several modalities can facilitate learning how to enter and adopt a deeply relaxed state, including instructional or mood-inducing tapes, concentration techniques such as meditation or creative imagery, or combining mind with movement techniques, such as yoga or tai chi.

Prescription remedies. There are several prescription options used to improve sleep.

- *Sedatives and hypnotics.* Sleeping pills may be used to break a cycle of insomnia, but preferably prescribed as a last resort.

  — *Short-acting nonbenzodiazepine hypnotic sleeping aids*, such as zolpidem (eg, Ambien, with 4-5 h duration), zaleplon (Sonata, or Starnoc in Canada, with 1-3 h duration), or eszopiclone (Lunesta, or Imovane in Canada, with 6 h duration) may be prescribed to improve sleep patterns. Compared with benzodiazepines, they show fewer withdrawal effects, less tolerance or addictive issues, and less loss of effectiveness over time, but long-term data are sparse and equivocal.

  — *Benzodiazepines*, such as diazepam (eg, Valium) or alprazolam (eg, Xanax), may be needed for women who have trouble staying asleep. However, side effects (such as next-day sedation, rebound insomnia when drug is discontinued, tolerance, and dependence) underlie recommendations that they be used periodically at most (a maximum of 3 nights/wk).

  — *Ramelteon*, a melatonin receptor agonist marketed as Rozerem, is a newer hypnotic sleep aid; it is FDA approved to assist in falling asleep.

  — *Indiplon*, a nonbenzodiazipine hypnotic that acts on the γ-aminobutyric acid-A receptor for promoting sleep, is in development.

- *Trazodone.* Approved as an antidepressant (eg, Desyrel), this nonaddictive treatment is often prescribed off label as a sleep aid at a lower dose (25-50 mg/d).

- *Menopausal hormone therapy.* Neither ET nor EPT is government approved as a treatment for insomnia. However, oral ET has been shown to improve nighttime restlessness and awakening. Both ET and EPT seem to affect perceived and polysomnographic sleep positively, mainly in conjunction with reducing hot flash and night sweat activity. However, reducing hot flashes may not treat the underlying sleep disturbance. Because many sleep disorders can result in significant morbidity and mortality, they require careful attention.

EPT has been observed to lessen SDB, although small-sample studies have not confirmed these effects. Using progesterone instead of progestin may improve sleep, as progesterone is a mild soporific. Bedtime dosing of progesterone is advised.

Nonprescription remedies. Botanical sedatives and melatonin are sometimes considered as nonprescription options to improve sleep. OCT products containing these ingredients are government regulated in the United States as dietary supplements; in Canada, they are regulated as natural health products (see Section H for more about this type of product).

- *Botanicals.* Some sufferers use botanical sedatives to improve sleep quality. Valerian has been observed to promote sleep onset and deeper sleep (see Section I, page 271, for more about valerian). German chamomile, lavender, hops, lemon balm, and passion flower are said to be mild sedatives, although there are few scientific data.

- *Melatonin.* Some women self-medicate with melatonin, an endogenous pineal gland hormone, but its effects on sleep and behavioral sedation are inconsistent in studies. Moreover, there are no data demonstrating that melatonin provides relief from menopause-related sleep disturbances. Although melatonin is a hormone, it is not government regulated as a drug. (See Section G, page 227, for more about melatonin.)

When to refer. Referral to sleep centers is warranted for women with SDB manifestations or other sleep-related disorders, such as restless leg syndrome (crawly and strong urge-to-move sensations), periodic limb movements during sleep (jerky, rhythmic movements of legs), or narcolepsy (uncontrollable sleep bouts during waking hours, loss of muscle tone known as cataplexy, hypnologic hallucinations, excessive daytime sleepiness, fragmented sleep, and automatic behaviors).

Headache

Headaches are one of the most common problems treated in both primary care and neurology settings. As many as 50 million people in North America suffer from severe headaches. However, about half of all headache sufferers do not seek treatment.

There are three common types of headache: tension-type, cluster, and migraine. Most patients who present to a primary care setting with a chief complaint of headache meet the criteria for migraines. Patients with tension-type headaches rarely seek help. Unfortunately, about half of those who request treatment for tension-type or migraine headaches either do not receive appropriate treatment or are dissatisfied with their treatment.

Although most headaches are not serious, the following characteristics may be an indication of a more serious problem, such as hypertension or a brain tumor:

- Occurrence of a new, "worst-ever" headache
- Progressively worsening headache
- More severe headache pain than usual
- Headache that causes nocturnal awakening
- Stiff neck accompanied by a high fever
- Confusion, dizziness, weakness
- Presence of a focal neurologic symptom

Causes. A variety of trigger factors are thought to produce headaches in susceptible individuals. Using a headache diary to identify (and avoid) triggers can be very helpful in headache management. Data to record include the time a headache was experienced, the symptoms, and the potential triggers (eg, particular foods, menses, or stress).

Causes of headaches include sinus infections, dental problems, allergies, or colds. Most presumed migraine triggers have not been well studied. However, there are common factors that may be triggers for susceptible individuals:

- Consumption of alcoholic beverages, caffeine, tyramine-containing foods (eg, chocolate, yogurt, sour cream, aged cheese, red wine), foods containing nitrite preservatives (eg, hot dogs, sausage, bacon, bologna, smoked fish), and foods containing monosodium glutamate (MSG; a flavor-enhancer sometimes added to Chinese food as well as to processed or frozen foods)
- Change in eating pattern (eg, fasting or skipping meals, not drinking enough water)
- Change in sleeping pattern (eg, getting too much or too little sleep)
- Emotional changes (eg, stress, anxiety, anger, or excitement)
- Environmental changes (eg, noise, bright lights, changes in barometric pressure, or inhaling fumes
- Endogenous hormone fluctuations (eg, menstrual migraines)
- Use of any type of systemic ovarian hormone (for menopause or contraception), especially with a progestin

Role of hormones. In the United States, migraines affect about 18% of women and 6% of men between the ages of 25 and 55. However, before puberty and after menopause, the incidence of headaches is approximately the same in both men and women, suggesting some role for ovarian hormones.

Hormonal fluctuations, such as those that occur during menstrual periods and perimenopause, play a role in the incidence of headaches. Studies have clearly established a connection between headaches and menstrual periods (sometimes called *menstrual migraines*) in susceptible women. In these women, the incidence of migraines often declines during pregnancy when estrogen levels are more stable. The hormonal fluctuations that occur during the placebo week of oral contraceptives also have been shown to trigger headaches in susceptible women.

During perimenopause, the prevalence or intensity of headaches often increases, especially in women with a history of menstrual headaches. A link between increased rates of migraines and perimenopause is well accepted among neurologists, based on observational data and prospective studies.

Management of headache. The following describes headache types and their management.

Tension headache. This type of headache is described as a steady squeezing or pressing pain on both sides of the head. Tension-type headaches can be acute or chronic, last from 30 minutes to 1 week, and are not aggravated by exertion. Women reportedly experience them more frequently than men. Most tension-type headaches can be effectively treated with nonprescription analgesics (such as aspirin, acetaminophen) and NSAIDs (such as naproxen, ibuprofen).

Nonpharmacologic therapies, including physical therapy, stress management, relaxation therapy, and biofeedback, are also helpful for some people. For those who need prophylactic treatment, tricyclic antidepressants or SSRIs may be helpful. Muscle relaxants have not been found to be effective for tension-type headaches.

Migraine headache. Typically, migraines cause a moderate to severe throbbing pain that is worse on one side of the head and is usually aggravated by physical activity. Other symptoms, such as nausea, vomiting, and sensitivity to light and noise, are often present. Migraines usually last 4 to 72 hours and may occur rarely or up to several times a week.

There are two types of migraine headaches: those with aura and those without aura. An aura is typically visual, with flashing lights, wavy lines, or other visual changes, and begins less than an hour before the headache. A person may temporarily lose vision, have speech problems, or experience numbness, tingling, or weakness in an extremity, although this is rare. Migraines without aura are much more common than migraines with aura. Both types of migraines may have accompanying symptoms, such as mood changes, fatigue, nausea, vomiting, diarrhea, and facial congestion. These symptoms may occur up to several days before a headache. Individuals with facial congestion are often misdiagnosed with sinus headaches; many of these headaches meet the criteria for migraines. Research indicates that migraines may also be accompanied by cutaneous allodynia, or excessive skin sensitivity and/or skin pain (eg, pain with brushing the hair or touching the scalp). Patients with cutaneous allodynia should be treated as early as possible in the course of the migraine, as their headaches may be less responsive to medication if treatment is delayed.

Acute migraines can be difficult to treat. For mild to moderately painful migraines, nonprescription preparations such as aspirin or acetaminophen combinations with caffeine may be as effective as prescription medications. Paradoxically, caffeine can also be a migraine trigger for some individuals. Used primarily to treat acute migraines, Midrin (a nonprescription combination of isometheptene mucate, dichloralphenazone, and acetaminophen) has also been found to be effective in treating mixed tension-type/migraine headaches. It should be used with caution as it may be habit forming.

The advent of the triptan prescription medications, such as frovatriptan (Frova), rizatriptan (Maxalt), sumatriptan (Imitrex), eletriptan (Relpax), and zolmitriptan (Zomig), has greatly enhanced migraine treatment. Triptans have made it possible for many migraine sufferers to lead relatively normal productive lives despite severe or debilitating headaches. The triptans are extremely effective and safe, although they are contraindicated in individuals with coronary heart disease. NSAIDs are often recommended in combination with a triptan.

Migraines should be treated both acutely and, when appropriate, preventively. Preventive medication should be considered when an individual has headaches more than two to three times per week, or if headache severity affects quality of life. Any preventive medication is about 60% likely to be effective for a given individual. Prescription drugs found to be most effective in preventing migraines include beta-blockers such as propranolol (Inderal), antidepressants such as amitriptyline (Elavil), and anticonvulsants such as topiramate (Topamax). With a preventive drug, starting doses should be low and increased slowly. Drugs should be taken for at least 2 months to judge effectiveness.

Magnesium, riboflavin, and/or coenzyme Q10 are nonprescription preventive medications that, when taken daily, are effective and safe for many migraine sufferers. They can be used as baseline preventive treatment that may diminish the need for other preventive medications. (See Section H, pages 248 and 250, for more about magnesium and coenzyme Q10, respectively.)

Any type of systemic ovarian hormone therapy has been found to exacerbate migraines in some women while easing them in others. Benefit is more likely if hormonal fluctuations with therapy can be avoided (eg, adding a low-dose estrogen supplement during the withdrawal phase of OCs; using continuous ET/EPT therapy, not cyclic; using continuous-release transdermal estrogen). No hormone product is government approved to prevent or treat headaches. Caution should be used when prescribing estrogen-containing contraceptives or menopausal HT for a woman who has migraine with aura, as studies suggest that these women have an increased risk of ischemic stroke. Migraine without aura has not been found to increase stroke risk. (See Section G for more.)

Some evidence suggests that progestogens can precipitate or aggravate headaches. If headaches are worsened by a progestin such as MPA in EPT, switching to micronized progesterone may help. Because of its long-term risks, menopausal HT should not be the first choice for treating migraines, but should be considered only after an individual assessment of risks and benefits.

For many women, migraines occur around their menses in a way that is predictable. An NSAID or a triptan may be used preventively, beginning up to 2 days before expected onset of menstrual migraines.

Cluster headache. Less common than tension-type or migraine headaches, cluster headaches are described as being very severe, with nonthrobbing pain felt behind one eye that may be accompanied by inflammation, watering of the eye, and/or severe pain on that side of the face. Cluster headaches usually last up to 3 hours and occur periodically over several weeks or months, sometimes disappearing for months to years. Treatment of an acute attack includes the inhalation of oxygen or a triptan-type medication often given by self-administered injection. Daily use of a prescription corticosteroid or calcium channel blocker can help prevent or reduce the frequency of cluster attacks.

Ongoing treatment. Both over-the-counter (OTC) and prescription drugs used for acute treatment can result in rebound headaches. Care should be taken to monitor their use and, if headaches occur more than twice a week, preventive medications should be considered. For many women, headaches are debilitating and frustrating, greatly interfering with quality of life at a time when career and family responsibilities are already stressful. A supportive relationship between the chronic headache sufferer and her healthcare provider can be extremely effective in determining the appropriate individual interventions.

Cognition

The term *cognition* describes the group of mental processes by which knowledge is acquired or used. It encompasses such mental skills as concentration, learning and memory, language, spatial abilities, judgment, and reasoning.

From a neuropsychological perspective, concentration is closely related to concepts of awareness, attention, and vigilance. Concentration refers to the ability to focus on the task at hand while at the same time suppressing awareness of potential distractions. Impaired concentration is a common symptom of brain damage. Even among healthy people, the ability to concentrate is influenced by fatigue, mood, stress, and a variety of physical symptoms.

Concentration affects memory. Typically, memory refers to the ability to learn new information and to recall this information after time. Another kind of memory involves the memory for words, names, and general facts. Poor concentration means that new information is learned less efficiently and that recall strategies are applied less effectively.

Steroid hormones—including the sex hormones estrogen, progesterone, and androgen, and the adrenal hormone cortisol—modulate aspects of brain function. Subsets of nerve cells within the brain have receptors for these steroid hormones. Effects of estrogen on several neurotransmitter systems, including acetylcholine, serotonin, norepinephrine, and dopamine, can potentially influence processes involved in concentration, memory, and other cognitive functions. Other estrogen actions within the hippocampus (a brain region essential to the formation of new conscious memories) might affect learning and memory. However, the clinical importance of these brain effects is not always clear.

Cognitive aging and dementia. Memory and other cognitive abilities change throughout life. With advancing age, performance tends to decline on many, but not all, cognitive tests.

Difficulty concentrating and remembering are common complaints during the menopause transition and early postmenopause. Sleep disturbances, hot flashes, and various midlife stressors may contribute to these symptoms. However, most studies fail to show a clear association between hot flashes and difficulty with concentration and memory.

Importantly, there is no firm evidence that memory or other cognitive skills actually decline during the natural menopause transition, despite the frequency of symptoms of cognitive challenges in midlife. Some problems that women encounter may be more related to aging than to the menopause transition.

Rapid transition to menopause may have an effect on cognitive performance. Speculatively, neuronal systems influenced by estrogen might be compromised by an abrupt decline in ovarian estrogen production, such as that occurring with surgical menopause. Menopause-related symptoms are more frequent and intense following surgical menopause than natural menopause, and there is some evidence that cognitive skills such as memory for verbal information can be compromised in the immediate period after surgical menopause.

Dementia refers to the loss of memory and other intellectual abilities severe enough to interfere substantially with usual daily activities. It is perhaps the most-feared consequence of aging. Alzheimer's disease (AD), the most common cause of dementia, accounts for well over one half of cases. More women are affected than men, primarily because women tend to live longer. AD and other forms of dementia may be preceded by a period of moderate difficulty with memory or other cognitive abilities. The term *mild cognitive impairment* is sometimes used to refer to excessive cognitive difficulty that falls short of dementia but may presage its development.

Management of cognition symptoms. Observational data indicate that some activities, such as attaining higher education, maintaining an extensive social network, increasing intake of omega-3 fatty acids and certain vitamins, consuming alcohol in moderation, and remaining physically and mentally active, may benefit memory or help protect against dementia. Only a few of the various activities and medications touted to improve cognitive skills or reduce the risk of dementia have been assessed in RCTs.

High antioxidant intake from food and supplement sources has been associated with delaying cognitive decline in the elderly. However, the large Women's Health Study of generally healthy US women aged 65 and older found that long-term use of 600 IU vitamin E on alternate days did not provide cognitive benefits compared with placebo. Other clinical trials have reached similar conclusions. Neither does vitamin E prevent progression from mild cognitive impairment to AD. Higher doses are associated with a slight increase in mortality. (See Section H, page 242, for more about vitamin E.)

Vitamins B_6, B_9 (folic acid), and B_{12} have been associated with cognitive function in some studies. A systematic review found that levels of folic acid showed significant correlation with poor test performance in the global cognitive domain, although data supporting this association were limited. The review revealed no association of vitamin B_6 and vitamin B_{12} blood concentrations with cognitive-test performance or AD, nor was vitamin-B dietary intake associated with cognitive function. In an RCT (N = 818) of older individuals (50-70 y), 800 µg of daily oral folic acid intake for 3 years significantly improved some domains of cognitive function that tend to decline with age, while a 2-year RCT (N = 276) of healthy participants with elevated homocysteine concentrations found no effect on cognition for a combined daily supplement of folic acid (500 µg), B_6 (10 mg), and B_{12} (500 µg). (See Section H, page 239, for more about vitamin B.)

One RCT found that omega-3 fatty acids had no effect on AD.

Clinical trials evaluating the benefits of soy protein and botanicals such as *Ginkgo biloba* on cognitive effects in middle age or old age have provided inconsistent and generally disappointing results. (See Section I, pages 264 and 267, for more about soy and botanicals, respectively.)

Hypertension is a direct risk factor for vascular dementia and studies have suggested hypertension also impacts upon prevalence of AD. Two antihypertensive trials published in 2002 and 2003—one just in individuals with a prior stroke or transient ischemic attack—showed significant reductions in dementia risk. A Cochrane systematic review published in 2006 concluded that there was no convincing evidence from the trials identifed that BP lowering prevents the development of dementia or cognitive impairment in hypertensive patients with no apparent prior cerebrovascular disease.

It is still unclear to what extent HT affects cognitive abilities after menopause (see Section G, page 205, for more about HT). Some observational studies of healthy, older postmenopausal women found that those using HT had higher scores on cognitive tasks than women not using HT. Other studies found the opposite. The Women's Health Initiative Memory Study (WHIMS), an RCT conducted in relatively healthy postmenopausal women aged 65 to 79 years, reported that risk of dementia was doubled for women using EPT and was increased by half for women without a uterus who used ET.

Based on evidence from the WHIMS trial, initiating ET/EPT after age 65 should not be recommended for primary prevention of dementia. The evidence is insufficient to know whether HT might help prevent—or might contribute to—late-life dementia when therapy is initiated during perimenopause or early postmenopause. For younger women undergoing surgical menopause, there is limited clinical trial evidence that HT begun soon after surgery may benefit cognitive skills such as verbal memory. Regardless, HT is not approved for this indication. Fortunately, the absolute risk of dementia before age 65 is quite low.

Few studies have focused on HT and vascular dementia. Clinical trial data indicate either no long-term effect on cerebrovascular disease (stroke) or an increase in ischemic stroke risk.

For women with dementia caused by AD, there are still no therapies that lead to persisting improvement in symptoms or halt the degenerative course of the illness. In a trial of men and women with mild cognitive impairment, donepezil (Aricept, a drug indicated to treat AD) was not found to prevent progression to AD.

Several medications for treating patients with symptoms of AD are government approved in the United States and Canada. One class of drugs (cholinesterase inhibitors) that increases levels of acetylcholine (a chemical transmitter) in the brain by blocking its breakdown includes donepezil (Aricept), rivastigmine (Exelon), and galantamine (Razadyne or Reminyl in Canada). These agents can have a modest beneficial impact on the disease. Memantine (Namenda or Ebixa in Canada), a drug thought to reduce nerve damage caused by excitatory neurotransmitters, is approved for patients with moderate or severe Alzheimer symptoms. The clinical impact of this medication is modest.

Limited clinical trial evidence suggests that HT does not have a role in the treatment of women with AD. Other agents or medications that do not seem to have a clear effect in AD include prednisone (a steroid), the NSAIDs rofecoxib and naproxen, and omega-3 fatty acids.

Psychological symptoms

While most perimenopausal women do not experience major depressive disorder, many report symptoms of depressed mood, anxiety, stress, and a decreased sense of well-being. Cognitive symptoms such as decreased memory and attention are also commonly reported. (See page 45 in this section for more about cognition.)

Mood changes have been observed in up to 10% of perimenopausal women participating in longitudinal, community-based studies. Epidemiologic studies suggest a greater incidence of mood disturbances in perimenopausal women than in postmenopausal women. Some perimenopausal women report distressing symptoms of irritability, tearfulness, insomnia, fatigue, decreased memory and concentration, and depression.

The term *depression* can sometimes be misleading because it may refer to a symptom or a number of syndromes, each of which is managed differently. Depression includes the following three conditions:

- *Depressed mood.* Sometimes called *dysphoria*, this is a normal, brief period of feeling blue or sad that is commonly experienced and rarely requires treatment.

- *Depression as a symptom.* Sometimes called an *adjustment reaction*, this type of depression may be due to a wide variety of medical or psychological problems, or to intense reactions to life events (eg, divorce, losing a job, death of a loved one). It is usually short term and most often does not require treatment, although it can progress to clinical depression. Depression that occurs most of the day, more days than not, for at least 2 years is called a *dysthymic disorder* or *dysthymia*.

- *Clinical depression.* Sometimes called a *major depression* (in contrast to dysphoria and adjustment reactions, which are classified as *minor depression*), this is a pathologic disorder believed to result from a chemical imbalance in the brain. A clinical depression requires treatment. Women with a history of clinical depression seem to be particularly vulnerable to recurrent depression during perimenopause.

Most women present to their primary care clinicians with symptoms of psychological problems instead of or before they consult a mental health professional. Therefore, it is the responsibility of the primary care clinician to conduct an initial assessment of psychological health, screening for clinical depression. Even minor depression is associated with social dysfunction and disability, and any symptoms should be carefully assessed. *The Diagnostic and Statistical Manual of Mental Disorders (DSM IV-TR)* outlines valid and reliable criteria for determining diagnoses.

A psychosocial history is the first step in identifying mental health problems. This assessment includes asking about changes in mood, appetite, sleep, energy, sexual function, concentration, memory, and suicidal thoughts. Symptoms such as depressed mood, prolonged tiredness, low energy, loss of interest in normal activities, increased levels of guilt, anhedonia (inability to experience pleasure in normally pleasurable acts), irritability, psychomotor retardation or agitation, or other symptoms that may persist 2 weeks or longer may be the result of a depressive disorder.

Use of alcohol or other illegal substances may mask mood problems. Information on family or past history of depression, other psychiatric disorders, substance abuse or suicide attempts, as well as previous responses to psychopharmacologic medication and psychotherapy, is also useful.

A medical history, physical examination, and routine laboratory tests can rule out nutritional deficiencies and medical illnesses that are frequently associated with depression (eg, hypothyroidism). Depression may also be a side effect of medications (see Table 6). Only when the exact cause of depression is determined can an appropriate treatment plan be developed.

The most predictive factor for depression during midlife and beyond is a prior history of depression. Women who have been diagnosed with depression in their younger reproductive years may experience exacerbation of symptoms during perimenopause. Taking a history of depression at other times related to hormonal fluctuations (eg, premenstrual, pregnancy, or postpartum) or during the use of hormonal contraception may help to determine whether a woman is vulnerable to depressive episodes caused by changes in hormone levels.

If a perimenopausal woman does not have a history of depression and she develops mood changes or minor depressive symptoms after experiencing menopausal symptoms, her primary problem may be what some have proposed as the "domino effect" of menopausal symptoms. According to this model, estrogen fluctuations result in vasomotor symptoms, leading to sleep disturbance which, in turn, precipitates psychological and cognitive symptoms of depression. Women experiencing induced menopause may be especially vulnerable to this sort of emotional distress.

In addition, an evaluation of anxiety is needed to differentiate normal day-to-day anxiety from pathologic states. Anxiety conditions such as obsessive-compulsive and posttraumatic stress disorders may benefit from pharmacologic and/or psychotherapy interventions. Anxiety may also be a warning symptom of a panic disorder (distinguished by shortness of breath, chest pain, dizziness, heart palpitations, and/or feelings of "going crazy" or being "out of control") as well as depression.

Table 6. Medications associated with depression

- Antihypertensives (eg, reserpine, clonidine, thiazides, beta-blockers, hydralazine)
- Sedatives (eg, alcohol, barbiturates, benzodiazepines, chloral hydrate)
- Steroids (eg, corticosteroids, oral contraceptives)
- Dopamine agonists (eg, levodopa, bromocriptine, amantadine)
- Anticonvulsants (eg, phenytoin, carbamazepine)
- Analgesics (eg, ibuprofen, indomethacin, opiates)
- H_2-receptor antagonists (eg, cimetidine, ranitidine)
- Stimulant withdrawal (eg, amphetamines, cocaine)

Source: Landau *Menopause* 1996.

Perimenopausal mood disorders. Most women become accustomed to their own hormonal rhythm during their reproductive years. During perimenopause, however, this rhythm changes. Hormonal fluctuations, although a normal consequence of the decline in ovarian activity, may still provoke stress. Many women find that the unexpected timing and extent of these changes create upset and a sense of loss of control, and reports of irritability, fatigue, and blue moods (dysphoria) are common. Women often do not recognize that the onset of the numerous physical and psychological symptoms may be associated with perimenopause. Because perimenopausal symptoms may occur as early as age 35, education and anticipatory guidance about common perimenopausal symptoms are best addressed with women in their early to mid-thirties.

Transient depressed mood during perimenopause is often associated with a history of depression, a longer perimenopause, or more severe menopause-related symptoms. Compared with perimenopausal women without mood changes, perimenopausal women seeking help for mood changes are usually less healthy, have more hot flashes and psychosomatic complaints, and are more likely to have a history of premenstrual symptoms.

Some women of reproductive age sometimes report symptoms such as irritability, tension, dysphoria, and lability of mood that could be the beginning of perimenopause—or the beginning or worsening of premenstrual syndrome (PMS) or, if symptoms are extreme, premenstrual dysphoric disorder (PMDD). Table 7 presents the diagnostic criteria for PMDD.

There has been considerable controversy in the scientific literature regarding the direct impact of changing estrogen levels on perimenopausal mood symptoms, and the interaction between estrogen and mood is complex. Some studies have suggested that as estrogen levels decline, susceptibility to major depression increases, whereas other studies have found an association between high estrogen levels and dysphoric mood in perimenopause. It remains unclear whether mood symptoms are related to the gradual decline in estrogen or to the abrupt fluctuations in estrogen concentrations caused by intermittent ovulatory cycles. Recent longitudinal studies, however, found an association between depression and greater FSH, luteinizing hormone, and estradiol variability during the menopause transition compared with premenopausal levels. This association remains significant even when adjustments are made for confounding factors such as vasomotor symptoms and sleep disturbances.

Table 7. DSM-IV-TR criteria for PMDD

PMDD is confirmed when Criteria A, B, C, and D are met.

Criteria A: Five or more of the following symptoms are present:

1. Distinct depressed mood, feeling hopeless or insecure
2. Distinct anxiety, tension, feeling "on edge"
3. Instability (eg, suddenly feeling sad or tearful)
4. Persistent anger or irritability
5. Decreased interest in everyday activities
6. Difficulty concentrating
7. Lethargy, fatigue, lack of energy
8. Distinct change in appetite, overeating, or food cravings
9. Hypersomnia or insomnia
10. Feeling overwhelmed or out of control
11. Physical symptoms, such as breast tenderness or swelling, headaches, joint or muscle pain, bloated feeling, or weight gain

Criteria B: The symptom interferes with work, school, or social activities and relationships.

Criteria C: The symptom is not associated with another disorder, such as clinical depression, panic disorder, dysthymia, or a personality disorder.

Criteria D: Criteria A, B, and C must be confirmed during at least two consecutive symptomatic cycles.

Source: Adapted from American Psychiatric Association 1994.

In a 1998 NAMS/Gallup Poll of recently postmenopausal US women, respondents indicated that they felt happier and more fulfilled at this time of their life than at any other. Nevertheless, growing older may be difficult for some women. Often, hormone-related changes coincide with other stressors and losses in their lives (see Table 8).

Many women begin to think about their own mortality and become introspective about the meaning and purpose of their lives. Although these changes may provide an opportunity for positive transformation and growth, some women may need supportive assistance to adapt. Healthcare providers may be able to diminish or prevent some minor psychological symptoms by counseling women on what to expect at menopause, both physically and psychologically.

Table 8. Potential stressors at midlife

- Undesired childlessness
- Difficulties in relationship with a partner
- Development of personal or family medical problems
- Changes in self-concept, self-esteem, and body image
- Divorce or widowhood
- Care of young children, struggles with adolescents, or return of grown children to the home
- Concerns about aging parents or other family members
- "Sandwich generation" phenomena (ie, responsibility for both children and elders)
- Career and education issues
- Socioeconomic status

Management of perimenopausal mood disorders. Relaxation and stress-reduction techniques, including lifestyle modification, may help women cope with stress-producing factors in their lives during this time of hormonal fluctuations (see Table 9).

Some women attempt to self-treat their depression (mild or major) by using OTC products, such as St. John's wort or vitamin B_6. (For more about herbal therapies, see Section I, page 267; and for more about vitamins, see Section H, page 238.) Always ask what medications and OTC products women are taking and for what reason.

If the diagnosis is PMDD, four prescription drugs are FDA approved to treat the condition: three SSRIs—fluoxetine (Sarafem), controlled-release paroxetine (Paxil CR), and sertraline (Zoloft)—and the OC with ethinyl estradiol plus drospirenone (Yaz). Refer to the product labeling before prescribing. OTC pain medications will not relieve the most extreme physical symptoms of PMDD.

Table 9. Nonpharmacologic methods for coping with stress

- Deep breathing exercises and muscle relaxation training
- Daily exercise (yoga may be particularly helpful)
- Healthy diet (ie, plant-based, low-fat, low-caffeine, and low-alcohol)
- Sufficient self-care and enjoyable self-nurturing activities (eg, massage)
- Psychological support/therapy (eg, psychotherapy, menopause support group)
- Creative outlets that enhance quality of life

Hormone-based contraceptives affect mood in healthy women and in women with mood disorders. For example, positive effects on premenstrual symptoms have been observed with low-dose OCs. A study among 241 Brazilian women with premenstrual disorders requesting contraception concluded that the ethinyl estradiol plus drospirenone oral contraceptive (Yaz) improved symptoms of premenstrual disorder. Hormone-based contraceptives are also associated with improving mood in women with clinical depression. In a study by Young et al of women younger than 40 years of age with major depressive disorder, those using combined estrogen-progestin contraception were significantly less depressed than those with no hormone treatment, as determined by the 16-item Quick Inventory of Depressive Symptomatology–Self-Rated. These women also demonstrated better physical functioning and less obsessive-compulsive disorder comorbidity than women using progestin-only contraception or no hormone treatment.

Women may also experience symptoms of mild depression, such as depressed mood, irritability, poor concentration, and fatigue, because of sleep deprivation resulting from hot flashes and night sweats. These symptoms often improve when hot flashes are treated and sleep patterns return to baseline. There are a variety of treatment options for hot flashes, including nonpharmacologic approaches and prescription drugs, such as menopausal HT or, used off label, hormonal contraceptives or antidepressants (see vasomotor symptoms on page 35).

Antidepressants used for hot flashes may also provide a mood-stabilizing effect during perimenopause. Hormonal contraceptives or HT may have the same effect for women whose mood is affected by hormonal fluctuations (perhaps manifested earlier as PMDD or postpartum depression). To minimize hormone fluctuations, transdermal HT may be a better choice than oral HT.

There is evidence that estrogen has a positive impact on neural functions involved in the regulation of mood and behavior, which suggests a mood-enhancing effect. Many women using estrogen report a feeling of well-being, whereas its absence has the opposite effect. In prospective, controlled trials in postmenopausal women, HT has been shown to be consistently effective in relieving dysphoric mood.

Other studies of HT use in peri- and postmenopausal women who have generalized complaints of depressive symptoms but not major depression also found improvement in mood associated with HT. However, in some of these studies, the placebo recipients also showed evidence of improved mood over time, indicating that the significant advantage of HT over placebo in short-term mood enhancement (≥ 1 mo) did not persist in the long term. It may be that, although depressive symptoms naturally improve in perimenopausal women over time, this improvement is hastened by treatment with estrogen.

Small-sample observational studies and an open-label clinical trial provided preliminary evidence that in some perimenopausal women with depression (including minor depression, mild-type clinical depression, and dysthymia), HT may have an antidepressant effect, although the extent of this effect remains to be elucidated. In contrast, estrogen has not been shown to be more effective than placebo in treating postmenopausal women with depression. Given these different findings, it has been suggested that the antidepressant response to estrogen may be effective during the changing hormonal milieu but not when hormonal levels have finally stabilized.

The potential antidepressant effects of HT were examined in the Rancho Bernardo Study. Women aged 50 to 59 years using ET had higher Beck Depression Inventory scores than non-ET users. After age 60, the rate of depression increased significantly in non-ET users, but remained the same for ET users. In a preliminary study of ET for the treatment of depression in perimenopausal women, transdermal 17β-estradiol therapy effectively treated depression independent of its salutary effects on vasomotor symptoms. However, the findings were not sufficient to suggest that estrogen alone is effective in alleviating the totality of symptoms that constitute a depressive syndrome. Additional clinical trials are still needed to confirm these observations.

Some evidence suggests that estrogen potentiates the effect of some antidepressants, allowing lower doses of antidepressants. In a similar fashion, some women who have not responded to antidepressants may benefit from the addition of estrogen to their treatment regimen. HT may also accelerate the antidepressant response.

The administration of HT or hormonal contraceptives in doses that are conventionally used to treat hot flashes will often reduce or eliminate mood swings, tearfulness, irritability, and feelings of sadness. However, while HT or hormonal contraceptives might have a positive effect on mood and behavior, these drugs are not antidepressants and should not be considered as such. The government-approved product labeling for estrogen-containing HT products includes a statement that there is no adequate evidence that estrogen is effective for nervous symptoms or depression without associated vasomotor symptoms, and it should not be used to treat these conditions.

Progestogens (particularly progestins) in menopausal EPT may worsen mood in some women, particularly those with a history of PMS, PMDD, or depression. In these women, clinicians can try switching to another progestin, using a continuous-combined EPT regimen in which the dose of progestin is lower than in cyclic therapy, using oral micronized progesterone instead of progestin, or using vaginal progestogen. In the absence of contraindications, a short trial of unopposed estrogen (with appropriate endometrial surveillance) may be considered.

If emotional symptoms persist after hormone treatment has alleviated the vasomotor symptoms, consideration should be given to a trial with an antidepressant or mental health evaluation, or both. In many cases, referral to a healthcare professional with psychiatric training is appropriate.

Clinical depression. A number of clinical findings may indicate that a woman requires further psychiatric or psychosocial evaluation. Table 10 presents the symptoms of clinical depression.

Women exhibiting relevant symptoms should be screened for clinical depression using tools such as the Beck Depression Inventory or the Zung Self-Rating Depression Scale.

Table 10. DSM-IV-TR criteria for clinical depression

Clinical depression is confirmed when five or more of the following symptoms have been present during the same 2-week period and represent a change from previous functioning, and at least one of the symptoms is Item #1 (depressed mood) or Item #2 (loss of interest or pleasure). Symptoms that are clearly due to a general medical condition, mood-incongruent delusions, or hallucinations should not be counted.

1. Depressed mood most of the day, nearly every day, as indicated by either subjective report (eg, feels sad or empty) or observation made by others (eg, seems tearful)

2. Markedly diminished interest or pleasure in all, or almost all, activities most of the day, nearly every day (as indicated by either subjective account or observation made by others)

3. Significant weight loss when not dieting, or weight gain (eg, a change of more than 5% of body weight in a month), or decrease or increase in appetite nearly every day

4. Insomnia or hypersomnia nearly every day

5. Psychomotor agitation or retardation nearly every day (observable by others, not merely subjective feelings of restlessness or being slowed down)

6. Fatigue or loss of energy nearly every day

7. Feelings of worthlessness or excessive or inappropriate guilt (which may be delusional) nearly every day (not merely self-reproach or guilt about being sick)

8. Diminished ability to think or concentrate or indecisiveness nearly every day (either by subjective account or as observed by others)

9. Recurrent thoughts of death (not just fear of dying), recurrent suicidal ideation without a specific plan, a suicide attempt, or a specific plan for committing suicide

Source: American Psychiatric Association 2000.

Dysthymic disorder is also a prevalent condition. This chronic (ie, persisting for >2 years) mood disorder is in contrast to the more acute and more severe symptomatology of clinical depression, and is generally more difficult to treat. Treatment of dysthymic disorder is outside the scope of this textbook.

Management of clinical depression. Any time a woman meets the criteria for depression, regardless of where she is in the menopause transition, treatment is indicated with antidepressant medication, psychotherapy, or a combination of the two. SSRIs are shown to improve both mood and cognition in clinically depressed peri- and postmenopausal women. Recent clinical studies have implicated SSRIs in both reduced bone mass and clinical fragility fractures. Because depression is also associated with lower bone mass, a more judicious use of SSRIs in depressed patients with low bone mass or at risk of fragility fracture may be warranted. It is beyond the scope of this textbook, however, to present a complete discussion of management of clinical depression.

Vulvovaginal symptoms

Approximately one third of US women experience some vulvovaginal symptoms during their lifetimes. These symptoms include unusual vaginal discharge (often with an unpleasant odor) that may cause redness, irritation, and itching of the vulva (outer genital area). Discharge and itching can be caused by both infectious and noninfectious vaginitis (inflammation of the vagina). There are multiple possible causes of these symptoms (see Table 11). This textbook focuses primarily on menopause-related causes.

Vaginitis and vaginal atrophy. In the premenopausal woman, normal vaginal fluid may appear clear or white, or even flocculent, but it is odorless and does not cause pruritus or irritation. As women reach menopause and estrogen levels decline, vaginal fluid becomes yellowish and scant. During sexual activity, women may notice reduced vaginal lubrication. Sexually inactive women may present with uncomfortable vaginitis. Not all women develop troublesome symptoms or their symptoms may not become problematic until several years after menopause. However, for those women who experience premature menopause, vulvovaginal symptoms can occur at a younger age. Elderly women may also present with uncomfortable symptoms that require treatment.

Estrogen loss causes vaginal epithelial thinning, which leads to increasingly fragile vaginal mucosa characterized by pallor, decreased elasticity, and disappearance of rugae (the small folds of the mucous membrane). Vaginal blood flow and cervical and vaginal secretions diminish, resulting in decreased lubrication. In addition, vaginal shortening and narrowing occur. Pruritus and irritation may subsequently ensue. Cytologic examination of the vaginal epithelium reveals a loss of superficial cells and an increase of basal

Table 11. Possible causes of vulvovaginal complaints
• Vaginal infection, including candidiasis (yeast) and trichomoniasis
• Bacterial vaginosis (overgrowth of certain vaginal bacteria)
• Sexually transmitted diseases
• Allergic reactions to chemicals in soaps, bubble baths, spermicides, condoms, feminine hygiene sprays, deodorant tampons/pads
• Douching
• Irritation from tampons or birth control devices (eg, diaphragm or cervical cap) left inside the vagina too long
• Trauma
• Foreign body
• Skin conditions, such as eczema or lichen sclerosus
• Certain diseases (eg, inflammatory bowel disease, diabetes mellitus, lupus erythematosus)
• Benign and malignant tumors
• Psychological causes
• Injury to pelvic nerve fibers, leading to persistent vulvar pain
• Vulvodynia
• Certain endocrine therapies (eg, aromatase inhibitors)
• Certain medications (eg, antibiotics) which contribute to candidiasis
• Hypoestrogenic states (eg, peri- and postmenopause, premature ovarian failure)
• Medically induced menopause (eg, cancer treatment)

and parabasal cells compared to the characteristics of the reproductive years.

Loss of estrogen at menopause also results in an increase in the vaginal pH from a healthy acidic environment to an unhealthy alkaline one, creating a more susceptible habitat for vaginal infection. In reproductive-age women, the vaginal flora are dominated by lactobacilli. In postmenopausal women, diverse flora may colonize the vagina, including pathogenic organisms commonly found in urinary tract infections.

Vaginal health may progressively worsen in susceptible women. The term *vaginal atrophy* describes vaginal walls that are thin, pale, dry, and sometimes inflamed (ie, atrophic vaginitis). They can exhibit small petechiae (ie, pinpoint, nonraised, round, purple-red spots caused from intradermal or submucous hemorrhage). These changes increase the likelihood of trauma and pain. This can result in dyspareunia and/or pain during a pelvic examination, as well as tears and bleeding from vaginal penetration. These effects are less likely to occur in women who experience regular sexual stimulation, which promotes blood flow to the genital area.

Peri- and postmenopausal reductions in ovarian estrogen production are not, however, the only potential causes of vulvovaginal symptoms, including vaginal atrophy. Additional causes—including other hypoestrogenic states (eg, premature ovarian failure, hypothalamic amenorrhea, hyperprolactinemia, and possibly prolonged lactation), some endocrine therapies (eg, selective estrogen-receptor modulators, aromatase inhibitors, and gonadotropin-releasing hormone agonists or antagonists), and medically induced menopause (eg, cancer treatment)—must be ruled out. Similar symptoms can be experienced by postmenopausal women suffering from vaginal infection, trauma, foreign body, allergic reaction, inflammatory conditions of the vulva, certain medical disorders (eg, inflammatory bowel disease [Crohn's disease], diabetes mellitus [DM], lupus erythematosus), and psychological causes. Infections of the sebaceous, Bartholin's, or Skene's glands are also possible, along with benign or cancerous vaginal tumors.

Symptomatic vaginal atrophy can be associated with cancer treatments such as surgery, pelvic radiation therapy, chemotherapy, and endocrine therapy, as these interventions may result in changes in the vaginal epithelium, impaired vascular supply, and anatomic alterations in the vaginal canal. Many cancer treatments also cause either temporary or permanent ovarian failure, which in the premenopausal woman will result in adverse vaginal changes. The effects of cancer treatments may be associated with painful pelvic examinations, dyspareunia, increased risk of vaginal infections, and a narrower and shortened vagina. Vaginal symptoms related to an abrupt menopause induced by chemotherapy are associated with significantly greater sexual dysfunction and distress, as well as poorer quality-of-life outcomes.

Endocrine therapy for breast cancer is also associated with vaginal symptoms. Drugs called selective estrogen-receptor modulators (SERMs) vary in their effect on vaginal tissue. One SERM, tamoxifen, exerts predominantly antiestrogenic effects in the breast; however, it also produces estrogen-agonistic effects in the uterus and vagina. Vaginal discharge is the most common vaginal complaint, and there is a slightly increased incidence of vaginal moniliasis. Another SERM, raloxifene, has been found to have fewer adverse vaginal effects. Compared with tamoxifen, aromatase inhibitors have a significantly greater incidence of vaginal dryness and dyspareunia. (Note that the FDA has disallowed the term "selective estrogen-receptor modulator" [SERM], preferring "estrogen agonist/antagonist.")

Vulvar disorders. Included among the benign disorders of the vulva (external genitals, including the labia and clitoris) are contact dermatitis, dermatoses, vulvodynia, and vulvar dystrophy—all of which need to be diagnosed and treated.

Although estrogen receptors are found in the vulva, whether estrogen deprivation contributes to these conditions is not confirmed. Diminished estrogen levels result in a decrease in the size of the vulva.

Vulvar disorders can be categorized according to their predominent presenting characteristics (see Table 12). A high index of suspicion for preinvasive carcinoma of the vulva is necessary whenever a vulvar lesion is evaluated.

Vulvodynia. Although the term "vulvar dysesthesia" has been used in the past, there is now consensus to use the term *vulvodynia* when describing chronic vulvar pain and discomfort (not itching) in the absence of gross anatomic or neurologic findings (other than erythema and, occasionally, "paper cuts" or erosions in the skin). The clinican is advised to clearly describe the symptoms (eg, vulvar burning, stinging, irritation, rawness, knifelike pain) rather than simply notate a term. Pain with intercourse may linger for minutes to days.

Table 12. Typical presentation of vulvar disorders

Most common causes	*Less common causes*
Cystic mass	
Epidermal inclusion cyst	Inguinal hernia
Bartholin's gland cyst	Pilonidal cyst
Follicular cyst	Cysts of embryonic origin
	Hidradenoma
	Urethral diverticulum
Solid mass	
Condylomata acuminatum	Seborrheic keratosis
Acrochordon (skin tags)	Nevi
	Fibromas and lipomas
	Urethral caruncle
	Endometriosis
	Carcinoma
Pruritis	
Atrophic vaginitis	Carcinoma
Infectious vulvitis	Scabies
(*Candida, Trichomonas*)	Sjögren's syndrome
Human papillomavirus	Vulval intraepithelial neoplasia
Bacterial vaginosis	
Squamous hyperplasia	
Lichen sclerosus	
Contact dermatitis	
Irritant vulvitis	
Pain	
Atrophic vaginitis	Vulvodynia
Herpes genitalis	Postherpetic neuralgia
Human papillomavirus	Pudendal neuralgia
Lichen planus	Herpes zoster
Vulvar vestibulitis	

Source: Adapted from Michlewitz et al. *Primary Care of Women* 1995.

Vulvodynia was previously thought to be rare, but studies in a variety of populations now suggest that the prevalence ranges from 3% to 15% of women from diverse backgrounds and ethnicities. These women often suffer in silence, with an accurate diagnosis established only after years of pain, distress, and frustration.

Vulvodynia is not caused by commonly identified infection (eg, herpes), inflammation (eg, lichen planus), neoplasia (eg, Paget's disease), or a neurologic disorder (eg, herpes neuralgia). Several potential causes have been proposed (eg, genetic or immune factors), although a single cause is not likely.

According to the 2005 guidelines of the International Society for the Study of Vulvovaginal Disease (ISSVD), the classification of vulvodynia is based on the site of the pain; whether it is provoked, unprovoked, or mixed; and whether it is generalized or localized. Generalized vulvodynia, which involves chronic, often non-localized vulvar pain that occurs with or without stimulation, is thought to differ from *vulvar vestibulitis syndrome* (VVS) in which pain is localized or confined to the vulvar vestibule (an oval area that includes the urethral and vaginal openings). However, these may be two different manifestations of the same disease process. The cotton swab test is used to distinguish these conditions, guiding appropriate treatment.

When presented with a woman with one or more of these symptoms, alternate causes should be excluded. These include vulvitis from irritants such as soap, panty liners, synthetic underwear, moistened wipes, deodorants, douches, lubricants, spermicides, excessive vaginal discharge, urine, and feces; allergic contact dermatitis from sanitary napkins, colored toilet paper, vaginal sprays, laundry detergents, bubble baths, fragrances, and topical medications; parasites such as scabies; and diseases such as candidiasis, recurrent herpes infection, herpes zoster and postherpetic neuralgia, lichen sclerosus, erosive lichen planus, Sjögren's syndrome, vulval intraepithelial neoplasia, and carcinoma. Similar symptoms can also result from low estrogen levels.

Vulvar dystrophies. The term *vulvar dystrophy* describes a degeneration of the vulvar tissue that can develop at any age, but is mostly found in peri- and postmenopausal women. Vulvar dystrophies are nonneoplastic epithelial disorders of the vulvar skin and mucosa.

Vulvar dystrophy may be characterized by thinning of squamous epithelium, termed *lichen sclerosus*; older terms include kraurosis vulvae, atrophic leukoplakia, and lichen sclerosus et atrophicus. The cause is unknown. Pruritis is usually present and worsens with time. The lesion is white and wrinkled, frequently involving the entire vulva. The labia minora first adhese to the majora, then atrophy and disappear. The vaginal opening can shrink in size (kraurosis).

Vulvar dystrophy may also be *squamous cell hyperplasia,* characterized by thickened lesions, usually the result of chronic irritation or infection. Older terms include hyperplastic dystrophy, lichen simplex chronicus, hypertrophic vulvitis, chronic reaction vulvitis, and neurodermatitis. The skin develops a white, thickened surface with some cracking. Bleeding and pruritis may also occur. Unlike lichen sclerosus, the labia minora do not disappear and the lesion is usually localized.

Lichen planus affects the mucosal surfaces of the vulva, especially the vestibule. This condition is characterized by thickening of all layers of the epithelium. Painful erosive areas may be present and adhesions of opposite mucosal surfaces can cause marked stenosis of the introitus and vagina. The lesion bleeds on contact and is associated with severe dyspareunia. Lichen planus appears as a white, raised lesion with a reticular, lacy pattern; the erosive variant has the appearance of a desquamation bordered by reticular white epithelium. The external labia may resemble lichen sclerosus, but the mucosal changes are quite characteristic.

With all vulvar disorders, sources of cutaneous irritation should be identified and discontinued, and neoplasia and infection should be ruled out.

Vulvar masses. Several subcutaneous vulvar lesions are possible.

- The most common subcutanous vulvar lesion is the *epidermal inclusion cyst*—a smooth, yellowish cyst typically 5 to 15 mm in diameter. It is usually nontender and slow-growing. Multiple lesions may occur. These must be distinguished from inguinal hernias.

- *Bartholin's gland cysts* arise in the labia minora in the greater vestibular gland (ie, Bartholin's gland), resulting in swelling in the posterior labia minora and deep to the perineal body. Noninfected cysts are usually compressible and not tender. Infection produces an extremely tender mass along with swelling that may extend to the labia majora. In a postmenopausal woman, a mass at the site of the Bartholin's gland may arise from a benign or malignant neoplasm.

- *Folliculitis* is the term describing subcutaneous masses of the labia majora resulting from infections at the base of the hair follicle. The tender lesions vary in size from 5 mm up to several centimeters.

- *Condylomata acuminatum* (a genital wart) is caused by human papilloma virus (HPV). Benign genital warts can be asymptomatic, minute, or grow to the 8 to 10 cm in size. Inspection of genitals with the use of a magnifying glass is recommended so that warts are not overlooked. An association with malignancy has been observed; studies show that most cervical cancers are related to infection by sexually transmitted, high-risk types of HPV. (See Section C, page 156, for more about sexually transmitted infection and Section E, page 149, for more about cervical cancer.)

Management of vulvovaginal symptoms. All women at menopause and beyond should have a thorough evaluation of vulvovaginal health during the pelvic examination, regardless of whether they are symptomatic or sexually active.

The pelvic examination should include an assessment for vaginal atrophy, whether or not vulvovaginal problems have been disclosed. Friability and pallor of the vaginal epithelium should be noted, along with any bleeding from low levels of trauma (eg, speculum insertion).

Vaginal fluid should also be examined, noting the amount, character, and pH. An increase in vaginal pH of 5 or above is one sign of estrogen loss and atrophic changes, provided presence of pathogens (eg, *Trichomonas*) has been ruled out. One common vaginal pathogen is *Candida albicans* (yeast). Women often recognize recurrent infections and treat them empirically with over-the-counter medications. Clinicians should question women about these symptoms and be prepared to investigate the cause or causes, as other conditions can imitate yeast infections. The reader should refer to standard medical texts for the differential diagnosis and management of vaginal pathogens. (Also see Section E, page 156, for more about sexually transmitted diseases.)

Many clinicians support instructing women in vulvar self-examination, performed once a month with breast self-examination; a hand-held mirror is necessary in order to detect moles, warts, ulcers, sores, or changes in pigmentation. During the clinical examination, subtle vulvar changes require close observation, often via a magnifying glass. The toluidine blue dye test can be useful to direct a biopsy, but this test is not absolute; biopsy is recommended to investigate any questionable finding. White lesions of the vulva should always be biopsied.

Vulvodynia, a pain syndrome with no other identified cause, is a diagnosis of exclusion. The history should identify the duration of pain, previous treatments, allergies, medical and surgical history, and sexual history. Cotton swab testing (at the 2-, 4-, 6-, 8-, and 10-o'clock positions) is used to identify areas of localized pain and to classify the areas where there is mild, moderate, or severe pain. A diagram of pain locations may be helpful in assessing the pain over time. The vagina should be examined and tests, including wet mount, vaginal pH, fungal culture, and Gram stain, should be performed, as indicated.

If the reported complaint from a peri- or postmenopausal woman includes a gradual reduction in vaginal secretions during sexual activity, the cause is probably vaginal atrophy from estrogen loss. When the problem is acute, especially associated with vaginal discharge, pelvic pain, and/or following sexual activity with a new partner, the cause is more likely to be a sexually transmitted infection or a vulvar dystrophy. If the symptoms are unexplained, treatment should be chosen carefully with the understanding that there are few consistent data from trials to support any particular intervention.

Vaginal atrophy. Between 10% and 40% of all postmenopausal women may have symptoms related to vaginal atrophy, but only about 25% of them seek medical help. Although it is rarely a serious condition, vaginal atrophy can be distressing and typically does not resolve on its own. Estrogen treatment is often required.

Regular sexual stimulation, which promotes blood flow to the genital area, can help maintain vaginal health. Many women with vaginal atrophy have developed, with their partner, an expanded view of sexual pleasure through massage, extended caressing, and mutual masturbation. Women without a partner may employ self-stimulation or masturbation.

• *Nonprescription therapy.* Mild vaginal dryness can often be managed with vaginal lubricants and moisturizers available without a prescription (see Section H, page 252, for more about vaginal moisturizers and lubricants). During sexual activity, both lubricants and moisturizers can decrease the friction on atrophic vulvovaginal structures. Improvements in vaginal dryness and elimination of dyspareunia may allow many postmenopausal women to resume premenopausal levels of sexual function. In contrast to vaginal lubricants, vaginal moisturizers can also reduce uncomfortable symptoms of mild vaginal atrophy by maintaining adequate vaginal moisture and lower vaginal pH.

Water-soluble (not oil) products are recommended, although vitamin E or olive oil is reported to provide lubrication without adverse effects. Inadequate data exist to evaluate the effect on vaginal dryness, if any, of herbal supplements and isoflavone-containing foods and supplements.

• *Estrogen therapy.* If vaginal atrophy is moderate or severe and nonprescription remedies are inadequate, estrogen therapy (ET) can be recommended. Estrogen has been proven to restore vaginal blood flow, decrease vaginal pH, and improve the thickness and elasticity of these tissues. Judging estrogen need or dosage is not possible through assessment of vaginal cytology through the maturation index.

A list of the various types of estrogen and modes of delivery that are government approved in the United States and Canada for the treatment of vaginal atrophy (ie, vulval and vaginal atrophy, atrophic vaginitis, kraurosis vulvae) is found in Table 13. Those delivering a localized estrogen dose are an estradiol cream (Estrace Vaginal Cream, available in the United States but not Canada), a conjugated estrogen (CE) vaginal cream (Premarin Vaginal Cream), a sustained-release Silastic ring that delivers estradiol (Estring), and a micronized estradiol hemihydrate vaginal tablet (Vagifem). The optimal treatment regimen and minimum effective dose for each preparation, however, have not yet been established, so the regimens used clinically reflect the treatment protocols used in the studies, commercial product availability, and government-approved labeling.

Another vaginal estrogen product that is available in the United States but not Canada is the estradiol acetate ring (Femring); this product delivers a systemic dose of estrogen.

Systemic ET products (oral tablets, transdermal patches, topical lotions and gels, and Femring) are government approved for treating hot flashes and vaginal atrophy. Because systemic ET is associated with greater side effects than localized ET, its use is not recommended for treating vaginal atrophy unless other symptoms require management and benefits outweigh risks.

Improvements in vulvovaginal health usually occur within a few weeks of starting low-dose vaginal ET; however, some women may need to use vaginal estrogen for 4 to 6 weeks before adequate improvement is observed. Women can use vaginally administered estrogen as needed; no time limits for therapy use have been established. Vaginal estrogen is not generally used in combination with systemically delivered estrogen. However, some women using systemic low-dose ET who experience persistent vaginal atrophy may benefit from the addition of localized ET, provided that the systemic adverse effects are closely monitored.

Localized ET with a vaginal cream (Estrace Vaginal Cream, Premarin Vaginal Cream) typically consists of a loading dose of 2 to 4 g/day for 2 weeks. After the initial therapeutic response is attained, the frequency and dose can be reduced to maintain the response. A maintenance schedule of one to three doses per week is usually sufficient, but it should be titrated to the lowest dose and frequency of vaginal estrogen that provides the desired effect for each woman.

The sustained-release estradiol ring (Estring) releases 7.5 µg of estradiol every 24 hours for up to 90 days. One study has shown that the ring provides therapeutic efficacy for vaginal atrophy without an increase in serum estradiol levels above the normal postmenopausal range. The estradiol acetate vaginal ring (Femring) (marketed in the United States, not Canada) is a systemic-dose device available in formulations releasing either 50 or 100 µg/day. Both doses are approved for the treatment of moderate to severe symptoms of vulvar and vaginal atrophy associated with menopause.

Table 13. Vaginal estrogen therapy products for postmenopausal use in the United States and Canada

Composition	Product Name	Dosing
Vaginal Creams		
17β-estradiol	Estrace Vaginal Cream*	initial: 2-4 g/d for 1-2 wk maintenance: 1 g/d (0.1 mg active ingredient/g)
conjugated estrogens (formerly conjugated equine estrogens)	Premarin Vaginal Cream	0.5-2 g/d (0.625 mg active ingredient/g)
esterified estrogens	Neo-Estrone Vaginal Cream**	2-4 g/d (1 mg active ingredient/g)
Vaginal Rings		
17β-estradiol	Estring	device containing 2 mg releases 7.5 µg/d for 90 d
estradiol acetate	Femring*	device containing 12.4 mg or 24.8 mg estradiol acetate releases 0.05 mg/d or 0.10 mg/d estradiol for 90 d (systemic levels)
Vaginal Tablet		
estradiol hemihydrate	Vagifem	initial: 1 tablet/d for 2 wk maintenance: 1 tablet twice/wk (tablet containing 25.8 µg estradiol hemihydrate equivalent to 25 µg of estradiol)

* Available in the United States but not Canada.
** Available in Canada but not the United States.
Products not marked are available in both the United States and Canada.

The vaginal tablet containing 25 µg estradiol may be preferred by some women who find using a vaginal cream messy and difficult to insert. One tablet is inserted once daily for 2 weeks, followed by a maintenance dose twice weekly. In a 2000 trial by Rioux et al, the vaginal tablet had greater patient acceptance than estrogen cream and lower withdrawal rates (10% vs 32%) than estrogen cream.

All low-dose, local vaginal ET products that are government approved in the United States and Canada differ slightly in their adverse-event profiles. In general, creams are thought to be associated with more adverse effects than the ring or tablets, perhaps because there is greater potential for patients to apply higher-than-recommended dosing with cream. However, a Cochrane review of trials reported no significant differences among the delivery methods in terms of hyperplasia, endometrial thickness, or the proportion of women with adverse events.

All these approved products are equally effective at the doses recommended in labeling. The choice is dependent on clinical experience and patient preference.

Progestogen is generally not indicated when low-dose estrogen is administered locally for vaginal atrophy.

There are insufficient data to recommend annual endometrial surveillance in asymptomatic women using low-dose, local vaginal ET. If a woman is at high risk for endometrial cancer, is using a greater dose of vaginal ET, or is having symptoms (spotting, breakthrough bleeding), closer surveillance may be required.

- *Vulvodynia.* No treatment is government approved in the United States or Canada for the treatment of vulvodynia, and few randomized trials are available to guide treatment. Current recommendations are based mainly on clinical experience.

Multiple treatments have been used, including vulvar care measures (eg, avoiding vulvar irritants); topical medications (eg, lidocaine ointment 5%, plain petrolatum, but not topical steroids); oral medications (eg, antidepressants, anticonvulsants); biofeedback and physical therapy; intralesional injections; and surgery.

Off-label use of oral tricyclic antidepressants (amitriptyline [Elavil], nortriptyline [Pamelor], and desipramine [Norpramin]) and anticonvulsants (gabapentin [Neurontin] and carbamazepine [Tegretol]) can decrease neural hypersensitivity and have yielded good clinical results. Treatment should begin at the lowest dosage, typically much less than the dose required for the approved indications (see respective Package Inserts for a full discussion of contraindications, side effects, and guidance on safely discontinuing treatment). Only one drug should be prescribed at a time. Both therapies require time to achieve adequate pain control, perhaps up to 3 weeks. Tolerance to their side effects (eg, sedation, dry mouth, dizziness) is usually achieved over time.

Biofeedback and physical therapy may also be used in the treatment of both localized and generalized vulvar pain. These techniques are particularly helpful of there is concomitent vaginismus (inability to tolerate vaginal penetration for any reason).

Topical therapies have not proved highly effective and are primarily used as an adjunct to other approaches. Analgesics such as acetaminophen, NSAIDs, and narcotics are likewise ineffective.

There is evidence that many cases of vulvodynia improve with time, with or without treatment. For generalized vulvar burning unresponsive to previous behavioral and medical treatments, referral to a pain specialist may be helpful. Surgery should be reserved for women with localized symptoms who do not respond to other treatments.

- *Other vulvar disorders.* White lesions of the vulva should always be biopsied. Treatment of lichen sclerosus consists of topical application of corticosteroid cream or ointment twice daily for 1 to 2 months. Laser vaporization and total vulvectomy are not recommended due to the high recurrence rate. With squamous cell hyperplasia, topical application of corticosteroid preparations is the treatment in the absence of severe atypia. Unlike lichen sclerosus, once effectively treated, recurrence is uncommon, but recurrence does occur after vulvectomy. High-potency topic corticosteroids may control lichen planus as well.

All dark lesions of the vulva should be excised regardless of their appearance. Melanoma and Paget's disease are among the potential diagnoses.

Asymptomatic epidermal inclusion cysts should be carefully followed and excised if significant enlargement is observed or if the cyst causes discomfort. Aspiration of fluid is not advised, due to the risk of inoculating the cyst with bacteria, leading to abcess formation.

With Bartholin's gland cysts, incision and drainage are usually required, performed under no or local anesthesia. Maintaining drainage is essential for satisfactory resolution. Treatment with antibiotics is necessary only with associated cellulitis.

Folliculitis typically drain spontaneously as a result of warm compresses or sitz baths. Larger masses require incision and drainage.

Genital warts are treated with topical agents such as trichloroacetic acid, podophyllum, or imiquimod (Aldara 5% cream) to affected area every other day. A side effect of treatment is temporary intense burning, less with popophyllum. Regrowth of lesions may reflect inadequate treatment of resistence, with the latter demanding histological examination to rule out cancer before resuming local treatment. Intralesional interferon may be effective for resistent or recurrent warts. Larger lesions (>2 cm) require laser or surgical removal. Examination and treatment of the sexual partner are advised.

Sexual function effects

Sexual desire decreases with age in both sexes, and low desire is particularly common in women in their late 40s and 50s. Sexual concerns are often an issue for women at midlife and beyond, although they frequently are not reported to healthcare providers. Data from the National Health and Social Life Survey indicate that nearly one half of US women, including those at midlife, have a problem in one or more aspects of sexual functioning.

Menopause contributes to sexual function changes through the decreases in ovarian hormone production. The impact of the lower hormone levels varies from woman to woman, presumably because changes in sexual function are multifactorial in cause. A range of psychological, socio-cultural, interpersonal, and biologic factors can contribute to sexual dysfunction (see Table 14).

With sexual arousal, lubrication occurs as a result of secretions from the vaginal glands and transudate from the subepithelial vasculature. Changes in the epithelial lining of the vagina occur relatively rapidly as estrogen levels decline (see page 51 for more). Subsequent vascular, muscular, and connective tissue changes occur over time. Decreased vascularization of surrounding tissue makes engorgement and lubrication more difficult. These effects may impair touch and vibration perception, which could cause a delay or absence of orgasm and a reduction in perceived sexual satisfaction. The vagina also loses its elasticity, which can result in discomfort during sexual activity.

Decreased estrogen is responsible for most of these changes, but testosterone, too, is an important factor in midlife sexual changes affecting women. Testosterone is necessary for a normal sex drive in both men and women, playing a role in motivation, desire, and sexual sensation. By the time most women reach their 60s, their testosterone levels are one half of what they were before age 40.

During perimenopause, as estrogen levels decrease, women also experience a decrease in levels of sex hormone-binding globulin (SHBG), which binds both estrogen and testosterone. As a result, some women may notice an increase in sexual desire and activity, perhaps because the declining levels of SHBG free up more testosterone.

Desire and other components of sexual health. One of the most significant and universal changes that occurs with age is a decrease in the drive component of sexual desire.

Table 14. Potential factors influencing women's sexual function

- Previous attitudes. In general, women who enjoyed sex in their younger years will continue to do so during peri- and postmenopause. Those who have not enjoyed sex previously may view any midlife reduction in sexual activity as a relief rather than a loss. Some women, however, have an increased interest in sex as they reach menopause.
- No available partner.
- Partners may lose interest in sex or have decreased capacity for sexual activity (especially men with erectile dysfunction).
- A male partner's ability to once again achieve erections through erectile dysfunction therapy (eg, sildenafil [Viagra], tadalafil [Cialis]) could cause extreme vaginal discomfort for the woman due to her lack of vaginal lubrication and elasticity resulting from having no intercourse for months or years.
- Age-related changes. With age, sexual drive generally decreases gradually in both men and women. However, a decline does not mean an abrupt halt, and the rate and extent of any decline is individual.
- A woman's perception of her body. Menopause usually occurs at a time when women are experiencing changes in their physical appearance. Women who accept these changes and maintain a positive outlook about their bodies usually have a strong sense of self-esteem that contributes to sexual health. In contrast, those who perceive aging as unattractive often feel undesirable.
- Health concerns. Following surgical procedures such as removal of a breast or uterus, a woman may feel unattractive and may avoid initiating sexual encounters. Also, her partner may be fearful that sexual activity will cause her pain.
- Incontinence. This syndrome can lead to sexual avoidance.
- Sleep disturbances. These often result in fatigue and irritability, thereby affecting sexual desire.
- Stressors, such as family, work, and relationship issues.
- Medications. Some drugs, such as antihypertensives or antidepressants, can decrease sexual desire and orgasmic capacity.
- Diminished androgen levels.

Desire refers to an individual's interest in being sexual and is determined by the interaction of three related but separate components: drive; beliefs, values, and expectations; and motivation.

Drive. The biologic component of desire is drive, resulting from neuroendocrine mechanisms. Drive is typically manifested by sexual thoughts, feelings, fantasies, or dreams; increased erotic attraction to others in proximity; seeking out sexual activity (alone or with a partner); and genital tingling or increased genital sensitivity. Drive declines in both men and women as a function of aging, although the exact neuroendocrine mechanisms responsible for drive are not fully understood.

For some women, lower levels of free testosterone, related to reduced ovarian and adrenal function or surgical menopause, may result in a noticeable decrease in sexual drive.

Beliefs, values, and expectations. The second component of desire reflects an individual's beliefs, values, and expectations about sexual activity. The more positive the individual's beliefs and values are about sexuality, the greater the individual's desire to behave sexually.

Motivation. The third component, psychological and interpersonal motivation, is driven by emotional or interpersonal factors, and is characterized by the willingness of a person to behave sexually with a given partner. This component tends to have the greatest impact overall on desire and is the most complex and elusive.

For many women, particularly postmenopausal women, drive diminishes and may no longer be the initial step in the response cycle. The classic Masters and Johnson model first developed in 1966 suggested a linear model of the sexual response cycle—desire leading to arousal and plateau, then to orgasm and resolution. More recently, an alternative model to understanding the sexual response cycle has suggested that for many women, desire comes after arousal and that many women begin from a point of sexual neutrality. Arousal may come from a conscious decision or as a result of seduction or suggestion from a partner.

Hypoactive sexual desire disorder (HSDD) is the most prevalent of the six female sexual dysfunctions in the *Diagnostic and Statistical Manual of Mental Disorders (DSM-IV-TR)*. HSSD is defined as persistently or recurrently deficient (or absent) sexual fantasies and/or desire for sexual activity that causes personal distress. Often, a woman with deficient or absent sexual desire is diagnosed with HSDD when she does not have personal distress regarding her condition; this component is essential to the diagnosis. For peri- and postmenopausal women, decreased desire is a common problem, as are vaginal dryness and discomfort with intercourse.

The term *androgen insufficiency* (rather than *deficiency*) is defined as a pattern of clinical symptoms in the presence of decreased bioavailable testosterone and normal estrogen status. The clinical symptoms include impaired sexual function, mood alterations, and diminished energy and well-being. There is not enough is known about normal levels of androgens in women to define a deficiency. There are no consistent laboratory assessments. Most commercially available methods are inaccurate or unreliable. Equilibrium dialysis is the current gold standard, but it is not readily available in most laboratories.

Although this androgen insufficiency syndrome has been proposed, a clear association between decreased androgen levels and impaired sexual function is not supported by evidence. Not all women with low testosterone levels experience symptoms, and many women with sexual problems have normal androgen levels. Several large studies using quality hormone assays and validated sexual function measures have not identified an association between testosterone levels and sexual problems.

This lack of an association should not be unexpected, as female sexuality and HSDD are complicated and cannot be summed up by a single biologic marker. Even when androgen insufficiency may be involved, several other psychosocial factors are at least as important, if not more important, in understanding the problem.

The Massachusetts Women's Health Study (WHS), a large, population-based trial, showed that a woman's menopause status has a smaller impact on sexual functioning than other factors, such as health, sociodemographic variables, psychological aspects, a partner's health and sexual dysfunction, and lifestyle. Although menopause (but not serum estrogen levels) was significantly associated with decreases in several sexual function measurements, including lower sexual desire and declines in arousal, the impact was not as great as the other factors mentioned above. The Melbourne Women's Midlife Health Project found the major factors affecting women's sexuality were their feelings for their partner and any sexual difficulties experienced by their partner. Other social variables such as stress at work or interpersonal stress and educational level affect sexual function indirectly via effects on symptoms and well-being.

Lower estrogen levels have been associated with a decline in sexual function. The menopause-associated estrogen loss may lead to vaginal dryness, urogenital atrophy, and dyspareunia. These changes may appear during perimenopause, but they are more common during the first few years after menopause. During perimenopause, hot flashes can result in chronic sleep disturbance, which may affect psychologic function. Negative changes in mood and well-being as well as poor self-esteem may also be relevant to sexual dysfunction associated with menopause.

Other studies have illustrated that for younger postmenopausal women, dyspareunia (painful intercourse) plays an important role. As the time since menopause lengthens, delayed orgasm and reduced libido begin to become more common concerns. During peri- and postmenopause, any untreated anxiety disorder or depression, whether new or chronic, may have a negative impact on sexual function.

Some experts believe that changes in sexual desire, frequency, and responsiveness may be a result of either diminished estrogen effects on the cardiovascular system (impairing arterial blood flow) or decreased estrogenic effects on the central and peripheral nervous systems (impairing touch and vibration perception).

Lower endogenous progesterone levels appear to have no adverse effects on sexual function, although some types of progestogen therapy can indirectly affect sexual function and/or sexual activity by negatively influencing mood or by causing frequent uterine bleeding.

Most experts agree that a woman's libido (sex drive) is more associated with androgen (testosterone) than other hormones, but libido and sexual function are strongly influenced by nonhormonal factors. Conditions that accelerate declining androgen production are shown in Table 15.

Table 15. Conditions that accelerate declining androgen production in women

- *Bilateral oophorectomy.* Surgical removal of both ovaries decreases circulating levels of testosterone by 40% to 50%.
- *Pituitary/adrenal insufficiency.* Androgen depletion is seen with Sheehan's syndrome and Addison's disease. In addition to decreased libido, symptoms may include muscle wasting, loss of pubic and axillary hair, osteoporosis, and immune disorders.
- *Corticosteroids and ET.* Androgen levels are decreased with the suppression of adrenocorticotrophic hormone or luteinizing hormone that occurs with corticosteroid or oral ET use.
- *Chronic illness.* Low androgen concentration also occurs in those with anorexia nervosa, advanced cancer, and burn trauma

---

Evaluation of sexual function. A sexual history should focus on the conditions or circumstances that affect sexual function and should be confidential and nonjudgmental (see Table 16). In addition, clinicians should be sensitive to a woman's specific conditions, issues related to sexual orientation, and should not assume that all women are heterosexual.

The NAMS Menopause Health Questionnaire contains several questions addressing sexuality and may assist practitioners in gathering this information (see http://www.menopause.org/edumaterials/pquestionnaire.htm).

It is important that healthcare providers encourage their patients to discuss any sexual concerns. Epidemiologic data indicate that between one third and one half of peri- and postmenopausal women experience a problem with one or more aspects of sexual functioning. These include hypoactive sexual desire disorder, sexual arousal disorder, orgasmic disorder, and sexual pain disorders.

In addition to a thorough history, clinicians may obtain more detailed sexual function information by utilizing one of a wide variety of validated instruments. The Watts Sexual Function Questionnaire (used in the Postmenopausal Estrogen/Progestin Interventions [PEPI] trial) focuses on four subscales: desire, arousal, orgasm, and satisfaction. The Personal Experiences Questionnaire (PEQ) collects data on six factors: feelings for the partner, sexual responsivity, frequency of sexual activities, libido, partner problems, and vaginal dryness and/or dyspareunia. The Female Sexual Function Index (FSFI) is a brief, self-reported measure of six domains, including desire, subjective arousal, lubrication, orgasm, satisfaction, and pain associated with intercourse. Several other instruments to measure sexual function, interest, or desire are available, but their reliability and validity vary. Some provide reliable assessments only for the specialized populations for which they were developed.

Table 16. Areas of focus for a sexual history

- Menstrual history
- Obstetric history
- Gynecologic history
- Safe sex practices
- Drug-related side effects
- Relationship history
- Sexual orientation
- Substance abuse and alcohol history
- Psychosocial issues
- History of physical or sexual abuse
- Age-related issues
- Sexual satisfaction

An assessment of all potential physical, psychological, or social factors amenable to intervention should be the primary therapeutic consideration for women who express a specific complaint of loss of libido. Clinicians should evaluate potential causes of decreased libido such as depression, anxiety, fatigue, stress, relationship conflicts, or sexual dysfunction in the woman's partner. It is also important to evaluate the potential side effects of medications, herbal remedies, or other over-the-counter supplements.

Often, the first noticeable vulvovaginal change associated with menopause is reduced vaginal lubrication during sexual arousal. All women of perimenopausal age and beyond should have a thorough evaluation of vaginal health, regardless of symptoms or sexual activity. Some women using low-dose estrogen therapy may have sexual problems related to inadequate estrogenization of the vulvovaginal tissues despite systemic estrogen use.

Management of sexual dysfunction. If sexual dysfunction is present, a physical examination is required to identify any physical causes. Many sexual problems can be successfully treated. Nonprescription vaginal lubricants and moisturizers are available to treat mild vaginal dryness and resulting dyspareunia (see page 54 for more). Prescription ET is a viable option for moderate to severe vaginal atrophy (see page 54 for more). Vaginal ET (cream, tablet, or ring) may ameliorate or prevent other sexual problems from developing. These include delayed or less robust orgasm and dyspareunia.

Various treatment strategies for decreases in sexual desire are listed in Table 17.

Nonpharmacological interventions. A variety of over-the-counter (OTC) agents (eg, Zestra Feminine Arousal Fluid) are promoted to increase sexual pleasure when topically applied to the female genitalia (see Section H, page 253, for more).

Counseling and sex therapy are effective interventions for many women and couples with sexual concerns. Referrals for therapy should be considered even when pharmacological interventions are indicated. Continued sexual activity is a realistic and expected part of aging. Healthcare professionals must be sensitive and informed about sexuality issues to better counsel women about recognizing and adjusting to the changes. Confidentiality is a special concern when discussing sexual function.

Women without sexual partners have similar counseling requirements. As they age, they also will need more time and stimulation to reach an orgasm.

A study by the UMDNJ-Robert Wood Johnson Medical School found that only 3% of US women with sexual problems initiated discussion with their physicians. However, when asked specifically about sexual function, 19% reported a problem.

A survey published in 1999 reinforced the importance of clinicians' initiating a discussion about sexual health. This survey showed that 71% of patients believed that their physician would dismiss any mention of sexual concerns, 68% believed their physician would be embarrassed by any discussion regarding sexual problems, and 76% did not think there were any treatments available to help with sexual problems.

For a woman undergoing a hysterectomy, both she and her partner need to be assured that losing the uterus does not mean losing sexual desire and femininity. Following hysterectomy, some women may notice a change in sensation during intercourse and orgasm, but, in general, these changes do not interfere with sexual functioning or achieving orgasm. Most women report improved sex lives after a hysterectomy due to relief of pain, loss of uterine bleeding, and/or the lack of need for birth control. Some women, however, may experience a significant adverse change in sexual response if surgery is extensive. Women facing chemotherapy or pelvic radiation therapy should also be counseled about the special effects that these therapies have on sexual function (see Section D, page 103, for more about premature menopause and Section E, page 139, for more about cancer therpies).

General recommendations regarding sex-related counseling are found in Table 18.

Table 17. Strategies for treatment of sexual dysfunction

Nonpharmacological interventions

- Allow more time for manual or oral stimulation
- Experiment with erotic materials, sexual fantasies, vibrators, dildos
- Try a sensual massage or a warm bath
- Change the sexual routine, such as the location or the time of day
- Use vaginal lubricants or moisturizers (water-based)
- Explore noncoital sexual activity, such as oral sex or mutual masturbation
- Increase communication about sexual and other concerns between the woman and her partner
- Seek counseling and/or sex therapy, if needed

Pharmacological interventions

- Systemic or local ET
- Androgen therapy
- Consider modification of type or dose of drugs that adversely affect sexual function (eg, antidepressants)

Table 18. Suggestions for sexual counseling

- First, treat any vaginal atrophy.
- Counsel women regarding normal, age-related, sexual response changes, including diminished lubrication, need for increased time and stimulation for arousal, decreased orgasmic contractions, decreased breast fullness and nipple erection, reduced clitoral sensitivity.
- Counsel male partners regarding normal, age-related, sexual response changes, including decreased penile rigidity, need for increased time and stimulation for erection and orgasm, longer refractory time.
- Educate couples regarding normal age-related changes in sexual function.
- Try warm baths before genital sexual activity.
- Extend foreplay time to accommodate longer sexual arousal time.
- Use sexual fantasies, erotic clothing or materials (eg, movies, literature), vibrators.
- Experiment with noncoital activities such as massage, oral stimulation.
- Use masturbation as an alternative to intercourse.
- Change the sexual routine, such as having sex in the morning when energy levels are higher.
- Experiment with positions other than the standard "missionary" position.

Pharmacological interventions. Although ET improves vaginal health and may improve sexual function by restoring vaginal lubrication and reducing dyspareunia, its effect on libido is uncertain. No studies have confirmed a beneficial effect of ET on sexual desire. Oral estrogens, unlike transdermal estrogens, increase SHBG levels, resulting in decreased levels of free testosterone. Women who experience decreased libido after initiating oral ET may benefit from switching to transdermal ET.

Androgen therapy is receiving increasing attention for treating postmenopausal women with sexual dysfunction. (See Section G, page 223, for more about androgen treatments for women.)

In addition to androgen therapies, devices have been developed that may be helpful for some women with sexual dysfunction. A suction vacuum device, EROS CTD, is approved by the US Food and Drug Administration (FDA) for female sexual dysfunction. Its design is similar to that of vacuum devices used for male erectile dysfunction. Theoretically, it may improve arousal and response by improving clitoral blood flow. The device is expensive and likely no more effective than less costly devices available to women without a prescription.

Sildenafil (Viagra) at daily doses of 10, 50, and 100 mg did not improve sexual response in peri- or postmenopausal women with sexual dysfunction. Headaches and flushing are side effects of sildenafil use.

Treatment of a male partner's sexual dysfunction may be critically important in improving a woman's sexual satisfaction. Alternatively, a couple's sexual problems may be exacerbated when the male partner is successfully treated for erectile dysfunction, after the couple has not had intercourse for months or years. The woman may have extreme vaginal discomfort due to lack of lubrication and elasticity.

Urinary concerns

Urinary complaints, including urinary incontinence and overactive bladder syndrome, become more common during perimenopause and beyond. However, these urinary complaints are not an inevitable result of aging and should not be considered normal.

Urinary incontinence. Urinary incontinence is a common, debilitating, and costly problem, particularly in middle-aged and older women. Prevalence estimates in midlife women range from about 5% for severe incontinence to 60% for mild incontinence. Cross-sectional epidemiological studies have reported an increase in the prevalence of incontinence among women aged 45 to 55 years, an age range that coincides with the menopause transition. Traditionally, incontinence has been considered a symptom of urogenital atrophy related to the menopausal reduction in endogenous estrogens. Estrogen receptors are found throughout the lower urinary tract. However, estrogen treatment in postmenopause has been shown to worsen incontinence in some randomized trials. Whether the transition from pre- to postmenopause, independent of age or other factors, increases the risk for developing incontinence remains unclear.

Some factors that have been associated with incontinence include age, DM, obesity, parity, smoking/chronic cough, hysterectomy, and family history. Urinary incontinence can be classified into different types as follows:

- *Stress incontinence.* The symptom of stress incontinence is involuntary loss of urine that occurs with an activity that increases intra-abdominal pressure, such as coughing or sneezing. Leakage is usually in drops, unless it is severe. Stress incontinence is thought to be related to poor urethral support (urethral hypermobility) and/or urethral sphincter weakness (intrinsic sphincter deficiency).

- *Urge incontinence.* The symptom of urge incontinence is involuntary loss of urine preceded by a sensation of urgency to urinate. Urge incontinence is associated with losses of larger volumes of urine that soak through pads and clothing. It is caused by detrusor instability/overactivity—uninhibited contractions of the detrusor muscle (smooth muscle of the bladder wall).

- *Mixed incontinence.* Mixed incontinence is diagnosed when a woman reports both stress and urge incontinence symptoms.

- *Overflow incontinence.* Overflow incontinence is uncommon and is really a symptom of urinary retention. Leakage occurs because the bladder does not empty and cannot continue to accommodate the storage of large volumes of urine. Symptoms of overflow incontinence may include frequent insensible loss of urine or may mimic stress or urge leakage.

- *Extraurethral incontinence.* This type of incontinence is rare, occurring when there is an abnormal opening from the bladder, such as a vesicovaginal fistula that might occur as a complication of bladder injury during a hysterectomy.

Diagnosing the cause(s) and type(s) of a woman's urinary incontinence requires a careful assessment of her symptoms, medical history (including medications), surgical history, sexual history, a physical examination (including a pelvic examination), and a urinalysis and urine culture. In some cases, additional specialized studies such as urodynamic testing may be indicated.

Every woman with incontinence should be asked specific questions about her symptoms (see Table 19). Other conditions and symptoms associated with pelvic floor dysfunction should be investigated, including pelvic organ

---

Table 19. Standard questions regarding urinary incontinence

- How long have you had urinary incontinence/leaking urine?
- How many times do you urinate during the day? (frequency)
- How often do you wake up at night to urinate? (nocturia)
- Do you worry that you can't get to the bathroom in time? (urgency)
- Do you ever have the urge to urinate and lose your urine before you are able to reach the toilet? (urge incontinence)
- Do you leak urine when coughing, sneezing, walking, or lifting? (stress incontinence)

---

prolapse (the presence of a vaginal bulge) and bowel dysfunction (eg, constipation, fecal urgency, and anal incontinence).

One of the best tools to evaluate a woman's complaint of urinary incontinence is a 3-day urinary diary. The diary can help the clinician determine the frequency and type of incontinence, associated symptoms such as urinary frequency and exacerbating factors such as excessive consumption of fluids or caffeine (see Table 20).

Table 20. Information to include in a urinary diary

- Type and amount of fluid intake and time of day
- Circumstances of each leakage episode (eg, urgency on the way to the toilet or leakage with coughing/sneezing/exercise) and time of day
- Amount of urine leaked (eg, a few drops, wet underwear, soaked clothing) with each episode
- Use of external protection (pads), including quantity and how wet the pad is when changed
- Amount of urine voided and time of day can be helpful in some situations (normal total 24-hr urine volume is 1-1.5 liters)

Other important information, particularly for the frail elderly who may be at risk of falling, includes proximity to toilet facilities both during the day and at night.

The following should be included in the physical examination:

- Assessment of mental status
- Assessment of mobility (immobility may contribute to a woman's inability to reach the toilet)
- Neurological screening examination focusing on the sacral nerves, including perineal sensation and assessment of anal sphincter tone (to rule out rare neurological causes of incontinence)

- Inspection and palpation of the anterior vaginal wall and urethra (screen for urethral abnormalities such as a diverticulum)
- Inspection of the vulva/vagina for infection, discharge and pelvic organ prolapse
- Assessment of strength and ability to isolate the levator ani muscles (ability to do a Kegel exercise)
- Assessment for urine leakage with provocation, such as coughing or sneezing

Measuring a postvoid residual within 15 minutes of voiding is recommended, especially with concomitant pelvic organ prolapse or abnormal neurological signs and symptoms, to evaluate for urinary retention and overflow incontinence. A urinalysis can help identify potential medical causes for incontinence. For example, the presence of hematuria may suggest bladder pathology (eg, bladder stone or bladder cancer) and should be investigated. A urine culture can identify the presence of infection, which can be a cause of or can worsen incontinence symptoms.

Chronic dampness of underwear is sometimes mistaken for incontinence when the cause is an increase or change in vaginal secretions or perineal perspiration. A trial of phenazopyridine HCl (Pyridium), which will color the urine orange, may help differentiate urine from watery vaginal secretions.

Most incontinence can be successfully treated or managed based on the clinician's impression of incontinence type from an initial history and physical exam.

Management of urinary incontinence. Although up to half of midlife and older women report having urinary incontinence, less than 50% of them seek evaluation and treatment. Embarrassment, the misconception that incontinence is a normal part of aging, and lack of awareness about effective treatment options are the main reasons women cite for not seeking care. Even if a cure is not possible, clinicians can offer treatments or advice that can significantly improve incontinence symptoms.

After neurological and intrinsic bladder etiologies for urinary incontinence have been ruled out by a screening neurological exam and urinalysis, and after any bladder infection has been treated, most treatments for urinary incontinence can be initiated on the basis of patient-reported symptoms. Treatments are targeted to type of incontinence and are listed in Table 21. For women with mixed incontinence, the most troublesome symptoms should be addressed first. Treatment also depends on the significance of incontinence to the woman's quality of life, not necessarily how often she leaks or if she needs to wear pads for protection. Modifiable factors that cause or worsen incontinence should be considered and addressed first or at least early in treatment.

Table 21. Strategies for managing and treating urinary incontinence

Behavior modification for managing/treating both stress and urge incontinence

- *Pads.* Women with severe incontinence should be encouraged to use incontinence pads over menstrual pads. They provide better absorbency and better skin protection.

- *Fluid restriction.* For women who consume large volumes of fluid, limiting fluid intake to about 64 oz/ day can significantly reduce the number of leakage episodes. However, there is a theoretical risk that concentrated urine is irritating to the bladder, so overrestriction should be discouraged.

- *Weight loss.* For obese women, weight loss can reduce incontinence by up to 60%.

- *Timed voiding.* A woman is instructed to void at regular intervals by the clock, rather than waiting for the physical sensation of the urge to urinate. This can avoid the urge incontinence episodes and reduces the amount of urine in the bladder, which may decrease the frequency of stress incontinence episodes. This technique is especially useful for women who void infrequently or who have dementia.

Strategies and treatments for stress incontinence

- *Cough suppression.* Smokers should be encouraged to quit smoking and women with poorly controlled asthma or allergies should have these conditions optimally treated.

- *Incontinence pessaries.* Some women have excellent results from being fitted with incontinence pessaries. These can be worn all the time or just during the activities that induce incontinence (eg, running or aerobics).

- *Pelvic floor exercises.* Pelvic floor muscle (levator ani) strengthening exercises, commonly called Kegels, can improve stress incontinence by increasing the strength, bulk, and coordination of the levator ani. Women have reported up to 70% improvement in incontinence episodes. For Kegel instruction, women should not be asked to stop their urine flow but rather to contract the muscles they would use to delay a bowel movement. To help women who have difficulty isolating the pelvic floor muscles, Kegels can also be taught by trained clinicians (eg, physical therapists or nurse practitioners) with the use of biofeedback, electrical stimulation, or with vaginal cones. Women should also be taught to coordinate a pelvic floor muscle contraction at the time of a cough or sneeze. This maneuver can also prevent stress incontinence episodes.

- *Medications.* There is no medication approved by the FDA or Health Canada for the treatment of stress incontinence. Duloxetine (Cymbalta), a serotonin and noradrenaline reuptake inhibitor (SNRI), is approved in other countries and has been used off label; the effectiveness of this medication is limited. Systemic menopausal HT does not help stress incontinence and may exacerbate it if therapy increases uterine volume.

- *Surgery.* For women who have diagnosed stress incontinence and have failed more conservative treatments, surgery is an option. There are a number of surgical procedures currently being performed. The best surgical treatment has approximately an 85% success rate (either cured or significantly improved). The long-term outcomes (beyond 5 y) of stress incontinence surgeries have not been well studied.

Strategies and treatments for urge incontinence

- *Avoid bladder irritants.* Certain foods and beverages high in caffeine or acid (eg, coffee, cola soft drinks, grapefruit juice, tomatoes) can contribute to urge incontinence by irritating the bladder.

- *Improving mobility or toilet access.* In the frail elderly, urge incontinence has been associated with falls and fractures. Working to either improve mobility or providing a bedside commode may help reduce leaking accidents and prevent other morbidity.

- *Bladder retraining.* First, women must be able to isolate and contract their pelvic floor muscles, so training in Kegel exercises is required. Women are then taught to contract these muscles at the first sensation of urge. Because a Kegel sends negative feedback to the detrusor (bladder) muscle, this technique can suppress the detrusor contraction and prevent leakage. Women who have urinary frequency can also suppress the urge to urinate, thus extending the intervals between voids. Bladder retraining has been found to be the most effective method for treating urge incontinence.

- *Medications.* The most effective medications to treat urge incontinence are anticholinergic agents (see Table 22), all government approved for this indication. These agents work to decrease the frequency and intensity of detrusor contractions. The main side effects of these medications are dry mouth and constipation. Imipramine HCl (eg, Tofranil in US; Apo-imipramine in Canada) (10-25 mg 1-3 times/d) is a medication used off label to control nocturnal urge incontinence. Local vaginal estrogen therapy may benefit some women with urge incontinence who have atrophy.

- *Sacral neuromodulation stimulation.* For women whose urge incontinence does not respond to other treatments, sacral neuromodulation stimulation (InterStim) is another option. This system stimulates the sacral nerve root to modulate neural reflexes influencing bladder storage and emptying. An impulse generater is surgically implanted under the skin in the upper buttock area and attached to four leads that are placed into the sacral nerve space at S3. The effectiveness of InterStim for urge incontinence ranges from about 39% to 65%, depending on the definition of improvement.

If urge incontinence is not adequately controlled, the drug dose can be increased every 3 to 5 days until clinical improvement is seen or until the woman experiences adverse side effects. Caution should be used when prescribing anticholinergic drugs to elderly women, as they have been shown to increase cognitive impairment.

Table 22. Medications approved in North America for the treatment of urge urinary incontinence

Medication	Dosage
darifenacin (Enablex)	7.5-15 mg/d
oxybutynin chloride	
Ditropan	2.5-5 mg 1-3 times/d
Ditropan XL	5-15 mg/d
Oxytrol (patch)**	Change twice weekly
solifenacin (Vesicare)	5-10 mg/d
tolterodine tartrate	
Detrol	1-2 mg 1-2 times/d
Detrol LA**	2-4 mg/d
Detrol Unidet*	2-4 mg/d
trospium chloride (Sanctura)**	20 mg 1-2 times/d

* Available in Canada but not the United States.
** Available in the United States but not Canada.
Products not marked are available in both the United States and Canada.

Referral to a urologist or urogynecologist is appropriate for women with the following:

- Complex problems, such as neurologic conditions, pelvic organ prolapse, or a history of previous incontinence surgery
- Combined incontinence and recurrent bladder infections
- Extreme personal distress secondary to incontinence
- Failure of nonsurgical treatments

Overactive bladder syndrome, urinary tract infection, and interstitial cystitis. Overactive bladder (OAB) is a syndrome of idiopathic urinary urgency (with or without incontinence) usually with urinary frequency (>8 voids/24 hr) and nocturia (awakening to urinate >2 times/night) without a clear etiology. Because OAB is a diagnosis based on patient-reported symptoms and by exclusion of other etiologies, the evaluation includes ruling out specific causes of urgency, frequency, and nocturia symptoms.

The estimated prevalence of these symptoms in population-based studies of men and women is about 17%, with more women affected. OAB increases with age and is associated with urinary incontinence; up to 50% of women over the age 50 with urinary incontinence also report OAB symptoms. These symptoms have an important negative impact on women's quality of life and lead to coping behaviors such as mapping out toilets and decreased fluid intake. Women with nocturia can have poor sleep. Because OAB is a diagnosis

based on symptoms, it can have a number of etiologies including idiopathic and neurological (see Table 23).

Table 23. Differential diagnoses for urinary urgency, frequency, and nocturia symptoms

- *Behavioral.* Excessive fluid intake (often associated with dieting) or caffeine intake can cause or exacerbate OAB symptoms. Caffeine is both a diuretic and seems to act as a bladder irritant. Drinking prior to bedtime can lead to nocturia.

- *Neuromuscular disorders.* Although not well understood, the fact that women with OAB symptoms respond to pelvic floor physical therapy suggests a musculoskeletal etiology. Rarely, neurological diseases such as multiple sclerosis can present with urgency and frequency symptoms.

- *Urinary tract infection.* Recurrent lower urinary tract infections (UTI), bladder infection, and infectious cystitis comprise the most common diagnoses for urgency and frequency symptoms. After menopause, the vaginal pH increases, leading to greater colonization of bacteria that can act as bladder pathogens. Aging and loss of estrogen are thought to be the main factors associated with these changes. Important risk factors for recurrent UTIs are DM and increasing age.

- *Interstitial cystitis (IC).* Also called *painful bladder syndrome* (PBS), this condition, which most commonly presents in women aged 30 to 40 years, is characterized by bladder pain in conjunction with urgency and frequency symptoms. The etiology for this condition is unclear, though many treatments are targeted at what appears to be a deficient bladder mucosa. With IC, bladder capacity is often small (maximum <350 cc) and the bladder walls can become noncompliant. Often, evidence of inflammation or bleeding into the bladder walls can be seen on cystoscopy.

- *Urethral causes.* Urethral diverticulum is a rare cause of urinary symptoms. Isolated urethritis is also uncommon in women; causes of urethritis include infections (particularly STIs) and trauma (such as after catheterization). Also, the urethra shortens with age, decreasing its defense against bacteria. *Urethral syndrome* is a diagnosis given for chronic urethral irritation without a clear etiology and can include symptoms of urinary urgency and frequency.

- *Polyuria.* Causes of excessive urine production include diuretic use, uncontrolled DM, psychogenic polydipsia, and hypercalcemia.

- *Other bladder causes.* Other rare causes to consider include bladder stones, intrinsic bladder tumors, or extrinsic pelvic masses (eg, uterine fibroids, ovarian tumors) that may be causing compression of the bladder.

Evaluation for OAB is similar to the evaluation for urinary incontinence (see Table 24).

Table 24. Standard questions to evaluate for OAB

- How many times do you urinate during the day? (frequency)
- How often do you wake up at night to urinate? (nocturia)
- Do you worry that you can't get to the bathroom in time? (urgency)
- Do you ever have the urge to urinate and lose your urine before you are able to reach the toilet? (urge incontinence)

A urinary diary that details type and amount of fluid intake, number of voids during the day and night, and measures the amount of urine produced in a day can help diagnose urgency and frequency symptoms related to behavior such as excessive fluid and/or caffeine intake. Asking women about bladder pain can help to distinguish OAB from IC. Women with IC can have chronic midline pelvic pain or pain with a full bladder (see Table 25).

Table 25. Physical exam to screen for other causes of urgency and frequency symptoms

- Neurological screening examination focusing on the sacral nerves, including perineal sensation and assessment of anal sphincter tone (to rule out rare neurological causes of incontinence)
- Inspection and palpation of the anterior vaginal wall and urethra (screen for urethral abnormalities such as a diverticulum and urethritis)
- Inspection of the urethra/vulva/vagina for infection, discharge, and pelvic organ prolapse
- A bimanual exam to rule out a pelvic mass
- Assessment of pelvic floor muscles: tenderness, strength, and ability to isolate the levator ani muscles (ability to do a Kegel exercise)

As with incontinence, measuring a postvoid residual within 15 minutes of voiding is recommended, especially with concomitant pelvic organ prolapse or abnormal neurological signs and symptoms, to evaluate for urinary retention. A urinalysis can help identify potential medical causes for the symptom of urinary urgency. For example, the presence of hematuria may suggest bladder pathology (eg, stone or bladder cancer) and should be investigated. A urine culture can identify the presence of infection, which can be a cause of urgency and frequency symptoms or worsen OAB. Other investigations, such as cystoscopy, may be used in some women who do not respond to treatment or who have unusual symptoms or signs.

Management of OAB and recurrent UTIs. Once a woman has been screened for common and serious causes of urinary urgency, frequency, and nocturia symptoms, treatment of OAB can be initiated. Since urge incontinence is considered a symptom of OAB (sometimes referred to "OAB wet"), refer to specific treatments for urge incontinence on page 64. Treatment for OAB without incontinence (sometimes referred to as "OAB dry") has similar treatment recommendations.

Nonpharmacologic strategies for managing OAB without incontinence are found in Table 26.

Table 26. Nonpharmacological strategies for managing OAB without incontinence.

- *Fluid restriction.* For women who consume large volumes of fluid, limiting fluid intake to about 64 oz/day. However, there is a theoretical risk that concentrated urine is irritating to the bladder, so overrestriction should be discouraged.
- *Avoid bladder irritants.* Certain foods and beverages high in caffeine or acid (eg, coffee, cola soft drinks, grapefruit juice, tomatoes) can contribute to OAB by irritating the bladder lining.
- *Pelvic floor physical therapy.* Expert opinion and small case series suggest that myofascial treatments such as massage, stretching, and muscle training (including learning to isolate and contract the levator ani muscles) can improve OAB symptoms.
- *Bladder retraining.* First, women must be able to isolate and contract their pelvic floor muscles, so training in Kegel exercises is required (see page 63). Women are then taught to contract these muscles at the first sensation of urge. Because a Kegel sends negative feedback to the detrusor (bladder) muscle, this technique can suppress the detrusor contraction that causes the sense of urgency. Women who have urinary frequency can also suppress the urge to urinate, thus extending the intervals between voids.
- *Acupuncture.* At least one randomized clinical trial suggests that acupuncture may improve OAB symptoms.
- *Medications.* All of the anticholinergic medications available for urge urinary incontinence can be used for OAB without incontinence in the same dosages and schedule. Whether estrogen by any route is effective in treating OAB is not clear.
- *Sacral neuromodulation stimulation.* For women whose OAB does not respond to other treatments, sacral neuromodulation stimulation (InterStim) may be considered.

For women whose urgency and frequency symptoms are attributable to recurrent UTIs, the goal after initial antibiotic treatment is to help prevent UTIs. Clinicians should first emphasize the importance of nonpharmacologic approaches (see Table 27). Although voiding, hygiene, and dietary measures have not been conclusively proven to

> **Table 27. Nonpharmacological strategies for preventing UTIs**
>
> - Void after intercourse.
> - Wipe from front to back after a bowel movement to prevent spreading bacteria.
> - Do not use perfumed or feminine hygiene products that can irritate the urethra or change the normal vaginal bacterial environment of the vagina.
> - Consuming cranberry extract or pure unsweetened cranberry juice may decrease the rate of UTI recurrences.

prevent UTIs, they involve little risk or cost and may be beneficial to many women.

The use of local vaginal estrogen may also help reduce the risk of recurrent UTI by helping to restore the acidic environment and normal lactobacillus-predominant flora of the vagina, thus discouraging colonization of the vagina by UTI-associated pathogens. Clinically, only estrogen administered by the vaginal route has been shown in a randomized clinical trial to be effective in reducing the risk of recurrent UTI. Oral estrogen has not been found to have the same benefits. (See Section G for more.)

In the postmenopausal woman presenting with recurrent, symptomatic, lower UTI caused by common pathogens such as *E. coli*, therapeutic options include vaginal estrogen or prophylactic antibiotics. Postmenopausal women who present with unusual bacterial pathogens, or whose infection cannot be cleared, may require further evaluation. Asymptomatic bacteriuria, on the other hand, most often requires no treatment.

Fecal incontinence. Approximately 11% of all women report anal incontinence—defined as the loss of anal sphincter control leading to involuntary leakage of gas or solid or liquid stool sufficient enough to impair the individual's quality of life. Up to 17% of midlife women with other pelvic floor dysfunction, such as urinary incontinence, also report fecal incontinence.

Both anatomic defects (incompletely healed anal sphincter tears usually from third- or fourth-degree obstetrical lacerations) and neurologic damage (denervation of the anal sphincter related to childbirth and aging) can lead to anal incontinence. Loss of solid or liquid stool may also arise from intrinsic bowel problems such as inflammatory bowel disease, malabsorption syndromes, colonic polyps, and hemorrhoids.

In midlife women, evaluation of fecal incontinence starts with a diet review and may include colonoscopy, endoanal ultrasonography and evaluation for anal sphincter denervation.

Treatment for fecal incontinence may be as simple as dietary changes (bulking stool with fiber) and pelvic floor physical therapy, or may require anal sphincter repair.

Pelvic pain

Pelvic pain may be acute, recurrent, or chronic. Acute pelvic pain is considered to be a symptom of a disease. Recurrent pelvic pain is the term used to describe cyclic pain (eg, dysmenorrhea) or episodic pain (eg, dyspareunia). Chronic pelvic pain (CPP) is defined as noncyclical pelvic pain that lasts for more than 6 months, with no evidence of an organic cause after thorough evaluation (including laparoscopy), and that is serious enough to cause disability or lead to medical care. CPP is best viewed as a disease in itself.

CPP is most prominent in reproductive-age women (mean age, 30 y), yet peri- and postmenopausal women are not immune. Approximately 15% to 20% of women ages 18 to 50 have CPP of more than a year's duration. Pain can appear in locations such as the pelvis, anterior abdominal wall, lower back, or buttocks. Constant severe pain over an extended time takes a significant toll. At least one study indicates that 25% of women with CPP may spend 2 to 3 days in bed each month. More than half of women with CPP curtail daily activities 1 or more days each month. CPP may lead to years of disability and suffering, as well as requiring a significant amount of medical care and associated costs. CPP has been estimated to account for 10% of the referrals to a gynecologist.

The contributing factors and possible diagnoses in addition to CPP are numerous and varied (see Table 28).

Finding the exact cause(s) of a woman's pelvic pain can be difficult. Often the woman with CPP has been told by her clinician that there is nothing wrong and referred to a mental health specialist, or that there is nothing that can be done and she must live with the pain. Not unexpectedly, such turmoil often results in the woman moving from provider to provider in an attempt to find one she can trust and who can promise relief. To cope, the woman may make emotional and behavioral changes, resulting in *chronic pelvic pain syndrome*.

Women with CPP present, therefore, with a combination of physical symptoms (eg, pain, trouble sleeping, loss of appetite, muscle tension), psychological symptoms (eg, depression), and changes in behavior (eg, changes in relationships due to the physical and psychological problems, such as sexual dysfunction). The diagnosis and treatment of CPP are best approached from a biopsychologic perspective involving multidisciplinary healthcare providers. The high prevalence of a history of sexual and physical abuse in women with CPP highlights the importance of psychological factors as causes of this pain syndrome.

Rather than attempting to distinguish physical from psychological causes of pain, it is more useful to address all physical diseases or abnormalities that require medical or surgical treatment plus all emotional or psychological distress that requires treatment. Typically, women with CPP have more than one problem or diagnosis. For example, bladder irritability, irritable bowel syndrome, poor posture, and emotional stresses may all be contributing factors in a single woman, with the need for simultaneous urologic, gastroenterologic, and psychological treatment, and physical therapy. The challenge in diagnosing CPP is to identify causes that, inadequately treated, may lead to serious short-term sequelae or long-term complications.

Management of pelvic pain is complex and goals of treatment must be realistic. With CPP, research on treatments has been difficult due to the heterogenicity of patients. The American College of Obstetricians and Gynecologists (ACOG) reports that good and consistent scientific evidence supports a number of options:

- Combined estrogen-progestin contraceptives are a treatment option for decreasing primary dysmenorrhea.

- Nonsteroidal anti-inflammatory drugs should be considered for moderate pain, and are particularly effective for menstrual pain.

Table 28. Diseases that may cause or contribute to chronic pelvic pain in women

Gynecologic—extrauterine
Adhesions
Adnexal cysts
Chronic ectopic pregnancy
Chlamydial endometriosis or salpingitis
Endometriosis
Endosalpingiosis
Ovarian retention syndrome
Ovarian remnant syndrome
Ovarian dystrophy
Ovulatory pain
Pelvic congestion syndrome
Postoperative peritoneal cysts
Residual accessory ovary
Subacute salpingooophoritis
Tuberculosis salpingitis

Gynecologic—uterine
Adenomyosis
Atypical dysmenorrhea
Ovulatory pain
Cervical stenosis
Chronic endometritis
Endometrial or cervical polyps
Intrauterine contraceptive device
Leiomyomata
Symptomatic pelvic relaxation

Urologic
Bladder neoplasm
Chronic urinary tract infection
Interstitial cystitis
Radiation cystitis
Recurrent acute cystitis
Recurrent acute urethritis
Stone/urolithiasis
Uninhibited bladder contractions
Urethral diverticulum
Urethral syndrome
Urethral caruncle

Gastrointestinal
Carcinoma of the colon
Chronic intermittent bowel obstruction
Colitis
Constipation
Diverticular disease
Hernias
Inflammatory bowel disease
Irritable bowel syndrome

Musculoskeletal
Abdominal wall myofascial pain
Chronic coccygeal pain
Compression of lumbar vertebrae
Degenerative joint disease
Faulty or poor posture
Fibromyositis
Hernias
Low back pain
Muscular strains and sprains
Neoplasia of spinal cord or sacral nerve
Neuralgia of iliohypogastric, ilioinguinal, and/or genitofemoral nerves
Pelvic floor myalgia (levator ani spasm)
Piriformis syndrome
Rectus tendon strain
Spondylosis

Other
Abdominal cutaneous nerve entrapment in surgical scar
Abdominal epilepsy
Abdominal migraine
Bipolar personality disorders
Depression
Familial Mediterranean fever
Neurologic dysfunction
Porphyria
Shingles
Sleep disturbances
Somatic referral

Source: Adapted from Howard et al. *Pelvic Pain: Diagnosis & Management* 2000.

- GnRH agonists are effective in relieving pelvic pain associated with endometriosis and irritable bowel syndrome.

- Progestins in daily, high doses are effective in treating CPP associated with endometriosis and pelvic congestion syndrome.

- Laparoscopic surgical destruction of endometriosis lesions should be considered to decrease pelvic pain associated with stages I-III endometriosis.

ACOG indicates that the following recommendations are based on more limited or inconsistent evidence:

- Sacral nerve stimulation may decrease pain in up to 60% of women with CPP.

- Injection of local anesthesia into various trigger points of the abdominal wall, vagina, and sacrum may provide temporary of prolonged relief of CPP.

- Nutritional supplements with vitamin B_1 or magnesium may decrease pain of dysmenorrhea.

- Acupuncture, acupressure, and transcutaneous nerve stimulation therapies may help decrease pain of primary dysmenorrhea.

- Magnetic field theory, which involves applying magnets to abdominal trigger points, may improve disability and reduce pain.

- In women who choose hysterectomy for pain associated with reproductive tract symptoms, pain relief is found in 75% to 95% of cases.

Women with CPP can be counseled that CPP is similar to a computer program gone awry. The body is "wired" to feel pain in order to protect itself from harm, but chronic pain no longer serves that purpose. Thus, the strategy for management entails "rewiring" the computer (ie, the central nervous system) so the patient's system no longer interprets normal physiologic functions and structures as pain.

Weight gain

Many women gain weight during the menopause transition. Although neither menopause nor HT is responsible for the added pounds, a recent study found that postmenopausal women are less likely to lose visceral adipose tissue than premenopausal women during a weight reduction program. Consequently, postmenopausal women may find it more difficult to overcome the increased risk of certain serious diseases, such as cardiovascular disease (CVD).

In the United States, more than 70% of women aged 55 to 75 years and 65% of women aged 45 to 55 years are overweight, defined as a BMI greater than 25 kg/m². Approximately 40% of those age groups are obese, defined as a BMI at or above 30 kg/m². More than 40% of Canadian women are estimated to be overweight or obese. The prevalence of obesity among Canadian women increases with age and peaks at ages 55 to 59. The incidence of both overweight and obesity has been increasing.

During the menopause transition, many women gain weight, averaging approximately 5 lb (2.27 kg). This increase is sometimes attributed to menopause or to treatment for menopause-related conditions, including use of menopausal HT. However, the notion that menopause or HT is responsible for weight gain is not supported by scientific evidence.

Weight gain during the menopause transition seems to be related mostly to aging and lifestyle. Several pieces of evidence support this conclusion. Body fat accumulates throughout adult life and, thus, any fat accumulated during perimenopause will add to the existing fat deposits. Also, lean body mass decreases with age, which is compounded by the more sedentary lifestyle of older women. Burning fewer calories through less physical activity also increases fat mass and weight gain.

Sleep deprivation has also been associated with weight gain. The mechanisms are unclear, but women with sleep deprivation may experience daytime fatigue and reduced activity. In addition, studies show that sleep deprivation can cause changes in serum leptin and ghrelin levels, subsequently increasing hunger and appetite. A 2006 study reported an association between reduced sleep and increased weight gain in over 68,000 women followed in the Nurses' Health Study (median follow-up, 12 y). Investigators found that women who slept 5 hours or less gained 2.5 lb (1.14 kg) more than those sleeping 7 hours. Women sleeping 6 hours gained 1.6 lb (0.71 kg) more than those sleeping 7 hours.

Although research suggests that age, rather than menopause, is associated with weight gain, there is some evidence that menopause may be related to changes in body composition and/or fat distribution. Several studies have shown that menopause is associated with increased fat in the abdominal region. Some current research is focusing more on changes in body composition and placement of body fat than on actual weight gain.

In the PEPI trial, women using estrogen with or without progestogen weighed, on average, 2.2 lb (1 kg) less than placebo recipients at the end of the 3-year trial. No weight change difference was noted between the groups using ET alone or estrogen plus progestogen (EPT). However, women using EPT were more likely than placebo recipients to note weight loss and decreased appetite, whereas women who used unopposed ET did not perceive more weight gain than placebo recipients.

Regardless of gender, higher levels of body weight and body fat are associated with increased risk for numerous adverse health consequences, such as CVD, type 2 DM, hypertension, some cancers, osteoarthritis, and premature mortality. Obese postmenopausal women also have a higher rate of breast cancer than nonobese postmenopausal women. One study found that gaining 15 to 20 lb (6.8-9.0 kg) after age 18 increases the risk of myocardial infarction later in life. Conversely, overweight women who lose just 10% of their body weight can reap many health benefits, including a significant lowering of blood pressure.

The *metabolic syndrome* is a combination of medical disorders that increases a patient's risk for CVD and DM. According to the National Cholesterol Education Program Adult Treatment Panel (ATP III), the definition includes the presence of any three of the following five traits:

- central obesity (waist circumference ≥35 in [85 cm])
- elevated triglycerides (≥150 mg/dL; 1.70 mmol/L) or drug treatment for elevated triglycerides
- reduced high-density lipoprotein cholesterol (HDL-C) (<50 mg/dL in women; 0.90 mmol/L) or drug treatment for low HDL-C
- elevated blood pressure (≥130/85 mm Hg) or use of antihypertensive medication
- elevated fasting glucose levels (≥100 mg/dL; 5.6 mmol/L) or use of medication for hyperglycemia.

Diagnosing women with this syndrome is crucial as it helps identify those who need aggressive lifestyle modification, focusing on weight reduction and increased physical activity, and medication if necessary.

Evidence from community-based, cross-sectional studies indicates that a high BMI predisposes women to more frequent or severe hot flashes. However, whether losing excess weight reduces hot flash risk has not been studied.

Moderating factors—including age, sex, family history, body fat distribution, diet, and physical activity—can affect an individual's risk of becoming overweight.

Being underweight can also be unhealthy. Very thin women are at increased risk for osteoporosis. Premenopausal women who overdiet or overexercise can become so underweight that their menstrual cycles stop temporarily, placing them at higher risk for osteoporosis later in life.

Management of weight gain. Efforts to manage weight in peri- and postmenopausal women are essential. The advice to eat a healthy diet, increase physical activity, and avoid further weight gain is appropriate for almost all women at or above a healthy weight. For those who are overweight or obese, weight loss is indicated. Underweight individuals also need counseling to maintain a healthy body weight.

Physical activity can help balance caloric intake with energy expenditure. Both physical activity and controlled caloric intake are necessary to achieve or maintain a healthy body weight. In the Women's Healthy Lifestyle Project, women prevented weight gain (and minimized low-density lipoprotein cholesterol [LDL-C] elevations) during the menopause transition by increasing physical activity and consuming a low-fat diet with moderate caloric restrictions.

No single diet or eating regimen is right for all women. Women seeking to shed weight should be encouraged to set realistic goals achieved through long-term lifestyle change. Emphasis should be placed on changing eating habits rather than relying on diets, especially faddish diets. Support can be obtained from family members, coworkers, and friends. Various organization and support groups (eg, Weight Watchers, Overeaters Anonymous) offer help with dieting, although no single program has been proven superior. A 2007 randomized trial compared adherence rates and effectiveness of four popular diets: Atkins (carbohydrate restriction), Zone (macronutrient balance), Weight Watchers (calorie restriction), and Ornish (fat restriction). Results showed that all four diets modestly decreased body weight and significantly decreased the LDL/HDL ratio, although overall adherence rates were low. Discontinuation rates were slightly higher in the more extreme diet groups (Atkins and Ornish), although this was not statistically significant. All four diets showed greater weight loss and reductions in cardiac risk factors in patients with increased adherence.

The WHI Dietary Modification Trial examined the long-term benefits and risks of a low-fat diet as well as increasing vegetable, fruit, and grain intake. The intervention group included group and individual sessions to promote decreased fat intake and increased vegetable, fruit, and grain consumption without weight loss or calorie restriction goals. In comparison, the control group received diet-related educational materials. Results showed that women in the intervention group lost weight in the first year and maintained a lower weight than the control-group women during an average 7.5-year follow-up period. These findings refuted claims that low-fat eating results in weight gain in postmenopausal women.

The benefits of eating at regular intervals (every 4-5 hr) and engaging in a regular exercise program—perhaps the most important element—must be emphasized. Regular exercise appears to have the most beneficial effect on minimizing weight gain in midlife women at menopause. Although both aerobic and resistance exercises will consume calories and eventually decrease weight, evidence suggests that peri- and postmenopausal women striving for a lower body fat ratio will benefit more from resistance-type exercise. This type of exercise builds more lean body muscle tissue and creates a more slender phenotype. Since lean muscle mass is more metabolically active, muscle building allows women to lose weight without excessively decreasing food consumption.

Recommendations from the US Preventive Services Task Force are to offer intensive counseling to obese adults to promote weight loss or refer them for counseling. Intensive counseling includes at least two individual or group counseling sessions on diet and exercise monthly for at least 3 months. The level of intervention required depends on the woman's BMI and the presence of comorbidities (see Table 29). The benefits and risks of obesity treatment must be assessed on an individual basis, as recommended in the National Heart, Lung, and Blood Institute's obesity education initiative.

Table 29. Intervention by BMI category	
BMI (in kg/m²)	Intervention
<18.5	Lifestyle changes*
18.5-24.9	No treatment needed
25-26.9	Lifestyle changes, if comorbidities are present**
27-29.9	Lifestyle changes plus drug therapy, if comorbidities are present
30-34.9	Lifestyle changes plus drug therapy
35-39.9	Lifestyle changes plus drug therapy; surgery needed if comorbidities are present
>40	Lifestyle changes, drug therapy, and surgery indicated

*Lifestyle changes are diet, exercise, and behavior therapy.
**Comorbidities include hypertension, DM, hyperlipidemia.

Source: National Heart, Lung, and Blood Institute 1998.

For overweight women, the initial goal should be to reduce body weight by approximately 10% over 6 to 12 months. This can be accomplished through a management program that includes a controlled diet with a deficit of 500 to 1,000 calories per day, reducing dietary fat intake to less than 30% of total energy intake, and participating in regular physical activity.

Nonpharmacological inteventions. Various herbal remedies and nutritional supplements are advertised to promote weight loss by boosting the metabolic rate; however, controlled clinical studies have not been conducted. Chromium picolinate is touted to help burn fat and build muscle. Studies are conflicting regarding chromium's effect on weight, although at least one study found that, when combined with a diet and exercise program, chromium produced favorable changes in body composition (more lean tissue and less fat). However, toxic effects are not well known. Remedies containing ephedra should be avoided. This plant contains the stimulant ephedrine, which can cause adverse effects on the central nervous system, heart rate, and blood pressure.

For more about counseling for weight management and nutrition, see Section J, page 286.

Pharmacological interventions. Pharmacologic therapy can be offered to obese patients who have failed to achieve their weight loss goals through an adequate trial of diet, exercise, and lifestyle changes. The amount of weight loss that can be attributed to medications is modest (approximately 5 kg in 1 y), but this may be enough to halt progression of some comorbid conditions. For example, medication may prevent or slow the progression of impaired glucose tolerance to type 2 DM, improving lipid profiles, and decreasing blood pressure levels.

Prescription drug therapies often used for the treatment of obesity include phentermine HCl (generics), diethylpropion (Tenuate), sibutramine (Meridia), and orlistat (Xenical). Half-strength orlistat (Alli) has been approved by the FDA for sale without a prescription, to be used in combination with a reduced-calorie, low-fat diet.

Phentermine and diethylpropion are sympathomimetic drugs that work as appetite suppressants. Due to the abuse potential associated with these medications, they are only approved for short-term use (widely interpreted as 12 wk).

Sibutramine is a norepinephrine, serotonin, and dopamine reuptake inhibitor, which works by inhibiting food intake. As a sympathomimetic drug, it can increase blood pressure and heart rate, and should be avoided in patients with heart disease and stroke. The recommended starting dose is 10 mg/day and can be titrated up to a maximum of 15 mg/day based on response.

Orlistat works by inhibiting pancreatic lipases, preventing absorption of dietary fat (30% with 120 mg Xenical and 25% with 60 mg Alli). A 16-wk controlled trial of 60 mg orlistat TID with meals in overweight (not obese) patients (avg BMI 26.8 kg/m²) on a reduced-calorie, low-fat diet found that patients taking the drug lost 2.5 lb (1.15 kg) more than those taking placebo. Orlistat causes flatulence with oily spotting, loose stools, and fecal urgency in 2%-40% of patients on a low-fat diet. Side effects would presumably increase with higher doses or higher fat intake. Fat-soluble vitamins and beta-carotene absorption are often decreased and supplementation may be necessary. The drug possibly interferes with the absorption of other drugs, and may increase the anticoagulant effect of warfarin.

Two prescription drugs used off label for obesity treatment include fluoxetine (Prozac) and bupropion (Wellbutrin). Fluoxetine and bupropion are approved for the treatment of depression, but may also facilitate weight loss. Bupropion is also approved to prevent weight gain during smoking cessation.

Surgery. Surgery should be considered for patients with a BMI greater than or equal to 40 kg/m² who have failed an adequate trial of diet, exercise, and lifestyle modification, and who suffer from comorbid conditions, such as hypertension, impaired glucose tolerance, DM, hyperlipidemia, and/or obstructive sleep apnea. The goal of surgery is to reduce the morbidity and mortality associated with obesity. The National Institutes of Health also suggest that adults with a BMI greater than 35 kg/m² with serious comorbidities, such as severe DM, sleep apnea, or joint disease, may also be candidates.

Bariatric surgery refers to surgical procedures used to promote weight loss, and can be divided into three groups: restrictive, malabsorptive, or mixed procedures. Restrictive procedures reduce the size of the stomach thereby limiting the amount of food that can be consumed. This includes vertical banded gastroplasty ("stomach stapling"), laparoscopic gastric banding, or sleeve gastrectomy. These restrictive procedures promote more gradual weight loss than the malabsorptive procedures; however, they are often simpler to perform. Malabsorptive surgery, such as the biliopancreatic diversion with or without duodenal switch, decreases the effective length of the small intestine, reducing absorption and inducing weight loss. These malabsorptive procedures can result in profound weight loss; however, significant metabolic complications such as protein calorie malnutrition and various micronutrient deficiencies can occur. Mixed procedures combine both restrictive and malabsorptive components, and include gastric bypass. Literature has shown that patients experience better surgical outcomes when referred to high-volume centers with experienced surgeons.

Two meta-analyses have summarized data on the effectiveness of bariatric surgery. One group in 2004 reviewed 136 studies in which patients underwent a variety of bariatric procedures. The mean overall percentage of excess weight loss was 61% and varied among procedure performed, with the most weight loss occurring after malabsorptive surgery (70.1%) and the least weight loss following gastric banding (47.5%). The 30-day mortality was 0.1% for restrictive procedures, 1.1% for malabsorptive procedures, and 0.5% for mixed procedures. Comorbidity resolution and improvement rates were excellent in these surgical patients. A 2005 meta-analysis included 147 studies and found the largest benefit of bariatric surgery in patients with a BMI greater than 40 kg/m², while benefits in patients with BMIs of 35 to 39 kg/m² were less clear. Greater weight loss was observed with gastric bypass as opposed to gastroplasty. Adverse events occurred in approximately 20% of patients and overall mortality was less than 1%. However, very long-term outcomes of bariatric surgery have not yet been evaluated as the procedures are usually performed on younger patients. This treatment has not yet been proven to decrease mortality.

Cardiovascular effects

Cardiovascular disease (CVD), including coronary heart disease (CHD) and stroke, remain the leading cause of death and disability in US and Canadian women. Among US women, the mortality rate from CVD is greater than the next 14 causes of death combined. Since 1984, CVD has caused more deaths in women than in men.

The median age of mortality from CVD in women is 74 years. The age-adjusted mortality rate for CVD per 100,000 women is 140 in white women and 160 in black women.

After age 50, more than one half of all deaths in women are caused by some form of CVD. Many more women die from heart disease than from breast cancer, although before age 65, more lives are lost to breast cancer. In part because women suffer myocardial infarctions (MIs; occlusion of coronary arteries) at older ages than men, women are more likely to die from an MI within a few weeks. About 38% of women will die within 1 year after having a recognized MI. Within 6 years of an MI, 35% of women will have another MI, 6% of women will experience sudden death, and 46% of women will be disabled with heart failure.

Mortality numbers provide only part of the picture. For example, nearly 25% of Canadian adults older than age 70 (and nearly 6% of all adults) have CVD and they report feeling less healthy than the rest of the Canadian population; many need help with activities of daily living.

Cardiovascular disease is an inclusive term used to describe many conditions:

- Hypertension
- Atherosclerosis (plaque deposits in blood vessels that reduce vascular flow)
- CHD (also called coronary artery disease), which can cause an MI or angina pectoris. In 2004, CHD was the single leading cause of death in the United States, causing over 450,000 deaths.
- Strokes (arterial occlusion in the brain) were responsible for the second greatest percentage; in 2004, strokes caused 1 out of every 16 deaths in the United States.
- Arrhythmias (abnormal rhythm of heart beats)
- Valvular heart disease including rheumatic fever and rheumatic heart disease
- Congenital cardiovascular defects
- Congestive heart failure

Proper function of the myocardium depends on a positive balance of oxygen and nutrient supply and demand. Angina is most often associated with the narrowing of coronary arteries, caused by the formation of atherosclerotic plaques in the proximal coronary arteries. Chronic narrowing of the lumen of the coronary artery is the result of a continuous process of plaque formation, disruption, reorganization, and reformation that begins early in life, and it may lead to stable angina. Genetic, metabolic, behavioral, and environmental factors can all contribute to the process. An MI usually occurs when a previously narrowed artery suddenly becomes completely occluded with a thromboembolism.

Diseased blood vessels outside the heart can lead to conditions such as stroke and hypertension. In addition, poor circulation can lead to peripheral vascular disease resulting in difficulty walking and, if severe, amputation of the affected limb.

For a detailed discussion of CVD, see Section E, page 129.

Palpitations. Medical literature has suggested that decreased estrogen levels slow the rate of ventricular repolarization, possibly rendering peri- and postmenopausal women more susceptible to cardiac arrhythmias. Measures of atrioventricular conduction time and cardiac repolarization time after hysterectomy and bilateral oophorectomy are not modified by HT.

During vasomotor episodes, heart rate increases of 7 to 15 beats per minute can occur, and some women may interpret the perceived increase as palpitation. Palpitations also are a common symptom in anxiety disorders including generalized anxiety, phobias, panic disorder, and agitated depression.

Management of palpitations. Although it is unlikely that palpitations in peri- and postmenopausal women are related to serious cardiac abnormalities, caution should be exercised. A stress test should be conducted if symptoms are accompanied by exercise intolerance, shortness of breath, or chest pain. Women with a high personal risk of coronary disease or with a strong family history of early cardiac death (ie, males who have died under age 50 or females who have died under the age of 60) should also be assessed.

Menopause and risk of CVD and CHD. CVD is less common in premenopausal women. After menopause, however, a woman's risk increases (especially after age 65), leading some to suggest that estrogen provides cardioprotective benefits. The extent to which diminished estrogen levels increase CVD risk in women has not been established.

There does seem to be a relationship between premature menopause and increased incidence of CVD morbidity and mortality. Menopause before age 35 has been associated with a two- to threefold increased risk of MI. The Nurses' Health Study (NHS) found an overall significant association between younger age at menopause and higher risk of CVD among women who experienced natural menopause and never used HT. An increased risk was observed only among current smokers, not among participants who never smoked. New data suggest that risk for CVD may be the determinant of menopausal age rather than the presumed reverse scenario. A 2006 report from the American College of Cardiology showed that for each 1% increase in premenopausal Framingham Risk score, there was a decrease in menopausal age of 1.8 years. This association may explain some of the conflicting data regarding the relationships CVD rates, menopausal age, and the effects of HT.

When examining the possible reasons for the increase in CVD in postmenopausal women, the most prevalent finding is that cholesterol levels change after menopause. LDL-C and very low LDL-C increase, and there is enhanced oxidation of LDL. In a cross-sectional analysis of 9,309

women who had never used HT, the increases in total cholesterol, LDL-C, and triglycerides from premenopause to postmenopause were 4.4%, 4.0%, and 3.2%, respectively, after adjusting for covariates such as smoking and age. Ongoing prospective studies are expected to provide more definitive results. Levels of HDL-C may decrease over time, but these changes are relatively insignificant compared with LDL-C increases.

The Women's Healthy Lifestyle Project, however, found that the menopause-related rise in LDL-C can be reduced through a lifestyle intervention program that focuses on two factors: decreasing saturated fat and cholesterol intake, and preventing excess weight gain through increased physical exercise and reduced caloric and fat intake.

The direct vascular effects of menopause-related hormone changes are considered important. Estrogen and progesterone receptors have been found in vascular tissues, including coronary arteries. Coagulation balance may also play a role in the hormone/vascular interaction and menopause changes. Certain fibrinolytic factors (eg, antithrombin III and plasminogen) increase along with some procoagulation factors (eg, factor VII and fibrinogen). After menopause, blood flow in all vascular beds decreases, prostacyclin decreases, endothelin levels increase, and vasoconstriction occurs in response to acetylcholine challenges. Circulating plasma levels of nitric oxide increase and levels of angiotensin-converting enzyme decrease.

Postmenopausal women who are healthy and not obese experience a decrease in carbohydrate tolerance as insulin resistance increases. Stress reactivity is exaggerated in postmenopausal women compared with younger women. However, the role of diminished estrogen in these results has not been determined.

See Section E, page 129, for information about management of CVD.

Skeletal system effects

Osteoporosis is a very common condition in aging populations. It is characterized by a reduction in bone mass and bone strength and results in an increased risk of fracture from a relatively minor trauma. Most cases of fracture occur more frequently in the elderly, but the pathogenesis of the disease begins earlier. Although bone loss starts in the fourth decade at the hip, loss from the spine is more closely related to estrogen deficiency and starts about 2 years before the last menses.

Pathophysiology. In normal bone remodeling, bone resorption is coupled tightly to bone formation. Bone loss occurs when there is an uncoupling of the process. On average, a bone remodeling cycle lasts 6 to 9 months. The primary function of bone remodeling is to repair microfractures in bones and replace old bone with new bone. At the cellular level, osteoclasts promote bone resorption by stimulating the production of enzymes that dissolve bone mineral and proteins. Osteoblasts promote bone formation by creating a protein matrix consisting primarily of collagen, which is soon calcified, resulting in remineralization of bone.

As women approach menopause, the remodeling process becomes uncoupled. The level of bone resorption increases much more than the level of bone formation and remains so for about 5 years; although resorption decreases with age, it still remains higher than formation.

Role of menopause. The increased rate of bone resorption immediately after menopause clearly indicates a hormonal influence on bone mineral density (BMD) in women. The most likely explanation for this increased resorption is the drop in ovarian estrogen production that accompanies menopause.

BMD loss begins to accelerate approximately 2 to 3 years before the last menses and this acceleration ends 3 to 4 years after menopause. For an interval of a few years around menopause, women lose 2% of bone annually. Afterward, bone loss slows to about 1% to 1.5% per year. A prospective, longitudinal study of white women reported BMD losses during this 5- to 7-year interval of 10.5% for the spine, 5.3% for the femoral neck, and 7.7% for the total body. Although some of the decline can be attributed to age-related factors, lower estrogen levels were implicated as the cause for approximately two thirds of the bone loss. Lower estrogen levels have also been significantly associated with increased fracture risk in older women (mean age, 75 y).

Women experiencing menopause at or before age 40—either naturally or induced (eg, through bilateral oophorectomy, chemotherapy, or pelvic radiation therapy)—are at greater risk of low BMD and fracture than other women of the same age who have not reached menopause. However, by age 70, when fractures are more likely to occur, women with early menopause have the same risk for fracture as women who reached menopause at the average age.

At a cellular level, the decline in circulating levels of 17β-estradiol is the predominant factor that leads to increased bone resorption, although evidence suggests that follicle-stimulating hormone may also play a role. Estrogen deficiency results in increases in the activity of the marrow and stromal cells of the marrow which secrete cytokines, particularly interleukins (IL-1, IL-6), tumor necrosis factor (TNF-α), and macrophage colony-stimulating factor (M-CSF). These cytokines lead to an increase in the activity of the "final" active cytokine, RANK ligand (RANKL), which promotes osteoclast activity by increasing both activity and numbers of osteoclasts that cause bone resorption. The loss of estrogen also reduces the secretion of osteoprotegerin, which is a natural antagonist of RANKL. Estrogen administration reduces bone resorption by increasing osteoprotegerin and reducing RANKL activity.

Clinically, the decrease in bone mass can be measured by dual energy x-ray absorptiometry (DXA). As BMD decreases, every standard deviation of reduction in BMD results in a twofold or greater risk of fracture compared with other women of the same age. However, increased fracture risk depends on many factors, including age (>65 y) and changes in bone quality and bone strength which are affected by risk factors (see Section E, page 113, for more about osteoporosis risk and Section H, page 244, for more about calcium).

Deciding when to initiate preventive treatment for low bone mass (osteopenia) is a controversial issue. Based on the National Osteoporosis Risk Assessment study (NORA), fractures become more prevalent when the T-score of a peripheral BMD value is about –2.0. The decision when to treat will become easier when BMD and risk factor analysis are combined together in the DXA software (see Section F, page 189, for more about screening).

Fractures. Within 10 years of menopause, the only significant fracture of consequence is the radial/ulna fracture (Colles fracture). There is a marked postmenopausal rise while, in contrast, most vertebral fractures start to occur 15 to 20 years past menopause and prevalence at age 80 is about 25% to 30%. Hip fractures start to occur 25 to 30 years past menopause and the prevalence at age 85 is about 35%. Clinically, two thirds of osteoporotic fractures occur after age 75. The Colles fracture may be the first sign of osteoporosis because many patients in later life are found to have a combination of Colles, vertebral, and hip fractures. All patients with a Colles fracture, regardless of age, should have the benefit of a DXA scan to look for significant osteopenia or osteoporosis in the spine or hip.

Prevention and treatment of osteopenia and osteoporosis also are important factors in maintaining postmenopausal dental health (see below for more about dental changes).

Dental and oral cavity changes

After menopause, tooth loss (and thus the need for dentures) has been associated with osteoporosis through a sequence that begins with atrophy of bony tooth sockets, leading to gum retraction and exposure of nonenameled tooth surfaces, periodontal pocket development, bacterial invasion, and clinical periodontitis.

The rate of systemic bone loss in postmenopausal women is a predictor of tooth loss. For each 1% per year decrease in whole-body BMD, the risk for tooth loss more than quadruples. A study of women with severe osteoporosis found them to be three times more likely than healthy, age-matched controls to have no teeth. In HT users, longitudinal studies have found higher tooth counts, reduced risk of tooth loss, and reduced alveolar bone loss from periodontal disease progression, thereby implying a relationship to menopause.

A number of studies also suggest a relationship between low BMD and periodontal disease. Most studies that enrolled osteoporotic and/or osteopenic women show a higher frequency of alveolar bone height and crestal/subcrestal loss than in normal controls.

Prevention and treatment of osteoporosis are important factors in maintaining postmenopausal dental health. Patients who are using long-term oral bisphosphonate therapy should be cautioned about reported cases of altered bone healing and bone necrosis (see Section E, page 124, for more about osteonecrosis risk with bisphosphonates), and should have frequent periodontal/dental maintenance and meticulous home care.

Fluctuations of sex hormones during menopause have been implicated in inflammatory changes in gingiva. Estrogen affects cellular proliferation, differentiation, and keratinization of the gingival epithelium. Thinning of the oral epithelium is reflected in increased gingival recession, enhanced susceptibility to tissue injury, and sensitivity (eg, burning mouth and tongue, root sensitivity, generalized increased tissue sensitivity). Hormone receptors have been identified in basal and spinous layers of the epithelium and connective tissue, implicating gingival and other oral tissues as targets manifesting hormone deficiencies.

A burning sensation in the mouth can be a symptom of another disease (such as anemia or type 2 DM) or a syndrome in its own right. It has been suggested that, when no underlying dental or medical causes are identified and no oral signs are found, the term *burning mouth syndrome* (BMS) should be used. The prominent feature is burning pain that is usually localized to the tongue and/or lips but can involve the entire oral cavity. A Cochrane Review reports that prevalence rates in general populations vary from 0.7% to 15%. Many of these patients show evidence of anxiety, depression, and personality disorders, which has led to treating BMS as an emotional problem. However, research shows that BMS may be the result of nerve damage. When nerves that carry taste signals are damaged, especially in people with sensitive taste buds, the brain seems to magnify mouth pain. Although a small percentage of women reaching menopause report BMS, it has not been associated with menopause.

Management of dental changes. Clinicians are urged to stress the importance of regular dental visits and encourage their women patients to floss and brush with fluoride-containing toothpaste daily.

Skin changes

The skin is composed of three layers: the epidermis, dermis, and subcutis. The top layer is the epidermis. The stratum corneum, the outermost part of the epidermis, consists of dead keratinocytes (squamous cells) that are continually shed. Below the stratum corneum are layers of living keratinocytes that produce keratin, sulfur-containing fibrous proteins that form the chemical basis of horny epidermal tissues such as hair and nails. At the lowest part of the epidermis are basal cells that continually divide to produce new keratinocytes. Also present in the epidermis are melanocytes, cells that produce melanin, the protective brown pigment that makes skin tan or brown. Melanin is formed to protect the deeper layers of the skin from the harmful effects of the sun.

The dermis forms the main bulk of the skin. The fibers present in the dermis consist primarily of two types of fibrous protein: collagen (97.5%) and elastin (2.5%). Collagen fibers are responsible for the main mass and the resilience of the dermis.

Skin ages relatively well. It is only with exposure to extrinsic factors, primarily sunlight, that a more marked aging of the skin occurs. In sun-damaged locations in the dermis, elastin becomes fragmented as a direct consequence of ultraviolet light absorption. Dark clumps can be seen in stained specimens of elastin, giving it an appearance that clearly differs from that of fine elastin fibers seen in young skin. Skin changes are also influenced by subcutaneous fat, which is diminished or redistributed with age. This change adds to increases in skin laxity. Weight fluctuations can also increase laxity because as skin elasticity is reduced with aging, the skin does not retract after loss of body fat, leaving excess skin. Loss of underlying muscle mass contributes to sagging skin because muscle acts as a skin-filler, especially on the face.

Role of hormones. Hormones play an important role in skin physiology. The androgen hormones modulate sebum (oil) production. Acne can result from androgen-induced excessive sebum production. The effects of androgens on acne are more evident in adult women than in adolescents. Clinically, the adult variety of acne occurs mostly on the lower face, particularly along the chin, jaw line, and neck. Lesions are predominantly papulonodular and are often tender. Levels of circulating androgens, although typically in the normal range, are significantly higher in women with acne than in women without acne.

Estrogen has a number of functions in the skin, where estrogen receptors are present in significant numbers. Cross-sectional data have shown a highly significant correlation between the declines in skin collagen and skin thickness and the years since menopause. The decline in skin collagen after menopause occurs at a much more rapid rate in the early postmenopausal years. Some 30% of skin collagen is lost during the first 5 years after menopause, followed by an average decline of 2% per postmenopausal year over 20 years. These statistics are similar to those for bone loss after menopause. Increases in skin laxity and wrinkling, as well as decreases in skin elasticity, also are seen after menopause. No significant correlation has been found between skin thickness and skin collagen content and a woman's actual chronologic age, which adds to the evidence suggesting that years since menopause is a more important factor than age in affecting skin parameters.

Photoaging. Exposure to the sun induces clinical and histological changes to the skin, commonly called photoaging. Clinically, photoaging can be manifested as wrinkles, skin roughness and dryness, irregular pigmentation, sallowness, and solar lentigines (brown spots). Benign conditions of vascular proliferation, including linear telangiectasia, cherry angiomas, and spider angiomas, often occur with aging and cutaneous photodamage. Other common age-related skin changes include seborrheic keratoses (tan, brown, or black raised spots with a waxy texture or rough surface); actinic keratoses (premalignant, sun-induced growths that are sometimes burning and tender); and "frown lines," which result from changes due to muscle hypertonicity.

Risk factors of photoaging and skin cancer include fair skin, difficulty tanning, ease of sunburning, sunburns before the age of 20, and advancing age. Smoking is an independent risk factor for wrinkling, telagiectasia, and squamous-cell cancer. Women with substantial photoaging should be examined periodically for actinic keratoses and skin cancers.

Most changes that occur as a result of photoaging have similar causes and risk factors, but the extent and consequences of these changes vary among women. The decision about whether to recommend treatment depends on the nature of the changes, their severity, the degree to which they bother the woman, and the patient's willingness to accept the risks and costs of treatment, which most insurance plans do not cover.

Although skin collagen content and skin thickness decline significantly with age, it is only with exposure to extrinsic factors, such as sunlight and tobacco smoke, that aging of the skin occurs in a more marked fashion. While this problem is often medically insignificant, it is of profound cosmetic concern and will detract from the quality of life for many women at midlife and beyond.

Management of photoaging. At any age, protection from the sun reduces the risk of actinic keratoses and squamous-cell cancer and the progression of photoaging. (Reducing the risk of basal-cell cancer depends primarily on reducing sun exposure during childhood.)

- *Sunscreen.* Ample use of a moisturizing sunscreen will have the greatest impact in protecting and improving the appearance of aging skin. Data support the importance of preventing both ultraviolet A (UVA) and B (UVB) radiation. For optimal skin protection, women should use a sunscreen throughout the year. Tanning should be discouraged.

UVB radiation (wavelengths from 290 to 320 nm) is much more important for the induction of nonmelanoma skin cancer and actinic keratoses than ultraviolet UVA radiation (320 to 400 nm). Both UVA and UVB radiation contribute to changes in pigment and wrinkles. Controlled studies have assessed the daily use (for up to 4.5 years) of broad-spectrum sunscreens with a sun protection factor (SPF) of 15 or higher. The incidence of actinic keratoses was reduced by about 40% versus no sunscreen use, and about 24% as compared with irregular use of sunscreen. The incidence of squamous-cell cancer was reduced by 25%, but the risk of basal-cell cancer was not reduced.

About 17% of individuals using a sunscreen with an SPF of 15 or higher over a 7-month period had irritation reactions, a major barrier to compliance.

Sunscreens that provide protection against UVB radiation may encourage increased exposure to the sun and to UVA radiation. However, sunscreen use has not been found to increase the risk of melanoma.

Sunscreens that provide protection against UVB radiation decrease the synthesis of vitamin D. Women using sunscreen coverage should take a vitamin D supplement to obtain the recommended amount. (See Section H, page 240, for more about vitamin D.)

- *Other treatments.* Antioxidants, alphahydroxy acids, and topical retinoids (vitamin A derivatives) have been used to repair photoaged skin. Only topical retinoids have demonstrated a well-documented ability to repair skin at the clinical, histologic, and molecular level. Two topical retinoid products (tretinoin [Retin-A] and tazarotene [Avage, Tazorac, Zorac]) have been FDA approved for the palliation of fine wrinkles and irregular pigmentation of photoaging. No good evidence supports the efficacy of other vitamin A derivatives often found in OTC preparations, including retinol and retinaldehyde.

Many products and procedures are advocated for facial rejuvenation. For example, injections of collagen or botulinum toxin type A (Botox) are popular wrinkle treatments. Long-term data on efficacy and safety for these products and procedures are not available.

- *Hormone therapy.* Clinical trial evidence indicates that systemic ET and combined EPT have some beneficial effects on skin. Systemic ET/EPT (HT) has been shown to limit skin-collagen loss, maintain skin thickness, improve skin elasticity and firmness, increase skin moisture, and decrease wrinkle depth and pore size. Systemic HT also appears to limit skin extensibility during perimenopause, exerting a preventive effect on skin slackness, although no effect on skin viscoelasticity has been noted. Although the data are not convincing enough to initiate HT for skin benefits alone, the potential facial skin benefits may appeal to some women. HT is not FDA approved for any skin benefit.

HT neither alters the effects of genetic aging or sun damage, nor does it affect the risk of skin cancer. Some women taking high doses of estrogen may experience increased pigmentation (melasma or cloasma) that may not be reversible.

Dry skin. Xerosis (dry skin), the most common condition of aging skin, is a consequence of the skin's reduced oil production. Xerosis is usually more pronounced on the back and the ankles, and can cause significant itching and discomfort. It tends to be more marked in dry climates and during winter months.

Xerosis is best prevented by avoiding hot, soapy showers and baths, which overdry the skin. Women should be advised to use a bath oil or heavy lotion on wet skin immediately after showering or bathing. Products that have an oily feel, such as petroleum jelly and baby oil, are most effective, since common hand lotions often contain alcohol and little oil. Skin will become more resistant to physical and chemical insults if it is kept lubricated.

Management of dry skin. It is important to keep skin hydrated by drinking adequate amounts of water. Most women consume far too little water. (Liquids like coffee, tea, and caffeinated soft drinks may quench thirst, but their diuretic action decreases hydration.) Avoidance of excessive alcohol consumption will also contribute to skin health. Other skin-healthy habits include getting adequate exercise and sleep, and avoiding stress and smoking. Because underlying muscle mass acts as a skin filler to reduce sagging, especially on the face, there is merit to exercising the facial muscles for bulk.

Acne. Some women will develop acne around menopause, usually due to an increase in the ratio of androgen to estrogen. Circulating androgens are typically in the normal range, but levels have been shown to be significantly higher in women with acne than in women without acne. Women who had acne during their teen years will almost always have acne in midlife. The effects of androgens on acne are most evident in adult women.

Management of acne. The net effect of systemic hormonal treatment for acne is a reduction of sebum production from the sebaceous gland. Neither topical acne preparations nor oral antibiotics influence sebum production. The first FDA-approved estrogen-containing contraceptive for the treatment of acne was norgestimate plus ethinyl estradiol (Ortho Tri-Cyclen). Efficacy has been demonstrated in two multicenter, double-blind, placebo-controlled trials. At least two other estrogen-progestin contraceptives—norethindrone acetate and ethinyl estradiol (Estrostep) and drospirenone and ethinyl estradiol (Yaz)—have also been approved for acne treatment. These brands are not available in Canada.

DIANE-35 (cyproterone acetate and ethinyl estradiol) is approved in Canada for the treatment of severe acne in women who have associated symptoms of androgenization, including seborrhea and mild hirsutism. It also provides reliable contraception.

Formication. Women presenting with formication (tactile sensation of insects crawling on the skin) may respond to treatment with HT and/or with psychopharmacologic therapies. However, no clinical studies have addressed this problem, and no therapy has been identified as effective.

When to refer. A referral to a dermatologist is recommended for treating any skin condition with which the menopause practitioner is inexperienced. Effective procedures to treat benign conditions are available from the dermatologist, including those utilizing lasers, cryosurgery, electrosurgery, and microdermabrasion. Any serious skin disease, including suspicion of precancerous lesions and skin carcinoma, should be referred to a dermatologist.

Hair changes

Some women experience thinning of hair on the scalp (androgenic alopecia) and/or unwanted growth of hair on the face (hirsutism) in midlife and associate these hair changes with menopause. The actual causes of both scalp hair thinning and growth of unwanted hair in women are unknown, but both appear to be caused by multiple factors, including genetic predisposition, local androgen metabolism, growth factors (especially cytokines), hormones, and stress. It has been postulated that the increase in the ratio of androgen to estrogen during the midlife transition may influence hair changes in some women. This is evidenced by the reduction in hair density that can be attained with antiandrogen treatments. The cause of the variable physiologic responses of hair follicles in different sites from the identical hormonal signal remains unknown. Hair growth aberrations can have significant psychological consequences that affect body image, self-esteem, and quality-of-life issues, underscoring the importance of effective medical management.

Androgenic alopecia. Androgenic alopecia and hair thinning are typically genetically determined and respond to the shift in the androgen-to-estrogen ratio. Hair follicles in balding skin differ from those in nonbalding skin with respect to androgen metabolism.

Thinning of the hair usually begins between the ages of 12 and 40 years in both sexes. Approximately 50% of women express this trait to some degree before age 50. Alopecia occurs as often in women as in men. Frequently, alopecia is first observed as an increased shedding of scalp hair, which can be acute or chronic. In rare cases, it can result in balding.

Most women with androgenic alopecia have normal menses, pregnancies, and endocrine function, including normal serum androgen levels. Hormonal evaluation is indicated if hair loss is sudden or if other symptoms of androgen excess are present, such as irregular menses (in reproductive years), a history of infertility, hirsutism, severe cystic acne, virilization, or galactorrhea.

After menopause, hyperandrogenic symptoms may worsen. Surgical menopause may result in an improvement of symptoms, since a significant amount of endogenous androgen is decreased.

Hair loss may also be associated with excessive dieting, iron deficiency, hypothyroid dysfunction, lupus, sudden hormonal shift (eg, bilateral oophorectomy), scalp wounds, burns or infections, intense prolonged stress, and, possibly, vitamin B_{12} deficiency.

Some medications, such as cancer chemotherapy agents, cause hair thinning or loss. Thinning can occasionally be associated with antihyperlipidemic agents, beta-blockers, or systemic retinoids. Although rare, use of testosterone preparations, dehydroepiandrosterone, and possibly oral contraception with high androgenicity can be a factor in androgenic alopecia in women.

Management of androgenic alopecia. Topical minoxidil solution (Rogaine) is the only drug available for promoting hair growth in women with androgenic alopecia. It is available in 2% and 5% formulations, which can be purchased over the counter (OTC). Trials with premenopausal women (18-45 y) have demonstrated improved scalp coverage and have slowed hair loss. No trials have been completed with postmenopausal women. Minoxidil therapy must be continued indefinitely because the condition may return to its pretreatment condition or worsen when the drug is stopped. It may take 3 to 4 months for hair growth to be noticed.

Finasteride (Propecia), a government-approved treatment for androgenic alopecia in men, is not recommended for women. A clinical trial in postmenopausal women found it was no more effective than placebo in treating hair loss.

Treatment for women with alopecia and excess circulating androgen levels focuses on combined treatment, including hormonal contraceptives and antiandrogens (for ovarian suppression) and low-dose corticosteroids (for adrenal suppression). For women with androgen excess and type 2 DM, therapies to reduce insulin resistance, such as weight reduction and metformin, may reduce ovarian testosterone.

Vitamin and mineral supplements with some effectiveness in treating hair loss generally have some antiandrogen activity (eg, zinc, vitamin B_6, green tea, saw palmetto). A shampoo containing hyaluronic acid has retarded hair loss in European clinical trials. Shampoos that treat scalp dermatitis can reduce cytokines, which can enhance or restore hair growth. None of these products are government approved in the United States or Canada for treating hair loss, although some are recommended by pharmacists and dermatologists based on clinical experience. Some licensed acupuncturists use herbal therapies to stimulate hair growth, with mixed success. These therapies, like pharmaceuticals, generally take 3 to 4 months before a change is noted.

If hormones (eg, menopausal HT, hormonal contraceptives) are prescribed for a woman with androgenic alopecia, care should be taken to select a progestogen with little androgenic activity. Additionally, testosterone or androgen precursors, such as dehydroepiandrosterone (DHEA), may worsen androgenic alopecia. However, HT has no recognized role in alopecia treatment. With all hair growth aberrations, photographs may be useful in monitoring therapeutic results.

Hirsutism. The presence of coarse facial hairs in females typically occurs in areas of the body where the hair follicles are the most androgen-sensitive, including the chin, upper lip, and cheeks. It affects between 5% and 15% of women. Except for rare cases of virilizing tumors or adrenal hyperplasia due to enzymatic defects, hirsutism is caused mainly by ovarian androgen overproduction (the polycystic ovarian syndrome) or by peripheral hypersensitivity to normal levels of circulating androgen (idiopathic hirsutism). The role of androgens in women with hirsutism is further evidenced by the reduction in hair density that can be attained with antiandrogen treatments, including hormonal contraceptives with low androgenicity.

Most women with hirsutism have an exaggerated utilization of androgens as a result of enhanced local 5α-reductase activity. Other clinical disorders that have been observed with acute or transient androgen excess include alopecia (female pattern), seborrhea (oily face and scalp, frequently with associated seborrheic dermatitis), and acne. If chronic androgen excess exists, the polycystic ovarian syndrome is the most common cause (40% of cases); insulin resistance, androgen-secreting tumors, and androgenic drug intake are less frequent causes.

Another hair-growth phenomenon of concern to many women is the appearance of fine hairs ("peach fuzz") on the face, most commonly on the upper lip and chin but sometimes generalized in appearance. Rapidly growing, large "rogue hairs" can sometimes be found on the chin. The growth of unwanted hair is common, and sometimes occurs long before menopause.

Management of hirsutism. The diagnostic evaluation of women with hirsutism first focuses on confirming the condition and the presence of excess levels of androgen. Other associated abnormalities and conditions need to be ruled out, including ovulatory dysfunction, adrenal hyperplasia, DM, and thyroid-hormone abnormalities.

Treatment for hirsutism focuses on a combination of therapies including hormonal drugs, peripheral androgen blockage, and mechanical depilation. A woman can remove hair by plucking, waxing, or shaving. Shaving is less traumatic than the other methods, but it may lead to folliculitis and ingrown hairs. Bleaching is also useful, particularly for mild conditions. Chemical depilatory agents may irritate the skin, especially facial skin. Electrolysis can usually destroy terminal hairs after 6 months of treatment. Laser treatment is effective for large areas.

Eflornithine HCl cream (Vaniqa; not available in Canada) is a prescription topical enzyme inhibitor of hair growth. It is indicated for reducing unwanted facial hair in women. The cream is applied twice daily.

HT may delay the progression of hirsutism, but it will not change coarse terminal hairs into softer and less noticeable vellus hairs. Off-label treatment options include estrogen-containing contraceptives and antiandrogens (eg, spironolactone) as well as 5α-reductase inhibitors (eg, finasteride).

To avoid progression of hirsutism symptoms, treatment of androgen excess should begin as soon as the diagnosis is established. Response to therapy may require 6 to 8 months. Hormonal suppression may need to be continued indefinitely. Androgen levels should be measured at regular intervals.

Ocular changes

Various ocular changes may occur during the menstrual cycle, during pregnancy, and at menopause. Ocular complaints reported by postmenopausal women include dry eye syndrome, blurred vision, increased lacrimation, tired eyes, and swollen and reddened eyelids. Presbyopia often starts just prior to menopause and requires many women to wear reading glasses.

Visual performance may be altered by increased corneal, lid, and conjunctival edema during certain phases of the menstrual cycle and during perimenopause. These effects may reduce contact lens tolerance. In addition, hormonal and menopausal status may adversely affect clinical outcomes following refractive surgery, which is now recognized to cause dry eye (keratoconjunctivitis sicca) in a segment of people, both male and female.

Dry eye syndrome. One of the most common ocular complaints associated with menopause is dry eye syndrome. It is characterized by symptoms of ocular irritation such as dryness, pressure, foreign-body sensation, scratchiness, and burning as well as photophobia (ie, light intolerance). The signs of ocular surface damage include redness, aberrant mucus production, and even corneal scarring. Any event that contributes to abnormalities of tear stability or flow can induce or exacerbate dry eye, such as environmental triggers (eg, low humidity or wind) and autoimmune diseases (eg, Sjögren's syndrome or rheumatoid arthritis). Drugs, such as diuretics, antihistamines, or psychotropics, may also be a factor.

Management of dry eye. Women presenting with symptoms of dry eye can be advised to use ocular lubricants such as drops, gels, and ointments. This treatment is palliative at best, resulting in temporary reduction of ocular surface-to-eyelid shear forces and transient symptomatic relief. Plugging of the lacrimal punctae, the openings through which tears drain from the surface of the eye into the nose, can increase the volume of tears on the ocular surface despite a decreased rate of tear production. This can be accomplished with temporary collagen plugs or with silicone plugs or cauterization; however, it may not relieve symptoms in all women.

Although there are many causes of dry eye, an underlying cytokine/receptor-mediated inflammatory process is common to all ocular surface diseases. By treating this process, it may be possible to normalize the ocular surface/lacrimal neural reflex and facilitate ocular surface healing. Anti-inflammatory medications are now recognized as a more appropriate therapeutic strategy for dry eye than are ocular drops. In women with moderate to severe dry eye, topical cyclosporine A has been shown to significantly increase tear production and significantly decrease ocular surface damage. Histopathologic evidence indicates that cyclosporine A (Restasis) treatment significantly reduces the numbers of activated T lymphocytes within the conjunctiva.

Similarly, there have been reports of symptomatic relief and reduction of signs of dry eye with the use of topical corticosteroids. Corticosteroids may have significant adverse effects, such as cataract formation and increased intraocular pressure, making them unsuitable for chronic use. Oral pilocarpine (Salagen), a parasympathomimetic, and cevimeline HCl (Evoxac; not available in Canada), a selective muscarinic cholinergic agonist, are indicated to treat dry mouth in Sjögren's syndrome. These drugs may also have beneficial effects in treating severe dry eye. A clinical trial studying the effect of topical cyclosporine A in the treatment of moderate to severe dry eye in patients with Sjögren's syndrome and in postmenopausal women is in progress.

Role of hormones. Sex-hormone receptors have been identified in many ocular tissues, including the meibomian glands, the lacrimal gland, the lens, the cornea, and conjunctiva, suggesting involvement of sex hormones in the maintenance of ocular surface homeostasis.

Studies in animal models have revealed that lacrimal gland function is significantly influenced by sex hormones. Androgens specifically have been shown to exert essential and specific effects on maintaining normal glandular functions and suppressing inflammation. Researchers found that topical androgen treatment (19-nortestosterone) improved signs of dry eye when administered to dogs.

It has been proposed that the pathology of dry eye may be initiated when systemic androgen levels fall below the threshold necessary to support secretory function and maintain an anti-inflammatory environment. The decrease in systemic androgen levels that comes with aging may have a direct effect on dry eye syndrome. These studies have since been supported clinically with studies in humans comparing tear production in peri- and postmenopausal women in which both quality and amount of tear production were reduced in the postmenopausal group.

The effects of topical application of estrogens or androgens in humans, however, have not been completely identified, although studies are being conducted. A few studies have reported improvement in dry eye signs and symptoms with ET, but these have involved relatively few patients. A review of data on 25,665 women from the WHS suggested that ET is actually associated with an increased risk of either clinically diagnosed dry eye or severe symptoms of both ocular dryness and irritation. Treatment with EPT was associated with an intermediate risk. Women who had never used estrogen had the lowest risk. Although several smaller studies have confirmed the finding that unopposed estrogen use may worsen dry eye, a separate small study showed that treatment with combined esterified estrogens and methyltestosterone resulted in improvement in dry eye symptoms.

Cataracts. Cataracts (lens opacity) become more common with age in men and women, although there is conflicting information regarding any sex predilection. There are no well-documented gender differences in cataract formation, which rarely occurs during women's reproductive years. However, administration of estrogen was protective against cataract formation in several animal models. Furthermore, retrospective analyses of large population-based studies suggest that ET has a protective effect in postmenopausal women.

Management of cataracts. Two large cross-sectional studies with postmenopausal women, the Beaver Dam Eye Study and the Blue Mountain Study, reported a protective effect of current menopausal HT use on cataract formation. The Salisbury Eye Evaluation also showed a protective association between the use of HT and both nuclear and posterior subcapsular cataract. In the Framingham Heart Study, 10 or more years of HT use was inversely associated with nuclear cataract. Women who have undergone surgical menopause are more likely to develop posterior subcapsular cataract than women who reach menopause spontaneously. Women with breast cancer treated with tamoxifen have an increased risk of cataract, which is consistent with a protective role for estrogen in lens opacification.

Data from the NHS indicate that vitamin C supplements may diminish the risks for cortical cataracts in women younger than age 60, and for posterior subcapsular cataracts in women who have never smoked.

Glaucoma. Glaucoma is another ocular condition for which age is an independent risk factor, regardless of gender. Some studies have demonstrated a hormonal effect on intraocular pressure, and increased intraocular pressure is in itself a risk factor for development of glaucoma.

Management of glaucoma. One large population-based study among postmenopausal women found that early menopause is associated with a higher risk of open-angle glaucoma. HT users showed improved ocular vascular-ization when compared to non-users. The clinical significance of this finding requires further study; however, it may play a role in glaucoma progression.

Although HT in postmenopausal women was found to decrease intraocular pressure, it is not used for this purpose in glaucoma patients.

Management of glaucoma includes use of ocular anti-hypertensive medications such as topical beta-blockers, alpha-agonists, prostaglandin analogues, and topical or oral carbonic anhydrase inhibitors.

Retina and vitreous. Several changes in the retina and vitreous have been found to be more prevalent in postmenopausal women when compared to age-matched men. One study showed a possible increased risk of posterior-vitreous detachment (PVD) in postmenopausal women. PVD in itself is not a vision-threatening condition; however, it may cause new floaters and slightly increase the risk of retinal tears or detachment in the acute phase. PVD also is a risk factor for macular hole formation, which would help to explain the higher incidence of macular hole in postmenopausal women when compared to age-matched men. The exact mechanism by which sex hormones influence these retinal and vitreous changes is not yet known.

Also among these conditions is neovascular age-related macular degeneration. Some researchers have suggested that HT may help to prevent macular degeneration in postmenopausal women. The 2006 WHI Sight Exam Study assesed possible protective effects of HT against progression of macular degeneration. Aside from HT, antioxidants such as vitamins C and E, beta-carotene, and zinc were found to reduce the risk of progression to late macular degeneration in patients with high-risk features. Other treatment modalities for exudative macular degeneration include laser photocoagulation, photodynamic therapy, and intravitreal anti-VEGF (vascular endothelial growth factor).

Other ocular changes. The effects of postmenopausal hormone changes have been further studied in ocular tissues other than the lacrimal gland, lens, retina, and vitreous. Sex hormone receptors have been found in conjunctiva, iris, and ciliary body, but the role of these receptors has yet to be determined.

Hearing changes

The impact of the menopause transition and lowered levels of estrogen on nervous system function is well known. There have been many studies about brain effects relating ovarian function to causes of vasomotor symptoms, mood changes, depression, sleep, cognition, and sexual response. Peripheral sensation has also been shown to respond to changes in estrogen levels. Indeed, two-point discrimination, an excellent clinical test of peripheral sensitivity, increases inversely to circulating estrogen levels.

Hearing impairment increases beyond age 50 with presbycusis (ie, progressive hearing impairment associated with aging, characterized by hearing loss and degeneration of cochlear structures) being the most important contributor to this increase. About 25% of individuals aged 51 to 65 years have decreased hearing in at least one ear, and objective hearing loss can be identified in over 33% of those aged 65 years and older.

There is some evidence of a relationship between gender, menopause, estrogens, and hearing. The question is whether sex steroids, specifically estrogen, preserve hearing during aging. Hultcrantz et al concluded that physiological levels of estrogen would appear to have a possible protective effect on hearing function. It is known that women with Turner's syndrome have earlier presbycusis, and that women using HT have slightly better hearing than those who are not. HT has a positive effect on auditory brain stem response in postmenopausal women, an important objective measure of hearing. More recently, HT was shown to improve conduction auditory pathways at the brain stem and thalamocortex. Estrogen-only users benefited more, and the addition of progestin to estrogen did not have a negative or potentiating effect. On the other hand, there is a report that progestin as a component of HT resulted in poorer hearing abilities in aged women taking HT, affecting both the peripheral (ear) and central (brain) auditory systems, interfering with the perception of speech in background noise.

The US Preventive Services Task Force confirms that the incidence of hearing impairment, largely presbycusis, rises quickly beyond age 50. They also report that self-assessment questionnaires to identify hearing impairment probably represent the most rapid and least expensive way to screen for hearing loss in the adult, being up to 70% to 80% accurate depending upon the audiometric criteria. Although no controlled study has proven the effectiveness of screening for hearing impairment in the adult population, there is evidence for measured improvement in social, cognitive, emotional, and communication function from hearing aid use.

Management of hearing changes. The Institute of Medicine recommends audiometric testing once during ages 40 and 59, 60 and 74, and 75 and over. The Canadian Task Force on the Periodic Health Examination recommends screening the elderly for hearing impairment by asking a single question about hearing difficulty whispered out of the field of vision or audioscope. The American Academy of Family Physicians recommends evaluation of hearing in persons aged 65 years and older, and recommends hearing aids for patients found to have hearing deficits, although these recommendations are under review.

Arthritis and arthralgia

There are over 100 causes of arthritis, many of which affect women at midlife and beyond.

Osteoarthritis. The most common form of joint disease is *osteoarthritis* (OA) or degenerative arthritis, which occurs in almost everyone with advancing age. A form of this condition, erosive OA, is of particular significance to this discussion because it affects predominantly women in their mid-40s and beyond. There is a major hereditary component to erosive OA; 90% of affected women will have a first-degree relative with the condition. The small joints of the fingers, particularly the PIP (mid-finger) and DIP (fingertip) joints, are the target of involvement. Initially, these joints may be inflamed with redness, warmth, and pain mimicking other forms of arthritis, but over months and years the inflammation resolves, leaving the typical gnarled, knobby joint that is most often relatively pain-free. The first CMC joint (at the base of the thumb) is another frequent area of involvement and can be exceptionally disabling. To date, there is no convincing explanation as to why women are targeted by erosive OA, although overuse may play a small role.

Other joints frequently affected by OA include the knees, hips, and feet as well as the cervical and lumbosacral spine. Although simplistic, it is useful to think of OA in these joints as a "wearing out." Men and women are equally affected, and joint disease tends to occur sooner and more often in the overweight and following injury and overuse. Perhaps because of better mechanics primary, OA rarely affects the wrists, elbows, ankles, or shoulders, and when found in these joints one should look for other causes such as rotator cuff tear or tendinitis (eg, tennis elbow). OA, for the most part, is noninflammatory.

Physical findings typically include joint tenderness, limitation, and crepitus. Joint swelling may be present, but significant warmth and redness should prompt concern about the diagnosis. Chondrocalcinosis (ie, deposition of calcium pyrophosphate dehydrate) is frequently found on x-ray of the osteoarthritic joint, particularly the knee and wrist. Release of these crystals into the joint space causes pseudogout, an intense inflammatory response. This is always a prime consideration in an older woman with acute joint pain and swelling.

Following menopause, there is an increase in the frequency and severity of OA—leading researchers to evaluate the role of estrogen within the disease. The role of HT in reducing the risk for OA has not been established. An epidemiologic review of the literature, published from 1989 to 1998, found some suggestion that menopausal HT decreases OA risk, but found no consistent association by joint site or symptomatology. However, no studies have directly linked menopause and joint pain.

Management of OA. To date, there is no means of either preventing or curing OA. Maintaining ideal weight has been shown to delay and reduce the severity of degeneration of the lumbar spine and weight-bearing joints. Exercise to strengthen periarticular muscles and improve posture also seems to be beneficial. Physical therapy can be useful for getting patients started on appropriate exercise, for aerobic conditioning and balance as well as strengthening. Applications of heat or cold and splinting of affected joints can be useful for exacerbation. Often, however, medication is necessary to try to control symptoms.

- *Nonprescription therapy.* Acetaminophen is the first-line treatment for relatively minor OA pain. If inadequate, nonsteroidal anti-inflammatry drugs (NSAIDs), such as ibuprofen, are often prescribed. Side effects of these drugs include fluid retention and secondary hypertension and reversible decreases in renal function. Serious cardiovascular events are also increased in frequency. The most common adverse effect of NSAIDs as a group is gastrointestinal (GI) irritation and bleeding, which can be life-threatening.

  It is important to maintain adequate vitamin D levels in patients with osteoarthritis as many are vitamin D deficient and restoring this vitamin may help with arthralgias. In addition, OTC glucosamine may provide improvement in knee OA in postmenopausal women. (See Section H, pages 240 and 251, for more about vitamin D and glucosamine, respectively.)

- *Prescription therapy.* Cyclooxygenase-2 (COX-2) selective inhibitors, such as celecoxib (Celebrex) and meloxicam (Mobic), have a lower incidence of GI bleeding and may be safer, especially in an older population.

  Systemic steroids are rarely, if ever, indicated for treatment of pure OA, but intraarticular injection of a long-acting corticosteroid agent, such as triamcinolone, can be effective for alleviating symptoms. Intraarticular hyalgans given as a series of injections may provide fairly long-term relief for selected patients with OA of the knee.

- *Joint replacement.* Finally, joint replacement remains the option of choice for those patients in whom joint pain affects daily activity and even sleep.

Rheumatoid arthritis. The next most common form of systemic joint disease is *rheumatoid arthritis* (RA). It occurs three times as often in women as men, and peak age of onset is between ages 35 and 55, commonly affecting peri- and postmenopausal women. The etiology of RA remains an enigma. There is a genetic association with the genotype HLA B7, and a somewhat higher incidence of disease in first-degree relatives, but in most cases hereditary factors are absent. RA often goes into remission during pregnancy, but there appears to be no direct connection to hormone levels.

RA typically affects multiple peripheral joints in a symmetric pattern producing the classic findings of inflammation, pain, swelling, heat, and erythema. Patients complain of prolonged morning stiffness and generalized symptoms of fatigue and low-grade fever. At times, vasculitis and involvement of lungs, eyes, and other organs emphasize the systemic nature of the disease. Laboratory studies reveal elevated acute phase reactants; rheumatoid factor is found in about 80% of individuals with RA, but is also present in a sizable percentage of those without RA. Recently, antibodies to cyclic citrullinated peptide antibody have been discovered to be a more reliable disease marker.

Rheumatoid inflammation, over time, leads to the growth of pannus, a destructive immune/inflammatory tissue within affected joints. The release of damaging enzymes and cytokines by infiltrating lymphocytes and macrophages leads to loss of cartilage and bony erosion. Joint limitation, instability, and functional impairment are the end result.

Management of RA. Enormous advances in the treatment of RA have now made it possible to prevent this progression, and make early diagnosis and aggressive treatment vital. While NSAIDs and low-dose corticosteroids can provide symptomatic improvement, use of disease-modifying antirheumatic drugs (such as low-dose methotrexate [generics] and leflunomide [Arava]) and biologic agents (such as etanercept [Enbrel] and adalimumab [Humira]) have been proven to prevent cartilage and bone damage as well as control clinical manifestations.

Arthralgia. Another frequent clinical presentation is *arthralgia*, joint pain without swelling or other signs of inflammation. The most common cause of acute arthralgias is viral infection. Infection with parvovirus B19, the agent of the childhood exanthem erytherma infectiosum, may be the etiology in up to 12% of patients presenting with recent onset arthralgia/arthritis. Rash may be minor or absent in adults with parvovirus infection, but arthralgias and even frank arthritis involving peripheral joints occur frequently, and may mimic early RA. Viral serologies confirm the diagnosis.

Rubella infection also causes joint symptoms in a high percentage of infected adults. Symptoms may precede the typical rash, and most often involve peripheral joints in a symmetric pattern. A similar clinical picture can follow rubella immunization.

Arthralgias and arthritis are often seen in the prodrome of hepatitis B infection. In this stage, a significant immune response is being mounted against the virus leading to large-scale production of circulating immune complexes. Deposition of these complexes within the synovium produces an intense response with severe polyarthralgias and frank arthritis. Rash (frequently urticarial) and fever are often observed in association with the joint symptoms. This systemic serum sickness-type prodrome resolves as the hepatitis becomes more obvious.

Chronic arthralgia and myalgia are the defining features of *fibromyalgia*. Pain tends to be primarily axial, with diffuse aching in the neck, shoulders, back, and pelvis. There is no joint swelling or synovitis, and muscle strength is normal. The key finding is the characteristic tender points, though patients with fibromyalgia tend to display heightened pain sensitivity diffusely as well. Arthralgias and myalgias in these patients are typically accompanied by other subjective symptoms of poor sleep, chronic fatigue, headache, and irritable bowel and bladder symptoms. It is likely that there is a common pathogenesis to these manifestations. Recent investigations have suggested that changes in central nervous system neurotransmitters may be the cause of aberrant pain sensitivity, and that sleep abnormalities may be an underlying cause in many patients.

Management of arthralgia. Treatment of fibromyalgia is often unsatisfying. Patient education and institution of an aerobic conditioning program can help in some cases. Minor analgesics and anti-inflammatory medications such as ibuprofen can also provide modest relief; other pharmacologic interventions are beyond the scope of this discussion.

Suggested reading

Decline in fertility

Bopp BL, Seifer DB. Oocyte loss and the perimenopause. *Clin Obstet Gynecol* 1998;41:898-911.

Burger HG, Dudley EC, Hopper JL, et al. Prospectively measured levels of serum follicle-stimulating hormone, estradiol, and the dimeric inhibins during the menopausal transition in a population-based cohort of women. *J Clin Endocrinol Metab* 1999;84:4025-4030.

Essure Permanent Birth Control. Essure clinical data. Available at http://www.essuremd.com/Home/bTheEssureProcedureb/bClinicalDatab/tabid/58/Default.aspx. Accessed September 17, 2007.

Kerin JF, Cooper JM, Price T, et al. Hysteroscopic sterilization using a micro-insert device: results of a multicentre Phase II study. *Hum Reprod* 2003;18:1223-1230.

Klein J, Sauer MV. Assessing fertility in women of advanced reproductive age. *Am J Obstet Gynecol* 2001;185:758-770.

Klein NA, Houmard BS, Hansen KR, et al. Age-related analysis of inhibin A, inhibin B, and activin a relative to the intercycle monotropic follicle-stimulating hormone rise in normal ovulatory women. *J Clin Endocrinol Metab* 2004;89:2977-2981.

Klein NA, Soules MR. Endocrine changes of the perimenopause. *Clin Obstet Gynecol* 1998;41:912-920.

Litta P, Cosmi E, Sacco G, Saccardi C, Ciavattini A, Ambrosini G. Hysteroscopic permanent tubal sterilization using a nitinol-dacron intratubal device without anaesthesia in the outpatient setting: procedure feasibility and effectiveness. *Hum Reprod* 2005;20:3419-3422.

Nugent D. The effects of female age on fecundity and pregnancy outcome. *Hum Fertil* 2001;4:43-48.

Pal L, Santoro N. Age-related decline in fertility. *Endocrinol Metab Clin North Am* 2003;32:669-698.

Pollack A, for the ACOG Committee on Practice Bulletins-Gynecology. Benefits and risks of sterilization: ACOG Practice Bulletin (no. 46). *Obstet Gynecol* 2003;102:647-658.

Soules MR. Endocrine changes of the perimenopause. *Clin Obstet Gynecol* 1998;41:912-920.

Soules MR, Sherman S, Parrott E, et al. Executive summary: stages of reproductive aging workshop (STRAW) Park City, Utah, July 2001. *Menopause* 2001;8:402-407.

Speroff L, Darney D, eds. *A Clinical Guide for Contraception*, 3rd ed. Philadelphia, PA: Lippincott Williams & Wilkins, 2001.

Speroff L, Glass RH, Kase NG, eds. *Clinical Gynecologic Endocrinology and Infertility*, 6th ed. Philadelphia, PA: Lippincott Williams & Wilkins, 1999.

Tarlatzis BC, Zepiridis L. Perimenopausal conception. *Ann N Y Acad Sci* 2003;997:93-104.

Ubeda A, Labastida R, Dexeus S. Essure: a new device for hysteroscopic tubal sterilization in an outpatient setting. *Fertil Steril* 2004;82:196-199.

Yen SC, Jaffe RB, eds. *Reproductive Endocrinology: Physiology, Pathophysiology, and Clinical Management*, 3rd ed. St. Louis, MO: WB Saunders, 1999.

Uterine bleeding changes

The American College of Obstetricians and Gynecologists. Endometrial ablation. ACOG Practice Bulletin No. 81. *Obstet Gynecol* 2007;109:1233-1248.

The American College of Obstetricians and Gynecologists. Noncontraceptive uses of the levonorgestrel intrauterine system. ACOG Committee Opinion No. 337. *Obstet Gynecol* 2006;107:1479-1482.

American Institute of Ultrasound in Medicine; American College of Obstetricians and Gynecologists; American College of Radiology. AIUM standard for the performance of saline infusion sonohysterography. *J Ultrasound Med* 2003;22:121-126.

Anderson FD, Hait H. A multicenter, randomized study of an extended cycle oral contraceptive. *Contraception* 2003;68:89-96.

Anderson GL, Judd HL, Kaunitz AM, et al. Effects of estrogen plus progestin on gynecologic cancers and associated diagnostic procedures: the Women's Health Initiative randomized trial. *JAMA* 2003;290:1739-1748.

Archer D. Duration of progestin use. *Menopause* 2001;8:245.

Association of Professors of Gynecology and Obstetrics. *Clinical Management of Abnormal Uterine Bleeding: Educational Series on Women's Health Issues*. Crofton, MD: Association of Professors of Gynecology and Obstetrics, 2002.

Baak JP, Mutter GL, Robboy S, et al. The molecular genetics and morphometry-based endometrial intraepithelial neoplasia classification system predicts disease progression in endometrial hyperplasia more accurately than the 1994 World Health Organization classification system. *Cancer* 2005;103:2304.

Bayer SR, DeCherney AH. Clinical manifestations and treatment of dysfunctional uterine bleeding. *JAMA* 1993;269:1823-1828.

Bonduelle M, Walker JJ, Calder AA. A comparative study of danazol and norethisterone in dysfunctional uterine bleeding presenting as menorrhagia. *Postgrad Med J* 1991;67:833-836.

Breitkopf D, Goldstein SR, Seeds JW, for the ACOG Committee on Gynecologic Practice. ACOG technology assessment in obstetrics and gynecology. Number 3, September 2003. Saline infusion sonohysterography. *Obstet Gynecol* 2003; 102:659-662.

Burger HG, Dudley EC, Hopper JL, et al. The endocrinology of the menopausal transition: a cross-sectional study of a population-based sample. *J Clin Endocrinol Metab* 1995;80:3537-3545.

Chuong CJ, Brenner PF. Management of abnormal uterine bleeding. *Am J Obstet Gynecol* 1996;175(pt 2):787-792.

Colacurci N, De Placido G, Mollo A, Perino A, Cittadini E. Short-term use of goserelin depot in the treatment of dysfunctional uterine bleeding. *Clin Exp Obstet Gynecol* 1995;22:212-219.

Crosignani PG, Vercellini P, Mosconi P, Oldani S, Cortesi I, De Giorgi O. Levonorgestrel-releasing intrauterine device versus hysteroscopic endometrial resection in the treatment of dysfunctional uterine bleeding. *Obstet Gynecol* 1997;90:257-263.

Davis A, Godwin A, Lippman J, Olson W, Kafrissen M. Triphasic norgestimate-ethinyl estradiol for treating dysfunctional uterine bleeding. *Obstet Gynecol* 2000;96:913-920.

Dietel M. The histological diagnosis of endometrial hyperplasia. Is there a need to simplify? *Virchows Arch* 2001;439:604.

Dockeray CJ, Sheppard BL, Bonnar J. Comparison between mefanamic acid and danazol in the treatment of established menorrhagia. *Br J Obstet Gynaecol* 1989;96:840-844.

Farquhar CM, Lethaby A, Sowter M, et al. An evaluation of risk factors for endometrial hyperplasia in premenopausal women with abnormal menstrual bleeding. *Am J Obstet Gynecol* 1999;181:525-529.

Fraser IS. Treatment of ovulatory and anovulatory dysfunctional uterine bleeding with oral progestogens. *Aust N Z J Obstet Gynaecol* 1990;30:353-356.

Fraser IS, McCarron G. Randomized trial of 2 hormonal and 2 prostaglandin-inhibiting agents in women with a complaint of menorrhagia. *Aust N Z J Obstet Gynaecol* 1991;31:66-70.

Friedman AJ, Hoffman DI, Comite F, Browneller RW, Miller JD, for the Leuprolide Study Group. Treatment of leiomyomata uteri with leuprolide acetate depot: a double-blind, placebo-controlled, multicenter study. *Obstet Gynecol* 1991;77:720-725.

Gambrell RD Jr. Strategies to reduce the incidence of endometrial cancer in postmenopausal women. *Am J Obstet Gynecol* 1997;177:1195-1204.

Gervaise A, Fernandez H, Capella-Allouc S, et al. Thermal balloon ablation versus endometrial resection for the treatment of abnormal uterine bleeding. *Hum Reprod* 2000;15:1424-1425.

Goldstein RB, Bree RL, Benson CB, et al. Evaluation of the woman with postmenopausal bleeding: Society of Radiologists in Ultrasound-Sponsored Consensus Conference statement. *J Ultrasound Med* 2001;20:1025-1036.

Goldstein SR, Monteagudo A, Popiolek D, Mayberry P, Timor-Tritsch I. Evaluation of endometrial polyps. *Am J Obstet Gynecol* 2002;186:669-674.

Good AE. Diagnostic options for assessment of postmenopausal bleeding. *Mayo Clin Proc* 1997;72:345-349.

Grigorieva V, Chen-Mok M, Tarasova M, Mikhailov A. Use of a levonogestrel-releasing intrauterine system to treat bleeding related to uterine leiomyomas. *Fertil Steril* 2003;79:1194-1198.

Gurtcheff SE, Sharp HT. Complications associated with global endometrial ablation: the utility of the MAUDE database. *Obstet Gynecol* 2003; 102:1278-1282.

Hale GE, Fraser IS. Changes in the menstrual pattern during the perimeno-pause. In: Lobo RA, ed. *Treatment of the Postmenopausal Woman: Basic and Clinical Aspect*, 3rd ed. San Diego, CA: Academic Press, 2007:149-156.

Harlow SD, Cain K, Crawford S, et al. Evaluation of four proposed bleeding criteria for the onset of late menopausal transition. *J Clin Endocrinol Metab* 2006;91:3432-3438.

Higham JM, Shaw RW. A comparative study of danazol, a regimen of decreasing doses of danazol, and norethindrone in the treatment of objectively proven unexplained menorrhagia. *Am J Obstet Gynecol* 1993;169:1134-1139.

Hurskainen R, Teperi J, Rissanen P, et al. Clinical outcomes and costs with the levonorgestrel-releasing intrauterine system or hysterectomy for treatment of menorrhagia: randomized trial 5-year follow-up. *JAMA* 2004; 291:1456-1463.

Hurskainen R, Teperi J, Rissanen P, et al. Quality of life and cost-effectiveness of levonorgestrel-releasing intrauterine system versus hysterectomy for treatment of menorrhagia: a randomized trial. *Lancet* 2001;357:273-277.

Irvine GA, Campbell-Brown MB, Lumsden MA, Heikkila A, Walker JJ, Cameron IT. Randomised comparative trial of the levonorgestrel intrauterine system and norethisterone for treatment of idiopathic menorrhagia. *Br J Obstet Gynaecol* 1998;105:592-598.

Kaunitz AM. Gynecologic problems of the perimenopause: evaluation and treatment. *Obstet Gynecol Clin North Am* 2002;29:455-473.

Kurman RJ, Kaminski PF, Norris HJ. The behavior of endometrial hyperplasia. A long term study of "untreated" hyperplasia in 170 patients. *Cancer* 1985; 56:403-412.

Lamb MP. Danazol in menorrhagia: a double blind placebo controlled trial. *J Obstet Gynecol* 1987;7:212-216.

Milsom I, Andersson K, Andersch B, Rybo G. A comparison of flurbiprofen, tranexamic acid, and a levonorgestrel-releasing intrauterine contraceptive device in the treatment of idiopathic menorrhagia. *Am J Obstet Gynecol* 1991;164:879-883.

Munro MG. Abnormal uterine bleeding: surgical management. Part III. *J Am Assoc Gynecol Laparosc* 2001;8:18-44.

Munro MG. Endometrial ablation with a thermal balloon: the first 10 years. *J Am Assoc Gynecol Laparosc* 2004;11:8-22.

Munro MG. Abnormal uterine bleeding in the reproductive years. Part II: Medical management. *J Am Assoc Gynecol Laparosc* 2000;7:17-35.

The North American Menopause Society. Clinical challenges of peri-menopause: consensus opinion of The North American Menopause Society. *Menopause* 2000;7:5-13.

Oriel KA, Schrager S. Abnormal uterine bleeding. *Am Fam Physician* 1999; 60:1371-1380.

Pickar JH, Thorneycroft I, Whitehead M. Effects of hormone replacement therapy on the endometrium and lipid parameters: a review of randomized clinical trials, 1985 to 1995. *Am J Obstet Gynecol* 1998;78:1087-1099.

Preston JT, Cameron IT, Adams EJ, Smith SK. Comparative study of tranexamic acid and norethisterone in the treatment of ovulatory menorrhagia. *Br J Obstet Gynaecol* 1995;102:401-406.

Raudaskoski T, Tapanainen J, Tomas E, et al. Intrauterine 10 microg and 20 microg levonorgestrel systems in postmenopausal women receiving oral oestrogen replacement therapy: clinical, endometrial and metabolic response. *BJOG* 2002;109:136-144.

Richter HE, Learman LA, Lin F, et al. Medroxyprogesterone acetate treatment of abnormal uterine bleeding: factors predicting satisfaction. *Am J Obstet Gynecol* 2003;189:37-42.

Seltzer VL, Benjamin F, Deutsch S. Perimenopausal bleeding patterns and pathologic findings. *J Am Med Womens Assoc* 1990;45:132-134.

Stabinsky SA, Einstein M, Breen JL. Modern treatments of menorrhagia attributable to dysfunctional uterine bleeding. *Obstet Gynecol Surv* 1999; 54:61-72.

Townsend DE, Fields G, McCausland A, Kauffman K. Diagnostic and operative hysteroscopy in the management of persistent postmenopausal bleeding. *Obstet Gynecol* 1993;82:419-421.

Treloar AE, Boynton RE, Behn BG, et al. Variation of the human menstrual cycle through reproductive life. *Int J Fertil* 1967;12(1 pt 2):77-126.

Varila E, Wahlstrom T, Rauramo I. A 5-year follow-up study on the use of a levonorgestrel intrauterine system in women receiving hormone replacement therapy. *Fertil Steril* 2001;76:969-973.

Vilos GA, Lefebvre G, Graves GR. Guidelines for the management of abnormal uterine bleeding. *J SOCG* 2001;23:704-709.

Weber AM, Belinson JL, Piedmonte MR. Risk factors for endometrial hyperplasia and cancer among women with abnormal bleeding. *Obstet Gynecol* 1999;93:594-598.

Williams DB, Voight BJ, Fu YS, Schoenfeld MJ, Judd HL. Assessment of less than monthly progestin therapy in postmenopausal women given estrogen replacement. *Obstet Gynecol* 1994;84:787-793.

Vasomotor symptoms

Al-Azzawi F, Buckler HM, for the United Kingdom Vaginal Ring Investigator Group. Comparison of a novel vaginal ring delivering estradiol acetate versus oral estradiol for relief of vasomotor menopausal symptoms. *Climacteric* 2003;6:118-127.

Albrecht BH, Schiff I, Tulchinsky D, Ryan KJ. Objective evidence that placebo and oral medroxyprogesterone acetate therapy diminish menopausal vasomotor flushes. *Am J Obstet Gynecol* 1981;139:631-635.

Amato P, Christophe S, Mellon PL. Estrogenic activity of herbs commonly used as remedies for menopausal symptoms. *Menopause* 2002;9:145-150.

Avis NE, Crawford SL, McKinlay SM. Psychosocial, behavioral, and health factors related to menopause symptomatology. *Womens Health* 1997;3:103-120.

Baber RJ, Templeman C, Morton T, Kelly GE, West L. Randomized placebo-controlled trial of an isoflavone supplement and menopausal symptoms in women. *Climacteric* 1999;2:85-92.

Bachmann GA. Vasomotor flushes in postmenopausal women. *Am J Obstet Gynecol* 1999;180(3 pt 2):S312-S316.

Barton D, Loprinzi C, Quella S, Sloan J, Pruthi S, Novotny P. Depomedroxy-progesterone acetate for hot flashes. *J Pain Symptom Manage* 2002;24:603-607.

Barton DL, Loprinzi CL, Quella SK, et al. Prospective evaluation of vitamin E for hot flashes in breast cancer survivors. *J Clin Oncol* 1998;16:495-500.

Bergmans MG, Merkus JM, Corbey RS, Schellekens LA, Ubachs JM. Effect of Bellergal Retard on climacteric complaints: a double-blind, placebo-controlled study. *Maturitas* 1987;9:227-234.

Blatt MHG, Wiesbader H, Kupperman HS. Vitamin E and climacteric syndrome. *Arch Intern Med* 1953;91:792-796.

Boothby LA, Doering PL, Kipersztok S. Bioidentical hormone therapy: a review. *Menopause* 2004;11:356-367.

Buckler H, Al-Azzawi F, for the UK VR Multicentre Trial Group. The effect of a novel vaginal ring delivering oestradiol acetate on the climacteric symptoms in postmenopausal women. *Br J Obstet Gynecol* 2003;110:753-759.

Bullock JL, Massey FM, Gambrell RD Jr. Use of medroxyprogesterone acetate to prevent menopausal symptoms. *Obstet Gynecol* 1975;46:165-168.

Burke GL, Legault C, Anthony M, et al. Soy protein and isoflavone effects on vasomotor symptoms in peri- and post-menopausal women: the Soy Estrogen Alternative study. *Menopause* 2003;10:147-153.

Chenoy R, Hussain S, Tayob Y, et al. Effect of oral gamolenic acid from evening primrose oil on menopausal flushing. *BMJ* 1994;308:501-503.

Dalais FS, Rice GE, Wahlqvist ML, et al. Effects of dietary phytoestrogens in postmenopausal women. *Climacteric* 1998;1:124-129.

Davis SR, Briganti EM, Chen RQ, Dalais FS, Bailey M, Burger HG. The effects of Chinese medicinal herbs on postmenopausal vasomotor symptoms of Australian women: a randomised controlled trial. *Med J Aust* 2001;174:68-71.

Faure ED, Chantre P, Mares P. Effects of a standardized soy extract on hot flushes: a multicenter, double-blind, randomized, placebo-controlled study. *Menopause* 2002;9:329-334.

Feldman BM, Voda A, Gronseth E. The prevalence of hot flash and associated variables among perimenopausal women. *Res Nurs Health* 1985;8:261-268.

Fitzpatrick LA, Good A. Micronized progesterone: clinical indications and comparison with current treatments. *Fertil Steril* 1999;72:389-397.

Freedman RR. Hot flashes: behavioral treatments, mechanisms, and relation to sleep. *Am J Med* 2005;118:124-130.

Freedman RR. Biochemical, metabolic, and vascular mechanisms in menopausal hot flushes. *Fertil Steril* 1998;70:1-6.

Freedman RR, Krell W. Reduced thermoregulatory null zone in post-menopausal women with hot flashes. *Am J Obstet Gynecol* 1999;181:66-70.

Freedman RR, Roehrs TA. Lack of sleep disturbance from menopausal hot flashes. *Fertil Steril* 2004;82:138-144.

Freedman RR, Woodward S. Behavioral treatment of menopausal hot flushes: evaluation by ambulatory monitoring. *Am J Obstet Gynecol* 1992;167:436-439.

Freeman EW, Sammel MD, Lin H, Gracia CR, Kapoor S, Ferdousi T. The role of anxiety and hormonal changes in menopausal hot flashes. *Menopause* 2005;12:258-266.

Freeman EW, Sherif K. Prevalence of hot flushes and night sweats around the world: a systematic review. *Climacteric* 2007;10:197-214.

Gallicchio L, Miller SR, Visvanathan K, et al. Cigarette smoking, estrogen levels, and hot flashes in midlife women. *Maturitas* 2006;53:133-143.

Gold EB, Sternfeld B, Kelsey JL, et al. Relation of demographic and lifestyle factors to symptoms in a multi-racial/ethnic population of women 40-55 years of age. *Am J Epidemiol* 2000;152:463-473.

Goldberg RM, Loprinzi CL, O'Fallen JR, et al. Transdermal clonidine for ameliorating tamoxifen-induced hot flashes. *J Clin Oncol* 1994;12:155-158.

Gordon PR, Kerwin JP, Boesen KG, Pharm D, Senf J. Sertraline to treat hot flashes: a randomized controlled, double-blind, crossover trial in a general population. *Menopause* 2006;13:568-575.

Guthrie JR, Dennerstein L, Hopper JL, Burger HG. Hot flushes, menstrual status, and hormone levels in a population-based sample of midlife women. *Obstet Gynecol* 1996;88:437-442.

Guttuso T Jr, Kurlan R, McDermott MP, Kieburtz K. Gabapentin's effects on hot flashes in postmenopausal women: a randomized controlled trial. *Obstet Gynecol* 2003;101:337-345.

Hammar M, Berg G, Lindgren R. Does physical exercise influence the frequency of postmenopausal hot flushes? *Acta Obstet Gynecol Scand* 1990;69:409-412.

Hammond MG, Hatley L, Talbert LM. A double blind study to evaluate the effect of methyldopa on menopausal vasomotor flushes. *J Clin Endocrinol Metab* 1984;58:1158-1160.

Han KK, Soares JM, Haidar MA, de Lima GR, Baracat EC. Benefits of soy isoflavone therapeutic regimen on menopausal symptoms. *Obstet Gynecol* 2002;99:389-394.

Hendrix SL. Bilateral oophorectomy and premature menopause. *Am J Med* 2005;118:131-135.

Hirata JD, Swiersz LM, Zell B, Small R, Ettinger B. Does dong quai have estrogenic effects in postmenopausal women? A double-blind, placebo-controlled trial. *Fertil Steril* 1997;68:981-986.

Hlatky MA, Boothroyd D, Vittinghoff E, Sharp P, Whooley MA, for the HERS Research Group. Quality-of-life and depressive symptoms in postmenopausal women after receiving hormone therapy: results from the Heart and Estrogen/Progestin Replacement Study (HERS) trial. *JAMA* 2002;287:591-597.

Huang MI, Nir Y, Chen B, Schnyer R, Manber R. A randomized controlled pilot study of acupuncture for postmenopausal hot flashes: effect on nocturnal hot flashes and sleep quality. *Fertil Steril* 2006;86:700-710.

Huntley A, Ernst E. A systematic review of the safety of black cohosh. *Menopause* 2003;10:58-64.

Irvin JH, Domar AD, Clark C, Zuttermeister PC, Friedman R. The effects of relaxation response training on menopausal symptoms. *J Psychosom Obstet Gynaecol* 1996;17:202-207.

Ivarrson T, Spetz AC, Hammar M. Physical exercise and vasomotor symptoms in postmenopausal women. *Maturitas* 1998;29:139-146.

Kimmick GG, Lovato J, McQuellon R, Robinson E, Muss HB. Randomized, double-blind, placebo-controlled, crossover study of sertraline (Zoloft) for the treatment of hot flashes in women with early stage breast cancer taking tamoxifen. *Breast J* 2006;12:114-122.

Knight DC, Howes JB, Eden JA. The effect of Promensil, an isoflavone extract, on menopausal symptoms. *Climacteric* 1999;2:79-84.

Knight DC, Howes JB, Eden JA, Lowes LG. Effects on menopausal symptoms and acceptability of isoflavone-containing soy powder dietary supplementation. *Climacteric* 2001;4:13-18.

Komesaroff PA, Black CV, Cable V, Sudhir K. Effects of wild yam extract on menopausal symptoms, lipids and sex hormones in healthy menopausal women. *Climacteric* 2001;4:144-150.

Kronenberg F. Hot flashes. In: Lobo RA, ed. *Treatment of the Postmenopausal Woman: Basic and Clinical Aspects*, 2nd ed. Philadelphia, PA: Lippincott Williams & Wilkins, 1999:157-177.

Kronenberg F. Hot flashes: epidemiology and physiology. *Ann NY Acad Sci* 1990;592:52-86.

Laufer LR, Erlik Y, Meldrum DR, Judd HL. Effect of clonidine on hot flushes in postmenopausal women. *Obstet Gynecol* 1982;60:583-589.

Leonetti HB, Longo S, Anasti JN. Transdermal progesterone cream for vasomotor symptoms and postmenopausal bone loss. *Obstet Gynecol* 1999;94:225-228.

Lobo RA. Clinical aspects of hormonal replacement: routes of administration. In: Lobo RA, ed. *Treatment of the Postmenopausal Woman: Basic and Clinical Aspects*, 2nd ed. Philadelphia, PA: Lippincott Williams & Wilkins, 1999:125-139.

Lobo RA, McCormick W, Singer F, Roy S. Depo-medroxyprogesterone acetate compared with conjugated estrogens for the treatment of postmenopausal women. *Obstet Gynecol* 1984;63:1-5.

Loprinzi CL, Barton D, Rummans T. Newer antidepressants inhibit hot flashes. *Menopause* 2006;13:546-548.

Loprinzi CL, Kugler JW, Barton DL, et al. Phase III trial of gabapentin alone or in conjunction with an antidepressant in the management of hot flashes in women who have inadequate control with an antidepressant alone: NCCTG N03C5. *J Clin Oncol* 2007;25:308-312.

Loprinzi CL, Michalak JC, Quella SK, et al. Megestrol acetate for the prevention of hot flashes. *N Engl J Med* 1994;331:347-352.

Loprinzi CL, Sloan JA, Perez EA, et al. Phase III evaluation of fluoxetine for treatment of hot flashes. *J Clin Oncol* 2002;20:1578-1583.

MacLennan A, Lester S, Moore V. Oral oestrogen replacement therapy versus placebo for hot flushes. *Cochrane Database Syst Rev* 2004;4:CD002978.

Miller SR, Gallicchio LM, Lewis LM, et al. Association between race and hot flashes in midlife women. *Maturitas* 2006;54:260-269.

Morrison JC, Martin DC, Blair RA, et al. The use of medroxyprogesterone acetate for relief of climacteric symptoms. *Am J Obstet Gynecol* 1980;138:99-104.

Murkies AL, Lombard C, Strauss BJG, Wilcox G, Burger HG, Morton MS. Dietary flour supplementation decreases post-menopausal hot flushes: effect of soy and wheat. *Maturitas* 1995;21:189-195.

Nagamani M, Kelver ME, Smith ER. Treatment of menopausal hot flashes with transdermal administration of clonidine. *Am J Obstet Gynecol* 1987;156:561-565.

Nelson HD, Vesco KK, Haney E, et al. Nonhormonal therapies for menopausal hot flashes; systemic review and meta-analysis. *JAMA* 2006;295:2057-2071.

Nesheim BI, Saetre T. Reduction of menopausal hot flashes by methyldopa: a double-blind crossover trial. *Eur J Clin Pharmacol* 1981;20:413-416.

Newton KM, Reed SD, LaCroix AZ, Grothaus LC, Ehrlich K, Guiltinan J. Treatment of vasomotor symptoms of menopause with black cohosh, multibotanicals, soy, hormone therapy, or placebo. *Ann Intern Med* 2006;145:869-879.

Nikander E, Kilkkinen A, Metsa-Heikkila M, et al. A randomized placebo-controlled crossover trial with phytoestrogens in treatment of menopause in breast cancer patients. *Obstet Gynecol* 2003;101:1213-1220.

The North American Menopause Society. Clinical challenges of perimenopause: consensus opinion of The North American Menopause Society. *Menopause* 2000;7:5-13.

The North American Menopause Society. Estrogen and progestogen use in peri- and postmenopausal women: March 2007 position statement of The North American Menopause Society *Menopause* 2007;14:168-182.

The North American Menopause Society. Role of progestogen in hormone therapy for postmenopausal women: position statement of The North American Menopause Society. *Menopause* 2003;10:113-132.

The North American Menopause Society. The role of isoflavones in menopausal health: consensus opinion of The North American Menopause Society. *Menopause* 2000;7:215-229.

The North American Menopause Society. Treatment of menopause-associated vasomotor symptoms: position statement of The North American Menopause Society. *Menopause* 2004;11:11-33.

Notelovitz M, Lenihan JP, McDermott M, Kerber IJ, Nanavati N, Arce J. Initial 17beta-estradiol dose for treating vasomotor symptoms. *Obstet Gynecol* 2000;95:726-731.

Ockene JK, Barad DH, Cochrane BB, Larson JC, et al. Symptom experience after discontinuing use of estrogen plus progestin. *JAMA* 2005;294:183-193.

Pandya KJ, Morrow GR, Roscoe JA, et al. Gabapentin for hot flashes in 420 women with breast cancer: a randomised double-blind placebo-controlled trial. *Lancet* 2005;366:818-824.

Penotti M, Fabio E, Modena AB, Rinaldi M, Omodei U, Vigano P. Effect of soy-derived isoflavones on hot flushes, endometrial thickness, and the pulsatility index of the uterine and cerebral arteries. *Fertil Steril* 2003;79:1112-1117.

Pinkerton JV, Santen R. Alternatives to the use of estrogen in postmenopausal women. *Endocr Rev* 1999;20:308-320.

Randolph JF, Sowers M, Gold EB, et al. Reproductive hormones in the early menopausal transition: relationship to ethnicity, body size, and menopausal status. *J Clin Endocrinol Metab* 2003;88:1516-1522.

Reddy SY, Warner H, Guttuso Jr T, et al. Gabapentin, estrogen, and placebo for treating hot flushes. *Obstet Gynecol* 2006;108:41-48.

Scambia G, Mango D, Signorile PG, et al. Clinical effects of a standardized soy extract in postmenopausal women: a pilot study. *Menopause* 2000;7:105-111.

Schiff I, Tulchinsky D, Cramer D, Ryan KJ. Oral medroxyprogesterone in the treatment of postmenopausal symptoms. *JAMA* 1980;244:1443-1445.

Schwingl PJ, Hulka BS, Harlow SD. Risk factors for menopausal hot flashes. *Obstet Gynecol* 1994;84:29-34.

Seidl MM, Stewart DE. Alternative treatments for menopausal symptoms: systematic review of scientific and lay literature. *Can Fam Physician* 1998;44:1299-1308.

Shargil AA. Hormone replacement therapy in perimenopausal women with a triphasic contraceptive compound: a three-year prospective study. *Int J Fertil* 1985;30:15-28.

St. Germain A, Peterson CT, Robinson JG, Alekel DL. Isoflavone-rich or isoflavone-poor soy protein does not reduce menopausal symptoms during 24 weeks of treatment. *Menopause* 2001;8:17-26.

Staropoli CA, Flaws JA, Bush TL, Moulton AW. Predictors of menopausal hot flashes. *J Womens Health* 1998;9:1149-1155.

Stearns V, Beebe KL, Iyengar M, Dube E. Paroxetine controlled release in the treatment of menopausal hot flashes: a randomized controlled trial. *JAMA* 2003;289:2827-2834.

Stearns V, Johnson MD, Rae JM, et al. Active tamoxifen metabolite plasma concentrations after coadministration of tamoxifen and the selective serotonin reuptake inhibitor paroxetine. *J Natl Cancer Inst* 2003;95:1758-1764.

Steingold KA, Laufer L, Chetkowski RJ, et al. Treatment of hot flashes with transdermal estradiol administration. *J Clin Endocrinol Metab* 1985;61:627-632.

Stoll W. Phytotherapy influences atrophic vaginal epithelium—double-blind study—*Cimicifuga* vs estrogenic substances [in German]. *Therapeutikon* 1987;1:23-31.

Thurston RC, Joffe H, Soares CN, Harlow BL. Physical activity and risk of vasomotor symptoms in women with and without a history of depression: results from the Harvard Study of Moods and Cycles. *Menopause* 2006; 13:553-560.

Tice JA, Ettinger B, Ensrud K, Wallace R, Blackwell T, Cummings SR. Phytoestrogen supplements for the treatment of hot flashes: the Isoflavone Clover Extract (ICE) Study: a randomized controlled trial. *JAMA* 2003; 290:207-214.

Upmalis DH, Lobo R, Bradley L, et al. Vasomotor symptom relief by soy isoflavone extract tablets in postmenopausal women: a multicenter, double-blind, randomized, placebo-controlled study. *Menopause* 2000;7:236-242.

Utian WU, Lederman SA, Williams BM, Vega RY, Koltun WD, Leonard TW. Relief of hot flushes with new plant-derived 10-component synthetic conjugated estrogens. *Obstet Gynecol* 2004;103:245-253.

Utian WH, Shoupe D, Bachmann G, Pinkerton J, Pickar JH. Relief of vasomotor symptoms and vaginal atrophy with lower doses of conjugated equine estrogens and medroxyprogesterone acetate. *Fertil Steril* 2001;75:1065-1079.

van de Weijer PHM, Barentsen R. Isoflavones from red clover (Promensil®) significantly reduce menopausal hot flush symptoms compared with placebo. *Maturitas* 2002;42:187-193.

Vincent A, Burton DL, Mandrekar JN, et al. Acupuncture for hot flashes: a randomized, sham-controlled clinical study. *Menopause* 2007;14:45-52.

Warnecke G. Influence of phytotherapy on menopausal syndrome: successful treatments with monoextract of *cimicifuga* [in German]. *Medizinische Welt* 1985;36:871-874.

Whiteman MK, Staropoli CA, Lengenberg PW, McCarter RJ, Kjerulff KH, Flaws JH. Smoking, body mass, and hot flashes in midlife women. *Obstet Gynecol* 2003;101:264-272.

Wiklund IK, Mattsson LA, Lindgren R, Limoni C, for the Swedish Alternative Medicine Group. Effects of a standardized ginseng extract on quality of life and physiological parameters in symptomatic postmenopausal women: a double-blind, placebo-controlled trial. *Int J Clin Pharmacol Res* 1999;19:89-99.

Williamson J, White A, Hart A, Ernst E. Randomised controlled trial of reflexology for menopausal symptoms. *BJOG* 2002;109:1050-1055.

Woods NF. Exercise and hot flashes: toward a research agenda. *Menopause* 2006;13:541-543.

Wren BG, Champion SM, Willetts K, Manga RZ, Eden JA. Transdermal progesterone and its effect on vasomotor symptoms, blood lipid levels, bone metabolic markers, moods, and quality of life for postmenopausal women. *Menopause* 2003;10:13-18.

Wuttke W, Seidlova-Wuttke D, Gorkow C. The Cimicifuga preparation BNO 1055 vs. conjugated estrogens in a double-blind placebo-controlled study: effects on menopause symptoms and bone markers. *Maturitas* 2003;44 (Suppl 1):S67-S77.

Wyon Y, Lindgren R, Lundeberg T, Hammar M. Effects of acupuncture on climacteric vasomotor symptoms, quality of life, and urinary excretion of neuropeptides among postmenopausal women. *Menopause* 1995;2:3-12.

Zaborowska E, Brynhildsen J, Damberg S, et al. Effects of acupuncture, applied relaxation, estrogens and placebo on hot flushes in postmenopausal women: an analysis of two prospective, parallel, randomized studies. *Climacteric* 2007;10:38-45.

Sleep disturbances

Barry NN, McGuire JL, van Vollenhoven RF. Dehydroepiandrosterone in systemic lupus erythematosus: relationship between dosage, serum levels, and clinical response. *J Rheumatol* 1998;25:2352-2356.

Carskadon MA, Bearpark HM, Sharkey KM, et al. Effects of menopause and nasal occlusion on breathing during sleep. *Am J Respir Crit Care Med* 1997;155:205-210

Collop NA, Adkins D, Phillips BA. Gender differences in sleep and sleep-disordered breathing. *Clin Chest Med* 2004;25:257-268.

Dancey DR, Hanly PJ, Soong C, Lee B, Hoffstein V. Impact of menopause on the prevalence and severity of sleep apnea. *Chest* 2001;120:151-155.

Da Silva I, Naftolin F. Clinical effects of sex steroids on the brain. In: Lobo RA, ed. *Treatment of the Postmenopausal Woman: Basic and Clinical Aspects*, 3rd ed. San Diego, CA: Academic Press, 2007:199-215.

Dockhorn RJ, Dockhorn DW. Zolpidem in the treatment of short-term insomnia: a randomized, double-blind, placebo-controlled clinical trial. *Clin Neuropharmacol* 1996;19:333-340.

Driver HS, Taylor SR. Exercise and sleep. *Sleep Med Rev* 2000;4:387-402.

Elie R, Ruther E, Farr I, Emilien G, Salinas E. Sleep latency is shortened during 4 weeks of treatment with zaleplon, a novel nonbenzodiazepine hypnotic. Zaleplon Clinical Study Group. *J Clin Psychiatry* 1999;60:536-544.

Erlik Y, Tataryn IV, Meldrum DR, Lomax P, Bajorek JG, Judd HL. Association of waking episodes with menopausal hot flushes. *JAMA* 1981;245:1741-1744.

Freedman RR. Hot flashes: behavioral treatments, mechanisms, and relation to sleep. *Am J Med* 2005;118:124-130.

Freedman RR. Laboratory and ambulatory monitoring of menopausal hot flashes. *Psychophysiology* 1989;26:573-579.

Freedman RR, Roehrs TA. Effects of REM sleep and ambient temperature on hot flash-induced sleep disturbance. *Menopause* 2006;13:576-583.

Freedman RR, Roehrs TA. Lack of sleep disturbance from menopausal hot flashes. *Fertil Steril* 2004;82:138-144.

Freedman RR, Roehrs TA. Sleep disturbance in menopause. *Menopause* 2007; 14:826-829.

Gambacciani M, Ciaponi M, Cappagli B, et al. Effects of low-dose, continuous combined hormone replacement therapy on sleep in symptomatic postmenopausal women. *Maturitas* 2005;50:91-97.

Garfinkel D, Loudon M, Nof D, Zisapel N. Improvement of sleep quality in elderly people by controlled-release melatonin. *Lancet* 1995;346:541-544.

Gislason T, Benediktsdottir B, Bjornsson JK, Kjartansson G, Kjeld M, Kristbjarnarson H. Snoring, hypertension, and the sleep apnea syndrome: an epidemiologic survey of middle-aged women. *Chest* 1993;103:1147-1151.

Haimov I, Laudon M, Zisapel N, et al. Sleep disorders and melatonin rhythms in elderly people. *BMJ* 1994;309:167.

Harvey AG. Sleep hygiene and sleep-onset insomnia. *J Nerv Mental Dis* 2000;188:53-55.

Huang MI, Nir Y, Chen B, Schnyer R, Manber R. A randomized controlled pilot study of acupuncture for postmenopausal hot flashes: effect on nocturnal hot flashes and sleep quality. *Fertil Steril* 2006;86:700-710.

Katz D, McHorney CA. Clinical correlates of insomnia in patients with chronic illness. *Arch Intern Med* 1998;158:1099-1107.

Keefe DL, Watson R, Naftolin F. Hormone replacement therapy may alleviate sleep apnea in menopausal women: a pilot study. *Menopause* 1999;6:196-200.

King AC, Oman RF, Brassington GS, Bliwise DL, Haskell WL. Moderate-intensity exercise and self-rated quality of sleep in older adults: a randomized controlled study. *JAMA* 1997;277:32-37.

Kravitz HM, Ganz PA, Bromberger J, Powell LH, Sutton-Tyrrell K, Meyer PM. Sleep difficulty in women at midlife: a community survey of sleep and the menopausal transition. *Menopause* 2003;10:19-28.

Landolt HP, Roth C, Dijk DJ, Borbely AA. Late-afternoon ethanol intake affects nocturnal sleep and the sleep EEG in middle-aged men. *J Clin Psychopharmacol* 1996;16:428-436.

Landolt HP, Werth E, Borbely AA, Dijk DJ. Caffeine intake (200 mg) in the morning affects human sleep and EEG power spectra at night. *Brain Res* 1995;675:67-74.

Leathwood PD, Chauffard F, Heck E, Munoz-Box R. Aqueous extract of valerian root (Valeriana officinalis L.) improves sleep quality in man. *Pharmacol Biochem Behav* 1982;17:65-71.

Lee KA. Sleep in midlife women. *Sleep Medicine Clinics* 2006;1:197-205.

Manber R, Kuo TF, Cataldo N, Colrain IM. The effects of hormone replacement therapy on sleep-disordered breathing in postmenopausal women: a pilot study. *Sleep* 2003;26:163-168.

Moline ML, Broch L, Zak R. Sleep in women across the life cycle from adulthood through menopause. *Med Clin N Am* 2004;88:705-736.

Morin CM, Hauri PJ, Espie CA, Spielman AJ, Buysse DJ, Bootzin RR. Nonpharmacologic treatment of chronic insomnia: an American Academy of Sleep Medicine review. *Sleep* 1999;22:1134-1156.

National Sleep Foundation. *2007 Sleep in America Poll*. Washington, DC: National Sleep Foundation, 2007. Available at: http://www.sleepfoundation.org/site/c.huIXKjM0IxF/b.2574229/k.14DA/2007_Sleep_in_America_Poll.htm. Accessed September 12, 2007.

Orentreich N, Brind J, Rizer R, Vogelmen JH. Age changes and sex differences in serum dehydroepiandrosterone sulfate concentration throughout adulthood. *J Clin Endocrinol Metab* 1984;59:551-555.

Owens JF, Matthews KA. Sleep disturbance in healthy middle-aged women. *Maturitas* 1998;30:41-50.

Parry BL. Sleep disturbances at menopause are related to sleep disorders and anxiety symptoms [editorial]. *Menopause* 2007;14:812-814.

Polo-Kantola P, Erkkola R, Helenius H, Irjala K, Polo O. When does estrogen replacement therapy improve sleep quality? *Am J Obstet Gynecol* 1998;178:1002-1009.

Polo-Kantola P, Erkkola R, Irjala K, Pullinen S, Virtanen I, Polo O. Effect of short-term transdermal estrogen replacement therapy on sleep: a randomized, double-blind crossover trial in postmenopausal women. *Fertil Steril* 1999;71:873-880.

Resta O, Caratozzolo G, Pannacciulli N, et al. Gender, age and menopause effects on the prevalence and the characteristics of obstructive sleep apnea in obesity. *Eur J Clin Invest* 2003;33:1084-1089.

Sarti CD, Chiantera A, Graziottin A, et al, and Gruppo di Studio IperAOGOI. Hormone therapy and sleep quality in women around menopause. *Menopause* 2005;12:545-551.

Shahar E, Redline S, Young T, et al. Hormone replacement therapy and sleep-disordered breathing. *Am J Respir Crit Care Med* 2003;167:1186-1192.

Shaver J, Giblin E, Lentz M, Lee K. Sleep patterns and stability in perimenopausal women. *Sleep* 1988;11:556-561.

Singh NA, Clements KM, Fiatarone MA. A randomized controlled trial of the effect of exercise on sleep. *Sleep* 1997;20:95-101.

Soares CN, Murray BJ. Sleep disorders in women: clinical evidence and treatment strategies. *Psychiatr Clin N Am* 2006;29:1095-1113.

Spitzer RL, Terman M, Williams JB, et al. Jet lag: clinical features, validation of a new syndrome-specific scale, and lack of response to melatonin in a randomized, double-blind trial. *Am J Psychiatry* 1999;156:1392-1396.

van Diest R. Subjective sleep characteristics as coronary risk factors: their association with type A behavior and vital exhaustion. *J Psychosom Res* 1990;34:415-426.

Young T, Rabago D, Zgierska A, Austin D, Finn L. Objective and subjective sleep quality in premenopausal, perimenopausal, and postmenopausal women in the Wisconsin Sleep Cohort Study. *Sleep* 2003;26:667-672.

Headache

Brandes JL. The influence of estrogen on migraine: a systematic review. *JAMA* 2006;295:1824-1830.

Burstein R, Collins B, Jakubowski M. Defeating migraine pain with triptans: a race against the development of cutaneous allodynia. *Annals of Neurology* 2004;55:19-26.

Dahlof CG, Dimenas E. Migraine patients experience poorer subjective well-being/quality of life even between attacks. *Cephalalgia* 1995;15:31-36.

Goadsby PJ, Lipton RB, Ferrari MD. Migraine—current understanding and treatment. *N Engl J Med* 2002;4:257-270.

Headache Classification Subcommittee of the International Headache Society. The international classification of headache disorders, 2nd ed. *Cephalalgia* 2004;24(Suppl 1):1-150. Available at: http://216.25.100.131/ihscommon/guidelines/pdfs/ihc_II_main_no_print.pdf. Accessed September 25, 2007.

Lipton RB, Stewart WF, Diamond S, Diamond ML, Reed M. Prevalence and burden of migraine in the United States: data from the American Migraine Study II. *Headache* 2001;41:646-657.

Loder EW. Menstrual migraine: Pathophysiology, diagnosis and impact. *Headache* 2006;46(Suppl 2):S55-S60.

Loder EW, Martin VT. *Headache: A Guide for the Primary Care Physician*. Philadelphia: American College of Physicians, 2004.

MacGregor EA. Menstruation, sex hormones, and migraine. *Neurol Clin* 1997; 15:125-141.

MacGregor EA, Barnes D. Migraine in a menopause clinic. *Climacteric* 1999;2:218-223.

Mattsson P. Hormonal factors in migraine: a population-based study of women aged 40 to 74 years. *Headache* 2003;43:27-35.

Misakian AL, Langer RD, Bensenor IM, et al. Postmenopausal hormone therapy and migraine headache. *J Womens Health* 2003;12:1027-1036.

Moloney M. Migraines and the perimenopause. *Menopause Management* 2000;9:8-15.

Neri I, Granella F, Nappi R, Manzoni GC, Facchinetti F, Genazzani AR. Characteristics of headache at menopause: a clinico-epidemiologic study. *Maturitas* 1993;17:31-37.

The North American Menopause Society. Estrogen and progestogen use in peri- and postmenopausal women: March 2007 position statement of The North American Menopause Society. *Menopause* 2007;14:168-182.

Rasmussen BK, Jensen R, Schroll M, Olesen J. Epidemiology of headache in a general population—a prevalence study. *J Clin Epidemiol* 1991;44:1147-1157.

Silberstein SD, Lipton RB. *Headache in Clinical Practice*. Oxford, UK: Isis Medical Media, 1998.

Silberstein S, Merriam G. Sex hormones and headache 1999 (menstrual migraine). *Neurology* 1999;53(4 Suppl 1):S3-S13.

Silberstein, SD, Saper, JR, Fretag, FG. Migraine diagnosis and treatment. In: Silberstein SD Lipton RB, Dalessio DE, eds. *Wolff's Headache and Other Head Pain*, 7th ed. Oxford, UK: Oxford University Press, 2001:121-237.

Snow V, Weiss K, Wall EM, Mottur-Pilson C, for the American Academy of Family Physicians and the American College of Physicians-American Society of Internal Medicine. Pharmacologic management of acute attacks of migraine and prevention of migraine headache. *Ann Intern Med* 2002;137:840-849.

Stewart W, Schechter I, Rasmussen BK. Migraine prevalence: a review of population-based studies. *Neurology* 1994;44(Suppl):S17-S23.

Tepper SJ. Tailoring management strategies for the patient with menstrual migraine: focus on prevention and treatment. *Headache* 2006;46(Suppl 2): S61-S68.

Wang SJ, Fuh JL, Lu SR, Juang KD, Wang PH. Migraine prevalence during menopausal transition. *Headache* 2003;43:470-478.

Cognition

Aisen PS, Davis KL, Berg JD, et al. A randomized controlled trial of prednisone in Alzheimer's disease. *Neurology* 2000;54:588-593.

Aisen PS, Schafer KA, Grundman M, et al. Effects of rofecoxib or naproxen vs placebo on Alzheimer disease progression: a randomized controlled trial. *JAMA* 2003;289:2819-2826.

Almeida OP, Lautenschlager NT, Vasikaran S, Leedman P, Gelavis A, Flicker L. 20-week randomized controlled trial of estradiol replacement therapy for women aged 70 years and older: effect on mood, cognition and quality of life. *Neurobiol Aging* 2006;27:141-149.

Asthana S, Baker LD, Craft S, et al. High-dose estradiol improves cognition for women with AD: results of a randomized study. *Neurology* 2001;57:605-612.

Bagger YZ, Tankó LB, Alexandersen P, Qin G, Christiansen C. Early postmenopausal hormone replacement therapy may prevent cognitive impairment later in life. *Menopause* 2005;12:12-17.

Carlson MC, Zandi PP, Plassman BL, et al. Hormone replacement therapy and reduced cognitive decline in older women: the Cache County study. *Neurology* 2001;57:2210-2216.

Colcombe S, Kramer AF. Fitness effects on the cognitive function of older adults: a meta-analytic study. *Psychol Sci* 2003;14:125-130.

Cummings JL. Alzheimer's disease. *N Engl J Med* 2004;351:56-67.

Dunn JE, Weintraub S, Stoddard AM, Banks S. Serum alpha-tocopherol, concurrent and past vitamin E intake, and mild cognitive impairment. *Neurology* 2007;68:670-676.

Durga J, van Boxtel MP, Schouten EG, et al. Effect of 3-year folic acid supplementation on cognitive function in older adults in the FACIT trial: a randomized, double blind, controlled trial. *Lancet* 2007;369:208-216.

Espeland MA, Rapp SR, Shumaker SA, et al, for the Women's Health Initiative Memory Study Investigators. Conjugated equine estrogens and global cognitive function in postmenopausal women: Women's Health Initiative Memory Study. *JAMA* 2004;291:2959-2968.

File SE, Hartley DE, Elsabagh S, Duffy R, Wiseman H. Cognitive improvement after 6 weeks of soy supplements in postmenopausal women is limited to frontal lobe function. *Menopause* 2005;12:193-201.

Forette F, Seux ML, Staessen JA, et al, for the Systolic Hypertension in Europe Investigators. The prevention of dementia with antihypertensive treatment: new evidence from the Systolic Hypertension in Europe (Syst-Eur) study. *Arch Intern Med* 2002;162:2046-2052.

Fratiglioni L, Wang HX, Ericsson K, Mayton M, Winblad B. Influence of social network on occurrence of dementia: a community-based longitudinal study. *Lancet* 2000;344:1315-1319.

Freund-Levi Y, Eriksdotter-Jonhagen M, Cederholm T, et al. Omega-3 fatty acid treatment in 174 patients with mild to moderate Alzheimer disease: OmegAD study: a randomized double-blind trial. *Arch Neurol* 2006; 63:1402-1408.

Fuh JL, Wang SJ, Lee SJ, Lu SR, Juang KD. A longitudinal study of cognition change during early menopausal transition in a rural community. *Maturitas* 2006;53:447-453.

Gauthier S, Reisberg B, Zaudig M, et al. Mild cognitive impairment. *Lancet* 2006;367:1262-1270.

Grady D, Yaffe K, Kristof M, Lin F, Richards C, Barrett-Connor E. Effect of postmenopausal hormone therapy on cognitive function: the Heart and Estrogen/Progestin Replacement Study. *Am J Med* 2002;113:543-548.

Heart Protection Study Collaborative Group. MRC/BHF Heart Protection Study of antioxidant vitamin supplementation in 20,536 high-risk individuals: a randomised placebo-controlled trial. *Lancet* 2002;360:23-33.

Henderson VW. Estrogen-containing hormone therapy and Alzheimer's disease risk: understanding discrepant inferences from observational and experimental research. *Neuroscience* 2006;138:1031-1039.

Henderson VW, Benke KS, Green RC, Cupples LA, Farrer LA. Postmenopausal hormone therapy and Alzheimer's disease risk: interaction with age. *J Neurol Neurosurg Psychiatry* 2005;76:103-105.

Henderson VW, Dudley EC, Guthrie JR, Burger HG, Dennerstein L. Estrogen exposures and memory at midlife: a population-based study of women. *Neurology* 2003;60:1369-1371.

Henderson VW, Paganini-Hill A, Miller BL, et al. Estrogen for Alzheimer's disease in women: randomized, double-blind, placebo-controlled trial. *Neurology* 2000;54:295-301.

Henderson VW, Sherwin BB. Surgical versus natural menopause: cognitive issues. *Menopause* 2007;14(Suppl 1):S72-S79.

Hendrix SL, Wassertheil-Smoller S, Johnson KC, et al. Effects of conjugated equine estrogen on stroke in the Women's Health Initiative. *Circulation* 2006;113:2425-2434.

Joffe H, Hall JE, Gruber S, et al. Estrogen therapy selectively enhances prefrontal cognitive processes: a randomized, double-blind, placebo-controlled study with functional magnetic resonance imaging in perimenopausal and recently postmenopausal women. *Menopause* 2006;13:411-422.

Kalmijn S, van Boxtel MP, Ocke M, Verschuren WM, Kromhout D, Launer LJ. Dietary intake of fatty acids and fish in relation to cognitive performance at middle age. *Neurology* 2004;62:275-280.

Kang JH, Cook N, Manson J, Buring JE, Grodstein F. A randomized trial of vitamin E supplementation and cognitive function in women. *Arch Intern Med* 2006;166:2462-2468.

Kang JH, Weuve J, Grodstein F. Postmenopausal hormone therapy and risk of cognitive decline in community-dwelling aging women. *Neurology* 2004;63:101-107.

Katzman R. Education and the prevalence of dementia and Alzheimer's disease. *Neurology* 1993;43:13-20.

Kok HS, Kuh D, Cooper R, et al. Cognitive function across the life course and the menopausal transition in a British birth cohort. *Menopause* 2006;13:19-27.

Kreijkamp-Kaspers S, Kok L, Grobbee DE, et al. Effect of soy protein containing isoflavones on cognitive function, bone mineral density, and plasma lipids in postmenopausal women: a randomized controlled trial. *JAMA* 2004;292:65-74.

Kritz-Silverstein D, Barrett-Connor E. Hysterectomy, oophorectomy, and cognitive function in older women. *J Am Geriatr Soc* 2002;50:55-61.

Kritz-Silverstein D, von Mühlen D, Barrett-Connor E, Bressel MA. Isoflavones and cognitive function in older women: the SOy and Postmenopausal Health in Aging (SOPHIA) Study. *Menopause* 2003;10:196-202.

Kuller LH, Lopez OL, Jagust WJ, et al. Determinants of vascular dementia in the Cardiovascular Health Cognition Study. *Neurology* 2005;64:1548-1552.

Lord C, Buss C, Lupien SJ, Pruessner JC. Hippocampal volumes are larger in postmenopausal women using estrogen therapy compared to past users, never users and men: a possible window of opportunity effect. *Neurobiol Aging* 2006 Oct 6 [Epub ahead of print].

MacLennan AH, Henderson VW, Paine BJ, et al. Hormone therapy, timing of initiation, and cognition in women aged older than 60 years: the REMEMBER pilot study. *Menopause* 2006;13:28-36.

Maki PM, Gast MJ, Vieweg AJ, Burriss SW, Yaffe K. Hormone therapy in menopausal women with cognitive complaints: A randomized, double-blind trial. *Neurology* 2007;69:1322-1330.

McGuinness B, Todd S, Passmore P, Bullock R. The effects of blood pressure lowering on development of cognitive impairment and dementia in patients without apparent prior cerebrovascular disease. *Cochrane Database Syst Rev* 2006;2:CD004034.

McMahon JA, Green TJ, Skeaff CM, Knight RG, Mann JI, Williams SM. A controlled trial of homocysteine lowering and cognitive performance. *N Engl J Med* 2006;354:2764-2772.

Meyer PM, Powell LH, Wilson RS, et al. A population-based longitudinal study of cognitive functioning in the menopausal transition. *Neurology* 2003; 61:801-806.

Miller ER, III, Pastor-Barriuso R, Dalal D, Riemersma RA, Appel LJ, Guallar E. Meta-analysis: high-dosage vitamin E supplementation may increase all-cause mortality. *Ann Intern Med* 2005;142:37-46.

Mitchell ES, Woods NF. Midlife women's attributions about perceived memory changes: observations from the Seattle Midlife Women's Health Study. *J Womens Health Gender-Based Med* 2001;10:351-362.

Mulnard RA, Cotman CW, Kawas C, et al. Estrogen replacement therapy for treatment of mild to moderate Alzheimer disease: a randomized controlled trial. *JAMA* 2000;283:1007-1015.

The North American Menopause Society. Estrogen and progestogen use in peri- and postmenopausal women: March 2007 position statement of The North American Menopause Society. *Menopause* 2007;14:168-182.

Petersen RC, Thomas RG, Grundman M, et al. Vitamin E and donepezil for the treatment of mild cognitive impairment. *N Engl J Med* 2005;352:2379-2388.

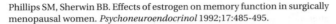

Phillips SM, Sherwin BB. Effects of estrogen on memory function in surgically menopausal women. *Psychoneuroendocrinol* 1992;17:485-495.

Polo-Kantola P, Portin R, Polo O, Helenuis H, Irjala K, Erkkola R. The effect of short-term estrogen replacement therapy on cognition: a randomized, double-blind, cross-over trial in postmenopausal women. *Obstet Gynecol* 1998;91:459-466.

Raman G, Tatsioni A, Chung M, et al. Heterogeneity and lack of good quality studies limit association between folate, vitamins B-6 and B-12, and cognitive function. *J Nutr* 2007;137:1789-1794.

Resnick SM, Maki PM, Rapp SR, et al. Effects of combination estrogen plus progestin hormone treatment on cognition and affect. *J Clin Endocrinol Metab* 2006;91:1802-1810.

Roberts RO, Cha RH, Knopman DS, Petersen RC, Rocca WA. Postmenopausal estrogen therapy and Alzheimer disease: overall negative findings. *Alzheimer Dis Assoc Disord* 2006;20:141-146.

Rozzini L, Chilovi BV, Bertoletti E, Conti M, Del Rio I, Trabucchi M, Padovani A. Angiotensin converting enzyme (ACE) inhibitors modulate the rate of progression of amnestic mild cognitive impairment. *Int J Geriatr Psychiatry* 2006;21:550-555.

Sano M, Ernesto C, Thomas RG, et al. A controlled trial of selegiline, alpha-tocopherol, or both as treatment for Alzheimer's disease. *N Engl J Med* 1997; 336:1216-1222.

Shaywitz SE, Naftolin F, Zelterman D, et al. Better oral reading and short-term memory in midlife, postmenopausal women taking estrogen. *Menopause* 2003;10:420-426.

Sherwin BB. Estrogen and cognitive function in women. *Endocr Rev* 2003; 24:133-151.

Shumaker SA, Legault C, Kuller L, et al, for the Women's Health Initiative Memory Study Investigators. Conjugated equine estrogens and incidence of probable dementia and mild cognitive impairment in postmenopausal women: Women's Health Initiative Memory Study. *JAMA* 2004;291:2947-2985.

Shumaker SA, Legault C, Rapp SR, et al, for the WHIMS Investigators. Estrogen plus progestin and the incidence of dementia and mild cognitive impairment in postmenopausal women: the Women's Health Initiative Memory Study: a randomized controlled trial. *JAMA* 2003;289:2651-2662.

Solomon PR, Adams F, Silver A, Zimmer J, DeVeaux R. Ginkgo for memory enhancement: a randomized controlled trial. *JAMA* 2002;288:835-840.

Stampfer MJ, Kang JH, Chen J, Cherry R, Grodstein F. Effects of moderate alcohol consumption on cognitive function in women. *N Engl J Med* 2005; 352:245-253.

Tzourio C, Anderson C, Chapman N, et al. Effects of blood pressure lowering with perindopril and indapamide therapy on dementia and cognitive decline in patients with cerebrovascular disease. *Arch Intern Med* 2003;163:1069-1075.

Viscoli CM, Brass LM, Kernan WN, Sarrel PM, Suissa S, Horwitz RI. Estrogen therapy and risk of cognitive decline: results from the Women's Estrogen for Stroke Trial (WEST). *Am J Obstet Gynecol* 2005;192:387-393.

Wassertheil-Smoller S, Hendrix S, Limacher M, et al. Effect of estrogen plus progestin on stroke in postmenopausal women: the Women's Health Initiative: a randomized trial. *JAMA* 2003;289:2673-2684.

Wengreen HJ, Munger RG, Corcoran CD, et al. Antioxidant intake and cognitive function of elderly men and women: the Cache County Study. *J Nutr Health Aging* 2007;11:230-237.

Wilson RS, Mendes De Leon CF, Barnes LL, et al. Participation in cognitively stimulating activities and risk of incident Alzheimer disease. *JAMA* 2002; 287:742-748.

Yaffe K, Barnes D, Nevitt M, et al. A prospective study of physical activity and cognitive decline in elderly women: women who walk. *Arch Intern Med* 2001;161:1703-1708.

Yaffe K, Clemons TE, McBee WL, Lendblad AS, for the Age-Related Eye Disease Study Research Group. *Neurology* 2004;63:1705-1707.

Yaffe K, Vittinghoff E, Ensrud KE, et al. Effects of ultra-low-dose transdermal estradiol on cognition and health-related quality of life. *Arch Neurol* 2006;63:945-950.

Zandi PP, Carlson MC, Plassman BL, et al, for the Cache County Memory Study Investigators. Hormone replacement therapy and incidence of Alzheimer disease in older women: the Cache County Study. *JAMA* 2002;288:2123-2129.

Psychological symptoms

Almeida OP, Lautenschlager NT, Vasikaran S, Leedman P, Gelavis A, Flicker L. A 20-week randomized controlled trial of estradiol replacement therapy for women aged 70 years and older: effect on mood, cognition and quality of life. *Neurobiol Aging* 2006;27:141-149.

Altshuler LL, Cohen LS, Moline ML, et al. Treatment of depression in women: a summary of the expert consensus guidelines. *J Psychiatr Pract* 2001;7:185-208.

American Psychiatric Association. *Diagnostic and Statistical Manual of Mental Disorders DSM-IV-TR*, 4th ed. Washington, DC: American Psychiatric Press, 2000.

Avis NE, Brambilla D, McKinlay SM, Vass K. A longitudinal analysis of the association between menopause and depression: results from the Massachusetts Women's Health Study. *Ann Epidemiol* 1994;4:214-220.

Avis NE, Crawford S, Stellato R, Longcope C. Longitudinal study of hormone levels and depression among women transitioning through menopause. *Climacteric* 2001;4:243-249.

Ballinger CB. Psychiatric aspects of menopause. *Br J Psychiatry* 1990; 156:773-787.

Bjorn I, Bixo M, Nojd KS, Nyberg S, Backstrom T. Negative mood changes during hormone replacement therapy: a comparison between two progestogens. *Am J Obstet Gynecol* 2000;183:1419-1426.

Borges LE, Andrade RP, Aldrighi JM, et al. Effect of a combination of ethinylestradiol 30 microg and drospireone 3 mg on tolerance, cycle control, general well-being and fluid-related symptoms in women with premenstrual disorders requesting contraception. *Contraception* 2006;74:446-450.

Boswell EB, Stoudemire A. Major depression in the primary care setting. *Am J Med* 1996;101:3S-9S.

Bromberger JT, Matthews KA. A longitudinal study of the effects of pessimism, trait anxiety, and life stress on depressive symptoms in middle-aged women. *Psychol Aging* 1996;11:207-213.

Bromberger JT, Matthews KA, Schott LL, et al. Depressive symptoms during the menopausal transition: The Study of Women's Health Across the Nation (SWAN). *J Affect Disord* 2007;[Epub ahead of print].

Burstein R, Collins B, Jakubowski M. Defeating migraine pain with triptans: a race against the development of cutaneous allodynia. *Annals of Neurology* 2004;55:19-26.

Cohen LS, Soares CN, Poitras JR, Prouty J, Alexander AB, Shifren JL. Short-term use of estradiol for depression in perimenopausal and postmenopausal women: a preliminary report. *Am J Psychiatry* 2003;160:1519-1522.

Cohen LS, Soares CN, Vitonis AF, Otto MW, Harlow BL. Risk for new onset of depression during the menopausal transition: The Harvard Study of Moods and Cycles. *Arch Gen Psychiatry* 2006;63:385-390.

Dahlof CG, Dimenas E. Migraine patients experience poorer subjective well-being/quality of life even between attacks. *Cephalalgia* 1995;15:31-36.

Dennerstein L, Dudley EC, Hopper JL, Guthrie JR, Burger HG. A prospective population-based study of menopausal symptoms. *Obstet Gynecol* 2000; 96:351-358.

Diem SJ, Blackwell TL, Stone KL, et al. Use of antidepressants and rates of hip bone loss in older women: the Study of Osteoporotic Fractures. *Arch Intern Med* 2007;167:1240-1245.

Ditkoff LC, Crary WG, Cristo M, Lobo RA. Estrogen improves psychological function in asymptomatic postmenopausal women. *Obstet Gynaecol* 1991; 178:991-995.

Dunkin J, Rasgon N, Wagner-Steh K, David S, Altshuler L, Rapkin A. Reproductive events modify the effects of estrogen replacement therapy on cognition in healthy postmenopausal women. *Psychoneuroendocrinology* 2005;30:284-296.

Freeman EW, Sammel MD, Lin H, Nelson DB. Associations of hormones and menopausal status with depressed mood in women with no history of depression. *Arch Gen Psychiatry* 2006;63:375-382.

Groeneveld FP, Bareman FP, Barentsen R, et al. Vasomotor symptoms and well being in the climacteric years. *Maturitas* 1996;23:293-299.

Halbreich U. Role of estrogen in postmenopausal depression. *Neurology* 1997;48(Suppl):S16-S19.

Halbreich U, Rojansky N, Palter S, Tworek H, Hissin P, Wang K. Estrogen augments serotonergic activity in postmenopausal women. *Biol Psychiatry* 1995;37:434-441.

Hallstrom T, Samuelsson S. Mental health in the climacteric: the longitudinal study of women in Gothenburg. *Acta Obstet Gynecol Scand* 1985;130(Suppl):13-18.

Hay AG, Bancroft J, Johnstone EC. Affective symptoms in women attending a menopause clinic. *Br J Psychiatry* 1994;164:513-516.

Henderson VW. *Hormone Therapy and the Brain: A Clinical Perspective on the Role of Estrogen.* New York, NY: Parthenon Publishing, 2000.

Henderson VW, Dudley EC, Guthrie JR, Burger HG, Dennerstein L. Estrogen exposures and memory at midlife: a population-based study of women. *Neurology* 2003;60:1369-1371.

Hlatky MA, Boothroyd D, Vittinghoff E, Sharp P, Whooley MA, for the Heart and Estrogen/Progetin Replacement Study (HERS) Research Group. Quality-of-life and depressive symptoms in postmenopausal women after receiving hormone therapy: results from the Heart and Estrogen/Progestin Replacement Study (HERS) trial. *JAMA* 2002;287:591-597.

Hunter M. The south-east England longitudinal study of the climacteric and postmenopause. *Maturitas* 1992;14:117-126.

Judd LL, Rapaport MH, Paulus MP, Brown JL. Subsyndromal symptomatic depression: a new mood disorder? *J Clin Psychiatry* 1994;55:18-28.

Kaufert PA, Gilbert P, Tate R. The Manitoba Project: a re-examination of the link between menopause and depression. *Maturitas* 1992;14:143-155.

Kessler RC. Gender differences in major depression. In: Frank E, ed. *Gender and Its Effects on Psychopathology.* Washington, DC: American Psychiatric Press, 2000.

Klein P, Versi E, Herzog A. Mood and menopause. *Br J Obstet Gynaecol* 1999;106:1-4.

Kuh DL, Wadsworth M, Hardy R. Women's health in midlife: the influence of the menopause, social factors and health in earlier life. *Br J Obstet Gynaecol* 1997;104:923-933.

Landau C, Milan FB. Assessment and treatment of depression during the menopause: a preliminary report. *Menopause* 1996;3:201-207.

Lyndaker C, Hulton L. The influence of age on symptoms of perimenopause. *J Obstet Gynecol Neonatal Nurs* 2004;33:340-347.

MacGregor EA. Menstruation, sex hormones, and migraine. *Neurol Clin* 1997;15:125-141.

Maoz B, Shiber A, Lazer S, Kopernik G. The prevalence of psychological distress among postmenopausal women attending a menopausal clinic and the effect of hormone replacement therapy on their mental state. *Menopause* 1994;1:137-141.

Matthews KA, Kuller LH, Wing RR, Meilahn EN. Biobehavioral aspects of menopause: lessons from the Healthy Women Study. *Exp Gerontol* 1994; 29:337-342.

McKinlay JB, McKinlay SM, Brambilla D. The relative contribution of endocrine changes and social circumstances to depression in mid-aged women. *J Health Soc Behav* 1987;28:345-363.

Meyer PM, Powell LH, Wilson RS, et al. A population-based longitudinal study of cognitive functioning in the menopausal transition. *Neurology* 2003;61:801-806.

Morrison MF, Kallan MJ, Ten Have T, Katz I, Tweedy K, Battistini M. Lack of efficacy of estradiol for depression in postmenopausal women: a randomized, controlled trial. *Biol Psychiatry* 2004;55:406-412.

Nathorst-Boos J, von Schoultz B. Psychological reactions and sexual life after hysterectomy with and without oophorectomy. *Gynecol Obstet Invest* 1992;4:97-101.

The North American Menopause Society. Clinical challenges of perimenopause: consensus opinion of The North American Menopause Society. *Menopause* 2000;7:5-13.

Ozturk O, Eraslan D, Elbe Mete H, Ozsener S. The risk factors and symptomatology of perimenopausal depression. *Maturitas* 2006;55:180-186.

Palinkas L, Barrett-Connor E. Estrogen use and depressive symptoms in postmenopausal women. *Obstet Gynecol* 1992;80:30-36.

Panay N, Studd JW. The psychotherapeutic effects of estrogens. *Gynecol Endocrinol* 1998;12:353-365.

Parikh SV, Lam RW, for the CANMAT Depression Work Group. Clinical guidelines for the treatment of depressive disorders: I. Definitions, prevalence, and health burden. *Can J Psychiatry* 2001;46(Suppl):13S-20S.

Pearce J, Hawton K, Blake F. Psychological and sexual symptoms associated with the menopause and the effects of hormone replacement therapy. *Br J Psychiatry* 1995;167:163-173.

Pearlstein TB. Hormones and depression: what are the facts about premenstrual syndrome, menopause, and hormone replacement therapy? *Am J Obstet Gynecol* 1995;173:646-653.

Pearlstein TB, Bachmann GA, Zacur HA, Yonkers KA. Treatment of premenstrual dysphoric disorder with a new drospirenone-containing oral contraceptive formation. *Contraception* 2005;72:414-421.

Rapkin AJ, Mikacich JA, Moatakef-Imani B, Rasgon N. The clinical nature and formal diagnosis of premenstrual, postpartum, and perimenopausal affective disorders. *Curr Psychiatry Rep* 2002;4:419-428.

Rasgon NL, Altshuler LL, Fairbanks L. Estrogen-replacement therapy for depression. *Am J Psychiatry* 2001;158:1738.

Rasgon NL, Dunkin J, Fairbanks L, et al. Estrogen and response to sertraline in postmenopausal women with major depressive disorder: a pilot study. *J Psychiatr Res* 2007;41:338-343.

Rubinow DR, Roca CA, Schmidt PJ. Estrogens and depression in women. In: Lobo RA, ed. *Treatment of the Postmenopausal Woman: Basic and Clinical Aspects,* 3rd ed. San Diego, CA: Academic Press, 2007:307-327.

Rubinow DR, Schmidt PJ. Androgens, brain, and behavior. *Am J Psychiatry* 1996;153:974-984.

Rubinow DR, Schmidt PJ, Roca CA. Estrogen-serotonin interactions: implications for affective regulation. *Biol Psychiatry* 1998;44:839-850.

Schmidt PJ, Daly RC, Bloch M, et al. Dehydroepiandrosterone monotherapy in midlife-onset major and minor depression. *Arch Gen Psychiatry* 2005; 62:154-162.

Schmidt PJ, Nieman L, Danaceau MA, Tobin MB, Roca CA, Murphy JH. Estrogen replacement in perimenopause-related depression: a preliminary report. *Am J Obstet Gynecol* 2000;183:414-420.

Schmidt PJ, Rubinow DR. Menopause-related affective disorders: a justification for further study. *Am J Psychiatry* 1991;148:844-852.

Schmidt PJ, Rubinow DR. Neuroregulatory role of gonadal steroids in humans. *Psychopharmacol Bull* 1997;33:219-220.

Schmidt PJ, Rubinow DR. Reproductive ageing, sex steroids and depression. *J Br Menopause Soc* 2006;12:178-185.

Sherwin BB. Affective changes with estrogen and androgen replacement therapy in surgically menopausal women. *J Affect Disord* 1988;14:177-187.

Sherwin BB. Estrogen and cognitive function in women. *Endocr Rev* 2003; 24:133-151.

Sherwin BB. Hormones and the brain: Canadian consensus on menopause and osteoporosis. *J SOGC* 2001;23:1102-1104.

Sherwin BB. Hormones, mood, and cognitive functioning in postmenopausal women. *Obstet Gynecol* 1996;87(Suppl):S20-S26.

Sherwin BB. Impact of the changing hormonal milieu on psychologic functioning. In: Lobo RA, ed. *Treatment of the Postmenopausal Woman: Basic and Clinical Aspects*, 3rd ed. San Diego, CA: Academic Press, 2007: 217-226.

Soares CN, Almeida OP, Joffe H, Cohen LS. Efficacy of estradiol for the treatment of depressive disorders in perimenopausal women: a double-blind, randomized, placebo-controlled trial. *Arch Gen Psychiatry* 2001;58:529-534.

Steiner M, Romano SJ, Babcock S, et al. The efficacy of fluoxetine in improving physical symptoms associated with premenstrual dysphoric disorder. *BJOG* 2001;108:462-468.

Stewart DE, Boydell K, Derzko C, Marshall V. Psychologic distress during the menopausal years in women attending a menopause clinic. *Int J Psychiatry Med* 1992;22:213-220.

Stewart W, Schechter I, Rasmussen BK. Migraine prevalence: a review of population-based studies. *Neurology* 1994;44(Suppl):S17-S23.

Studd JWW, Smith RNJ. Estrogens and depression in women. *Menopause* 1994;1:33-37.

Su TP, Schmidt PJ, Danaceau MA, et al. Fluoxetine in the treatment of premenstrual dysphoria. *Neuropsychopharmacology* 1997;16:346-356.

US Preventive Services Task Force. Screening for depression: recommendations and rationale. *Ann Intern Med* 2002;136:760-764.

Utian WH, Boggs PP. The North American Menopause Society 1998 Menopause Survey. Part I. Postmenopausal women's perceptions about menopause and midlife. *Menopause* 1999;6:122-128.

Wassertheil-Smoller S, Shumaker S, Ockene J, et al. Depression and cardiovascular sequelae in postmenopausal women: the Women's Health Initiative (WHI). *Arch Intern Med* 2004;164:289-298.

Woods NF, Mitchell ES. Patterns of depressed mood in midlife women: observations from the Seattle Midlife Women's Health Study. *Res Nurs Health* 1996;19:111-123.

Woods NF, Mitchell ES, Adams C. Memory functioning among midlife women: observations from the Seattle Midlife Women's Health Study. *Menopause* 2000;7:257-265.

Wren BG, Champion SM, Willetts K, Manga RZ, Eden JA. Transdermal progesterone and its effect on vasomotor symptoms, blood lipid levels, bone metabolic markers, moods, and quality of life for postmenopausal women. *Menopause* 2003;10:13-18.

Wroolie TE, Williams KE, Keller J, et al. Mood and Neuropsychological changes in women with mid-life depression treated with escitalopram. *J Clin Psychopharmacol* 2006;26:361-366.

Yonkers KA, Brown C, Pearlstein TB, Foegh M, Sampson-Landers C, Rapkin A. Efficacy of a new low-dose oral contraceptive with drospirenone in premenstrual dysphoric disorder. *Obstet Gyncol* 2005;106:492-501.

Young EA, Kornstein SG, Harvey AT, et al. Influences of hormone-based contraception on depressive symptoms in premenopausal women with major depression. *Psychoneuroendocrinology* 2007;32:843-853.

Zweifel JE, O'Brien WH. A meta-analysis of the effect of hormone replacement therapy upon depressed mood. *Psychoneuroendocrinol* 1997;22:189-212.

Vulvovaginal symptoms

The American College of Obstetricians and Gynecologists. Endometrial ablation. ACOG Practice Bulletin No 81. *Obstet Gynecol* 2007;109:1233-1248.

The American College of Obstetricians and Gynecologists. Genitourinary tract changes. *Obstet Gynecol* 2004;104(Suppl 4):56S-61S.

The American College of Obstetricians and Gynecologists. Vulvodynia. ACOG Committee Opinion No. 345. *Obstet Gynecol* 2006;108:1049-1052.

The Arimidex, Tamoxifen, Alone or in Combination Trialists' Group. Comprehensive side-effect profile of anastrozole and tamoxifen as adjuvant treatment for early-stage breast cancer: long-term safety analysis of the ATAC trial. *Lancet Oncol* 2006;7:633-643.

Ayton RA, Darling GM, Murkies AL, et al. A comparative study of safety and efficacy of continuous low dose oestradiol released from a vaginal ring compared with conjugated equine oestrogen vaginal cream in the treatment of postmenopausal urogenital atrophy. *Br J Obstet Gynaecol* 1996;103:351-358.

Bachmann G. Urogenital ageing: an old problem newly recognized. *Maturitas* 1995;22(Suppl):S1-S5.

Bachmann G, Cheng RF, Rovner E. Vulvovaginal complaints. In: Lobo RA, ed. *Treatment of the Postmenopausal Woman: Basic and Clinical Aspects*, 3rd ed. San Diego, CA: Academic Press, 2007:263-269.

Bachmann GA, Notelovitz M, Gonzalez SJ, Thompson C, Morecraft BA. Vaginal dryness in menopausal women: clinical characteristics and nonhormonal treatment. *Clin Pract Sex* 1991;7:25-32.

Barentsen R, van de Weijer PH, Schram JH. Continuous low dose estradiol released from a vaginal ring versus estriol vaginal cream for urogenital atrophy. *Eur J Obstet Gynecol Reprod Biol* 1997;71:73-80.

Bruner DW, Lanciano R, Keegan M, Corn B, Martin E, Hanks GE. Vaginal stenosis and sexual function following intracavitary radiation for the treatment of cervical and endometrial carcinoma. *Int J Radiat Oncol Biol Phys* 1993;27:825-830.

Bygdeman M, Swahn ML. Replens versus dienoestrol cream in the symptomatic treatment of vaginal atrophy in postmenopausal women. *Maturitas* 1996;23:259-263.

Byyny RL, Speroff L, eds. External genitalia after menopause. In: *A Clinical Guide for the Care of Older Women: Primary and Preventive Care*, 2nd ed. Baltimore, MD: Williams & Wilkins, 1996:385-395.

Casper F, Petri E. Local treatment of urogenital atrophy with an estradiol-releasing vaginal ring: a comparative and a placebo-controlled multicenter study. Vaginal Ring Study Group. *Int Urogynecol J Pelvic Floor Dysfunct* 1999;10:171-176.

Cella D, Fallowfield L, Barker P, Locker G, Howell A, for the ATC Trialists Group. Quality of life of postmenopausal women in the ATAC ("Arimidex," Tamoxifen, Alone or in Combination) trial after completion of 5 years' adjuvant treatment for early stage breast cancer. *Breast Cancer Res Treat* 2006;100:273-284.

Chen GD, Oliver RH, Leung BS, Lin LY, Yeh J. Estrogen receptor alpha and beta expression in the vaginal walls and uterosacral ligaments of premenopausal and postmenopausal women. *Fertil Steril* 1999;71:1099-1102.

Crandall C. Vaginal estrogen preparations: a review of safety and efficacy for vaginal atrophy. *J Womens Health* 2002;11:857-877.

Davies GC, Huster WJ, Lu Y, Plouffe L, Lakshmanan M. Adverse events reported by postmenopausal women in controlled trials with raloxifene. *Obstet Gynecol* 1999;93:558-565.

Davila GW, Singh A, Karapanagiotou I, et al. Are women with urogenital atrophy symptomatic? *Am J Obstet Gynecol* 2003;188:382-388.

Day R, Ganz PA, Costantino JP, Cronin WM, Wickerham L, Fisher B. Health-related quality of life and tamoxifen in breast cancer prevention: a report from the National Surgical Adjuvant Breast and Bowel Project P-1 study. *J Clin Oncol* 1999;17:2669-2695.

Drutz H, Bachmann G, Bouchard C, Morris B. Towards a better recognition of urogenital aging. *J SOGC* 1996;18:1017-1031.

Dugal R, Hesla K, Sordal T, Aase KH, Lilleeidet O, Wickstrom E. Comparison of usefulness of estradiol vaginal tablets and estriol vagitories for treatment of vaginal atrophy. *Acta Obstet Gynecol Scand* 2000;79:293-297.

Eriksen B. A randomized, open, parallel-group study on the preventive effect of an estradiol-releasing vaginal ring (Estring) on recurrent urinary tract infection in postmenopausal women. *Am J Obstet Gynecol* 1999;180:1072-1079.

Eriksen PS, Rasmussen H. Low-dose 17β-estradiol vaginal tablets in the treatment of atrophic vaginitis: a double-blind placebo controlled study. *Eur J Obstet Gynecol Reprod Biol* 1992;44:137-144.

Fallowfield L, Cella D, Cuzick J, Francis S, Locker G, Howell A. Quality of life of postmenopausal women in the Arimidex, Tamoxifen, Alone or in Combination (ATAC) adjuvant breast cancer trial. *J Clin Oncol* 2004;22:4261-4271.

Foidart JM, Vervliet J, Buytaert P. Efficacy of sustained-release vaginal oestriol in alleviating urogenital and systemic climacteric complaints. *Maturitas* 1991;13:99-107.

Foster DC, Palmer M, Marks J. Effect of vulvovaginal estrogen on sensorimotor response of the lower genital tract: a randomized clinical trial. *Obstet Gynecol* 1999;94:232-237.

Gorodeski GI. Vaginal-cervical epithelial permeability decreases after menopause. *Fertil Steril* 2001;76:753-761.

Greendale GA, Zibecchi L, Petersen L, Ouslander JG, Kahn B, Ganz PA. Development and validation of a physical examination scale to assess vaginal atrophy and inflammation. *Climacteric* 1999;2:197-204.

Haefner HK, Collins ME, Davis GD, et al. The vulvodynia guideline. *J Low Genit Tract Dis* 2005;9:40-51.

Handa VL, Bachus KE, Johnston WW, Robboy SJ, Hammond CB. Vaginal administration of low-dose conjugated estrogens: systemic absorption and effects on the endometrium. *Obstet Gynecol* 1994;84:215-218.

Henriksson L, Stjernquist M, Boquist L, Alander U, Selinus I. A comparative multicenter study of the effects of continuous low-dose estradiol released from a new vaginal ring versus estriol vaginal pessaries in postmenopausal women with symptoms and signs of urogenital atrophy. *Am J Obstet Gynecol* 1994;171:624-632.

Hillier SL, Lau RJ. Vaginal microflora in postmenopausal women who have not received estrogen replacement therapy. *Clin Infect Dis* 1997;25(Suppl):S123-S126.

Johnson S. Canadian consensus on menopause and osteoporosis: urogenital health. *J SOGC* 2001;23:973-977.

Johnston SL, Farrell SA, Bouchard C, et al. The detection and management of vaginal atrophy. *J Obstet Gynaecol Can* 2004;26:503-515.

Keil K. Urogenital atrophy: diagnosis, sequelae, and management. *Curr Womens Health Rep* 2002;2:305-311.

Land SR, Wickerham DL, Costantino JP, et al. Patient-reported symptoms and quality of life during treatment with tamoxifen or raloxifene for breast cancer prevention: the NSABP Study of Tamoxifen and Raloxifene (STAR) P-2 trial. *JAMA* 2006;295:2742-2751.

Lotery HE, McClure N, Galask RP. Vulvodynia. *Lancet* 2004;363:1058-1060.

Manonai J, Theppisai U, Suthutvoravut S, Udomsubpayakul U, Chittacharoen A. The effect of estradiol vaginal tablet and conjugated estrogen cream on urogenital symptoms in postmenopausal women: a comparative study. *J Obstet Gynaecol Res* 2001;27:255-260.

Michlewitz H. Benign vulvar disorders. In: Carlson KJ, Eisenstat SA, Frigoletto Jr FD, Schiff I, eds. *Primary Care of Women*. New York, NY: Mosby, 1995: 226-229.

Milsom I, Arvidsson L, Ekelund P, Molander U, Eriksson O. Factors influencing vaginal cytology, pH and bacterial flora in elderly women. *Acta Obstet Gynecol Scand* 1993;72:286-291.

Nachtigall L. Clinical trial of the estradiol vaginal ring in the U.S. *Maturitas* 1995;22(Suppl):S43-S47.

Nilsson K, Risberg B, Heimer G. The vaginal epithelium in the postmenopause—cytology, histology and pH as methods of assessment. *Maturitas* 1995;21:51-56.

The North American Menopause Society. Estrogen and progestogen use in peri- and postmenopausal women: March 2007 position statement of The North American Menopause Society. *Menopause* 2007;14:168-182.

The North American Menopause Society. The role of local vaginal estrogen for treatment of vaginal atrophy in postmenopausal women: 2007 position statement of The North American Menopause Society. *Menopause* 2007; 14:357-369.

Notelovitz M. Estrogen therapy in the management of problems associated with urogenital ageing: a simple diagnostic test and the effect of the route of hormone administration. *Maturitas* 1995(Suppl 22):S31-S33.

Pandit L, Ouslander JG. Postmenopausal vaginal atrophy and atrophic vaginitis. *Am J Med Sci* 1997;314:228-231.

Parsons A, Merritt D, Rosen A, Heath H, Siddhantis S, Plouffe L. Effect of raloxifene on the response to conjugated estrogen vaginal cream or nonhormonal moisturizers in postmenopausal vaginal atrophy. *Obstet Gynecol* 2003;101:346-352.

Rigg LA, Hermann H, Yen SSC. Absorption of estrogens from vaginal creams. *N Engl J Med* 1978;298:195-197.

Rioux JE, Devlin MC, Gelfand MM, Steinberg WM, Hepburn DS. 17β-estradiol vaginal tablet versus conjugated equine estrogen vaginal cream to relieve menopausal atrophic vaginitis. *Menopause* 2000;7:156-161.

Santen RJ, Pinkerton JV, Conaway M, et al. Treatment of urogenital atrophy with low-dose estradiol: preliminary results. *Menopause* 2002;9:179-187.

Scheinfeld N. The role of gabapentin in treating disease with cutaneous manifestations and pain. *Int J Dermatol* 2003;42:491-495.

Simunic V, Banovic I, Ciglar S, Jeren L, Pavicic Baldani D, Sprem M. Local estrogen treatment in patients with urogenital symptoms. *Int J Gynaecol Obstet* 2003;82:187-197.

Smith P, Heimer G, Lindskog M, Ulmsten U. Oestradiol-releasing vaginal ring for the treatment of postmenopausal urogenital atrophy. *Maturitas* 1993;16:145-154.

Sobel JD, Faro S, Force RW, et al. Vulvovaginal candidiasis: epidemiologic, diagnostic, and therapeutic considerations. *Am J Obstet Gynecol* 1998; 178:203-211.

Society of Obstetricians and Gynaecologists of Canada. SOCG clinical practice guidelines. The detection and management of vaginal atrophy. Number 145, May 2004. *Int J Gynaecol Obstet* 2005;88:222-228.

Suckling J, Lethaby A, Kennedy R. Local oestrogen for vaginal atrophy in postmenopausal women. *Cochrane Database Syst Rev* 2006;4:CD001500.

Tourgeman DE, Gentzchein E, Stanczyk FZ, Paulson RJ. Serum and tissue hormone levels of vaginally and orally administered estradiol. *Am J Obstet Gynecol* 1999;180:1480-1483.

Tourgeman DE, Slater CC, Stanczyk FZ, Paulson RJ. Endocrine and clinical effects of micronized estradiol administered vaginally or orally. *Fertil Steril* 2001;75:200-202.

Utian WH, Shoupe D, Bachmann G, Pinkerton JV, Pickar JH. Relief of vasomotor symptoms and vaginal atrophy with lower doses of conjugated equine estrogens and medroxyprogesterone acetate. *Fertil Steril* 2001; 75:1065-1079.

Vogel VG, Costantino JP, Wickerham DL, et al, for the National Surgical Adjuvant Breast and Bowel Project. Effects of tamoxifen vs raloxifene on the risk of developing invasive breast cancer and other disease outcomes: the NSABP Study of Tamoxifen and Raloxifene (STAR) P-2 trial. *JAMA* 2006;295:2727-2741.

Weisberg E, Ayton R, Darling G, et al. Endometrial and vaginal effects of low-dose estradiol delivered by vaginal ring or vaginal tablet. *Climacteric* 2005;8:83-92.

Whelan TJ, Pritchard KI. Managing patients on endocrine therapy: focus on quality-of-life issues. *Clin Canc Res* 2006;12(Suppl 3):S1056-S1060.

Willhite LA, O'Connell MB. Urogenital atrophy: prevention and treatment. *Pharmacotherapy* 2001;21:464-480.

Sexual function effects

The American College of Obstetricians and Gynecologists. *Clinical Updates in Women's Health Care: Sexuality and Sexual Disorders*. Washington, DC: American College of Obstetricians and Gynecologists, 2003.

American Psychiatric Association, Task Force on DSM-IV. *Diagnostic and Statistical Manual of Mental Disorders DSM-IV-TR*, 4th ed. Arlington, VA: American Psychiatric Association, 2000.

Andersen BL, Cyranowski JM. Women's sexuality: behaviors, responses and individual differences. *J Consult Clin Psychol* 1995;63:891-906.

Andrews WC. Approaches to taking a sexual history. *J Womens Health Gend Based Med* 2000;9(Suppl):S21-S24.

Avis NE, Stellato R, Crawford S, Johannes C, Longcope C. Is there an association between menopause status and sexual functioning? *Menopause* 2000;7:297-309.

Bachmann GA. Influence of menopause on sexuality. *Int J Fertil Menopausal Stud* 1995;40(Suppl):16-22.

Bachmann G, Bancroft J, Braunstein G, et al. Female androgen insufficiency: the Princeton consensus statement on definition, classification, and assessment. *Fertil Steril* 2002;77:660-665.

Basson R, ed. Update on sexuality at menopause and beyond: normative, adaptive, problematic, dysfunctional. *Menopause* 2004;11(2 Pt 2):707-788.

Basson R. Female sexual response: the role of drugs in the management of sexual dysfunction. *Obstet Gynecol* 2001;98:350-353.

Basson R, Berman J, Burnett A, et al. Report of the international consensus and development conference on female sexual dysfunction: definitions and classifications. *J Urol* 2000;163:888-893.

Buckler HM, Robertson WR, Wu FC. Which androgen replacement therapy for women? *J Clin Endocrinol Metab* 1998;83:3920-3924.

Buster JE, Casson PR. Where androgens come from, what controls them, and whether to replace them. In: Lobo RA, ed. *Treatment of the Postmenopausal Woman: Basic and Clinical Aspects*, 2nd ed. Philadelphia, PA: Lippincott Williams & Wilkins, 1999:141-154.

Buster JE, Kingsberg SA, Aguirre O, et al. Testosterone patch for low sexual desire in surgically menopausal women: a randomized trial. *Obstet Gynecol* 2005;105:944-952.

Caruso S, Intelisano G, Lupo L, Agnello C. Premenopausal women affected by sexual arousal disorder treated with sildenafil: a double-blind, cross-over, placebo-controlled study. *BJOG* 2001;108:623-628.

Daker-White G. Reliable and valid self-report outcome measures in sexual (dys)function: a systematic review. *Arch Sex Behav* 2002;31:197-209.

Davis SR, Davison SL, Donath S, Bell RJ. Circulating androgen levels and self-reported sexual function in women. *JAMA* 2005;294:91-96.

Davison SL, Bell R, Donath S, Montalto JG, Davis SR. Androgen levels in adult females: changes with age, menopause, and oophorectomy. *J Clin Endocrinol Metab* 2005;90:3847-3853.

Dennerstein L, Dudley EC, Hopper JL, Burger H. Sexuality, hormones and the menopausal transition. *Maturitas* 1997;26:83-93.

Dennerstein L, Lehert P, Burger H, Dudley E. Factors affecting sexual functioning of women in the mid-life years. *Climacteric* 1999;2:254-262.

Dessole S, Rubattu G, Ambrosini G, et al. Efficacy of low-dose intravaginal estriol on urogenital aging in postmenopausal women. *Menopause* 2004; 11:49-56.

Ferguson DM, Steidle CP, Singh GS, Alexander JS, Crosby MG. Randomized, placebo-controlled, double blind, crossover design trial of the efficacy and safety of Zestra for Women with and without female sexual arousal disorder. *J Sex Marital Ther* 2003;29(Suppl):33-44.

Gassman A, Santoro N. The influence of menopausal hormone changes on sexuality: current knowledge and recommendations for practice. *Menopause* 1994;1:91-98.

Gracia CR, Sammel MD, Freeman EW, Liu L, Hollander L, Nelson DB. Predictors of decreased libido in women during the late reproductive years. *Menopause* 2004;11:144-155.

Graves G, Lea R, Bourgeois-Law G. Menopause and sexual function: Canadian consensus on menopause and osteoporosis. *J SOGC* 2001;23:849-852.

Hallstrom T, Samuelsson S. Changes in women's sexual desire in middle life: the longitudinal study of women in Gothenburg. *Arch Sex Behav* 1990; 19:259-268.

Hawton K, Gath D, Day A. Sexual function in a community sample of middle-aged women with partners: effects of age, marital, socioeconomic, psychiatric, gynecological and menopausal factors. *Arch Sex Behav* 1994;23:375-395.

Hunter MS. Emotional well-being, sexual behaviour and hormone replacement therapy. *Maturitas* 1990;12:299-314.

Judd HL, Lucas WE, Yen SS. Effect of oophorectomy on circulating testosterone and androstenedione levels in patients with endometrial cancer. *Am J Obstet Gynecol* 1974;118:793-798.

Kaunitz AM. The role of androgens in menopausal hormonal replacement. *Endocrinol Metab Clin North Am* 1997;26:391-397.

Kolakowska T. The clinical course of primary recurrent depression in pharmacologically treated female patients. *Br J Psychiatry* 1975;126:336-345.

Laan E, Everaerd W, Van der Velde J, Geer JH. Determinants of subjective experience of sexual arousal in women: feedback from genital arousal and erotic stimulus content. *Psychophysiology* 1995;32:444-451.

Laumann EO, Paik A, Rosen RC. Sexual dysfunction in the United States: prevalence and predictors [erratum in: *JAMA* 1999;281:1117]. *JAMA* 1999;281:537-544.

Lieblum S, Koochaki P, Rodenberg C, Barton L, Rosen R. Hypoactive sexual desire disorder in postmenopausal women: US results from the Women's International Study of Health and Sexuality (WISHeS). *Menopause* 2006: 13:46-56.

Lobitz WC, Lobitz GK. Resolving the sexual intimacy paradox: a developmental model for the treatment of sexual desire disorders. *J Sex Marital Ther* 1996;22:71-84.

Lotery HE, McClure N, Galask RP. Vulvodynia. *Lancet* 2004;363:1058-1060.

Marwick C. Survey says patients expect little physician help on sex. *JAMA* 1999;281:2173-2174.

Meston CM, Derogatis LR. Validated instruments for assessing female sexual function. *J Sex Marital Ther* 2002;28(Suppl):155-164.

Montgomery JC, Appleby L, Brincat M, et al. Effect of oestrogen and testosterone implants on psychological disorders in the climacteric. *Lancet* 1987;1:297-299.

Nathorst-Boos J, von Schoultz B. Psychological reactions and sexual life after hysterectomy with and without oophorectomy. *Gynecol Obstet Invest* 1992;4:97-101.

The North American Menopause Society. The role of testosterone therapy in postmenopausal women: position statement of the North American Menopause Society. *Menopause* 2005;12:497-511.

Phillips NA, Rosen RC. Menopause and sexuality. In: Lobo RA, ed. *Treatment of the Postmenopausal Woman: Basic and Clinical Aspects*, 2nd ed. Philadelphia, PA: Lippincott Williams & Wilkins, 1999:437-443.

Rosen R, Brown C, Heiman J, et al. The Female Sexual Function Index (FSFI): a multidimensional self-report instrument for the assessment of female sexual function. *J Sex Marital Ther* 2000;26:191-208.

Sarrel PM. Sexuality and menopause. *Obstet Gynecol* 1990;75(Suppl): S26-S30.

Sherwin BB, Gelfand MM, Brender W. Androgen enhances sexual motivation in females: a prospective, crossover study of sex steroid administration in the surgical menopause. *Psychosom Med* 1985;47:339-351.

Shifren JL, Davis SR, Moreau M, et al. Testosterone patch for the treatment of hypoactive sexual desire disorder in naturally menopausal women: results from the Intimate NM1 study. *Menopause* 2006;13:770-779.

Simon J, Braunstein G, Nachtigall L, et al. Testosterone patch increases sexual activity and desire in surgically menopausal women with hypoactive sexual desire disorder. *J Clin Endocrinol Metab* 2005;90:5226-5233.

Utian WH, MacLean DB, Symonds T, Symons J, Somayaji V, Sisson M. A methodology study to validate a structured diagnostic method used to diagnose female sexual dysfunction and its subtypes in postmenopausal women. *Sex Marital Ther* 2005;31:271-283.

Warnock JK, Bundren JC, Morris DW. Female hypoactive sexual desire disorder due to androgen deficiency: clinical and psychometric issues. *Psychopharmacol Bull* 1997;33:761-766.

Wierman ME, Basson R, Davis SR, et al. Androgen therapy in women: an Endocrine Society clinical practice guideline. *J Clin Endocrinol Metab* 2006;91:2697-2710.

Urinary concerns

Bachmann G. Urogenital ageing: an old problem newly recognized. *Maturitas* 1995;22(Suppl):S1-S5.

Black NA, Downs SH. The effectiveness of surgery for stress incontinence in women: systematic review. *Br J Urol* 1996;78:497-510.

Brown JS, Grady D, Ouslander JG, Herzog AR, Varner RE, Posner SF. Prevalence of urinary incontinence and associated risk factors in postmenopausal women. Heart and Estrogen/Progestin Replacement Study (HERS) Research Group. *Obstet Gynecol* 1999;94:66-70.

Brown JS, Vittinghoff E, Kanaya AM, et al, for the Heart and Estrogen/progestin Replacement Study Group. Urinary tract infections in postmenopausal women: effect of HT and risk factors. *Obstet Gynecol* 2001;9:1045-1052.

Brubaker L. Urinary urgency and frequency: what should a clinician do? *Obstet Gynecol* 2005;105:661-667.

Burgio KL, Goode PS, Locher JL, et al. Behavioral training with and without biofeedback in the treatment of urge incontinence in older women: a randomized controlled trial. *JAMA* 2002;288:2293-2299.

Burgio KL, Locher JL, Goode PS, et al. Behavioral vs drug treatment for urge urinary incontinence in older women: a randomized controlled trial. *JAMA* 1998;280:1995-2000.

Cardozo L, Benness C, Abbott D. Low dose oestrogen prophylaxis for recurrent urinary tract infections in elderly women. *Br J Obstet Gynaecol* 1998;105:403-407.

Cardozo L, Lose G, McClish D, Versi E. A systematic review of the effects of estrogens for symptoms suggestive of overactive bladder. *Acta Obstet Gynecol Scand* 2004;3:892-897.

Cardozo LD, Kelleher CJ. Sex hormones, the menopause and urinary problems. *Gynecol Endocrinol* 1995;9:75-84.

Danforth KN, Townsend MK, Lifford K, Curhan GC, Resnick NM, Grodstein F. Risk factors for urinary incontinence among middle-aged women. *Am J Obstet Gynecol* 2006;194:339-345.

DeMarco EF. Urinary tract disorders in perimenopausal and postmenopausal women. In: Lobo RA, ed. *Treatment of the Postmenopausal Woman: Basic and Clinical Aspects*, 2nd ed. Philadelphia, PA: Lippincott Williams & Wilkins, 1999:213-227.

Diokno AC, Appell RA, Sand PK, et al. Prospective, randomized, double-blind study of the efficacy and tolerability of the extended-release formulations of oxybutynin and tolterodine for overactive bladder: results of the OPERA trial. *Mayo Clin Proc* 2003;78:687-695.

Drutz H, Bachmann G, Bouchard C, Morris B. Towards a better recognition of urogenital aging. *J SOGC* 1996;18:1017-1031.

Elia G, Bergman A. Pelvic muscle exercises: when do they work? *Obstet Gynecol* 1993;81:283-286.

Emmons SL, Otto L. Acupuncture for overactive bladder: a randomized controlled trial. *Obstet Gynecol* 2005;6:138-143.

Eriksen B. A randomized, open, parallel-group study on the preventive effect of an estradiol-releasing vaginal ring (Estring) on recurrent urinary tract infections in postmenopausal women. *Am J Obstet Gynecol* 1999;180:1072-1079.

Fantl JA, Bump RC, Robinson D, McClish DK, Wyman JF. Efficacy of estrogen supplementation in the treatment of urinary incontinence: the Continence Program for Women Research Group. *Obstet Gynecol* 1996;88:745-749.

Grady D, Brown JS, Vittinghoff E, Applegate W, Varner E, Snyder T. Postmenopausal hormones and incontinence: the Heart and Estrogen/progestin Replacement Study. *Obstet Gynecol* 2001;97:116-120.

Griebling TL, Nygaard IE. The role of estrogen replacement therapy in the management of urinary incontinence and urinary tract infection in postmenopausal women. *Endocrinol Metab Clin North Am* 1997;26:347-360.

Grodstein F, Lifford K, Resnick NM, et al. Postmenopausal hormone therapy and risk of developing urinary incontinence. *Obstet Gynecol* 2004;103:254-260.

Henalla SM, Kirwan P, Castleden CM, Hutchins CJ, Breeson AJ. The effect of pelvic floor exercises in the treatment of genuine urinary stress incontinence in women at two hospitals. *Br J Obstet Gynaecol* 1988;95:602-606.

Hannestad YS, Rortveit G, Sandvik H, et al, for the Norwegian EPINCONT study. A community-based epidemiological survey of female urinary incontinence: the Norwegian EPINCONT study. Epidemiology of Incontinence in the County of Nord-Trondelag. *J Clin Epidemiol* 2000;53:1150-1157.

Hendrix SL, Cochrane BB, Nygaard IE, et al. Effects of estrogen with and without progestin on urinary incontinence. *JAMA* 2005;293:935-948.

Holroyd-Leduc JM, Straus S. Management of urinary incontinence in women: scientific review. *JAMA* 2004;291:986-995.

Hunskaar S, Arnold EP, Burgio K, Diokno AC, Herzog AR, Mallett VT. Epidemiology and natural history of urinary incontinence. *Int Urogynecol J Pelvic Floor Dysfunct* 2000;11:301-319.

Iosif CS, Batra SC, Ek A, Astedt BI. Estrogen receptors in the human female urinary tract. *Am J Obstet Gynecol* 1981;141:817-820.

Jackson S, Shepherd A, Brookes S, Abrams P. The effect of oestrogen supplementation on post-menopausal urinary stress incontinence: a double-blind placebo-controlled trial. *Br J Obstet Gynaecol* 1999;106:711-718.

Jackson SL, Weber AM, Hull TL, Mitchinson AR, Walters MD. Fecal incontinence in women with urinary incontinence and pelvic organ prolapse. *Obstet Gynecol* 1997;89:423-427.

Janknegt RA, Hassouna MM, Siegel W, et al. Long-term effectiveness of sacral nerve stimulation for refractory urge incontinence. *Eur Urol* 2001;39:101-106.

Johnson S. Canadian consensus on menopause and osteoporosis: urogenital health. *J SOGC* 2001;23:973-977.

Kelada E, Jones A. Interstitial cystitis. *Arch Gynecol Obstet* 2007;275:223-229.

Khullar V, Damiano R, Toozs-Hobson P, Cardozo L. Prevalence of faecal incontinence among women with urinary incontinence. *Br J Obstet Gynaecol* 1998;105:1211-1213.

Klarskov P, Belving D, Bischoff N, et al. Pelvic floor exercise versus surgery for female urinary stress incontinence. *Urol Int* 1986;41:129-132.

Latini JM, Alipour M, Kreder KJ Jr. Efficacy of sacral neuromodulation for symptomatic treatment of refractory urinary urge incontinence. *Urology* 2006;67:550-554.

Long CY, Liu CM, Hsu SC, Chen YH, Wu CH, Tsai EM. A randomized comparative study of the effects of oral and topical estrogen therapy on the lower urinary tract of hysterectomized postmenopausal women. *Fertil Steril* 2006;5:155-160.

MacLennan AH, Taylor AW, Wilson DH, Wilson D. The prevalence of pelvic floor disorders and their relationship to gender, age, parity and mode of delivery. *BJOG* 2000;107:1460-1470.

Mariappan P, Alhasso A, Ballantyne Z, Grant A, N'Dow J. Duloxetine, a serotonin and noradrenaline reuptake inhibitor (SNRI) for the treatment of stress urinary incontinence: a systematic review. *Eur Urol* 2007;51:67-74.

Millard RJ, Moore K, Rencken R, et al. Duloxetine vs placebo in the treatment of stress urinary incontinence: a four-continent randomized clinical trial. *BJU Int* 2004;93:311-318.

Milsom I. Overactive bladder: current understanding and future issues. *BJOG* 2006;113 (Suppl 2):2-8.

Milsom I, Ekelund P, Molander U, Arvidsson L, Areskoug B. The influence of age, parity, oral contraception, hysterectomy and menopause on the prevalence of urinary incontinence in women. *J Urol* 1993;149:1459-1462.

Miner PB. Economic and personal impact of fecal and urinary incontinence. *Gastroenterology* 2004;126(Suppl):S8-S13.

Oliveria SA, Klein RA, Reed JI, Cirillo PA, Christos PJ, Walker AM. Estrogen replacement therapy and urinary tract infections in postmenopausal women aged 45-89. *Menopause* 1998;5:4-8.

Orlander JD, Jick SS, Dean AD, Jick H. Urinary tract infections and estrogen use in older women. *J Am Geriatr Soc* 1992;40:817-820.

Ouslander JG, Greendale GA, Uman G, et al. Effects of oral estrogen and progestin on the lower urinary tract among female nursing home residents. *J Am Geriatr Soc* 2001;49:803-807.

Privette M, Cade R, Peterson J, Mars D. Prevention of recurrent urinary tract infection in postmenopausal women. *Nephron* 1988;50:24-27.

Raz R, Stamm WE. A controlled trial of intravaginal estriol in postmenopausal women with recurrent urinary tract infections. *N Engl J Med* 1993; 329:753-756.

Rufford J, Hextall A, Cardozo L, Khullar V. A double-blind placebo-controlled trial on the effects of 25 mg estradiol implants on the urge syndrome in postmenopausal women. *Int Urogynecol J Pelvic Floor Dysfunct* 2003;14:78-83.

Sampselle CM, Harlow SD, Skurnick J, Brubaker L, Bondarenko I. Urinary continence predictors and life impact in ethnically diverse perimenopausal women. *Obstet Gynecol* 2002;100:1230-1238.

Subak LL, Johnson C, Whitcomb E, et al. Does weight loss improve incontinence in moderately obese women? *Int Urogynecol J Pelvic Floor Dysfunct* 2002;13:40-43.

Tyagi S, Thomas CA, Hayashi Y, Chancellor MB. The overactive bladder: epidemiology and morbidity. *Urol Clin North Am* 2006;33:433-438.

Van Voorhis BJ. Genitourinary symptoms in the menopausal transition. *Am J Med* 2005;118(Suppl 12B):47-53.

Waetjen LE, Liao S, Johnson WO, et al. Factors associated with prevalent and incident urinary incontinence in a cohort of midlife women: a longitudinal analysis of data: study of women's health across the nation. *Am J Epidemiol* 2007;165:309-318.

Wall LL. Drug therapy for incontinence: new agents, new applications. *OBG Management* 2006;18:42-53.

Walters MD. Evaluation of urinary incontinence: history, physical examination, and office tests. In: Walters MD, Karram MM, eds. *Urogynecology and Reconstructive Pelvic Surgery*, 2nd ed. St. Louis, MO: Mosby, 1999:45-54.

Wyman JF, Fantl JA, McClish DK, Bump RC. Comparative efficacy of behavioral interventions in the management of female urinary incontinence: Continence Program for Women Research Group. *Am J Obstet Gynecol* 1998;179:999-1007.

Pelvic pain

The American College of Obstetricians and Gynecologists. Chronic pelvic pain. ACOG Practice Bulletin No. 51. *Obstet Gynecol* 2004;103:589-605.

Howard FM, Perry CP, Carter JE, El-Minawi AM, Li R-Z, eds. *Pelvic Pain: Diagnosis and Management*. Philadelphia, PA: Lippincott Williams & Wilkins, 2000:5.

The International Pelvic Pain Society. Chronic pelvic pain. Available at: http://www.pelvicpain.org. Accessed August 13, 2007.

Petta CA, Ferriani RA, Abrao MS, et al. Randomized clnical trial of a levonorgestrel-releasing intrauterine system and a depot GnRH analogue for the treatment of chronic pelvic pain in women with endometriosis. *Hum Reprod* 2005;20:1993-1998.

Thurmond KF. Pelvic pain. In: Carlson KJ, Eisenstat SA, Frigoletto FD Jr, Schiff I, eds. *Primary Care of Women*. St. Louis, MO: Mosby, 1995:260-266.

Weight gain

AACE/ACE obesity statement. *Endocr Prac* 1997;3:164-188.

Anderson JW, Schwartz SM, Hauptman J, et al. Low-dose orlistat effects on body weight of mildly to moderately overweight individuals: a 16 week, double-blind, placebo-controlled trial. *Ann Pharmacother* 2006; 40:1717-1723.

Bjorkelund C, Lissner L, Andersson S, Lapidus L, Bengtssen C. Reproductive history in relation to relative weight and fat distribution. *Int J Obes Relat Metab Disord* 1996;20:213-219.

Bolton-Smith C, Woodward M, Fenton S, Brown CA. Does dietary trans fatty acid intake relate to the prevalence of coronary heart disease in Scotland? *Eur Heart J* 1996;17:837-845.

Buchwald H, Avidor Y, Braunwald E, et al. Bariatric surgery: a systematic review and meta-analysis. *JAMA* 2004;292:1724-1737.

Calle EE, Rodriguez C, Walker-Thurmond K, Thun MJ. Overweight, obesity, and mortality from cancer in a prospectively studied cohort of U.S. adults. *N Engl J Med* 2003;348:1625-1638.

Calle EE, Thun MJ, Petrelli JM, Rodriguez C, Heath CW. Body mass index and mortality in a prospective cohort of U.S. adults. *N Engl J Med* 1999; 341:1097-1105.

Canadian Society for Exercise Physiology. *Canada's Physical Activity Guide to Healthy Active Living*. Available at: http://www.phac-aspc.gc.ca/pau-uap/paguide/. Accessed June 27, 2007.

Crawford SI, Casey VA, Avis NE, McKinlay SM. A longitudinal study of weight and the menopause transition. *Menopause* 2000;7:96-104.

Dansinger ML, Gleason JA, Griffith JL, Selker HP, Schaefer EJ. Comparison of the Atkins, Ornish, Weight Watchers, and Zone diets for weight loss and heart disease risk reduction. *JAMA* 2005;293:43-53.

Drewnowski A, Warren-Mears VA. Does aging change nutrition requirements? *J Nutr Health Aging* 2001;5:70-74.

Elford RW, MacMillan HL, Wathen CN, with the Canadian Task Force on Preventive Health Care. Counseling for risky health habits: a conceptual framework for primary care practitioners. CTFPHC Technical Report #01-7. November, 2001. London, ON, Canada: Canadian Task Force.

Eliassen AH, Colditz GA, Rosner B, Cillett WC, Hankinson SE. Adult weight change and risk of postmenopausal breast cancer. *JAMA* 2006;296:193-201.

Godfrey JR. Toward optimal health: Robert Kushner, MD, offers a practical approach to assessment of overweight patients. *J Womens Health* 2006; 15:991-995.

Grundy SM, Cleeman JI, Daniels SR, et al. Diagnosis and management of the metabolic syndrome: an American Heart Association/National Heart, Lung, and Blood Institute Scientific Statement. *Circulation* 2005;112:2735-2752.

Han D, Nie J, Bonner MR, et al. Lifetime adult weight gain, central adiposity, and the risk of pre- and postmenopausal breast cancer in the Western New York exposures and breast cancer study. *In J Cancer* 2006;119:2931-2937.

Health Canada. *Physical Activity of Canadians: Baby Boomers Aged 40 to 54*. Ottawa, ON, Canada: National Population Health Survey Highlights, 1999.

Hu FB, Stampfer MJ, Manson JE, et al. Dietary fat intake and the risk of coronary heart disease in women. *N Engl J Med* 1997;337:1491-1499.

Jakicic JM, Marcus BH, Gallagher KI, Napolitano M, Lang W. Effect of exercise duration and intensity on weight loss in overweight, sedentary women: a randomized trial. *JAMA* 2003;290:1323-1330.

Koffman DM, Bazzarre T, Mosca L, Redberg R, Schmid T, Wattigney WA. An evaluation of Choose to Move 1999: an American Heart Association physical activity program for women. *Arch Intern Med* 2001;161:2193-2199.

Kris-Etherton P, Eckel RH, Howard BV, St. Jeor S, Bazzarre TL, for the Nutrition Committee, Population Science Committee, and Clinical Science Committee of the American Heart Association. AHA science advisory: Lyon Diet Heart Study. Benefits of a Mediterranean-style diet. National Cholesterol Education Program/American Heart Association step I dietary pattern on cardiovascular disease. *Circulation* 2001;103:1823-1825.

Kritz-Silverstein D, Barrett-Connor E. Long-term postmenopausal hormone use, obesity, and fat distribution in older women. *JAMA* 1996;275:987-988.

Kuller LH, Simkin-Silverman LR, Wing RR, Meilahn EN, Ives DG. Women's Healthy Lifestyle Project: a randomized clinical trial. *Circulation* 2001; 103:32-37.

Kushi LH, Meyer KA, Jacobs DR Jr. Cereals, legumes, and chronic disease risk reduction: evidence from epidemiologic studies. *Am J Clin Nutr* 1999; 70(Suppl):S451-S458.

Ley CJ, Lees B, Stevenson JC. Sex- and menopause-associated changes in body-fat distribution. *Am J Clin Nutr* 1992;55:950-954.

Lloyd T, Johnson-Rollings N, Eggli DF, Kieselhorst K, Mauger EA, Cusatis DC. Bone status among postmenopausal women with different habitual caffeine intakes: a longitudinal investigation. *J Am Coll Nutr* 2000;19:256-261.

Maggard MA, Shugarman LR, Suttorp M, et al. Meta-analysis: surgical treatment of obesity. *Ann Intern Med* 2005;142:547-559.

Mann T, Tomiyama AJ, Westling E, Lew AM, Samuels B, Chatman J. Medicare's search for effective obesity treatments: diets are not the answer. *Am Psychol* 2007;62:220-233.

Manson JE, Willett WC, Stampfer MJ, et al. Body weight and mortality among women. *N Engl J Med* 1995;333:677-685.

McTigue KM, Harris R, Hemphill B, et al. Screening and interventions for obesity in adults: summary of the evidence for the US Preventive Services Task Force. *Ann Intern Med* 2003;139:933-949.

Milewicz A, Tworowska U, Demissie A. Menopausal obesity—myth or fact? *Climacteric* 2001;4:273-283.

Montemuro S, Fluker M, Rogers J, Derzko C. Menopause: healthy living. Canadian consensus on menopause and osteoporosis. *J SOGC* 2001; 23:842-848.

Moore T, Conlin P, Ard J, Svetky L. DASH diet is effective treatment for stage 1 isolated systolic hypertension. *Hypertension* 2001;38:155-158.

National Cholesterol Education Program/American Heart Association step I dietary pattern on cardiovascular disease. *Circulation* 2001;103:1823-1825.

National Heart, Lung, and Blood Institute. *Clinical Guidelines on the Identification, Evaluation, and Treatment of Overweight and Obesity in Adults.* Available at: http://www.nblbi.nih.gov/guidelines/obesity/ob_gdlns.htm. Accessed October 10, 2007.

National Women's Health Report. Women and obesity. *Natl Womens Health Rep* 2006;28:1-4.

Norman RJ, Flight IH, Rees MC. Oestrogen and progestogen hormone replacement therapy for peri-menopausal and post-menopausal women: weight and body fat distribution. *Cochrane Database Syst Rev* 2000;2:CD001018.

The North American Menopause Society. The role of isoflavones in menopausal health: consensus opinion of The North American Menopause Society. *Menopause* 2000;7:215-229.

Park HS, Lee KU. Postmenopausal women lose less visceral adipose tissue during a weight reduction program. *Menopause* 2003;10:222-227.

Patel SR, Mahotra A, White DP, Gottlieb DJ, Hu FB. Association between reduced sleep and weight gain in women. *Am J Epidemiol* 2006;164:947-954.

Poehlman EAT, Tchernof A. Traversing the menopause: changes in energy expenditure and body composition. *Coron Artery Dis* 1998;9:799-803.

Province MA, Hadley EC, Hornbrook MC, et al. The effects of exercise on falls in elderly patients: a preplanned meta-analysis of the FICSIT trials. Frailty and injuries: cooperative studies of intervention techniques. *JAMA* 1995;273:1341-1347.

Reubinoff BE, Wurtman J, Rojansky N, et al. Effects of hormone replacement therapy on weight, body composition, fat distribution, and food intake in early postmenopausal women: a prospective study. *Fertil Steril* 1995; 64:963-968.

Rexrode KM, Carey VJ, Hennekens CH, et al. Abdominal adiposity and coronary heart disease in women. *JAMA* 1998;280:1843-1848.

Ricci TA, Chowdhury HA, Heymsfield SB, Stahl T, Pierson RN Jr, Shapses SA. Calcium supplementation suppresses bone turnover during weight reduction in postmenopausal women. *J Bone Miner Res* 1998;13:1045-1050.

Rimm EB, Willett WC, Hu FB, et al. Folate and vitamin B6 from diet and supplements in relation to risk of coronary heart disease among women. *JAMA* 1998;279:359-364.

Russell RM, Rasmussen H, Lichtenstein AH. Modified food guide pyramid for people over seventy years of age. *J Nutr* 1999;129:751-753.

Schatzkin A, Lanza E, Corle D, et al, for the Polyp Prevention Trial Study Group. Lack of effect of a low-fat, high-fiber diet on the recurrence of colorectal adenomas. *N Engl J Med* 2000;342:1149-1155.

Slavin JL, Jacobs D, Marquart L, Wiemer K. The role of whole grains in disease prevention. *J Am Diet Assoc* 2001;101:780-785.

Slemenda CW, Hui SL, Longcope C, et al. Cigarette smoking, obesity, and bone mass. *J Bone Miner Res* 1989;4:737-741.

Smith-Warner SA, Spiegelman D, Adami HO, et al. Types of dietary fat and breast cancer: a pooled analysis of cohort studies. *Int J Cancer* 2001; 92:767-774.

Snow V, Barry P, Fitterman N, Qaseem A, Weiss K, for the Clinical Efficacy Assessment Subcommittee of the American College of Physicians. Pharmacologic and surgical management of obesity in primary care: a clinical practice guideline from the American College of Physicians. *Ann Intern Med* 2005;142:525-531.

Sowers ME, Crutchfield M, Jannausch ML, Russel-Aulet M. Longitudinal changes in body composition in women approaching midlife. *Ann Hum Biol* 1996;23:253-265.

Thorneycroft IH, Lindsay R, Pickar JH. Body composition during treatment with conjugated estrogens with and without medroxyprogesterone acetate: analysis of the women's Health, Osteoporosis, Progestin, Estrogen (HOPE) trial. *Am J Obstet Gynecol* 2007;197:137.e1-137.e7.

US Department of Health and Human Services. *Healthy People 2010.* Washington, DC: US Department of Health and Human Services, 2000. Available at: http://www.health.gov/healthypeople/document/. Accessed June 27, 2007.

US Preventive Services Task Force. Screening for obesity in adults: recommendations and rationale. *Ann Intern Med* 2003;139:930-932.

Utian WH, Gass MLS, Pickar JH. Body mass index does not influence response to treatment, nor does body weight change with lower doses of conjugated estrogens and medroxyprogesterone acetate in younger, postmenopausal women. *Menopause* 2004;11:306-314.

Varenna M, Binelli L, Zucchi F, Ghiringhelli D, Sinigaglia L. Unbalanced diet to lower serum cholesterol level is a risk factor for postmenopausal osteoporosis and distal forearm fracture. *Osteoporos Int* 2001;12:296-301.

Velie E, Kulldorff M, Schairer C, Block G, Albanes D, Schatzkin A. Dietary fat, fat subtypes, and breast cancer in postmenopausal women: a prospective cohort study. *J Natl Cancer Inst* 2000;92:833-839.

Warren MP, Artacho CA. Role of exercise and nutrition. In: Lobo RA, ed. *Treatment of the Postmenopausal Woman: Basic and Clinical Aspects*, 3rd ed. San Diego, CA: Academic Press, 2007:655-682.

Wing RR, Matthews KA, Kuller LH, Meilahn EN, Plantinga PL. Weight gain at the time of menopause. *Arch Intern Med* 1991;151:97-102.

Wolff I, van Croonenborg JJ, Kemper HC, Kostense PJ, Twisk JW. The effects of exercise training programs on bone mass: a meta-analysis of published controlled trials in pre- and postmenopausal women. *Osteoporos Int* 1999; 9:1-12.

Wu AH, Pike MC, Stram DO. Meta-analysis: dietary fat intake, serum estrogen levels, and the risk of breast cancer. *J Natl Cancer Inst* 1999;91:529-534.

Wurtman JJ. Depression and weight gain: the serotonin connection. *J Affect Disord* 1993;29:183-192.

Yong LC, Brown CC, Schatzkin A, Schairer C. Prospective study of relative weight and risk of breast cancer: the Breast Cancer Detection Demonstration Project follow-up study, 1979 to 1987-1989. *Am J Epidemiol* 1996;143:985-995.

Zeigler RG, Mayne ST, Swanson CA. Nutrition and lung cancer. *Cancer Causes Control* 1996;7:157-177.

Cardiovascular effects

American Heart Association. Heart disease and stroke statistics—2007 update. *Circulation* 2007;115:e69-e171.

Gorodeski EZ, Gorodeski GI. Epidemiology and risk factors of cardiovascular disease in postmenopausal women. In: Lobo RA, ed. *Treatment of the Postmenopausal Woman: Basic and Clinical Aspects*, 3rd ed. San Diego, CA: Academic Press, 2007:405-452.

Heart and Stroke Foundation of Canada. *The Growing Burden of Heart Disease and Stroke in Canada 2003*. Ottawa, ON, Canada: Heart and Stroke Foundation of Canada, 2003.

Herrington DM. Sex hormones and normal cardiovascular physiology in women. In: Julian DG, Wenger NK, eds. *Women and Heart Disease*. London UK: Martin Dunitz Publishers, 1997:243-264.

Hu FB, Grodstein F, Hennekens CH, et al. Age at natural menopause and risk of cardiovascular disease. *Arch Intern Med* 1999;159:1061-1066.

Jensen J, Nilas L, Christiansen C. Influence of menopause on serum lipids and lipoproteins. *Maturitas* 1990;12:321-331.

Kok HS, van Asselt KM, Van der Schouw YT, et al. Heart disease risk determines menopausal age rather than the reverse. *J Am Coll Cardiol* 2006;47:1976-1983.

Kuller LH, Simkin-Silverman LR, Wing RR, Meilahn EN, Ives DG. Women's Healthy Lifestyle project: a randomized clinical trial: results at 54 months. *Circulation* 2001;103:32-37.

Poehlman ET, Toth MJ, Ades PA, Rosen CJ. Menopause-associated changes in plasma lipids, insulin-like growth factor I and blood pressure: a longitudinal study. *Eur J Clin Invest* 1997;27:322-326.

Saba S, Link MS, Homoud MK, Wang PJ, Estes NA. Effect of low estrogen states in healthy women on dispersion of ventricular repolarization. *Am J Cardiol* 2001;87:354-356.

Stampfer MJ, Colditz GA, Willett WC. Menopause and heart disease. *Ann N Y Acad Sci* 1990;592:193-203.

Skeletal system effects

Boyce BF, Hughes DE, Wright KR, et al. Recent advances in bone biology provide insight into the pathogenesis of bone diseases. *Lab Invest* 1999; 79:83-94.

Chez Z, Maricic M, Bassford TL, et al. Fracture risk among breast cancer survivors: results from the Women's Health Initiative Study. *Arch Intern Med* 2005;165:552-558.

Chrischilles EA, Butler CD, Davis CS, Wallace RB. A model of lifetime osteoporosis impact. *Arch Intern Med* 1991;151:2026-2032.

Coelho R, Silva C, Maia A, et al. Bone mineral density and depression: a community study in women. *J Psychosom Res* 1999;46:29-35.

Greendale GA, Barrett-Connor E, Ingle S, et al. Late physical and functional effects of osteoporotic fractures in women: the Rancho Bernardo Study. *J Am Geriatr Soc* 1995;43:955-961.

Hui SL, Perkins AJ, Zhou L, et al. Bone loss at the femoral neck in premenopausal white women: effects of weight change and sex hormone levels. *J Clin Endocrinol Metab* 2002;87:1539-1543.

Kado DM, Browner WS, Palermo L, Nevitt MC, Genant HK, Cummings SR, for the Osteoporotic Fractures Research Group. Vertebral fractures and mortality in older women: a prospective study. *Arch Intern Med* 1999;159:1215-1220.

Klotzbuecher CM, Ross PD, Landsman PB, Abbott TA, Berger M. Patients with prior fractures have an increased risk of future fractures: a summary of the literature and statistical synthesis. *J Bone Miner Res* 2000;15:721-739.

Lindsay R, Cosman F. Pathogenesis of osteoporosis. In: Lobo RA, ed. *Treatment of the Postmenopausal Woman: Basic and Clinical Aspects*, 3rd ed. San Diego, CA: Academic Press, 2007:323-330.

Lindsay R, Silverman SL, Cooper C, et al. Risk of new vertebral fracture in the year following a fracture. *JAMA* 2001;285:320-323.

Looker AC, Johnson C, Wahner HW, et al. Prevalence of low femoral bone density in older U.S. women from NHANES III. *J Bone Miner Res* 1995; 10:796-802.

Melton LJ III, Thamer M, Ray NF, et al. Fractures attributable to osteoporosis: report from the National Osteoporosis Foundation. *J Bone Miner Res* 1997; 12:16-23.

National Institutes of Health. Consensus Development Panel on Osteoporosis Prevention, Diagnosis, and Therapy. *JAMA* 2001;285:785-795.

National Osteoporosis Foundation. Disease statistics. Available at: http://www.nof.org/osteoporosis/stats.htm. Accessed June 19, 2007.

National Osteoporosis Foundation. *Osteoporosis: Physician's Guide to Prevention and Treatment of Osteoporosis*. Washington, DC: National Osteoporosis Foundation, 2003.

The North American Menopause Society. The management of osteoporosis in postmenopausal women: 2006 position statement of The North American Menopause Society. *Menopause* 2006;13:340-367.

The North American Menopause Society. The role of calcium in peri- and postmenopausal women: 2006 position statement of The North American Menopause Society. *Menopause* 2006;13:862-877.

Recker RR, Lappe J, Davies K, Heaney R. Characterization of perimenopausal bone loss: a prospective study. *J Bone Miner Res* 2000;15:1965-1973.

Seeman E. Pathogenesis of bone fragility in men and women. *Lancet* 2002: 359:1841-1850.

Siris ES, Miller PD, Barrett-Connor E, et al. Identification and fracture outcomes of undiagnosed low bone mineral density in postmenopausal women: results from the national osteoporosis risk assessment. *JAMA* 2001;286:2815-2822.

Tenenhouse A, Joseph L, Kreiger N, et al, for the CaMos Research Group. Estimation of the prevalence of low bone density in Canadian women and men using a population-specific DXA reference standard: the Canadian Multicentre Osteoporosis Study (CaMos). *Osteoporos Int* 2000;11:897-904.

US Congress Office of Technology Assessment. *Hip Fracture Outcomes in People Age 50 and Over—Background Paper*. Publication OTA-BP-H-120. Washington, DC: US Government Printing Office, 1994. Available at: http://www.princeton.edu/~ota/disk1/1994/9413/9413.PDF. Accessed September 25, 2007.

World Health Organization. *Assessment of Fracture Risk and Its Application to Screening for Postmenopausal Osteoporosis: Report of a WHO Study Group*. Geneva, Switzerland: World Health Organization, 1994.

Dental and oral cavity changes

American Dental Association. Dental management of patients receiving oral bisphosphonate therapy: expert panel recommendations. *J Am Dent Assoc* 2006;137:1144-1150.

Krall EA, Dawson-Hughes B, Hannan MT, Wilson PW, Kiel DP. Postmenopausal estrogen replacement and tooth retention. *Am J Med* 1997;102:536-542.

Krall EA, Dawson-Hughes B, Papas A, Garcia RI. Tooth loss and skeletal bone density in healthy postmenopausal women. *Osteoporos Int* 1994;4:104-109.

Krall EA, Garcia RI, Dawson-Hughes B. Increased risk of tooth loss is related to bone loss at the whole body, hip, and spine. *Calcif Tissue Int* 1996; 59:433-437.

Lerner UH. Inflammation-induced bone remodeling in periodontal disease and the influence of post-menopausal osteoporosis. *J Dent Res* 2006; 85:596-607.

Reinhardt RA, Payne JB, Maze CA, Patil KD, Gallagher SJ, Mattson JS. Influence of estrogen and osteopenia/osteoporosis on clinical periodontitis in postmenopausal women. *J Periodontol* 1999;70:823-828.

Tezal M, Wactawski-Wende J, Grossi SG, Ho AW, Dunford R, Genco RJ. The relationship between bone mineral density and periodontitis in postmenopausal women. *J Periodontol* 2000;71:1492-1498.

von Wowern N, Klausen B, Kollerup G. Osteoporosis: a risk factor in periodontal disease. *J Periodontol* 1994;65:1134-1138.

Wactawski-Wende J. Periodontal diseases and osteoporosis: association and mechanisms. *Ann Periodontol* 2001;6:197-208.

Woo SF, Hellstein JW, Kalmar JR. Narrrative review: bisphosphonates and osteonecrosis of the jaws. *Ann Intern Med* 2006;144:753-761.

Zakrzewska JM, Forssell H, Glenny AM. Interventions for the treatment of burning mouth syndrome. *Cochrane Database Syst Rev* 2005;1:CD002779.

Skin changes

Ashcroft GS, Ashworth JJ. Potential role of estrogens in wound healing. *Am J Clin Dermatol* 2003;4:737-743.

Autier P, Dore JF, Negrier S, et al. Sunscreen use and duration of sun exposure: a double-blind, randomized trial. *J Natl Cancer Inst* 1999;91:1304-1309.

Azziz R. The evaluation and management of hirsutism. *Obstet Gynecol* 2003;101:995-1007.

Brincat MP. Hormone replacement therapy and the skin. *Maturitas* 2000; 35:107-117.

Brincat MP, Galea R, Baron YM. Connective tissue changes in the menopause and with hormone replacement therapy. In: Lobo RA, ed. *Treatment of the Postmenopausal Woman: Basic and Clinical Aspects*, 3rd ed. San Diego, CA: Academic Press, 2007:227-235.

Brooke RC, Newbold SA, Telfer NR, Griffiths CE. Discordance between facial wrinkling and the presence of basal cell carcinoma. *Arch Dermatol* 2001;137:751-754.

Callens A, Vaillant L, Lecomte P, et al. Does hormonal skin aging exist? A study of the influence of different hormone therapy regimens on the skin of postmenopausal women using non-invasive measurement techniques. *Dermatology* 1996;193:289-294.

Cameron ST, Glasier AF, Gebbie A, et al. Comparison of a transdermal continuous combined and an interrupted progestin HRT. *Maturitas* 2006; 53:19-26.

Castelo-Branco C, Duran M, Gonzalez-Merlo J. Skin collagen changes related to age and hormone replacement therapy. *Maturitas* 1992;15:113-119.

Castelo-Branco C, Pons F, Gratacos E, Fortuny A, Vanrell JA, Gonzalez-Merlo J. Relationship between skin collagen and bone changes during aging. *Maturitas* 1994;18:199-206.

Crawford SI, Casey VA, Avis NE, McKinlay SM. A longitudinal study of weight and the menopause transition. *Menopause* 2000;7:96-104.

Creidi P, Faivre B, Agache P, Richard E, Hadiquet V, Sauvanet JP. Effect of a conjugated oestrogen (Premarin) cream on ageing facial skin: a comparative study with a placebo cream. *Maturitas* 1994;19:211-223.

Dunn LB, Damesyn M, Moore AA, Reuben DB, Greendale GA. Does estrogen prevent skin aging? Results from the First National Health and Nutrition Examination Survey (NHANES I). *Arch Dermatol* 1997;133:339-342.

Foote JA, Harris RB, Giuliano AR, et al. Predictors for cutaneous basal- and squamous-cell carcinoma among actinically damaged adults. *Int J Cancer* 2001;95:7-11.

Green A, Williams G, Neale R, et al. Daily sunscreen application and beta-carotene supplementation in prevention of basal-cell and squamous-cell carcinomas of the skin: a randomised controlled trial [erratum in: *Lancet* 1999;354:1038]. *Lancet* 1999;354:723-729.

Griffiths CE. Drug treatment of photoaged skin. *Drugs Aging* 1999;14:289-301.

Griffiths CEM, Russman AN, Majmudar G, Singer RS, Hamilton TA, Voorhees JJ. Restoration of collagen formation in photodamaged human skin by tretinoin (retinoic acid). *N Engl J Med* 1993;329:530-535.

Henry F, Pierard-Franchimont C, Cauwenbergh G, Pierard GE. Age-related changes in facial skin contours and rheology. *J Am Geriatr Soc* 1997; 45:220-222.

Huncharek M, Kupelnick B. Use of topical sunscreens and the risk of malignant melanoma: a meta-analysis of 9067 patients from 11 case-control studies. *Am J Public Health* 2002;92:1173-1177.

Kennedy C, Bastiaens MT, Bajdik CD, Willemze R, Westendorp RGJ, Bouwes Bavinck JN. Effect of smoking and sun on the aging skin. *J Invest Dermatol* 2003;120:548-554.

Kincade PW, Medina KL, Payne KJ, et al. Early B-lymphocyte precursors and their regulation by sex steroids. *Immunol Rev* 2000;175:128-137.

Kritz-Silverstein D, Barrett-Connor E. Long-term postmenopausal hormone use, obesity, and fat distribution in older women. *JAMA* 1996;275:987-988.

Leveque JL. Quantitative assessment of skin aging. *Clin Geriatr Med* 2001; 17:673.

Lucky A, Henderson T, Olson W, Robish DM, Lebwohl M, Swinger LJ. Effectiveness of norgestimate and ethinyl estradiol in treating moderate acne vulgaris. *J Am Acad Dermatol* 1997;37:746-754.

Maheux R, Naud F, Rioux M, et al. A randomized, double-blind, placebo-controlled study on the effect of conjugated estrogens on skin thickness. *Am J Obstet Gynecol* 1994;170:642-649.

Mercurio MG, Gogstetter DS. Androgen physiology and the cutaneous pilosebaceous unit. *J Gend Specif Med* 2000;3:59-64.

Milewicz A, Tworowska U, Demissie A. Menopausal obesity—myth or fact? *Climacteric* 2001;4:273-283.

Norman RJ, Flight IH, Rees MC. Oestrogen and progestogin hormone replacement therapy for peri-menopausal and post-menopausal women: weight and body fat distribution. *Cochrane Database Syst Rev* 2000;2:CD001018.

Park HS, Lee KU. Postmenopausal women lose less visceral adipose tissue during a weight reduction program. *Menopause* 2003;10:222-227.

Pierard GE, Letawe C, Dowlati A, Pierard-Franchimont C. Effect of hormone replacement therapy for menopause on the mechanical properties of skin. *J Am Geriatr Soc* 1995;43:662-665.

Pierard-Franchimont C, Cornil F, Dehavay J, et al. Climacteric skin ageing of the face: a prospective longitudinal comparative trial on the effect of oral hormone replacement therapy. *Maturitas* 1999;32:87-93.

Quatresooz P, Pierard-Franchimont C, Gaspard U, Pierard GE. Skin climacteric aging and hormone replacement therapy. *J Cosmet Dermatol* 2006;5:3-8.

Raine-Fenning NJ, Brincat MP, Muscat-Baron Y. Skin aging and menopause: implications for treatment. *Am J Clin Dermatol* 2003;4:371-378.

Redmond G, Olson W, Lippman J, et al. Norgestimate and ethinyl estradiol in the treatment of acne vulgaris: a randomized, placebo-controlled trial. *Obstet Gynecol* 1997;89:615-622.

Sauerbronn AV, Fonseca AM, Bagnoli VR, Saldiva PH, Pinotti JA. The effects of systemic hormonal replacement therapy on the skin of postmenopausal women. *Int J Gynaecol Obstet* 2000;68:35-41.

Schmidt JB, Binder M, Demschik G, Bieglmayer C, Reiner A. Treatment of skin aging with topical estrogens. *Int J Dermatol* 1996;35:669-674.

Seite S, Bredoux C, Compan D, et al. Histological evaluation of a topically applied retinol-vitamin C combination. *Skin Pharmacol Physiol* 2005; 18:81-87.

Sowers ME, Crutchfield M, Jannausch ML, Russel-Aulet M. Longitudinal changes in body composition in women approaching midlife. *Ann Hum Biol* 1996;23:253-265.

Thompson SC, Jolley D, Marks R. Reduction of solar keratoses by regular sunscreen use. *N Engl J Med* 1993;329:1147-1151.

Wines N, Willsteed E. Menopause and the skin. *Australas J Dermatol* 2001;42:149-159.

Hair changes

Azziz R. The evaluation and management of hirsutism. *Obstet Gynecol* 2003;101:995-1007.

Carmina E, Lobo RA. Treatment of hyperandrogenic alopecia in women. *Fertil Steril* 2003;79:91-95.

Dawn G, Holmes SC, Moffat D, Munro CS. Post-menopausal frontal fibrosing alopecia. *Clin Exp Dermatol* 2003;28:43-45.

DeVillez RL, Jacobs JP, Szpunar CA, Warner ML. Androgenetic alopecia in the female. Treatment with 2% topical minoxidil solution. *Arch Dermatol* 1994;130:303-307.

Georgala S, Gourgiotou K, Kassouli S, Stratigos JD. Hormonal status in postmenopausal alopecia. *Int J Dermatolol* 1992;31:858-859.

Georgala S, Katoulis AC, Georgala C, Moussatou V, Bozi E, Stavrianeas NG. Topical estrogen therapy for androgenetic alopecia in menopausal females. *Dermatology* 2004;208:178-179.

Jacobs JP, Szpunar CA, Warner ML. Use of topical minoxidil therapy for androgenetic alopecia in women. *Int J Dermatol* 1993;32:758-762.

Lucky AW, Piacquadio DJ, Ditre CM, et al. A randomized, placebo-controlled trial of 5% and 2% topical minoxidil solutions in the treatment of female pattern hair loss. *J Am Acad Dermatol* 2004;50:541-553.

Price VH. Treatment of hair loss. *N Engl J Med* 1999;341:964-973.

Price VH, Roberts JL, Hordinsky M, et al. Lack of efficacy of finasteride in postmenopausal women with androgenetic alopecia. *J Am Acad Dermatol* 2000;43:768-776.

Van Neste D. Thickness, medullation and growth rate of female scalp hair are subject to significant variation according to pigmentation and scalp location during ageing. *Eur J Dermatol* 2004;14:28-32.

Venning VA, Dawber MA. Patterned androgenic alopecia in women. *J Am Acad Dermatol* 1988;18:1073-1077.

Vexiau P, Chaspoux C, Boudou P, et al. Effects of minoxidil 2% vs. cyproterone acetate treatment on female androgenetic alopecia: a controlled, 12-month randomized trial. *Br J Dermatol* 2002;146:992-009.

Ocular changes

Affinito P, De Spiezio Sardo A, et al. Effects of hormone replacement therapy on ocular function in postmenopause. *Menopause* 2003;10:482-487.

Altintas O, Caglar Y, Yuksel N, et al. The effects of menopause and hormone replacement therapy on quality and quantity of tear, intraocular pressure and ocular blood flow. *Ophthalmologica* 2004;218:120-129.

Armaly MF. On the distribution of applanation pressure. I: Statistical features and the effect of age, sex, and family history of glaucoma. *Arch Ophthalmol* 1965;73:11-18.

Atalay E, Karaali K, Akar M, et al. Early impact of hormone replacement therapy on vascular hemodynamics detected via ocular Doppler analysis. *Maturitas* 2005;50:282-284.

Battaglia C, Mancini F, Regnani G, et al. Hormone replacement therapy and ophthalmic artery blood flow changes with primary open-angle glaucoma. *Menopause* 2004;11:69-77.

Barrett-Connor E. Postmenopausal estrogen therapy and selected (less-often-considered) disease outcomes. *Menopause* 1999;6:14-20.

Benitez del Castillo JM, del Rio T, Garcia-Sanchez J. Effects of estrogen use on lens transmittance in postmenopausal women. *Ophthalmology* 1997;104:970-973.

Bigsby RM, Cardenas H, Caperell-Grant A, et al. Protective effects of estrogen in a rat model of age-related cataracts. *Proc Natl Acad Sci USA* 1999;96:9328-9332.

Chuo J, Lee TY, Hollands H, et al. Risk factors for posterior vitreous detachment: a case-control study. *Am J Ophthalmol* 2006;142:931-937.

Cumming RG, Mitchell P. Hormone replacement therapy, reproductive factors, and cataract. The Blue Mountains Eye Study. *Am J Epidemiol* 1997;145:242-249.

Erdem U, Ozdegirmenci O, Sobaci E, et al. Dry eye in post-menopausal women using hormone replacement therapy. *Maturitas* 2007;56:257-262.

The Eye Disease Case-Control Study Group. Risk factors for neovascular age-related macular degeneration. *Arch Ophthalmol* 1992;110:1701-1708.

Foote JA, Harris RB, Giuliano AR, et al. Predictors for cutaneous basal- and squamous-cell carcinoma among actinically damaged adults. *Int J Cancer* 2001;95:7-11.

Freeman EE, Munoz B, Schein O, West SK. Hormone replacement therapy and lens opacities: the Salisbury Eye Evaluation Project. *Arch Ophthalmol* 2001;119:1687-1692.

Fuchsjage-Mayrl G, Nepp J, Schneeberger C, et al. Identification of estrogen and progesterone receptor mRNA expression in the conjunctiva of premenopausal women. *Invest Ophthalmol Vis Sci* 2002;43:2841-2844.

Guttridge NM. Changes in ocular and visual variables during the menstrual cycle. *Ophthalmic Physiol Opt* 1994;14:38-48.

Haan MN, Klein R, Klein BE. Hormone therapy and age-related macular degeneration: The Women's Health Initiative Sight Exam Study. *Arch Ophthalmol* 2006;124:988-992.

Hales AM, Chamberlain CG, Murphy CR, McAvoy JW. Estrogen protects lenses against cataract induced by transforming growth factor-beta (TGFbeta). *J Exp Med* 1997;185:273-280.

Hulsman CA, Westendorp IC, Ramrattan R, et al. Is open-angle glaucoma associated with early menopause? The Rotterdam Study. *Am J Epidemiol* 2001;154:138-144.

Kanda N, Tamaki K. Estrogen enhances immunoglobulin production by human PBMCs. *J Allergy Clin Immunol* 1999;103:282-288.

Khurana RN, LaBree LD, Scott G, et al. Esterified estrogens combined with methyltestosterone raise intraocular pressure in postmenopausal women. *Am J Ophthalmol* 2006;142:494-495.

Kincade PW, Medina KL, Payne KJ, Smith RE, Yiu SC. Early B-lymphocyte precursors and their regulation by sex steroids. *Immunol Rev* 2000; 175:128-137.

Klein BE, Klein R, Ritter LL. Is there evidence of an estrogen effect on age-related lens opacities? The Beaver Dam Eye Study. *Arch Ophthalmol* 1994;112:85-91.

Kramer P, Lubkin V, Potter W, et al. Cyclic changes in conjunctival smears from menstruating females. *Ophthalmology* 1990;97:303-307.

Kunert KS, Tisdale AS, Stern ME, et al. Analysis of topical cyclosporine treatment of patients with dry eye syndrome: effect on conjunctival lymphocytes. *Arch Ophthalmol* 2000;118:1489-1496.

Lee AJ, Mitchell P, Rochtchina E, Healey PR, for the Blue Mountains Eye Study. Female reproductive factors and open angle glaucoma: the Blue Mountains Eye Study. *Br J Ophthalmol* 2003;87:1324-1328.

Marcozzi G, Liberati V, Madia F, Pizzinga A, de Feo G. Effect of hormone replacement therapy on lacrimal fluid peroxidase activity in women. *Maturitas* 2003;45:225-229.

McCarthy CA, Ng I, Waldron B, et al. Relation of hormone and menopausal status to outcomes following excimer laser photorefractive keratectomy in women. Melbourne Excimer Laser Group. *Aust NZ J Ophthalmol* 1996; 24:215-222.

Metka M, Enzelsberger H, Knogler W, et al. Ophthalmic complaints as a climacteric symptom. *Maturitas* 1991;14:3-8.

Ogueta SB, Schwartz SD, Yamashita CK, Ferber DB. Estrogen receptor in the human eye: influence of gender and age on gene expression. *Invest Ophthalmol Vis Sci* 1999;40:1906-1911.

Paganini-Hill A, Clark LJ. Eye problems in breast cancer patients treated with tamoxifen. *Breast Cancer Res Treat* 2000;60:167-172.

Sall K, Stevenson OD, Mundorf TK, Reis BL, for the CsA Phase 3 Study Group. Two multicenter, randomized studies of the efficacy and safety of cyclosporine ophthalmic emulsion in moderate to severe dry eye disease. *Ophthalmology* 2000;107:631-639.

Sator MO, Akramian J, Joura EA, et al. Reduction of intraocular pressure in a glaucoma patient undergoing hormone replacement therapy. *Maturitas* 1998;29:93-95.

Schaumberg DA, Buring JE, Sullivan DA, Dana MR. Hormone replacement therapy and dry eye syndrome. *JAMA* 2001;286:2114-2119.

Schaumberg DA, Gulati A, Mathers WD, et al. Development and validation of a short global dry eye symptom index. *Ocul Surf* 2007;1:50-57.

Schaumberg DA, Sullivan DA, Buring JE, Dana MR. Prevalence of dry eye syndrome among US women. *Am J Ophthalmol* 2003;136:318-326.

Scott G, Yiu SC, Wasilewski D, et al. Combined esterified estrogen and methyltestosterone treatment for dry eye syndrome in postmenopausal women. *Am J Ophthalmol* 2005;139:1109-1110.

Smith JA, Vitale S, Reed GF, et al. Dry eye signs and symptoms in women with premature ovarian failure. *Arch Ophthalmol* 2004;122:151-156.

Stern ME, Beuerman RW, Fox RI, Gao J, Mircheff AK, Pflugfelder SC. The pathology of dry eye: the interaction between the ocular surface and lacrimal glands. *Cornea* 1998;17:584-589.

Sullivan DA, ed. *Lacrimal Gland, Tear Film, and Dry Eye Syndromes: Basic Science and Clinical Relevence.* New York: Springer, 2007.

Tanriverdi F, Silveira LF, MacColl GS, Boulox PM. The hypothalamic-pituitary-gonadal axis: immune function and autoimmunity. *J Endocrinol* 2003;176:293-304.

Taylor A, Jacques PF, Chylack LT Jr, et al. Long-term intake of vitamins and carotenoids and odds of early age-related cortical and posterior subcapsular lens opacities. *Am J Clin Nutr* 2002;75:540-549.

Toker E, Yenice O, Akpinar I, et al. The influence of sex hormones on ocular blood flow in women. *Acta Ophthalmol Scand* 2003;81:617-624.

Uncu G, Avci R, Uncu Y, et al. The effects of different hormone replacement therapy regimens on tear function, intraocular pressure and lens opacity. *Gynecol Endocrinol* 2006;22:501-505.

van Leeuwen, Boekhoorn S, Vingerling JR, et al. Dietary intake of antioxidants and risk of age-related macular degeneration. *JAMA* 2005;294:3101-3107.

Vecsei PV, Kircher K, Kaminski S, Nagel G, Breitenecker G, Kohlberger PD. Immunohistochemical detection of estrogen and progesterone receptor in human cornea. *Maturitas* 2000;36:169-172.

Worzola K, Hiller R, Sperduto RD, et al. Postmenopausal estrogen use, type of menopause, and lens opacities: the Framingham Studies. *Arch Intern Med* 2001;161:1448-1454.

Hearing changes

American Academy of Family Physicians. *Age Charts for Periodic Health Examination*. Kansas City, KS: American Academy of Family Physicians, 1994.

Canadian Task Force on the Periodic Examination. *Canadian Guide to Clinical Preventive Health Care*. Ottawa, ON, Canada: Canada Communication Group, 1994;258-266, 298-304, 954-963.

Davis A, Stephens D, Rayment A, et al. Hearing impairments in middle age; the acceptability, benefit, and cost of detection (ABCD). *Br J Audiol* 1992; 26:1-14.

Guimaraes P, Frisina ST, Mapes F, et al. Progestin negatively affects hearing in aged women. *Proc Natl Acad Sci USA* 2006;103:14246-14249.

Hederstierna C, Hultcrantz M, Collins A, Rosenhall U. Hearing in women at menopause. Prevalence of hearing loss, audiometric configuration and relation to hormone replacement therapy. *Acta Otolaryngol* 2007;127:149-155.

Hultcrantz M, Simonska R, Sternberg AE. Estrogen and hearing: a summary of recent investigations. *Acta Otolaryngol* 2006;126:10-14.

Khaliq F, Tandon OP, Goel N. Differential effects of estrogen-progesterone on auditory evoked potentials in menopausal women. *Indian J Physiol Pharmacol* 2005;49:345-352.

Mulrow CD, Aguilar C, Endicott JE, et al. Quality of life changes and hearing impairment: results of a randomized trial. *Ann Intern Med* 1990;113:188-194.

Mulrow CD, Lichtenstein MJ. Screening for hearing impairment in the elderly: rationale and strategy. *J Gen Intern Med* 1991;6:249-258.

National Academy of Sciences, Institute of Medicine. Ad Hoc Advisory Group on Preventive Services. *Preventive Services for the Well Population*. Washington DC: National Academy of Sciences, 1978.

Strachan D. Sudden sensineural deafness and hormone replacement therapy. *J Laryngol Otol* 1996;110:1148-1150.

US Preventive Services Task Force. *Guide to Clinical Preventive Services*, 2nd ed. Baltimore, MD: Williams & Wilkins, 1996:393-405.

Arthritis and arthralgia

American College of Rheumatology. Guidelines for the management of rheumatoid arthritis: 2002 update. *Arthritis Rheum* 2002;46:328-346.

Arthritis Foundation. *Alternative Therapies: Glucosamine Sulfate and Chondroitin* Available at: http://www.arthritis.org/conditions/alttherapies/glucosamine.asp. Accessed September 25, 2007.

Barrett-Connor E. Postmenopausal estrogen therapy and selected (less-often-considered) disease outcomes. *Menopause* 1999;6:14-20.

Bathon JM, Martin RW, Fleischmann AM, et al. A comparison of etanercept and methotrexate in patients with early rheumatoid arthritis. *N Engl J Med* 2000;343:1586-1593.

Bradley JD, Flusser D, Katz BP, et al. A randomized, double-blind, placebo controlled trial of intravenous loading with S-adenosylmethionine (SAM) followed by oral SAM therapy in patients with knee osteoarthritis. *J Rheumatol* 1994;21:905-911.

Brandt KD, Doherty M, Lohmander S, eds. *Osteoarthritis*, 2nd ed. New York: Oxford University Press, 2003.

Brennan P, Bankhead C, Silman A, Symmonds D. Oral contraceptives and rheumatoid arthritis: results from a primary care-based incident case-control study. *Semin Arthritis Rheum* 1997;26:817-823.

Bruyere O, Pavelka K, Rovati LC, et al. Glucosamine sulfate reduces osteoarthritis progression in postmenopausal women with knee osteoarthritis: evidence from two 3-year studies. *Menopause* 2004;11:138-143.

Clauw DJ, Chrousos GP. Chronic pain and fatigue syndromes: overlapping clinical and neuroendocrine features and potential pathogenic mechanisms. *Neuroimmunomodulation* 1997;4:134-153.

Clegg DO, Reda DJ, Harris CL, et al. Glucosamine, chondroitin sulfate, and the two in combination for painful knee osteoarthritis. *N Engl J Med* 2006;354:795-808.

Deal C, Moskowitz RW. Nutraceuticals as therapeutic agents in osteoarthritis: the role of glucosamine, chondroitin sulfate, and collagen hydrolysate. *Rheum Dis Clin North Am* 1999;25:379-395.

Felson DT, Nevitt MC. The effects of estrogen on osteoarthritis. *Curr Opin Rheumatol* 1998;10:269-272.

Felson DT, Zhang Y. An update on the epidemiology of knee and hip osteoarthritis with a view to prevention. *Arthritis Rheum* 1998;41:1343-1355.

Gabriel SE, Jaakkimainen L, Bombardier C. Risk for serious gastrointestinal complications related to use of nonsteroidal anti-inflammatory drugs: a meta-analysis. *Ann Intern Med* 1991;115:787-796.

Hall GM, Daniels M, Huskisson EC, Spector TC. A randomized controlled trial of the effect of hormone replacement therapy on disease activity in postmenopausal rheumatoid arthritis. *Ann Rheum Dis* 1994;53:112-116.

Hall GM, Spector TD, Delmas PD. Markers of bone metabolism in postmenopausal women with rheumatoid arthritis: effects of corticosteroids and hormone replacement therapy. *Arthritis Rheum* 1995;38:902-906.

Hernandez-Avila M, Liang MH, Willett WC, et al. Exogenous sex hormones and the risk of rheumatoid arthritis. *Arthritis Rheum* 1990;33:947-953.

Hochberg MC, Lethbridge-Cejku M, Scott WW, Reichle R, Plato CC, Tobin JD. The association of body weight, body fatness and body fat distribution with osteoarthritis of the knee: data from the Baltimore Longitudinal Study of Aging. *J Rheumatol* 1995;22:488-493.

Klippel JH, ed. *Primer on the Rheumatic Diseases*, 12th ed. Atlanta, GA: Arthritis Foundation, 2001.

Lowe CJ, Barker KL, Dewey M, Sackley CM. Effectiveness of physiotherapy exercise after knee arthroplasty for osteoarthritis: systematic review and meta-analysis of randomised controlled trials. *BMJ* 2007;[Epub ahead of print].

MacDonald AG, Murphy EA, Capell HA, Bankowska UZ, Ralston SH. Effects of hormone replacement therapy in rheumatoid arthritis: a double-blind placebo-controlled study. *Ann Rheum Dis* 1994;53:54-57.

McAlindon TE, LaValley MP, Gulin FP, Felson DT. Glucosamine and chondroitin for treatment of osteoarthritis: a systematic quality assessment and meta-analysis. *JAMA* 2000;283:1469-1475.

Najm WI, Reinsch S, Hoehler F, Tobis JS, Harvey PW. S-Adenosyl methionine (SAMe) versus celecoxib for the treatment of osteoarthritis symptoms: a double-blind cross-over trial. *BMC Musculoskelet Disord* 2004;5:6.

Nevitt MC, Cummings SR, Lane NE, et al, for the Study of Osteoporotic Fractures Research Group. Association of estrogen replacement therapy with the risk of osteoarthritis of the hip in elderly white women. *Arch Intern Med* 1996;156:2073-2080.

Oliveria SA, Felson DT, Klein RA, Reed JI, Walker AM. Estrogen replacement therapy and the development of osteoarthritis. *Epidemiology* 1996;7:415-419.

Pavelka K, Gatterova J, Olejarova M, Machacek S, Giacovelli G, Rovati LC. Glucosamine sulfate use and delay of progression of knee osteoarthritis: a 3-year, randomized, placebo-controlled, double-blind study. *Arch Intern Med* 2002;162:2113-2123.

Rao JK, Mihaliak K, Kroenke K, Bradley J, Tierney WM, Weinberger M. Use of complementary therapies for arthritis among patients of rheumatologists. *Ann Intern Med* 1999;131:409-416.

Reginster JY, Deroisy R, Rovati LC, et al. Long-term effects of glucosamine sulphate on osteoarthritis progression: a randomised, placebo-controlled clinical trial. *Lancet* 2001;357:251-256.

Richy R, Bruyere O, Ethgen O, Cucherat M, Henrotin Y, Reginster J-Y. Structural and symptomatic efficacy of glucosamine and chondroitin in knee osteoarthritis. *Arch Intern Med* 2003;163:1514-1522.

Ryan LM, McCarthy DJ. Calcium pyrophosphate disease; pseudogout; articular chondrocalcinosis. In: Koopman WJ, ed. *Arthritis and Allied Conditions.* Baltimore, MD: Williams & Wilkins, 2001.

Scroggie DA, Albright A, Harris MD. The effect of glucosamine-chondroitin supplementation on glycosylated hemoglobin levels in patients with type 2 diabetes mellitus: a placebo-controlled, double-blinded, randomized clinical trial. *Arch Intern Med* 2003;163:1587-1590.

Sergent JS. Extrahepatic manifestations of hepatitis B infection. *Bull Rheum Dis* 1983;33:1-6.

Spector TD, Nandra D, Hart DJ, Doyle DV. Is hormone replacement therapy protective for hand and knee osteoarthritis in women? The Chingford study. *Ann Rheum Dis* 1997;56:432-434.

Towheed TE, Maxwell L, Anastassiades T, et al. Glucosamine therapy for treating osteoarthritis. *Cochrane Database Syst Rev* 2005;2:CD002946.

van den Brink HR, van Everdingen AA, van Wijk MJ, Jacobs JW, Bijlsma JW. Adjuvant estrogen therapy does not influence disease activity in postmenopausal patients with rheumatoid arthritis. *Ann Rheum Dis* 1993;52:862-865.

von Muhlen D, Morton D, von Muhlen CA, Barrett-Connor E. Post-menopausal estrogen and increased risk of clinical osteoarthritis at the hip, hand, and knee in older women. *J Womens Health Gend Based Med* 2002;11:511-518.

Zhang Y, McAlindon TE, Hannan MT, et al. Estrogen replacement therapy and worsening of radiographic knee osteoarthritis: the Framingham Study. *Arthritis Rheum* 1998;41:1867-1873.

Menopause is a natural event for most women, occurring at around age 51. The usual range is 45 to 55 years. However, some women experience menopause earlier than usual. Ovarian insufficiency resulting in premature menopause is thought to affect approximately 1% of reproductive-age women in North America (approximately 0.1% before age 30). Most women with this diagnosis have remaining primordial follicles that do not adequately respond to gonadotropin stimulation. Those follicles, however, may still function sufficiently to produce estradiol. Ovulation (and thus potential pregnancy) may occur intermittently and unpredictably for years. Although menopausal hormone therapy (HT), either estrogen alone or with progestogen, is often prescribed to augment folliculogenesis, no treatment has proven effective in restoring fertility.

Premature menopause is a general term used to describe menopause that occurs at or before age 40. This can happen either naturally (spontaneously) or it can be induced through medical interventions (bilateral oophorectomy or ovarian damage from chemotherapy or pelvic radiation therapy).

The younger a woman is when she experiences menopause, the longer she is without reproductive-age levels of endogenous estrogen. This increases her risk for symptoms and diseases associated with low estrogen levels compared with women who reach menopause at the typical age. Menopause symptoms, the possible effects on sexual function and mental health, and prevention of osteoporosis and heart disease should be discussed.

Premature ovarian failure (POF) describes ovarian insufficiency leading to amenorrhea in women before age 40. Although most cases are permanent, POF can be transient. When POF is permanent, the term "premature menopause" applies.

Some cases of premature ovarian insufficiency or POF lead to temporary amenorrhea. Women who overexercise or overdiet may experience amenorrhea due to a hypo-estrogenic state, which is a typical premature secondary ovarian insufficiency as the problem is due to hypothalamic dysfunctions. Some women experience temporary amenorrhea after chemotherapy or pelvic radiation therapy. Certain drug therapies, such as gonadotropin-releasing hormone (GnRH) analogues—which inhibit secretion of gonadotropins by blocking GnRH receptors at the pituitary, causing the ovaries to temporarily stop hormone production, inducing a hypoestrogenic state—may also result in temporary amenorrhea.

Natural premature menopause

This section reviews the causes, evaluation, symptoms, and management of natural premature menopause.

Causes. It is estimated that between 5% and 25% of women with idiopathic or presumed autoimmune POF will experience at least one spontaneous remission. Among women with POF who have a normal karyotype, one half may still have ovarian follicles capable of functioning intermittently.

Because the ovaries of women with POF fail to function adequately in response to appropriate endogenous gonadotropin stimulation, the condition is also known as "primary ovarian insufficiency." In contrast, "secondary ovarian insufficiency" refers to the failure of the hypothalamus and pituitary glands to produce appropriate gonadotropin stimulation.

Two thirds of cases of POF are idiopathic. Known causes are listed below in Table 1.

Table 1. Known causes of premature ovarian failure
Karyotype abnormality
Pure gonadal dysgenesis
Iatrogenic treatments
Autoimmune disorders
• Polyglandular
• Immunoglobulin G, immunoglobulin A
Miscellaneous disorders
• Enzyme deficiency
• Metabolic syndromes
• Pseudohypoparathyroidism
• Thymic disorders
Pseudo causes
• Gonadotropin-producing pituitary adenoma
• Hypothyroidism
• Isolated gonadotropin deficiency

Familial clusters of POF clearly exist. In a large Italian study, early ovarian failure had a recognizable heritable association in nearly one third of the women evaluated. Although genetic or familial factors may influence ovarian aging, the prevalence of these factors, the relative expression, and the proportion of early ovarian failure attributed to genetic or familial causes are not known.

The gene locus on the X chromosome is related to ovarian failure. Women with a single X chromosome, such as those with Turner's syndrome, develop normal ovaries with a normal complement of primordial follicles. They experience accelerated atresia (degeneration of ovarian follicles) that often leads to ovarian failure. Most women with galactosemia (an autosomal-recessive condition) eventually develop POF, along with hepatocellular damage, renal cellular damage, the development of cataracts, and mental retardation.

Uterine artery embolization for symptomatic uterine fibroids is another possible cause of earlier ovarian failure with an iatrogenic basis. Women undergoing this procedure should be informed about the possible risk for ovarian failure earlier than expected.

With hysterectomy, the ovaries are not automatically removed. However, a hysterectomy alone is associated with earlier ovarian failure. In the experience of one institution, the mean age of ovarian failure in a group of women who had undergone hysterectomy was 45.4 ± 4.0 years—significantly younger than the mean age of 49.5 ± 4.04 years in women who had not had this surgery (see page 107 for more about induced menopause).

Inflammatory causes of ovarian failure are well known. These include many infectious etiologies. Classically, mumps infection is associated with POF. When a patient develops mumps parotitis, ovarian failure should be suspected when lower abdominal tenderness or ovarian pain occurs. Cause-and-effect relationships between febrile illness and ovarian failure have not been established in part because POF is relatively infrequent.

Lifestyle factors such as smoking, socioeconomic factors, and oral contraceptive use have not been associated with POF (although smoking is associated with earlier menopause). If primary amenorrhea is associated with pubertal delay, a chromosomal defect is much more likely.

Evaluation. Unfortunately, there is no characteristic menstrual history preceding either POF or premature menopause. Cessation of menses may be abrupt; it may manifest as oligomenorrhea (infrequent menstrual flow) or as abnormal uterine bleeding. These conditions can also occur postpartum or after cessation of oral contraceptive use.

Diagnosis of premature natural menopause (ie, hypergonadotropic amenorrhea in women aged 40 y or younger) is mainly clinical and, to a degree, retrospective. Studies have not determined which women with signs and symptoms of POF progress to premature menopause. Because estrogen deficiency has a cumulative negative effect on bone density and probably cardiovascular disease (CVD), a timely diagnosis is warranted.

Prognosis regarding progression from intermittent POF to premature menopause is poorly understood. This makes individual patient counseling regarding fertility prognosis very uncertain. Obtaining a karyotype in the workup to identify an X chromosome abnormality can be helpful. This will be more likely for women who are less than age 30 or have short stature.

In most women with premature menopause, the gynecologic history is unremarkable. The majority give a history of no prior problem with conception. Symptoms vary. As POF develops, many women have some type of menstrual disorder, such as oligomenorrhea, amenorrhea, or abnormal uterine bleeding. During the transition from normal to abnormal function, estrogen levels and follicle-stimulating hormone (FSH) levels fluctuate.

A careful history and physical examination are needed to rule out potential secondary causes of menstrual dysfunction, such as androgen excess, systemic disease (eg, hyperthyroidism, adrenal insufficiency, bleeding disorder), eating disorder, opiate abuse or use of a psychotropic drug, gonorrheal or chlamydial infection, or galactorrhea. The medical history should also identify any prior ovarian surgery, chemotherapy, or pelvic radiation, as well as a personal or family history of autoimmune disorders, such as hypothyroidism, Hashimoto's thyroiditis, Addison's disease, diabetes mellitus (DM), Graves' disease, vitiligo, systemic lupus erythematosus, rheumatoid arthritis, Sjögren's syndrome, or inflammatory bowel disease. The differential diagnosis of abnormal uterine bleeding includes common gynecologic disorders that can also be present, such as uterine fibroids, ovarian cysts, endometriosis, or pelvic inflammatory disease.

The physical examination should include evaluation for atrophic vaginal changes, such as vaginal pallor, increased vaginal pH, vaginal or cervical petechiae, decreased vaginal moisture, or friability, in addition to complete pelvic and rectal examinations when appropriate. Because intermittent estrogen stimulation is possible, these symptoms and signs are not definitive.

Laboratory tests should be performed to exclude other potential endocrine or genetic causes. (Potential tests are listed in Table 2.)

Table 2. Evaluation for premature ovarian failure and premature menopause

- Complete history and physical examination
- Luteinizing hormone, FSH, and estradiol levels on at least two occasions
- Maturation index
- Karyotype (most appropriate for women younger than age 30, particularly those with short stature)
- Complete blood cell count with differential cell count, sedimentation rate, total serum protein and albumin-globulin ratio, rheumatoid factor, antinuclear antibody
- Fasting blood sugar level, serum calcium and phosphorus concentrations, evaluation of adrenal status
- Free thyroxine, thyroid-stimulating hormone, thyroid peroxidase antibody, antithyroglobulin and thyroid-stimulating hormone receptor antibodies
- Bone mineral determination by dual-energy x-ray absorptiometry

---

In addition to evaluating clinical estrogen status, measuring circulating FSH, luteinizing hormone (LH), and estradiol concentrations at different times may help determine if any functional follicles are present. Vaginal pelvic ultrasound used to detect the presence of follicles can be helpful if accurate and precise ultrasound capability is available.

An estradiol concentration greater than 50 pg/mL (183 pmol/L) or an LH level greater than the FSH level suggests the presence of viable oocytes. Irregular uterine bleeding, indicative of continuing estrogen production, also suggests the presence of remaining functional oocytes.

When women are under age 40, particularly when they have short stature, obtaining a karyotype is recommended. This may be important in counseling if a Y chromosomal fragment is present, and it might be helpful in regard to familial syndromes that include POF. POF should be in the differential diagnosis when patients present with postpartum amenorrhea.

The progestogen-withdrawal challenge test can be misleading and is not routinely recommended. When 4 months of amenorrhea are encountered, an FSH level in the postmenopausal range (>30 mIU/mL), particularly if reconfirmed 1 month later, suggests ovarian failure. Premature menopause implies 12 months of amenorrhea.

Bone density testing by dual-energy x-ray (DXA) is now widely available to assess for bone loss. Many women with POF have osteopenia (decrease in bone density). Normative values for naturally postmenopausal women are available now for Caucasians, African Americans, and, in some centers, other racial groups. The norms, however, were developed for women who experienced natural menopause at the typical age. Extrapolation to younger women is problematic, with lack of precision and diminished accuracy. Because of the inability to discern signal from noise, serial bone density testing is recommended when clinically indicated, no more frequently than every 2 years. (For more about bone health, see Section E, page 113.)

It may be of value to assess ovarian reserve in women of increasing age as well as younger women who may be at risk for POF (previous ovarian surgery, pelvic radiation, exposure to cytotoxic drugs, autoimmune diseases, and smokers). There are a number of tests that seek to identify depleted ovarian reserve. Day-3 determination of FSH is widely used. Clinicians should be aware that assays for such testing often use different reference standards and there is no unanimity of normal cutoff values. It is important that the diagnosis of POF never be made based upon one elevated FSH level. Another test of ovarian reserve is the Clomid challenge test in which day-3 FSH is measured, 100 mg of clomiphene citrate is given on cycle days 5 through 9, and FSH remeasured on cycle day 10. An elevation of FSH on day 10 may indicate diminished ovarian reserve. Other tests sometimes employed include ultrasound examination to determine mean ovarian volume and number of antral follicles, as well as estradiol measurements on cycle day 3.

Symptoms. Women experiencing menopause earlier than usual may report more physical and psychological consequences than women who experience the transition to menopause at the usual age. If the premature menopause is natural, perimenopause can last for several years and will often resemble perimenopause that would occur at the typical age. If menopause is surgically induced, ovarian function ends abruptly, often resulting in more severe symptoms. If menopause is induced by medical treatments, severe symptoms can occur, particularly in young women who had high hormone levels before treatment. If menopause is the result of a disease or medical treatment of the disease, those effects must also be managed.

Compared with natural menopause at the typical age, premature menopause is associated with a higher risk of osteopenia. The younger a woman is when premature menopause occurs, the greater her potential risk of a fracture. Risk of CVD seems to be increased as well. Of those experiencing menopause at age 35 or younger, it has been estimated that there is a 2.8 greater relative risk of developing a myocardial infarction. Women with premature menopause are also more likely to develop dry eye syndrome.

Management. Although research to guide clinical management of some forms of premature menopause is lacking, the following management approaches to physical and emotional health issues are appropriate:

- Provide counseling regarding childbearing options before treatments or surgery that may induce menopause. Referral to an infertility specialist and discussion of potential for pregnancy using donated eggs may be appropriate.

- Offer psychological support (eg, for concerns about early loss of fertility, self-image, and sexual function).

- Offer menopausal HT, if not contraindicated, to treat acute menopause-related symptoms. For women undergoing chemotherapy or radiation therapy, it is also important to consider the diseases that led to those treatments and manage the adverse effects associated with those treatments.

- Discuss strategies to reduce long-term risks of diseases related to prolonged diminished levels of estrogen.

There are no definitive research data on treatment options for this population of women. Clinicians must choose from those approaches proven effective in trials among women reaching menopause at the typical age (see Section C).

Vasomotor and vaginal symptoms. Most women who experience premature menopause may consider estrogen therapy (ET) or, if their uterus is intact, estrogen plus progestogen therapy (EPT) to relieve acute vasomotor and vaginal symptoms associated with diminished estrogen. The latest NAMS position statement on HT advises that data from trials such as the Women's Health Initiative (WHI) should not necessarily be extrapolated to considerably younger women experiencing premature menopause. Some women will have persistent vaginal atrophy that becomes more severe with advancing age. Long-term use of low-dose local ET may be required to maintain a healthy vaginal epithelium. (See Section G, page 222.)

The guideline of using the lowest effective dose of HT applies, with periodic reevaluation focusing on weighing risks and benefits. However, in these women, long-term use until the typical age of menopause is indicated as they are deprived of normal circulating ovulatory levels, which are much higher than the doses useful to prevent symptoms, bone loss, and possible CVD. Higher doses may be required by some women for complete symptom relief. Oral contraceptives will supply this higher dose, and some women might find these pills more socially acceptable.

Although clinical trial data are lacking regarding the optimal length of HT for women with premature menopause, most healthcare professionals recommend continuing until at least age 50, provided no adverse effects are observed. Therapy can continue as long as the benefits outweigh the risks.

Sexual function. Since premature menopause occurs at an age when women usually engage in more frequent sexual activity, they may be more affected by any sexual function change than older women. After a period of adjustment, most women experiencing premature menopause are able to resume a fulfilling sex life. Clinicians can provide information regarding what to expect during this time of change to make coping easier. Treatment with methyltestosterone or compounded testosterone may also be considered, although there are no clinical data regarding safety and efficacy with long-term therapy (see Section G, page 223, for more about testosterone).

Bone loss. Women experiencing premature menopause will spend more years with lower levels of endogenous estrogen, increasing their lifetime risk for osteoporosis. The younger a woman is when she reaches menopause, the greater the potential long-term risk. A healthy lifestyle to reduce this health risk should be a part of the woman's counseling.

To help prevent bone loss, recommendations should include intake of calcium (1,200-1,500 mg/day) and vitamin D (at least 800 IU/d) as well as the need for weight-bearing exercises. (For more, see Section H, page 240.) Baseline and periodic bone density testing may be required.

Women who experience premature menopause, regardless of the cause, need long-term protection against bone loss. When lifestyle approaches alone are not adequate, clinicians may choose from several prescription options that have been proven effective in other populations of women (see Section E, page 119, for more). There are no trial data to determine whether any prescription therapy will reduce morbidity or mortality from osteoporosis in women with premature menopause. For women reaching menopause at an early age, the benefits of HT may outweigh the risks, even with lifelong therapy. However, some women as well as

clinicians may be concerned about the use of HT over the long term. They may prefer to manage the acute vasomotor and vaginal symptoms with HT, and then choose from among several bone-specific agents (eg, bisphosphonate) for long-term therapy, although none of these agents has been studied in young women with premature menopause, and their safety for more than 10 years is unknown. Also, these women should not use bisphosphonates if a pregnancy by ova donation is a consideration as these drugs are leached from the bone over time and their effect on the developing fetus is unknown.

Cardiovascular disease. Women experiencing premature menopause will probably have increased risk of CVD. To lower cardiovascular risk, testing for risk factors and changes in lipids is important, along with recommendations for a heart-healthy diet, weight loss (if needed), and aerobic exercise daily. Studies are lacking to determine whether any prescription therapy will reduce morbidity or mortality from CVD in women with premature menopause. Whether or not premature menopause has occurred, women who are at high risk for CVD should have all cardiovascular risk factors assessed. They should be appropriately screened for DM and practitioners should be proactive in prevention, including giving good dietary and exercise prescriptions. When risk factors for DM or heart disease are uncovered, the practitioner needs to assure adequate control of cholesterol, blood pressure, and blood sugar by lifestyle or prescription medication, or both, if indicated. (For more, see Section E.)

Autoimmune disease. If a woman has experienced premature menopause attributed to an autoimmune etiology, she should also be followed for the presence of associated autoimmune endocrine disorders, including thyroiditis, hypothyroidism, hypoparathyroidism, adrenal insufficiency, and DM.

Mental health. Because premature menopause means the end of "natural" childbearing, the psychological impact can be significant (see Table 3). Some women (and their partners) may benefit from professional counseling in dealing with their feelings.

Pregnancy. Due to the potential for spontaneous and unexpected pregnancy, women with POF should be counseled regarding their desire to conceive. If pregnancy is not desired, the full range of contraceptive choices should be offered, remembering that long-term use of contraceptives represents a pharmacologic dose that provides levels much higher than those in normally cycling woman (and much higher than the usual HT dose). If contraception is not desired, lower menopausal levels of EPT can be recommended. In this setting, cyclic EPT is preferred over continuous therapy, as cyclic therapy will induce regular menses. If a period is missed on this regimen, a pregnancy test should be performed and EPT stopped.

Table 3. Possible emotions linked to premature menopause
• Feeling old, regardless of actual age, in a society that values youth and fertility
• Embarrassment about going through menopause at a young age
• A feeling of losing control over bodily functions
• Grief and loss for the children the woman hoped to conceive, similar to that experienced after the death of a loved one
• A feeling of failure or of no longer being a "complete woman," that her inability to have children is her fault
• Concerns about her partner's and/or extended family's reaction to her inability to conceive and, sometimes, a feeling of uncertainty about whether her partner will continue to love her
• Concerns about relationships and sexuality, such as fear of losing the ability to elicit or feel sexual desire, fear of rejection by her sexual partner, and a fear of discomfort during intercourse
• Concerns about finding someone who will love her even though she is unable to have children
• Isolation and loneliness, as if no one understands what she is going through
• Concerns about the long-term effects of estrogen loss (eg, increased risk of osteoporosis, CVD)
• Jealousy, anger, and resentment when friends or family members become pregnant, and guilt over having those feelings
• Irritability and fatigue caused by menopause-related hot flashes that interfere with sleep, making coping more difficult

Before undergoing treatments or surgery that may cause premature menopause, all women should discuss their concerns about childbearing with their healthcare providers and partners. Options for preserving fertility include prior oocyte retrieval, oocyte cryopreservation, embryo cryopreservation, ovarian tissue cryopreservation, ovarian suppression with hormones, ovarian transposition, and conservative gynecologic surgery (eg, trachelectomy for cervical cancer). However, not all options are available for all women. Surrogacy or ovum donation may be another option. Whether a woman can use these options depends on factors such as age, general health, financial status, and the cause of premature menopause. Adoption is also an alternative to keep in mind.

Because the impact of pelvic radiation and/or chemotherapy on ovarian function is sometimes not readily apparent, sexually active, reproductive-age women facing these interventions should discuss fertility preservation or the need for birth control with their healthcare clinician.

Induced menopause

Induced menopause occurs as a result of bilateral oophorectomy or ovarian damage from other medical causes, such as chemotherapy or radiation therapy. With induced menopause, levels of ovarian hormones (including estrogen, progesterone, testosterone, and androstenedione) often drop rapidly, which may exacerbate symptoms, especially hot flashes. Some women can also experience mood changes, lack of energy, depression, and insomnia, although it is unclear whether these symptoms are due to the original disease process, comorbid conditions, the stress of treatment, or loss of hormone production.

This section reviews the different effects that induced menopause—from surgery, chemotherapy, or pelvic radiation—has on menopause symptoms, fertility, sexual function, and mental health.

Menopause symptoms. The frequency and severity of menopause symptoms in a woman experiencing premature menopause depend on her age and whether menopause was natural, surgically induced, induced by chemotherapy, or caused by pelvic radiation therapy. With induced menopause, ovarian hormone levels fall dramatically, typically resulting in more sudden and severe menopause symptoms such as hot flashes, insomnia, and vaginal atrophy (particularly after menopause induced by chemotherapy and pelvic radiation therapy), and changes in sexual function (particularly after some forms of medically induced menopause). Complaints of cognitive dysfunction are not unusual in women experiencing induced menopause.

Surgery. Hot flashes are experienced by most women after surgically induced menopause. Although little objective investigation has been conducted, anecdotal evidence reveals that surgically induced menopause causes more frequent and/or severe hot flash symptoms in association with the rapid lowering of sex steroids. Over time, however, the frequency and severity of symptoms seem to be about the same as those experienced by women who reach menopause naturally.

When postoperative HT is an option, women should receive information on potential risks and benefits of treatment before surgery. Patients should be informed that the WHI randomized clinical trial of oral HT demonstrated reduced risk of breast cancer and heart disease in hysterectomized women using estrogen alone compared with women using combination EPT. ET is sometimes initiated the day of bilateral oophorectomy, avoiding unnecessary hot flashes and night sweats. Often, transdermal estrogen is prescribed because oral therapy may be difficult to ingest immediately after surgery. Using a transdermal preparation also may be associated with less risk of thromboembolism during the immediate postoperative period—a time known to be of greater risk for an event. Some clinicians might recommend HT only after a woman has been discharged from the hospital. (See Section G for more.)

Women who should not or choose not to start HT after bilateral oophorectomy should be prepared preoperatively for symptoms they likely will experience and alternative approaches discussed.

Cancer therapy. Menopause-related symptoms may be more intense after high-dose pelvic radiation than after chemotherapy. With both types of therapy, symptoms may occur concurrently with treatment or within 3 to 6 months.

For women who experience induced menopause from chemotherapy or pelvic radiation therapy for hormone-sensitive cancer, all types of HT (eg, ET/EPT, hormonal contraception) might be contraindicated because of potential adverse effects on their tumors. These women may need to use alternative therapies for symptom relief. For vaginal symptoms, low-dose vaginal estrogen that exerts predominantly a local effect, not systemic, is considered a low-risk option.

There may also be other causes of symptoms. For example, hot flashes can result from medications, such as tamoxifen, often prescribed for breast cancer patients. Difficulty coping with cancer can lead to stress that, in turn, can have an adverse effect on sleep.

In addition to hot flashes, vaginal dryness, and diminished sex drive, women undergoing chemotherapy often experience a range of side effects, including extreme fatigue, nausea, and hair loss. There are many effective treatments for these side effects. Women should be advised to maintain a nutritious, protein-filled diet to guard against infection and support tissue rebuilding. Pelvic radiation therapy can result in side effects, but they vary greatly depending on the type and amount of radiation used.

Fertility. The causes of induced menopause affect fertility differently.

Surgery. With bilateral oophorectomy (with or without a hysterectomy), there is no oocyte pool available for fertilization. Fertility ends immediately and permanently, although pregnancy using previously fertilized embryos from the woman or a donor is still possible so long as the uterus is preserved. A hysterectomy with or without a bilateral oophorectomy ends menses and the ability to carry a fetus. If one or both ovaries remain and menopause does not occur, a woman has the potential to have her oocytes fertilized in vitro. The resulting zygote or blastocyst can potentially be implanted into a surrogate who has intact uterine function.

Cancer therapy. Fertility is often possible in women undergoing either chemotherapy or radiation treatment for cancer. The effect on fertility depends on the drug, the size of the radiation field, the dose, the dose intensity, the method of administration, the disease, the patient's age, and the pretreatment fertility of the patient. Female fertility may be impaired despite resumption of cyclic menses.

Systemic chemotherapy affects both normal and carcinogenic cells. The cells most likely to be affected are those of rapid cell turnover, including those in the reproductive system. These effects usually occur over time, not immediately. The more gradual the reduction in ovarian hormones, the more likely the menopause-related symptoms will be moderate as opposed to severe.

Radiation therapy affects the reproductive system only when it is used to treat the pelvic area. Pelvic radiation therapy is more likely to cause permanent menopause if the ovaries receive high doses of radiation (such as during the treatment for cervical cancer). Estrogen levels often decline quickly. If smaller doses of pelvic radiation are used (such as for Hodgkin's disease), the ovaries may recover.

After chemotherapy, the ovaries of younger women (<30 y) are more likely to recover. Some women may experience temporary ovarian failure, with subsequent resumption of menstruation and fertility. Women age 40 or older are more likely to have permanent ovarian damage. Certain chemotherapeutic agents, such as alkylating agents, seem to be more toxic.

Sexual function. The various causes of induced menopause are associated with differing effects on aspects of sexual function, including the following:

Surgery. Surgical procedures vary greatly in the effects on the vagina. Some do not directly affect vaginal tissues, whereas others can adversely affect coital function through a shortening of vaginal length or the development of a painful neuroma or fibroma at the vaginal vault incision.

As noted above, hysterectomy may lead to enjoyable sexual activity for the first time in many years, as women experience relief from pelvic pain, dyspareunia, heavy bleeding, and worries about contraception. During intercourse and orgasm, some women may notice a change in sensation but, in general, these changes do not interfere with sexual functioning.

Women with preexisting sexual problems or depression may continue to experience problems postoperatively. It is advisable to diagnose and treat preoperative depression, as well as to establish sexual function, before surgery.

Without exogenous estrogen, significantly lowered endogenous estrogen can cause severe vaginal symptoms, such as vaginal dryness, irritation, and atrophy. This may result in dyspareunia and increased risk of vaginal infections. The changes in the epithelial lining of the vagina occur relatively rapidly as estrogen levels decline. Subsequent vascular, muscular, and connective tissue changes also occur. Decreased vascularization of the surrounding tissues interferes with delivery of necessary nutrients to the vagina and inhibits engorgement and lubrication. The vagina also loses elasticity and narrows, particularly in women who are sexually abstinent. Induced menopause may also affect the clitoris. Possible changes include a decrease in clitoral perfusion, diminished engorgement during the desire and arousal phases, and a decline in the neurophysiologic response, including slowing of nerve impulses and decreased touch perception, vibratory sensation, and reaction time. In some women, the clitoris may noticeably diminish in size.

Cancer therapy. The side effects of chemotherapy can dramatically reduce sexual desire. Agents used for chemotherapy may irritate the vaginal and uterine linings, which often become dry and inflamed. Vaginal yeast infections are common during chemotherapy, especially in women using steroids or broad-spectrum antibiotics. In addition, fatigue, nausea, altered body image related to hair loss, and other physical changes related to cancer or chemotherapy can interfere with sexual interest.

Depending on the extent of the ovarian damage caused by chemotherapy, the ovaries may continue to produce low levels of testosterone after treatment. If testosterone levels decline significantly, a loss of sexual desire may occur.

Induced menopause is typically associated with an abrupt decline in androgen levels, which may reduce sexual drive. The side effects of chemotherapy can also reduce sexual drive. In addition, women who undergo cancer treatment often have additional emotional concerns that may affect their libido.

Pelvic radiation may cause vaginal itching, burning, and dryness. Vaginal tenderness may occur during treatment and persist for a few weeks afterward. The walls of the vagina may become tough and fibrous, and lose elasticity. Pelvic radiation may make the vaginal lining thin and fragile, and thus more prone to vaginal sores or ulcers. Vaginal scarring from radiation therapy may shorten the vagina, making intercourse impossible. Some women experience pain related to the vagina's decreased caliber or lack of fluid, which may result in vaginismus (the muscles around the opening of the vagina becoming tense and spasmodic, preventing penetration).

During pelvic radiation treatment, some women are advised not to have intercourse. Most women are able to resume intercourse within a few weeks after treatment ends. In this population, use of topical ET may enhance the healing process and sexual function. If estrogen is contraindicated, alternative treatments to support vaginal health and sexual function should be offered.

Mental health. For some women, particularly those who are younger, procedures that cause permanent infertility can precipitate a range of emotions. Women who undergo surgical menopause may have lingering feelings of doubt about the necessity of the surgery. Women who experience induced menopause as a result of treatment for a serious illness may have additional emotional concerns related to the illness and the treatment (see Table 4).

Table 4. Potential emotional concerns related to induced menopause

- Impact of illness
- Decline in sexual function
- Side effects of treatments
- Risk of disease recurrence
- Concerns about mortality (cancer patients)
- Disease risk related to lower ovarian hormone levels
- Infertility
- Emotional health
- More severe menopause symptoms

Surgery. In anticipation of surgical menopause, women often have significant concerns regarding the effects of surgery on psychological well-being and sexuality. The impact of hysterectomy (often with concurrent oophorectomy) on well-being and sexuality will vary depending on many factors. These include a woman's preoperative mental health and sexual function, the indications for surgery, and the specific procedure being performed. Whether or not HT is an option also will affect postoperative symptoms.

Early clinical reports from the 1940s to 1970s suggested that hysterectomy led to increased psychiatric disorders and other psychological problems for women. Those early studies supported the notion that hysterectomy might lead to increased psychological morbidity and psychiatric problems. These studies, however, had a number of methodologic limitations. Most of them assessed psychiatric functioning only after hysterectomy, few used standardized measures, and study groups were very heterogeneous in terms of reason for and type of surgery, especially as to whether ovaries were removed or kept intact. In addition, women who underwent hysterectomy were not compared with women in the general population.

More recent research that overcomes some of these methodologic limitations presents a different picture. Prospective studies of women undergoing hysterectomy show no evidence of increased psychological dysfunction after surgery. Most studies show that mental health and overall quality of life improve for most women after hysterectomy. Research that has examined factors related to outcomes has shown that women who have preexisting psychiatric problems are least likely to improve after surgery. There is some evidence that women who also undergo bilateral oophorectomy may have worse outcomes, but this may be due in part to preexisting differences. Likewise, a systematic review of the literature from 1985 to 2003 revealed that many of the studies addressing the important question of sexuality after hysterectomy were of limited quality. Well-designed, prospective studies generally demonstrate improved sexual function after hysterectomy. In the Maine Women's Health Study, a prospective cohort of approximately 400 women undergoing hysterectomy for benign disease, dyspareunia, as well as interest in and enjoyment of sexual activity, all improved significantly 1 year after surgery. In the Maryland Women's Health Study, investigators found that sexual functioning generally improved after hysterectomy, similar to the observed increase in overall health status and quality of life. The percentage of women who engaged in sexual relations increased significantly from 70% before hysterectomy to 78% and 77% at 12 and 24 months, respectively, postoperatively. Frequent dyspareunia decreased from 19% preoperatively to 4% after hysterectomy, and the likelihood of experiencing orgasms increased from 63% to 72%. Low libido also decreased significantly, from 10% before hysterectomy to 6% after surgery.

Now, most studies demonstrate improved sexual functioning after hysterectomy for benign disease. These benefits are seen whether the cervix is removed or retained, and even with concurrent bilateral oophorectomy. Several studies do suggest an adverse effect of bilateral oophorectomy on libido and orgasmic response, possibly owing to a decline in circulating androgen concentrations postoperatively. Women considering elective bilateral oophorectomy should be informed that although most studies identify no adverse effects of concurrent oophorectomy on sexuality, some women may be affected by the sudden and significant decline in ovarian hormones. Although many forms of HT are government approved to treat hot flashes and vaginal dryness, currently no androgen product is approved for the treatment of female sexual dysfunction. A transdermal testosterone patch has been shown to be effective in the treatment of hypoactive sexual desire disorder in surgically menopausal women, but approval in North America awaits confirmation of long-term safety. (See Section C, page 57, for more about sexual function.)

Cancer therapy. Emotional and physical health are closely linked. Physical illness or discomfort may cause emotional distress, which may negatively affect the body's ability to heal and remain healthy. Induced menopause that results from treatment or surgery for a benign condition will be associated with different concerns than menopause that result from treatment for a life-threatening disease, such as cancer. Women who have been treated for cancer are likely to have significant fears about disease recurrence or death (see Table 5).

Women who undergo cancer treatment often have a variety of emotional concerns that may affect sexual desire. Weight changes, hair loss, and physical changes may be perceived as disfigurement and may have a negative impact on body image. Some patients may express fear of rejection by their partners. Both women and their partners might fear that vaginal penetration will cause pain.

Alternatively, women who are psychologically healthy without sexual concerns may be reassured that they likely will have a quality of life that is the same, or better, after hysterectomy.

When counseling women regarding hysterectomy, healthcare professionals are advised to inform patients that most research shows improved psychological well-being and sexual function after hysterectomy for benign disease. However, women with depression or sexual problems preoperatively are at increased risk for experiencing a worsening of mood, libido, or sexual response postoperatively.

Table 5. Emotional concerns related to cancer and cancer therapy

- Fears about cancer returning or of developing a new cancer
- Fear of death
- Fear of pain or discomfort related to the illness and/or treatment
- Fear of being disabled or becoming dependent on others
- Feelings related to lack of information or "information overload"
- Concerns about body image due to changes caused by the illness or treatment; in some cases, women may grieve for a lost body part or organ
- Apprehension about sexual function, intimacy, and relationships (fear of rejection)
- Feelings of guilt about family members having to deal with the illness
- A feeling of hopelessness and uncertainty about the future after cancer treatment
- Anger about getting cancer
- Fears about using HT because of potential serious adverse effects

---

In summary, adequate patient counseling is especially important with induced menopause, no matter the cause, before the medical intervention occurs. Preoperative counseling is critical to ensure well-informed decisions regarding women's choices. Subsequent attention should be paid to local estrogenization of vulvar or vaginal tissues as well as to psychological factors, such as the impact of the illness or treatment and any possible concomitant depression.

Suggested reading

Aiman J, Smentek C. Premature ovarian failure. *Obstet Gynecol* 1985;66:9-14. American Diabetes Association. Standards of medical care in diabetes—2007. *Diabetes Care* 2007;30(Suppl):S4-S41.

American Heart Association. Third Report of the National Cholesterol Education Program (NCEP) Expert Panel on Detection, Evaluation, and Treatment of High Blood Cholesterol in Adults (Adult Treatment Panel III, or ATP III). 2001. Available at: http://www.americanheart.org/presenter.jhtml?identifier=11206. Accessed September 10, 2007.

American Society of Clinical Oncology. Fertility preservation in people treated for cancer: summary slide set. 2006. Available at: http://www.asco.org/ASCO/Downloads/Cancer%20Policy%20and%20Clinical%20Affairs/Clinical%20Affairs%20(derivative%20products)/Fertility%20slides-v1.pdf. Accessed September 10, 2007.

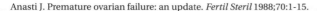

Anasti J. Premature ovarian failure: an update. *Fertil Steril* 1988;70:1-15.

Anasti JN, Kalantaridou SN, Kimzey LM, Defensor RA, Nelson LM. Bone loss in young women with karyotypically normal spontaneous premature ovarian failure. *Obstet Gynecol* 1998;91:12-15.

Anderson GL, Limacher M, Assaf AR, for the Women's Health Initiative Steering Committee. Effects of conjugated equine estrogen in post-menopausal women with hysterectomy: the Women's Health Initiative randomized controlled trial. *JAMA* 2004;291:1701-1712.

Bairey Merz CN, Johnson BD, Sharaf BL, et al, for the WISE Study Group. Hypoestrogenemia of hypothalamic origin and coronary artery disease in premenopausal women: a report from the NHLBI-sponsored WISE study. *J Am Coll Cardiol* 2003;41:413-419.

Brunner RL, Gass M, Aragaki A, et al, for the Women's Health Initiative Investigators. Effects of conjugated equine estrogen on health-related quality of life in postmenopausal women with hysterectomy. *Arch Intern Med* 2005; 165:1976-1986.

Bukman A, Heineman MJ. Ovarian reserve testing and the use of prognostic models in patients with subfertility. *Hum Reprod Update* 2001;7:581-590.

Carlson KJ, Miller BA, Fowler FJ. The Maine Women's Health Study: I. Outcomes of hysterectomy. *Obstet Gynecol* 1994;83:556-565.

Cawood EH, Bancroft J. Steroid hormones, the menopause, sexuality and well-being of women. *Psychol Med* 1996;26:925-936.

Chalmers C, Lindsay M, Usher D, Warner P, Evans D, Ferguson M. Hysterectomy and ovarian function: levels of follicle stimulating hormone and incidence of menopausal symptoms are not affected by hysterectomy in women under age 45 years. *Climacteric* 2002;5:366-373.

Conway GS, Kaltsas G, Patel A, Davies MC, Jacobs HS. Characterization of idiopathic premature ovarian failure. *Fertil Steril* 1996;65:337-341.

Coulam C. Immunology of ovarian failure. *Am J Reprod Immunol* 1991;25:169-174.

Couzinet B, Young J, Brailly S, Le Bouc Y, Chanson P, Schaison G. Functional hypothalamic amenorrhea: a partial and reversible gonadotropin deficiency of nutritional origin. *Clin Endocrinol* 1999;50:229-235.

Davis SR. Androgens and female sexuality. *J Gend Specif Med* 2000;3:36-40.

Farrell SA, Kieser K. Sexuality after hysterectomy. *Obstet Gynecol* 2000;95:1045-1051.

Gath D, Cooper P, Bond A, Edmonds G. Hysterectomy and psychiatric disorder: II. Demographic psychiatric and physical factors in relation to psychiatric outcome. *Br J Psychiatry* 1982;140:343-350.

Farquhar CM, Sadler L, Harvery SA, Stewart AW. The association of hysterectomy and menopause: a prospective cohort study. *BJOG* 2005; 112:956-962.

Gorodeski EZ, Gorodeski GI. Epidemiology and risk factors of cardiovascular disease in postmenopausal women. In: Lobo RA, ed. *Treatment of the Postmenopausal Woman: Basic and Clinical Aspects*, 3rd ed. San Diego, CA: Academic Press, 2007:405-452.

Grinspoon S, Miller K, Coyle C, et al. Severity of osteopenia in estrogen-deficient women with anorexia nervosa and hypothalamic amenorrhea. *J Clin Endocrinol Metab* 1999;84: 2049-2055.

Groff AA, Covington SN, Halverson LR, et al. Assessing the emotional needs of women with spontaneous premature ovarian failure. *Fertil Steril* 2005;83:1734-1741.

Heim C, Newport DJ, Heit S, et al. Pituitary-adrenal and autonomic responses to stress in women after sexual and physical abuse in childhood. *JAMA* 2000;284:592-597.

Hu FB, Grodstein F, Hennekens CH, et al. Age at natural menopause and risk of cardiovascular disease. *Arch Intern Med* 1999;159:1061-1066.

Hughes E, Fedorkow D, Collins J, Vandekerckhove P. Ovulation suppression for endometriosis. *Cochrane Database Syst Rev* 2007;3:CD000155.

Judd HL, Lucas WE, Yen SS. Effect of oophorectomy on circulating testosterone and androstenedione levels in patients with endometrial cancer. *Am J Obstet Gynecol* 1974;118:793-798.

Kalantaridou SN, Davis SR, Nelson LM. Premature ovarian failure. *Endocrinol Metab Clin North Am* 1998;27:989-1006.

Kannel WB, Hjortland MC, McNamara PM, Gordon T. Menopause and risk of cardiovascular disease: the Framingham study. *Ann Intern Med* 1976;85:447-452.

Kaunitz AM, Grimes DA, Kaunitz KK. A physician's guide to adoption. *JAMA* 1987;258:3537-3541.

Khastgir G, Studd J. Hysterectomy, ovarian failure, and depression. *Menopause* 1998;5:113-122.

Kjerulff K, Langenberg P, Rhodes J, et al. Effectiveness of hysterectomy. *Obstet Gynecol* 2000;95:319-326.

Kjerulff KH, Rhodes JC, Langenberg PW, Harvey LA. Patient satisfaction with results of hysterectomy. *Am J Obstet Gynecol* 2000;183:1440-1447.

Kuppermann M, Varner RE, Summitt RL, et al, for the Medicine or Surgery Research Group. Effect of hysterectomy vs medical treatment on health-related quality of life and sexual functioning: the medicine or surgery (Ms) randomized trial. *JAMA* 2004;291:1447-1455.

Laumann EO, Paik A, Rosen RC. Sexual dysfunction in the United States: prevalence and predictors. *JAMA* 1999;281:537-544.

Luborsky JL, Meyer P, Sowers MF, Gold EB, Santoro N. Premature menopause in a multi-ethnic population study of the menopause transition. *Hum Reprod* 2003;18:199-206.

Meirow D. Reproduction post-chemotherapy in young cancer patients. *Mol Cell Endocrinol* 2000;169:123-131.

Metka M, Holzer G, Heytmanek G, Huber J. Hypergonadotropic hypogonadic amenorrhea (World Health Organization III) and osteoporosis. *Fertil Steril* 1992;57:37-41.

Myers LS. Methodological review and meta-analysis of sexuality and menopause research. *Neurosci Biobehav Rev* 1995;19:331-341.

Nasir J, Walton C, Lindow S, Masson E. Spontaneous recovery of chemotherapy-induced primary ovarian failure: implications for management. *Clin Endocrinol* 1997;46:217-219.

Nathorst-Boos J, von Schoultz B. Psychological reactions and sexual life after hysterectomy with and without oophorectomy. *Gynecol Obstet Invest* 1992;4:97-101.

The North American Menopause Society. Estrogen and progestogen use in peri- and postmenopausal women: March 2007 position statement of The North American Menopause Society. *Menopause* 2007;14:168-182.

The North American Menopause Society. Management of osteoporosis in postmenopausal women: 2006 position statement of The North American Menopause Society. *Menopause* 2006;13:340-367.

The North American Menopause Society. The role of calcium in peri- and postmenopausal women: 2006 position statement of The North American Menopause Society. *Menopause* 2006;13:859-861.

Parker WH, Border MS, Liu Z, Shoupe D, Farquhar C, Berek JS. Ovarian conservation at the time of hysterectomy for benign disease. *Obstet Gynecol* 2005;106:219-226.

Pouilles JM, Tremollieres F, Bonneu M, Ribot C. Influence of early age at menopause on vertebral bone mass. *J Bone Miner Res* 1994;9:311-315.

Progetto Menopausa Italia Study Group. Premature ovarian failure, frequency and risk factors among women attending a network of menopause clinics in Italy. *BJOG* 2003;110:59-63.

Rebar RW. Premature ovarian failure. In: Lobo RA, ed. *Treatment of the Postmenopausal Woman: Basic and Clinical Aspects*, 3rd ed. San Diego, CA: Academic Press, 2007:99-109.

Rebar RW, Cedars MI, Liu JH. Premature ovarian failure: a model for the menopause? In: Lobo RA, ed. *Perimenopause*. New York, NY: Springer-Verlag, 1997:7-11.

Rebar RW, Connelly HV. Clinical features of young women with hypergonadotropic amenorrhea. *Fertil Steril* 1990;53:804-808.

Rhodes JC, Kjerulff KH, Langenberg PW, Guzinski GM. Hysterectomy and sexual functioning. *JAMA* 1999;282:1934-1941.

Rosenberg L, Hennekens CH, Rosner B, Belanger C, Rothman KJ, Speizer FE. Early menopause and the risk of myocardial infarction. *Am J Obstet Gynecol* 1981;139:47-51.

Rossouw JE, Anderson GL, Prentice RL, et al, for the Writing Group for the Women's Health Initiative investigators. Risks and benefits of estrogen plus progestin in healthy postmenopausal women: principal results from the Women's Health Initiative randomized controlled trial. *JAMA* 2002;288:321-333.

Ryan MM. Hysterectomy: social and psychosexual aspects. *Bailliere's Clin Obstet Gynaecol* 1997;11:23-36.

Ryan MM, Dennerstein L, Pepperell R. Psychological aspects of hysterectomy: a prospective study. *Br J Psychiatry* 1989;154:516-522.

Ryu RK, Chrisman HB, Omary RA, et al. The vascular impact of uterine artery embolization: prospective sonographic assessment of ovarian arterial circulation. *J Vasc Interv Radiol* 2001;12:1071-1074.

Schulman IH, Aranda P, Raij L, Veronesi M, Aranda FJ, Martin R. Surgical menopause increases salt sensitivity of blood pressure. *Hypertension* 2006;47:1168-1174.

Sherwin BB. Affective changes with estrogen and androgen replacement therapy in surgically menopausal women. *J Affect Disord* 1988;14:177-187.

Sherwin BB. Impact of the changing hormonal milieu on psychologic functioning. In: Lobo RA, ed. Treatment of the *Postmenopausal Woman: Basic and Clinical Aspects*, 3rd ed. San Diego, CA: Academic Press, 2007:217-226.

Sherwin BB, Gelfand MM. The role of androgen in the maintenance of sexual functioning in oophorectomized women. *Psychosom Med* 1987;49:397-409.

Sherwin BB, Gelfand MM, Brender W. Androgen enhances sexual motivation in females: a prospective, crossover study of sex steroid administration in the surgical menopause. *Psychosom Med* 1985;47:339-351.

Shifren JL, Braunstein GD, Simon JA, et al. Transdermal testosterone treatment in women with impaired sexual function after oophorectomy. *N Engl J Med* 2000;343:682-688.

Siddle N, Sarrel P, Whitehead M. The effect of hysterectomy on the age at ovarian failure: identification of a subgroup of women with premature loss of ovarian function and literature review. *Fertil Steril* 1987;47:94-100.

Simon J, Braunstein G, Nachtigall L, et al. Testosterone patch increases sexual activity and desire in surgically menopausal women with hypoactive sexual desire disorder. *J Clin Endocrinol Metab* 2005;90:5226-5233.

Smith JA, Vitale S, Reed GF, et al. Dry eye signs and symptoms in women with premature ovarian failure. *Arch Ophthalmol* 2004;122:151-156.

Testa G, Chiaffarino F, Vegetti W, et al. Case-control study on risk factors for premature ovarian failure. *Gynecol Obstet Invest* 2001;51:40-43.

Tibiletti MG, Testa G, Vegetti W, et al. The idiopathic forms of premature menopause and early menopause show the same genetic pattern. *Hum Reprod* 1999;14:2731-2734.

Tzafettas JM. Current and potential application of GnRH agonists in gynecologic practice. *Ann NY Acad Sci* 2000;900:435-443.

van der Vort DJ, van der Weijer PH, Barentsen R. Early menopause: increased fracture risk at older age. *Osteoporos Int* 2003;14:525-530.

van Kasteren YM, Schoemaker J. Premature ovarian failure: a systematic review on therapeutic interventions to restore ovarian function and achieve pregnancy. *Hum Reprod Update* 1999;5:483-492.

Vega EM, Egea MA, Mautalen CA. Influence of the menopausal age on the severity of osteoporosis in women with vertebral fractures. *Maturitas* 1994;19:117-124.

Vegetti W, Grazia Tibiletti M, Testa G, et al. Inheritance in idiopathic premature ovarian failure: analysis of 71 cases. *Hum Reprod* 1998;13:1796-1800.

Vegetti W, Marozzi A, Manfredini E, et al. Premature ovarian failure. *Mol Cell Endocrinol* 2000;161:53-57.

Veneman TF, Beverstock GC, Exalto N, Mollevanger P. Premature menopause because of an inherited deletion in the long arm of the X-chromosome. *Fertil Steril* 1991;55:631-633.

Wild RA, ed. Surgical menopause. *Menopause* 2007;14(Pt 2):555-597.

Zinn AR. The X chromosome and the ovary. *J Soc Gynecol Investig* 2001; 8(Suppl):S34-S36.

Women's Health Initiative Steering Committee. Effects of conjugated equine estrogen in postmenopausal women with hysterectomy: the Women's Health Initiative randomized controlled trial. *JAMA* 2004;291:1701-1712.

Zobbe V, Gimbel H, Andersen BM, et al. Sexuality after total vs subtotal hysterectomy. *Acta Obstet Gynecol Scand* 2004;83:191-196.

This section of the textbook addresses risk factors for common diseases of women at menopause and beyond, strategies to lower risk, and treatment recommendations. Included are diseases for which some data exist regarding a relationship to ovarian hormones. However, it should not be inferred that menopause or changes in ovarian hormones are responsible for all these diseases.

Osteoporosis

Osteoporosis—the most common bone disorder affecting humans—is a skeletal disorder characterized by compromised bone strength predisposing a person to an increased risk of fracture. Postmenopausal osteoporosis is a major health issue in Western countries, especially among thin Caucasian women who are older than age 65. Fractures of the spine and hip are the most significant complications of osteoporosis, but fractures of the distal forearm, pelvis, ribs, and other limb bones are also consequences of osteoporosis (see Section C, page 72, for more).

Bone strength (and hence fracture risk) depends on both bone quality and bone mineral density (BMD). Expressed as grams of mineral per area or volume, BMD at any given age is a function of peak bone mass (reached around age 30) and how much bone is subsequently lost. Qualities of bone other than BMD (including degree of mineralization, hydroxyapatite crystal size, collagen structure, heterogeneity of bone microstructure, connectivity of trabeculae, and microdamage) are difficult or impossible to measure in clinical practice.

To standardize values from different bone densitometry tests, results are reported as either a Z-score or a T-score, with both expressed as standard deviation (SD) units. (For more about Z-scores and T-scores, see Section F, page 193.)

- *T-score* is calculated by comparing current BMD to the mean peak BMD of a normal, young adult population of the same gender. For women, the reference database is Caucasian (non–race-adjusted) women aged 20 to 29 years. Use of T-scores is the preferred choice for postmenopausal women.
- *Z-score* is based on the difference between the woman's BMD and the mean BMD of a reference population of the same gender, age, and ethnicity.

NAMS supports the World Health Organization (WHO) definition of osteoporosis in a postmenopausal woman as a BMD T-score less than or equal to –2.5 at the total hip, femoral neck, or lumbar spine (posterior-anterior, not lateral) (see Table 1). If anatomic factors such as obesity or arthritis make measurements invalid, the distal one-third radius BMD may be considered a diagnostic site. However, the relationship between the T-score at this site and fracture risk has not been systematically examined.

In addition to diagnosis through densitometry, osteoporosis can be diagnosed clinically, regardless of the T-score.

Table 1. WHO criteria for defining bone mineral density
• Normal: T-score above –1.0
• Low bone mass (osteopenia): T-score between –1.0 and –2.5
• Osteoporosis: T-score below or equal to –2.5

Source: World Health Organization 1994.

Presence of a fragility fracture constitutes the clinical diagnosis of osteoporosis.

Risk factors. In determining risk factors, it is important to distinguish between risk factors for *osteoporosis as defined by BMD* (both primary and secondary causes) and risk factors for *osteoporotic fracture*. For BMD-defined osteoporosis, major risk factors in postmenopausal women are advanced age, genetics, lifestyle factors (eg, low calcium and vitamin D intake, smoking), thinness, and menopause status. Risk factors for osteoporotic fracture are listed in Table 2; the most common are advanced age, low BMD, and previous fracture (other than skull, facial bone, ankle, finger, and toe) as an adult.

Risk factors for BMD-defined osteoporosis and osteoporotic fracture overlap, given that BMD is a risk factor for fracture. Importantly, however, many fracture risk factors are not related to BMD.

Table 2. Risk factors for osteoporotic fracture
Advanced age
Low BMD
Previous fracture (other than skull, facial bone, ankle, finger, and toe) as an adult
History of hip fracture in a parent
Thinness (body weight <127 lb [57.7 kg] or low BMI [<21 kg/m^2])
Current smoking, any amount
Low calcium or vitamin D intake
More than two alcoholic drinks per day
Oral or intramuscular glucocorticoid use for >3 mo
Increased fall risk
Impaired vision
Dementia
Poor health/frailty
Low physical activity
History of recent falls

BMD, bone mineral density; BMI, body mass index.

BMD and fracture risk. BMD is an important determinant of fracture risk, especially in women aged 65 and older. In general, lower BMD scores indicate more severe osteoporosis and higher risk of fracture. A decrease of 1 SD in BMD represents a 10% to 12% decrease in BMD and an increase in fracture risk by a factor of 1.5 to 2.6. BMD and fracture risk are most closely related when BMD is used to predict the fracture risk at that same site. Risks for spine fracture and hip fracture increase 2.3-fold and 2.6-fold, respectively, for each decrease of 1 SD in age-adjusted BMD at spine and hip, respectively.

Fracture risk, however, depends largely on factors other than BMD. Furthermore, a reliable marker to predict fracture risk or determine fracture risk reduction from therapy is not currently available. The use of BMD scores to assess fracture risk can be markedly improved by combining BMD with information about other risk determinants, particularly the woman's age and fracture history. The WHO is currently developing a model to estimate the 10-year absolute fracture risk based on known risk factors. It will offer substantial benefits to healthcare providers compared with current methods.

Treatment-induced changes in BMD do not always correlate well with reductions in vertebral fracture risk. In addition, fracture risk reductions in response to antiresorptive therapy occur much more rapidly than discernible BMD changes. For example, significant fracture risk reduction has been reported after 6 months of risedronate therapy, although minimum BMD increases were observed at that time.

Advanced age. As women age, their risk for fracture increases. In general, the risk of osteoporotic fracture doubles every 7 or 8 years after age 50. The median age for hip fracture is 82 years. The median age for vertebral fracture is thought to occur in a woman's 70s.

Older women are at substantially greater risk for fracture at any given BMD value. For example, at the same T-score of −2.5, a 75-year-old woman has about 8 to 10 times the 10-year hip fracture risk of a 45-year-old woman.

Fracture history. In two analyses of studies, a peri- or postmenopausal woman who has had a fracture has approximately double the risk of sustaining another fracture; adjustment for BMD did not significantly affect the risk. A study of older women (mean age, 74 y) with recent vertebral fractures found that approximately 20% of these women experienced another vertebral fracture within 1 year of an incident vertebral fracture. However, the risk of recurrent fracture was significantly affected by the number of existing fractures—women with two or more vertebral fractures had a significantly increased risk (relative risk, 11.6) of another vertebral fracture within 1 year.

Genetics. The greatest influence on a woman's peak bone mass (ie, the maximal BMD gained during the skeletal development and maturation phase) is heredity. Studies have suggested that up to 80% of the variability in peak BMD might be attributable to genetic factors. Female children of women who have had osteoporotic fractures have lower BMD than would be expected for their age. First-degree relatives (ie, mother, sister) of women with osteoporosis also tend to have lower BMD than those with no family history of osteoporosis.

A history of fracture in a first-degree relative also significantly increases the fracture risk. In a meta-analysis, a family history of fracture was found to be associated with significant increases in any osteoporotic fracture. Hip fracture risks were nearly 50% higher—127% higher if a hip fracture had occurred in a parent.

Lifestyle factors. All postmenopausal women should be encouraged to employ lifestyle practices that reduce the risk of bone loss and osteoporotic fractures: maintaining a healthy weight, eating a balanced diet, obtaining adequate calcium and vitamin D, participating in appropriate exercise, avoiding excessive alcohol consumption, not smoking, and utilizing measures to prevent falls. Periodic reviews of calcium and vitamin D intake and lifestyle behaviors are useful, including risk of falls.

- *Weight.* Being thin—often cited as body weight under 127 lb (57.7 kg), the lower quartile of weight for US women over age 65, or a body mass index (BMI) less than 21 kg/m^2—is a risk factor for low BMD. Thinness has also been associated with increased fracture risk, especially in older women. In a meta-analysis of population-based cohort studies, a BMI of 20 kg/m^2 conferred nearly a twofold increased risk for fracture compared with a BMI at the upper range of normal (≥25 kg/m^2). Being thin seems to have its primary effect on fracture risk by its association with low BMD. Very thin women also are at increased risk for osteoporosis and fracture.

- *Nutrition.* A balanced diet is essential for overall health and is particularly important for bone development and maintenance of bone health throughout life. Many young women, especially women who diet frequently or have eating disorders, or elderly women with reduced appetites, may not consume adequate vitamins and minerals to support optimal bone mass. In addition, premenopausal women who overdiet or overexercise can become very thin, develop hypoestogenicity and amenorrhea, resulting in bone loss and a higher risk for osteopororsis later in life.

Both calcium and vitamin D have well-known roles in bone metabolism. Adequate intake of calcium and vitamin D is required throughout life for a woman to achieve her genetically determined peak bone mass and to maintain optimal bone mass and strength after peak bone mass is attained.

Low vitamin D intake has been linked to impaired muscle strength, increased fall risk, and increased fracture risk along with increased rates of bone loss. Furthermore, treatment with vitamin D has been found to reduce fracture risk in elderly postmenopausal women, although not in all studies. Elderly postmenopausal women have an increased risk of hip fracture associated with low dietary calcium intake.

Guidelines from the National Institutes of Health, NAMS, and the Osteoporosis Society of Canada call for total calcium intake of 1,500 mg/day for postmenopausal women, not 1,500 mg/day in addition to their normal diet.

The current recommended dietary intake for vitamin D from the National Academy of Sciences is 400 IU/day for women aged 51 to 70 years and 600 IU/day for women older than age 70. In addition, NAMS recommends intake of at least 700 to 800 IU/day for women at risk of deficiency because of inadequate sunlight exposure, such as older, frail, chronically ill, housebound, or institutionalized women, or those who live in northern latitudes. New (2007) guidelines from the National Osteoporosis Foundation recommend 800 to 1,000 IU/day of vitamin D_3 for adults age 50 and over. Doses as high as 2,000 IU/day are safe. Much higher doses may introduce risks such as hypercalciuria and hypercalcemia.

All osteoporosis prescription-drug therapies should be used in conjunction with adequate calcium and vitamin D intake. Dietary sources should be the primary source of calcium intake because of the other essentail nutrients found in high-calcium foods. Sunlight exposure is an ideal source of vitamin D. However, with both nutrients, supplementation with fortified foods and nonprescription therapies is often required to obtain the recommended amounts. (See Section H, page 237, for more about these nutrients.)

Another nutrient, magnesium, is sometimes mentioned as a necessary supplement for the protection of bone health and/or for the absorption of calcium. However, in most trials focused on BMD or osteoporotic fracture, the benefits of calcium were observed without magnesium supplementation. (See Section H, page 248, for more information about magnesium.)

Clinical trial data do not support the use of isoflavones (a class of phytoestrogens found in rich supply in soybeans and soy products as well as in red clover) to prevent or treat osteoporosis. Although some data suggest that isoflavones may favorably affect bone health, accumulating data from several more recent studies indicate a lack of bone benefits from isoflavones, regardless of the source (ie, extracted from red clover or soy or consumed in soy foods). (For more about isoflavones, see Section I, page 264.)

- *Exercise.* There is general agreement that weight-bearing exercises confer a positive effect on the musculoskeletal system and that weight-bearing exercises (eg, walking, running, step aerobics, gymnastics) provide the greatest osteogenic stimulus. The effects of exercise on bone mass could be caused by osteoblast activity.

Early in life, exercise promotes higher peak bone mass. During midlife, exercise provides many health benefits, although its effect on BMD has not been empirically established. In early postmenopausal women, strength training provides small but significant benefits on bone mass. A meta-analysis found that women who exercised increased spinal BMD by approximately 2%. For women who use menopausal hormone therapy (HT), strength training provides additional BMD benefits over HT alone. Later in life, exercise likely has a modest effect on slowing the decline in BMD, provided that calcium and vitamin D intakes are adequate. Long-term immobilization, such as prolonged bed rest, has been associated with rapid and significant bone loss.

Regular exercise has been associated with reduced fracture risk. Among women aged 75 and older, exercises that build muscle mass, strength, and balance have been shown to reduce the risk of falls and fall-related injuries by 75%, although it is unclear if exercise affects the risk for fracture from falls that do occur.

Most strength training studies have used progressive resistance obtained with machines designed for this purpose (eg, Nautilus). However, strength training can be performed as few times as twice a week and need not involve expensive equipment. Exercise for women with established osteoporosis should not include heavy weight-bearing exercises or activity so vigorous that it may trigger a fracture. (For more about physical activity, see Section J, page 285.)

- *Alcohol consumption.* Heavy alcohol consumption (defined in the Framingham Study as ≥7 oz/wk [200 mL/wk]) has been shown to increase the risk of falls and hip fracture. A recent meta-analysis showed that consuming as few as two drinks per day significantly increases fracture risk. Very heavy alcohol consumption also has detrimental effects on BMD. However, moderate alcohol consumption (1-2 oz/wk [30-60 mL/wk]) in women 65 years of age and older is associated with higher BMD and decreased risk of hip fracture. (See Section J, page 284, for patient counseling strategies about alcohol abuse.)

- *Cigarette smoking.* Compared with nonsmokers, women smokers tend to lose bone more rapidly, have lower bone mass, and reach menopause 2 years earlier, on average. In addition, some data show that postmenopausal women who currently smoke have significantly higher fracture rates than nonsmokers. The risk imparted by smoking remains significant even after adjusting for BMD.

- The mechanisms by which smoking might adversely affect bone mass are not known, although evidence suggests that cigarette smokers may have impaired calcium absorption and lower 17β-estradiol levels.

Smoking cessation should be encouraged for all women who are smokers (see Section J, page 282 for smoking cessation strategies).

• *Fall prevention.* Falls are the precipitating factor in nearly 90% of all fractures. In the United States and Canada, approximately one third of women over age 60 fall at least once a year. In nearly one half of these cases, it is a recurrent fall. The incidence of falls increases with age, rising to a 50% annual rate in people over age 80. Elderly women have a significantly higher risk for falls than do men of the same age. As a result, prevention of falls that can cause fractures should be an aspect of routine care for all postmenopausal women. After menopause, a woman's risk for falls should be assessed at least annually.

Several healthcare interventions have proven effective in reducing the risk of falls. These focus primarily on exercises to improve balance and muscle strength, adjusting medication use (especially psychotropic drugs), and reducing fall hazards in the home. Tapering or discontinuing use of benzodiazepines, neuroleptic agents, and antidepressants has been found to reduce the risk of falling by more than 60%. Implementing relatively inexpensive measures to eliminate safety hazards in the home may also reduce this risk (see Table 3), but home hazard intervention studies have failed to show significant reductions in fracture.

Menopause status. The increased rate of bone resorption immediately after menopause clearly indicates a hormonal influence on BMD in women. The most likely explanation for this increased resorption is the drop in ovarian estrogen production that accompanies menopause.

Bone loss begins to accelerate approximately 2 to 3 years before the last menses and this acceleration ends 3 to 4 years after menopause. For an interval of a few years around menopause, women lose 2% of bone annually. Afterward, bone loss slows to about 1% to 1.5% per year. A prospective, longitudinal study of Caucasian women reported BMD losses during this 5- to 7-year interval of 10.5% for the spine, 5.3% for the femoral neck, and 7.7% for the total body. Although some of the decline can be attributed to age-related factors, lower estrogen levels were implicated as the cause for approximately two thirds of the bone loss. Lower estrogen levels have also been significantly associated with increased fracture risk in older women (mean age, 75 y).

Women experiencing menopause at or before age 40—either naturally or induced (eg, through bilateral oophorectomy, chemotherapy, or pelvic radiation therapy)—are at greater risk of low BMD than other women of the same age who have not reached menopause. However, by age 70, when fractures are more likely to occur, these women have the same risk for low BMD or fracture as women who reached menopause at the average age.

Secondary causes of bone loss. The prevalence of secondary causes of osteoporosis in women is likely underappreciated. Common causes of low BMD in women with age-matched Z-scores of less than or equal to –1.5 include vitamin D

Table 3. Recommendations for fall prevention

Lighting
Provide ample lighting
Have easy-to-locate light switches for rooms and stairs
Use night lights to illuminate walkways

Obstructions
Remove clutter, low-lying objects
Remove raised door sills to ensure smooth transition

Floors and carpets
Provide nonskid rugs on slippery floors
Repair or replace worn, buckled, or curled carpet
Use nonskid floor wax

Furniture
Arrange furniture to ensure clear pathways
Remove or avoid low chairs and armless chairs
Adjust bed height if too high or low

Storage
Install shelves and cupboards at accessible height
Keep frequently used items at waist height

Bathroom
Install grab bars in tub and shower and near toilet
Use chair in shower and tub
Install nonskid strips or decals in tub and shower
Elevate low toilet seat or install safety frame

Stairways and halls
Install handrails on both sides of stairs
Remove or tape down throw rugs and runners
Repair loose and broken steps
Install nonskid treads on steps

deficiency, primary hyperparathyoidisms, and premature ovarian insufficiency.

Various medications, disease states, and genetic disorders are associated with bone loss (see Table 4). Oral glucocorticoid use causes the most common form of drug-related osteoporosis. Evidence suggests that high-dose inhaled glucocorticoids may cause bone loss. Other studies suggest that no effect occurs with the approved doses of inhaled steroids. In a meta-analysis of seven population-based cohort studies (N = 42,500 men and women), current and prior oral glucocorticoid use was found to be significantly associated with increased risk of osteoporotic fracture. This risk appears within 3 months of beginning corticosteroid use.

Current use of two drugs prescribed for premenopausal women—gonadotropin-releasing hormone (GnRH) and intramuscular medroxyprogesterone acetate (MPA)—has been associated with bone loss. GnRH contributes to bone loss by creating iatrogenic hypogonadism. Bone loss with short-term use of GnRH agonist therapy is reversible. Bone loss with long-term use can be ameliorated by "adding back" low-dose estrogen therapy (ET). Use of depot MPA (DPMA;

150 mg/3 mo) as a contraceptive has been associated with bone loss. This bone loss, which has never been linked to the occurrence of osteoporotic fracture, has been shown in some studies to be reversible; however, other studies have indicated that BMD recovers only partially.

Recent clinical studies have implicated selective serotonin reuptake inhibitors (SSRIs) in both reduced bone mass and clinical fragility fractures. Because depression, too, is associated with lower bone mass, a more judicious use of SSRIs in depressed patients with low bone mass or at risk of fragility fracture may be warranted.

Other medical conditions associated with bone loss include excess urinary calcium excretion, which may be caused by a renal calcium leak or hyperthyroidism. Vitamin D deficiency, an especially common condition in older women, is a correctable cause of secondary hyperparathyroidism and accelerated bone loss. Other conditions that can have a detrimental effect on bone include multiple myeloma, endocrine disorders such as hyperparathyroidism and Cushing's syndrome, and disorders of collagen structures. Renal failure can cause either increased bone resorption (secondary/tertiary hyperparathyroidism) or decreased bone formation, leading to renal osteodystrophy.

Evaluation. All postmenopausal women should be assessed for risk factors associated with osteoporosis and fracture. This assessment requires a history, physical examination, and any necessary diagnostic tests. The goals of this evaluation are to identify risk factors for fractures, including whether osteoporosis is present and, if so, assessing its severity; ruling out secondary causes for osteoporosis; and identifying modifiable risk factors for falls and injuries.

History and physical examination. The medical history and physical examination should focus on the detection of clinical risk factors for osteoporosis and fracture. This includes a personal history of fracture as well as a history of hip fracture in a parent. Most of these risks can be uncovered with a simple questionnaire. Although risk factors may help identify contributing causes of osteoporosis or help guide therapeutic recommendations, they cannot be used to diagnose osteoporosis.

Loss of height may be a sign of vertebral fracture. After achieving maximal height, women (and men) can lose up to 1.0 to 1.5 inches (2.5-3.8 cm) of height as part of the normal aging process, primarily as a result of shrinkage of intervertebral disks. Height loss greater than 1.5 inches (3.8 cm) increases the likelihood that a vertebral fracture is present. Height should be measured annually with an accurate method, such as a wall-mounted ruler or a stadiometer. Loss of 1.5 inches (3.8 cm) or more calls for evaluation by a lateral thoraco-lumbar radiograph to identify silent vertebral fractures.

Table 4. Secondary causes of bone loss
Medications
Oral or intramuscular use of glucocorticoids for >3 mo
Excessive thyroxine doses
Aromatase inhibitors
Long-term use of certain anticonvulsants (eg, phenytoin)
Heparin
Cytotoxic agents
Gonadotropin-releasing hormone agonists or analogues
Intramuscular depot medroxyprogesterone acetate contraceptive
Immunosuppressives (eg, cyclosporine)
Genetic disorders
Osteogenesis imperfecta
Thalassemia
Hypophosphatasia
Hemochromatosis
Disorders of calcium balance
Hypercalciuria
Vitamin D deficiency
Endocrinopathies
Cortisol excess
Cushing's syndrome
Gonadal insufficiency (primary and secondary)
Hyperthyroidism
Type 1 and type 2 diabetes mellitus
Primary hyperparathyroidism
Gastrointestinal diseases
Chronic liver disease (eg, primary biliary cirrhosis)
Malabsorption syndromes (eg, celiac disease, Crohn's disease)
Total gastrectomy
Billroth I gastroenterostomy
Other disorders and conditions
Multiple myeloma
Lymphoma and leukemia
Systemic mastocytosis
Nutritional disorders (eg, anorexia nervosa)
Rheumatoid arthritis
Chronic renal disease

Weight also should be recorded to identify those with a body weight of 127 lb (57.7 kg) or lower and to calculate BMI (see Section F, page 186, for details on calculating BMI).

The examination should include an assessment for acute or chronic back pain, especially in the middle back, which may indicate the presence of vertebral fractures. The mid-back vertebrae T11, T12, and L1 are the most common fracture sites, followed by T6 through T9. Multiple, severe vertebral compression fractures ultimately result in kyphosis (abnormal curvature of the thoracic spine), the most obvious sign of osteoporosis.

Because back pain, height loss, and kyphosis can occur without osteoporosis, and two thirds of vertebral fractures are asymptomatic, vertebral fracture must be confirmed, usually by lateral spine radiographs. In addition, some dual-energy x-ray absorptiometry (DXA) techniques (eg, instant vertebral assessment, morphometric x-ray absorptiometry) allow vertebral fracture assessment and can therefore be used to visualize a fracture at the same time that BMD is being measured. Height loss of more than 20% (or 4 mm) of the anterior, mid, or posterior dimension of a vertebra on spinal radiograph is also indicative of vertebral fracture.

After menopause, a woman's risk for falls should be assessed at least annually. Clinical factors related to an increased risk of falls include the following:

- A history of falls, fainting, or loss of consciousness
- Muscle weakness or coordination
- Dizziness or balance problems
- Difficulty standing or walking
- Arthritis
- Impaired vision

The risk of falls is also increased by use of medications that affect balance and coordination (eg, sedatives, narcotic analgesics, anticholinergics, antihypertensives) or by use of multiple medications.

The greater the number of risk factors, the greater the risk of falling. In one study, having four or more of these risk factors increased the risk of falls by nearly 80%.

Safety hazards in the home and work environment, such as obstacles and poor lighting, also contribute to the risk of falls. These hazards can be assessed by questioning the woman or through a home and/or workplace visit by an occupational therapist or other healthcare professional knowledgeable about fall prevention.

BMD measurement. BMD testing is the technical standard for diagnosing osteoporosis. Determinants of bone strength other than BMD cannot be measured in the clinical setting.

- *Indications for BMD testing.* Testing of BMD should be performed based on a woman's risk profile. Testing is not indicated unless the results will influence a treatment or management decision. Other factors such as availability of BMD testing equipment and reimbursement by insurance also affect the decision to measure BMD.

  NAMS recommends that BMD be measured in the following populations:
  — Postmenopausal women with medical causes of bone loss, regardless of age
  — Postmenopausal women at least 65 years of age, regardless of additional risk factors

Testing should be considered for healthy postmenopausal women younger than age 65 when one or more of the following risk factors for fracture have been identified (the greater the number of risk factors, the greater the need for testing):

- Fracture (other than skull, facial bone, ankle, finger, and toe) after menopause;
- Thinness (body weight <127 lb [57.7 kg] or BMI <21 kg/m^2)
- History of hip fracture in a parent
- Current smoker

- *BMD testing options.* Several tests to measure BMD are available. (For details regarding tests to measure BMD, see Section F, page 193.) DXA is the preferred technique for measuring central (eg, spine, hip) BMD and for diagnosing osteoporosis because it measures BMD at the important sites of osteoporotic fractures. When BMD testing is indicated, NAMS recommends measuring the total hip, femoral neck, and posterior-anterior lumbar spine, and using the lowest of the three BMD scores. In some older patients (>60 y), there can be artifacts of the spine that make measurements unreliable. The spine, however, is a useful site for BMD measurement in early postmenopausal women because they tend to lose bone faster in the spine than in the hip. Although tests at peripheral sites (eg, wrist, calcaneus) can identify women with low bone mass, they are not as useful as central-site tests because their prediction of risk is not well determined. WHO diagnostic criteria cannot be applied to peripheral sites except for the distal radius, although BMD measurement has been predictive of fracture risk Peripheral site measurements should be limited to the assessment of fracture risk when DXA is not available. They cannot be used to diagnose osteoporosis or to follow response to therapy.

- *Follow-up BMD testing.* In most cases, repeat DXA testing in untreated postmenopausal women is not useful until 3 to 5 years have passed, given the rate of bone loss of 1% to 1.5% per year. Postmenopausal women, after substantial BMD losses in early postmenopause, generally lose about 0.5 T-score units every 5 years.

For women receiving osteoporosis therapy, BMD monitoring may not provide clinically useful information until after 2 years of treatment. The lack of an increase in BMD is not evidence of treatment failure. In two randomized controlled trials (RCTs), most women who seemed to have lost more than 4% of BMD during the first year of treatment with either alendronate or raloxifene showed substantial gains the second and third years while remaining on the same therapy. This variability was seen despite excellent quality assurance programs and is a consequence of the imprecision of DXA testing.

A statistically *insignificant* decrease in BMD on treatment may be related to imprecision in the DXA measurement rather than to treatment failure. However, a statistically *significant* decrease in BMD (usually >4%-5%) would warrant further consideration of secondary causes of bone loss and evaluation of adherence to therapy.

Bone turnover markers. Biochemical markers of bone turnover cannot diagnose osteoporosis and have varying ability to predict fracture risk. Nevertheless, these tests have been studied as a means to assess therapeutic response earlier than through BMD changes, sometimes within a few months as opposed to the 1 to 3 years required with BMD. However, bone turnover markers vary from day to day, are affected by food intake and time of day, and lack assay standardization, limiting their clinical utility.

The value of bone turnover markers in routine clinical practice has not been established. Although some clinicians have found that these data can encourage adherence to therapy, several trials have found no difference in adherence when marker values are communicated to women.

Tests for secondary causes. Once osteoporosis is diagnosed, any secondary causes should be identified. Various laboratory tests can be useful (Table 5). Routine tests include a complete blood cell count plus serum levels of calcium, 25-hydroxyvitamin D, alkaline phosphatase, and albumin, as well as urinary calcium excretion to identify calcium malabsorption or renal calcium leak. If the clinical history, physical examination, or routine laboratory tests indicate a need, special tests that may be appropriate include measurement of thyroid-stimulating hormone, urinary cortisol, serum protein electrophoresis, and parathyroid hormone.

Pharmacologic interventions. In adults, the primary goal of osteoporosis management is to prevent fracture by slowing or preventing net bone loss, maintaining bone strength, and minimizing or eliminating factors that contribute to falls. Initiating preventive steps well into adulthood or old age may lessen a woman's risk of osteoporosis and fractures. A management strategy focused on lifestyle approaches may be all that is needed for postmenopausal women who are at low risk for osteoporotic fracture. NAMS recommends adding osteoporosis drug therapy in the following populations:

- All postmenopausal women who have had an osteoporotic vertebral fracture
- All postmenopausal women who have BMD values consistent with osteoporosis (ie, T-scores equal to or worse than −2.5)
- All postmenopausal women who have T-scores from −2.0 to −2.5 and at least one of the following risk factors for fracture: thinness (body weight <127 lb [57.7 kg] or low BMI [<21 kg/m²]), history of fragility fracture since menopause, or history of hip fracture in a parent

The diagnostic categorization should be based on the lowest of the BMD values among the three measured sites of total hip, femoral neck, and posterior-anterior lumbar spine. Current treatment guidelines are based on specific BMD thresholds and risk factors. Available in the near future will be an improved method from the WHO utilizing algorithms that incorporate estimates of absolute fracture risk.

Table 5. Routine laboratory tests for osteoporosis evaluation

Test	Diagnostic result	Possible secondary cause
Complete blood cell count	Anemia	Multiple myeloma
Serum calcium	Elevated	Hyperparathyroidism
	Low	Vitamin D deficiency, GI malabsorption
Serum 25-hydroxyvitamin D	Low	GI malabsorption, celiac disease
Serum albumin	Used to interpret serum calcium	
Serum alkaline phosphatase	Elevated	Vitamin D deficiency, GI malabsorption, hyperparathyroidism, Paget's disease
Urinary calcium excretion	Elevated	Renal calcium leak, multiple myeloma, metastatic cancer involving bone, hyperparathyroidism, hyperthyroidism
	Low	GI malabsorption, inadequate intake of calcium and vitamin D

GI, gastrointestinal.

Several pharmacologic options are government approved in the United States and Canada for the treatment and/or prevention of postmenopausal osteoporosis—including bisphosphonates, the selective estrogen-receptor modulator (SERM; now called estrogen agonist/antagonist) raloxifene, the anabolic agent parathyroid hormone, calcitonin, and HT, both estrogen alone and combination estrogen-progestogen regimens (ET/EPT). Lists of these options are found in Tables 6, 7, and 8. Although other marketed drugs in these categories have not obtained government approval for a postmenopausal osteoporosis indication, they are nonetheless prescribed off label by some clinicians who desire this outcome.

Treatment recommendations are based on both efficacy data and clinical parameters, which include magnitude of fracture risk, side effect profile, tolerability of specific drugs, extraskeletal risks and potential benefits, confounding diseases, cost, and patient preference, including choice of dosing. Selection of one therapy over another cannot be made on the basis of clinical evidence because head-to-head trials comparing the effectiveness of pharmacologic therapies to reduce fracture risk have not been conducted.

Adherence to postmenopausal osteoporosis therapy is poor. In studies of 6 months to 1 year, adherence rates for prescription drugs ranged from below 25% to 81%, depending on the therapy. Ensuring adherence to the treatment plan is perhaps the most important follow-up measure for clinicians.

Table 6. Bone-specific prescription drugs approved for postmenopausal osteoporosis in the United States and Canada

Composition	Product name	Availability	Indication	Recommended dose
Bisphosphonates				
alendronate	Fosamax	Oral tablet, oral solution*	Prevention Prevention + Treatment	5 mg/d or 35 mg/wk 10 mg/d or 70 mg/wk
alendronate + cholecalciferol (vitamin D_3)	Fosamax Plus D* Fosavance**	Both therapies in single tablet	Treatment	70 mg + 2,800 IU /wk; 70 mg + 5,600 IU/wk*
risedronate	Actonel	Oral tablet	Prevention + Treatment	5 mg/d; 35 mg/wk; 75 mg in 2 consecutive d/mo
risedronate + calcium carbonate	Actonel with Calcium	Packet of oral tablets (not combined therapies) with 4-wk supply	Prevention	35 mg/wk (day 1) + 1,250 mg Ca for no-risedronate days (days 2-7 of 7-d treatment cycle)
ibandronate	Boniva*	Oral tablet	Prevention + Treatment	150 mg/mo
		Intravenous injection	Treatment	3 mg every 3 mo
etidronate	Didrocal**	Oral tablet (packaged with calcium carbonate)	Prevention + Treatment	400 mg/d for 14 d every 3 mo, with calcium taken between cycles
zoledronic acid	Reclast*	Intravenous infusion	Treatment	5 mg/y
SERMs				
raloxifene	Evista	Oral tablet	Prevention + Treatment	60 mg/d
Calcitonin				
calcitonin-salmon	Fortical*	Nasal spray	Treatment (>5 y postmenopause)	200 IU/d
	Miacalcin	Nasal spray	Treatment (>5 y postmenopause)	200 IU/d
		Subcutaneous injection*	Treatment (>5 y postmenopause)	100 IU every other day
Parathyroid hormone				
teriparatide (recombinant human PTH 1-34)	Forteo	Subcutaneous injection	Treatment (high Fx risk)	20 µg/d

PTH, parathyroid hormone; Fx, fracture
* Available in the United States but not Canada.
** Available in Canada but not the United States.
Products not marked are available in both the United States and Canada.

Table 7. Estrogen-only prescription drugs approved for the prevention of postmenopausal osteoporosis in the United States and Canada

Composition	Product name	Availability	Available dosages
conjugated estrogens (formerly conjugated equine estrogens)	Premarin	Oral tablet	0.3, 0.45*, 0.645, 0.9, 1.25 mg/d
estropipate (formerly piperazine estrone sulfate)	Ogen	Oral tablet	0.625 (0.75 estropipate, calculated as sodium estrone sulfate 0.625), 1.25 (1.5), 2.5 (3.0) mg/d
17β-estradiol	Alora*	Matrix patch (twice weekly)	0.025, 0.05, 0.075, 0.1 mg/d
	Climara	Matrix patch (once weekly)	0.025, 0.375*, 0.05, 0.075, 0.1 mg/d
	Estrace	Oral tablet	0.5, 1.0, 2.0 mg/d
	Menostar*	Matrix patch (once weekly)	0.014 mg/d
	Vivelle	Matrix patch (twice weekly)	0.025*, 0.0375*, 0.05, 0.075*, 0.1* mg/d
	Vivelle-Dot* Estradot**	Matrix patch (twice weekly)	0.025, 0.0375, 0.05, 0.075, 0.1 mg/d
	Estraderm	Reservoir patch (twice weekly)	0.025, 0.05, 0.1 mg/d

* Available in the United States but not Canada.
** Available in Canada but not the United States.
Products not marked are available in both the United States and Canada.

Bisphosphonates. This class of drugs works by inhibiting the activity of osteoclasts and shortening their lifespan, thereby reducing bone resorption. Bisphosphonates do not have known beneficial effects on the body other than on bone.

Clinical trials have demonstrated that bisphosphonates significantly increase BMD at the spine and hip in a dose-dependent manner in both younger and older postmenopausal women. In women with osteoporosis, bisphosphonates have reduced the risk of vertebral fractures by 40% to 50% and reduced the incidence of nonvertebral fracture, including hip fracture, by about half this amount.

The NAMS 2006 position statement on the management of postmenopausal osteoporosis concludes that bisphosphonates are the first-line drugs for treating this condition. The paper further states that whether there are differences in fracture protection among the available bisphosphonates is uncertain, and that it is likely that all produce greater relative and absolute fracture risk reductions in women with more severe osteoporosis.

In North America, five bisphosphonates are government approved for the management of postmenopausal osteoporosis: alendronate, risedronate, ibandronate, etidronate, and zoledronic acid. However, not all are government approved for postmenopausal osteoporosis in both the United States and Canada (see Table 6).

- *Alendronate.* The first bisphosphonate approved for postmenopausal osteoporosis in the United States and Canada is alendronate (Fosamax oral tablets; an oral solution is also available in the United States but not Canada). A tablet dosage of 5 mg/day is approved for osteoporosis prevention. In women in early menopause without osteoporosis, 2 to 4 years of alendronate therapy (5 mg daily) increased BMD at the spine and hip by 1% to 4%, whereas those on placebo had declines of 2% to 4%. In a trial comparing alendronate with HT, the BMD effect was similar in both groups. Fracture risk reduction was not demonstrated on this dosage of alendronate.

A dosage of 10 mg/day alendronate is approved for prevention and treatment of postmenopausal osteoporosis. Several large clinical trials have documented its ability to increase BMD and reduce fracture risk in women with osteoporosis. Because bioequivalence of a dose of 70 mg per week on BMD was demonstrated, this dose is approved for treatment also, and in reality represents 98% of prescriptions.

In older women with low BMD or previous vertebral fractures, alendronate (5-10 mg/d) increased BMD in the spine and hip by 4% to 10% after treatment for 3 to 7 years. In this population, alendronate therapy reduced the risk of fracture at the hip and spine by approximately 50% and the occurrence of multiple vertebral fractures by approximately 90%. An effect on clinical (symptomatic) vertebral fractures was evident as early as 12 months after treatment was started. The reduction in nonvertebral fractures averages approximately 20%.

The efficacy of alendronate in decreasing fracture risk has been demonstrated only in postmenopausal women with osteoporosis. Similar to other bisphosphonates, alendronate has shown lesser effects in women without osteoporosis.

A single table of alendronate plus vitamin D_3 is approved for osteoporosis treatment, marketed in the United States as Fosamax Plus D, and in Canada as Fosavance (see Table 6 for more).

- *Risedronate.* Another bisphosphonate—risedronate (Actonel oral tablets)—is approved in the United States and Canada for the prevention and treatment of postmenopausal osteoporosis at doses of 5 mg/day, 35 mg/week, or 75 mg in 2 consecutive days/month.

In postmenopausal women, risedronate (5 mg/d for 3 y) suppressed bone turnover and increased BMD in the spine and hip by 3% to 6%, respectively. In women with previous vertebral fractures, risedronate therapy reduced subsequent vertebral fracture rates by 40% to 50% and the risk of experiencing multiple vertebral

Table 8. Estrogen-progestin prescription drugs approved for the prevention of postmenopausal osteoporosis (intact uterus) in the United States and Canada

Composition	Product name	Availability	Available dosages
conjugated estrogens (E) + medroxyprogesterone acetate (P) (continuous-cyclic: E alone for days 1-14, followed by E+P on days 15-28)	Premphase*	Oral	0.625 mg E + 5.0 mg P (2 tablets: E and E+P)
conjugated estrogens (E) + medroxyprogesterone acetate (P) (continuous-combined)	Prempro*	Oral	0.3 or 0.45 mg E + 1.5 mg P (1 tablet); 0.625 mg E + 2.5 or 5.0 mg P (1 tablet)
	Premplus**	Oral	0.625 mg E + 2.5 or 5.0 mg P (2 tablets: E and P)
ethinyl estradiol (E) + norethindrone acetate (P)	femhrt*	Oral	2.5 µg E + 0.5 mg P (1 tablet); 5 µg E + 1 mg P (1 tablet)
	femHRT**	Oral	5 µg E + 1 mg P (1 tablet)
17β-estradiol (E) + norethindrone acetate (P)	Activella*	Oral	0.5 mg E + 0.1 mg P (1 tablet); 1 mg E + 0.5 mg P (1 tablet)
17β-estradiol (E) + norgestimate (P) (intermittent-combined: E alone for 3 d, followed by E+P for 3 d, repeated continuously)	Prefest*	Oral	1 mg E + 0.09 mg P (2 tablets: E and E+P)
17β-estradiol (E) + levonorgestrel (P) (continuous-combined)	Climara Pro*	Patch	0.045 mg E + 0.015 mg P (22 cm² patch, once/wk)
17β-estradiol (E) + norethindrone acetate (P) (continuous-sequential: E alone for 2 wk, followed by E+P for 2 wk, repeated continuously)	Estracomb**	Patch	0.05 mg E twice/wk for 2 wk, then 0.05 mg E + 0.25 mg P for 2 wk

*   Available in the United States but not Canada.
** Available in Canada but not the United States.

fractures by 77% to 96%. This effect on vertebral fractures, as demonstrated by radiography, has been observed as early as 1 year after starting treatment. After 3 years, the risk of multiple vertebral fractures is reduced by approximately 90%, and nonverterbal fracture incidence is decreased by 20%. In a trial designed to evaluate the effect of risedronate on hip fracture risk, treatment for 3 years decreased the risk by 40% in women aged 70 to 79 years with established osteoporosis. However, no effect on hip fracture risk was observed in older women ($\geq$80 y) who were identified primarily on the basis of fall-related risk factors for hip fracture.

Convenient packets of separate risedronate and calcium carbonate tablets are also approved for osteoporosis prevention, marketed as Actonel with Calcium (see Table 6 for more).

- *Ibandronate.* This bisphosphonate is available in the United States but not Canada. Ibandronate, as an oral tablet (Boniva), is approved by the US Food and Drug Administration (FDA) for the prevention and treatment of postmenopausal osteoporosis at a once-monthly dose of 150 mg. Ibandronate is also approved at an intravenous dose (IV) of 3 mg every 3 months (given as an IV push administered by a healthcare professional) for postmenopausal osteoporosis treatment.

At an oral dose of 2.5 mg/day for 3 years in women with osteoporosis, ibandronate therapy decreased bone resorption, increased BMD in the spine by 3% to 5%, and reduced the incidence of new vertebral fractures by 52%. No effect was seen in reducing nonverterbal fractures, although later analysis of subgroups with lower BMD did show efficacy. Bioequivalence studies on BMD showed that 150 mg/month of the IV dose was equivalent to 2.5 mg/day of oral tablet therapy.

- *Etidronate.* This drug was the first bisphosphonate used clinically. In the United States, it is marketed as Didronel but it is FDA approved for treating Paget's disease, not the prevention or treatment of osteoporosis, because the submitted studies were small and did not demonstrate efficacy. Etidronate is approved in Canada for the prevention and treatment of postmenopausal osteoporosis.

For osteoporosis, etidronate is administered in cycles of 400 mg/day for 14 days, followed by 500 mg/day of calcium for the remainder of each 3-month cycle. (This is not the schedule for Paget's disease, the FDA-approved indication.) Administration is cyclic because daily use has been associated with osteomalacia (abnormal bone mineralization). In Canada, etidronate is packaged with calcium carbonate tablets and marketed in a dose pack as Didrocal.

Treatment with cyclic etidronate and calcium increased BMD by approximately 8% in the spine and 1% in the hip, and it reduced the incidence of vertebral fracture in older women with established osteoporosis. No effect on vertebral fracture has been observed in RCTs.

- *Zoledronic acid.* The most potent bisphosphonate is zoledronic acid. Administered as an IV infusion, it is the first and only once-yearly medicine for postmenopausal osteoporosis. Zoledronic acid is available in the United States and Canada, where it is approved for the treatment of certain types of cancer (marketed as Zometa), Paget's disease (marketed as Reclast in the United States; Aclasta in Canada), and for the treatment of postmenopausal osteoporosis (as Reclast in the United States; in Canada, Aclasta is not approved for osteoporosis).

In the Health Outcomes and Reduced Incidence with Zoledronic Acid Once Yearly (HORIZON) Pivotal Fracture Trial—a randomized, double-blind, placebo-controlled trial—a once-yearly IV infusion of a 5-mg dose of zoledronic acid significantly reduced the risk of vertebral fractures by 70%, hip fractures by 41%, and nonverterbal fractures by 25%. BMD increased at the total hip by 6%, lumbar spine 7%, and femoral neck 5%. Adverse events, including change in renal function, were similar in the two study groups.

Zoledronic acid is the first treatment shown to not only prevent new fractures in elderly patients with broken hips, but also reduce deaths. In the large (N = 2,127) HORIZON trial, a once-yearly IV infusion of a 5-mg dose of zoledronic acid was administered within 90 days after surgical repair of a low-trauma hip fracture. All patients (mostly women; mean age, 74.5 y) received supplemental vitamin D and calcium. After a median follow-up of 1.9 years, the rate of new fractures in the treatment group was 8.6%, compared with 13.9% in the placebo group. The risk of all-cause mortality was reduced by 28% in the treatment group, where 101 people died, compared with 141 in the placebo group.

Since zoledronic acid is administered as an IV infusion, treatment will typically not occur in the clinician's office, but rather in a clinic or an infusion center.

Other bisphosphonate issues include side effects, optimal duration of therapy, and anticipated effects after discontinuing therapy.

- *Side effects.* The most common adverse effect of oral bisphosphonate therapy approved for osteoporosis is esophageal and gastric irritation, characterized by heartburn or abdominal pain. These side effects may be less severe when not using the daily dosage schedule. Patients who have most difficulty are those who dose inappropriately. To minimize these symptoms, patients should take each dose with a full glass of plain water (not mineral water) to facilitate delivery to the stomach, and remain upright for 30 minutes after ingestion. Whether there is a difference in gastrointestinal (GI) tolerability among oral bisphosphonates is uncertain.

Therapy should be taken on an empty stomach, first thing in the morning. Bisphosphonates are poorly absorbed (eg, about 0.5% of an oral dose), even when taken in this manner. Food, drink, and medications (including supplements) must be avoided for at least 30 minutes (60 minutes with oral ibandronate). Refer to each drug's product labeling for specific advice.

Oral etidronate is somewhat different from other oral bisphosophates. Because upper GI side effects are uncommon with this therapy, it may be useful for women who experience these side effects with other oral bisphosphonate drugs. It should be taken several hours before and after meals. Mild diarrhea is the most common side effect.

IV ibandronate and zoledronic acid are well tolerated; labeling does not carry the warnings of the oral formulations regarding upper GI adverse events. Osteoporotic patients with such conditions as gastritis, hiatus hernia, and gastroesophageal reflex disease may be good candidates for these forms of therapy. Labeling for IV ibandronate and zoledronic acid includes an enhanced precaution on hypocalcemia and renal impairment.

The advent of once-weekly and once-monthly dosing options has been associated with improved tolerability, although adherence remains suboptimal. The once-yearly dosing regimen of zolendronic acid may realize better adherence.

A transient flu-like illness, often called an acute-phase reaction, occurs infrequently with large doses of oral or IV bisphosphonates. Symptoms are generally mild, most often occur with the first, but not subsequent doses, and are treated symptomatically.

Studies have shown that treatment with zoledronic acid has a favorable safety profile and is well tolerated. In one trial, atrial fibrillation was observed with the zoledronic acid treatment group (1.3%; 50 out of 3,862) compared to 0.4% (17 out of 3,852) in the placebo group. Over 90% of these events in both treatment groups occurred more than a month after the infusion; a subsequent substudy showed no difference in the incidence of atrial fibrillation between treatment groups, suggesting the events were not related to the acute infusions. This concern did not result in a labeling precaution or warning.

Before starting bisphosphonate therapy, serum creatinine should be used to estimate the glomerular filtration rate. Treatment may be initiated only if the rate is 30 mL/min or greater.

Over the past few years, the presence of osteonecrosis of the jaw (ONJ) has been identified in patients receiving bisphosphonate therapy, primarily high doses of IV bisphosphonate, prescribed to treat patients with cancer-related bone diseases. The diagnosis of ONJ is made when exposed bone in the mouth is present for 3 months or more. Many patients present with no symptoms, and the diagnosis is made by observing a nonhealing lesion of the jaw after an invasive dental procedure, such as tooth extraction or dental implant. In other patients, pain and swelling in the jaw occurs when the exposed bone becomes secondarily infected. ONJ is not a cause of periodontal bone loss, tooth loss, tooth pain, dental caries, or periodontal disease and is not present in most patients with jaw pain.

Several studies have suggested that ONJ develops in 2% to 10% of patients receiving IV bisphosphonate therapy for cancer, usually after 2 or more years of treatment. The risk seems to increase with longer-term treatment. In patients without cancer who receive the lower bisphosphonate doses for osteoporosis, the incidence of ONJ is not known but is estimated to be between 1:60,000 and 1:100,000. The risk is higher in patients who have dental procedures exposing the bone. It is unclear whether longer treatment is a risk factor in these patients. Whether the risk differs among the available bisphosphonate drugs is unknown.

Although ONJ seems to be a potential complication of oral bisphosphonate therapy for osteoporosis, the likelihood of its happening is very small and should not preclude therapy in patients at moderate to high risk of fracture. However, because of the risk of ONJ, a routine oral examination should be performed by the prescriber prior to initiation of bisphosphonate treatment. It would be appropriate to have any planned invasive dental procedures performed and the lesions healed before beginning treatment with a bisphosphonate.

Dental examination (by a dentist) with appropriate preventive dentistry should be considered prior to initiation of therapy in patients with a history of concomitant risk factors (eg, cancer, chemotherapy, corticosteroid use, poor oral hygiene). While on treatment, patients with concomitant risk factors should avoid invasive dental procedures, if possible.

For patients on bisphosphonate therapy for 2 or more years who require nonemergency invasive dental procedures, it is advised to stop therapy for 2 to 3 months and then wait until the lesions have healed before restarting treatment. There is no evidence that discontinuing therapy reduces the risk of ONJ, but there is very little risk in stopping therapy for a few months. There is no justification for these patients to avoid routine dental care such as cleaning, fillings, or placement of crowns or for stopping osteoporosis treatment before routine dental treatments. On the contrary, it is probably more important for patients on bisphosphonate therapy to receive regular dental care. If a patient receiving a bisphosphonate develops oral lesions consistent with ONJ, stopping therapy is advised, and referral to an oral surgeon experienced in managing this problem is appropriate.

- *Optimal duration.* NAMS believes that current evidence does not support recommendations regarding the optimal duration of bisphosphonate therapy. A 2007 review by Briot et al concluded that gains in BMD persisted throughout 10 years of treatment with alendronate or 7 years with risedronate. However, proof of long-term protection against fractures was obtained only for shorter treatment periods, 4 years and 5 years, respectively.

- *Discontinuation.* The persistence of treatment effects after drug discontinuation varies across medications. Following discontinuation of alendronate after 4 to 5 years of therapy, bone turnover remains relatively suppressed with BMD remaining stable or decreasing slowly. Bone turnover markers remain suppressed but return to pretreatment levels over time. A 10-year study (FLEX trial) compared fracture rates in patients who discontinued alendronate after 5 years with those who continued it for 10 years. There was no difference in nonvertebral or morphometric (measured) vertebral fracture rates; however, clinical vertebral fractures were 55% fewer in those who continued treatment.

Discontinuation of risedronate therapy after 2 years in young postmenopausal women (mean ages, 51-52 y) has been shown to result in significant bone loss at both the spine and hip during the first year after treatment is stopped. The effects of stopping therapy in older women or after longer treatment intervals are not known.

Ravn et al found that the bone loss that resumes after withdrawal of 1 year of ibandronate treatment is of a magnitude similar to that of normal postmenopausal bone loss.

Several studies have documented the effects after cyclical etidronate therapy is withdrawn. Both Fogelman et al and Brown et al found a residual protective effect in both the lumbar spine and femoral neck for up to 1 year posttreatment. Miller et al found bone mass was maintained for at least 2 years after treatment.

The review by Briot et al concluded that further studies are needed before this point can be incorporated into treatment decisions.

Selective estrogen-receptor modulators (SERMs). SERMs (now termed estrogen agonists/antagonists by the FDA) are estrogen-like compounds that act as weak estrogen agonists in some organ systems and as estrogen antagonists in others. The goal of SERM therapy is to provide the bone benefits of estrogen without an adverse effect on the endometrium or breast.

Raloxifene (Evista tablets) is the only SERM available in the United States and Canada that is approved for osteoporosis therapy. It is approved for the prevention and treatment of postmenopausal osteoporosis at a dose of 60 mg/day. SERMs in development include bazedoxifene and lasofoxifene.

In postmenopausal women, raloxifene reduced bone turnover and produced modest (1%-3%) increases in BMD in the spine, hip, and wrist. Results from the Multiple Outcomes of Raloxifene Evaluation (MORE) trial showed that in women (mean age, 67 y) with low BMD, with or without an existing vertebral fracture, treatment with raloxifene at 60 mg/day reduced spine fracture risk by 30% and 50%, respectively, and reduced the incidence of multiple vertebral fractures by 93%. The risk of clinical vertebral fractures was reduced by 68% after 1 year of treatment. Reduction in nonvertebral fractures has not been demonstrated.

Raloxifene may accentuate the frequency or severity of vasomotor symptoms. Leg cramps occur more frequently in raloxifene-treated women than in those receiving placebo. Raloxifene lowers total and LDL cholesterol (LDL-C) levels and does not raise HDL cholesterol (HDL-C) or triglyceride concentrations. Unlike HT, which increases C-reactive protein levels, raloxifene has no significant effect on those levels. The Raloxifene Use for The Heart (RUTH) trial, a large RCT, failed to show any reduction or any increase in cardiovascular disease.

In older women with osteopenia or osteoporosis, raloxifene therapy is associated with a significant reduction in the incidence of ER-positive breast cancer. The Study of Tamoxifen and Raloxifene (STAR) revealed that raloxifene is equivalent to tamoxifen in reducing the incidence of invasive breast cancer in postmenopausal women at high risk for the disease. Raloxifene also significantly reduced the incidence of ER-positive breast cancer in the RUTH trial. Unlike the SERM tamoxifen, indicated for breast cancer, raloxifene does not adversely affect the endometrium. In mid-2007, the FDA approved raloxifene for reducing invasive breast cancer risk (see page 145 for more about breast cancer and SERMs).

Raloxifene carries the same risk as HT and tamoxifen of venous thromboembolic (VTE) events, such as deep vein thrombosis (DVT) and stroke, although such events are rare. However, these drugs should not be prescribed to women experiencing periods of prolonged immobilization or to those with a history of clotting disorders. A black box warning in the raloxifene labeling emphasizes that the drug is contraindicated in women with an active or past history of VTE and that women at risk for stroke should use raloxifene only after evaluating the risk-benefit ratio.

The most commonly reported side effects are hot flashes, leg cramps, peripheral edema, athralgia, flu syndrome, and sweating.

The optimal duration of use of raloxifene has not been established. A 2007 review by Briot et al concluded that the BMD effect observed after 3 and 4 years persisted when the drug was given for 8 years, and the fracture risk reduction was similar. The long-term safety profile was also similar, with a significant decrease in the incidence of ER-positive breast cancer and a persistent increase in the risk of DVT. However, a sharp drop in BMD occurred upon raloxifene discontinuation.

The NAMS 2006 position statement on the management of postmenopausal osteoporosis concludes that raloxifene is most often considered in postmenopausal women with low bone mass or younger postmenopausal women with osteoporosis who are at greater risk of spine fracture than hip fracture. Extraskeletal risks and benefits are important when considering raloxifene therapy.

Anabolic agents. Unlike antiresorptive drugs such as bisphosphonates and estrogen, anabolic agents stimulate bone formation and result in the accumulation of new bone tissue.

- *Teriparatide.* One drug in this class—teriparatide (Forteo), a recombinant preparation of the first 34 amino acids of human parathyroid hormone (PTH)—is approved in the United States and Canada for the treatment of osteoporosis for up to 2 years in adults at high fracture risk. The approved dose is 20 µg/day by subcutaneous injection. Noninjectable forms of PTH 1-34, such as nasal, oral, and transdermal preparations, are in development.

In postmenopausal women with osteoporosis and previous spine fractures, teriparatide treatment via subcutaneous injection increased BMD in the spine by 9.2% after 21 months of treatment. A small increase occurred in hip BMD. Blood test levels of bone formation increased quickly, and markers of bone resorption increased somewhat later. The microarchitecture of trabecular bone was improved. Therapy reduced the vertebral fracture incidence by 65% and nontraumatic, nonvertebral fracture risk by 53%. Too few hip fractures occurred to evaluate the effect of teriparatide therapy in hip fracture risk.

Leg cramps occurred more frequently in the women who received teriparatide than placebo, and blood calcium levels increased transiently in a small number of patients.

In young rats treated with long-term, high doses of teriparatide throughout most of their lives, a dose-related increase in bone cancer (osteosarcoma) occurred. Women should be advised of this finding, although its significance for the use of teriparatide in humans is not known.

Contraindications to teriparatide use include abnormal serum calcium levels and the presence of risk factors for bone cancer, such as Paget's disease of bone, previous radiation to the skeleton (including radiation therapy for breast cancer), and unexplained elevations of alkaline phosphatase.

When PTH therapy is stopped, substantial bone loss has occurred within the first year.

The NAMS 2006 position statement on management of postmenopausal osteoporosis concludes that teriparatide is reserved for treating women at high risk for fracture, including those with very low BMD (T-score worse than –3.0) with a previous vertebral fracture. Dosage requirements (ie, daily subcutaneous injections) may limit use.

- *PTH 1-84.* This anabolic agent—a full-length (1-84) parathyroid hormone (Preos injection)—is approved for osteoporosis treatment in Europe. In a 2007 phase 3 randomized trial by Greenspan et al, PTH 1-84 significantly reduced vertebral fractures by 61%, but the incidence of hypercalcemia has delayed approval in North America.

Hormone therapy. Several systemic ET and EPT preparations are approved in the United States and Canada for the prevention of bone loss after menopause, but no ET or EPT preparation is approved for the treatment of women known to have osteoporosis.

The administration of estrogen, orally or transdermally, reduces bone resorption markers into the normal *premenopausal* range. The beneficial effects of systemic oral or transdermal ET/EPT at standard doses on BMD preservation are well established. A 2002 meta-analysis of 57 RCTs comparing ET/EPT against placebo in postmenopausal women found consistent BMD increases with ET/EPT at all sites. In trials of 2 years duration, the mean difference in BMD after ET/EPT was 6.8% at the lumbar spine and 4.1% at the femoral neck.

The two largest and best controlled trials support these findings. In the Postmenopausal Estrogen/Progestin Interventions (PEPI) trial (N = 875), standard daily doses of 0.625 mg conjugated estrogens (CE), with or without a progestogen (either MPA or micronized progesterone), for 3 years significantly increased spinal BMD by 3.5% to 5.0%, with a 1.7% increase in hip BMD. More recently, the Women's Health Initiative (WHI)—a 5-year RCT of 16,608 postmenopausal women aged 50 to 79 years—reported that standard doses of daily EPT (0.625 mg CE plus 2.5 mg MPA) significantly increased spine and total hip BMD by 4.5% and 3.7%, respectively, relative to placebo.) However, BMD was not systematically measured in the WHI, so whether participants had osteopenia or osteoporosis is unknown.

Effects of lower-than-standard doses of ET/EPT on BMD have been investigated. RCTs using doses as low as 0.3 mg/

day oral CE, 0.25 mg/day oral micronized 17β-estradiol, and 0.014 mg/day transdermal 17β-estradiol reported significant increases in spine and hip BMD relative to placebo. These trials were conducted either in populations of early postmenopausal women (mean age, 51-52 y) or in older postmenopausal women (mean ages, 67 and 74 y). Changes in lumbar spine BMD were in the range of 1% to 3%, significantly better than placebo.

Significant BMD improvements have also been noted with systemic estrogen doses delivered via a vaginal ring (Femring). In an RCT of 174 postmenopausal women younger than age 65, daily doses of 0.05 and 0.1 mg of estradiol acetate delivered via the ring significantly increased hip BMD (1.7% and 1.8%, respectively) and lumbar spine BMD (2.7% and 3.3%) compared with baseline.

Evidence from both RCTs and observational studies indicates that standard doses of ET/EPT (including 0.625 mg/d CE or the equivalent) not only improve BMD, but also reduce fracture risk in postmenopausal women. Two meta-analyses have found that ET/EPT significantly reduces the risk of fracture by up to 27%.

Two large observational studies support these data. The National Osteoporosis Risk Assessment (NORA) study examined 200,160 postmenopausal women and reported that current estrogen use was associated with a significantly reduced risk for new fracture. Participants were at least 50 years old and had no previous diagnosis of osteoporosis. The Million Women Study, a prospective observational study of 138,737 postmenopausal women, reported that current ET/EPT use provided a significant relative risk reduction in incidence of fracture.

In postmenopausal women in the WHI, both EPT and ET significantly reduced the risk of both spine and hip fractures by 34%; ET reduced hip fractures by 35% to 40%.

The Million Women Study, although observational in design, addressed issues related to ET/EPT and the risk of fracture that could not be ascertained in the WHI trials, such as comparisons between different EPT formulations, doses, and routes of administration. When the overall fracture-risk reduction was examined by type of hormone, no difference was found between ET and EPT. Sequential or continuous progestin use also did not significantly affect the results. Furthermore, the relative risk of fracture was not different when specific estrogen or progestin products were compared (ie, CE versus estradiol; MPA versus norethisterone or norgestrel/levonorgestrel). This study did not specifically report on the possible fracture protection afforded by a low estrogen dose (ie, 0.3 mg), but found that similar risk reductions for doses greater than 0.625 mg were similar to those for doses 0.625 mg or less.

The primary indication for systemic ET/EPT is for women experiencing moderate to severe menopause symptoms (eg, vasomotor symptoms, vaginal atrophy). Long-term use is associated with increased risks (see Section G, page 218). In a 2007 position statement on the role of HT, NAMS recommended that, because of the potential risks associated with HT, women who require drug therapy for osteoporosis risk reduction (including women at high risk for fracture in the next 5-10 y), should consider both HT and alternatives, weighing the risks and benefits of each. NAMS recommends use of ET/EPT at the lowest effective dose for the shortest time period consistent with treatment goals. Lower-than-standard doses of ET/EPT, however, have not been examined with regard to fracture efficacy. The optimal time to initiate ET/EPT and the optimal duration of therapy have not been established. For hysterectomized women aged 50 to 60 years, use of estrogen only is a minimal risk and many clinicians believe it should be the first choice. Women experiencing premature menopause have an increased osteoporosis risk and are candidates for longer-term hormone use.

Some studies show that hormone withdrawal accelerates bone loss. Evidence from the NORA trial found that women who stopped using HT more than 5 years previously had similar hip fracture risk to never users. However, a recent study from Denmark found that hormones administered in the early postmenopausal years maintained significantly higher BMD and resulted in fewer fractures than placebo even many years after stopping therapy.

Calcitonin. Salmon calcitonin is government approved in the United States and Canada for osteoporosis treatment more than 5 years postmenopause, but not for osteoporosis prevention. It is available in the United States as a nasal spray (Miacalcin Nasal Spray, Fortical Nasal Spray) and a subcutaneous injection (Miacalcin Injection). Available in Canada are a nasal spray (Miacalcin Nasal Spray) and an injectable form (Calcimar Solution, Caltine), although these injectables are not indicated for osteoporosis.

Salmon calcitonin is a potent inhibitor of osteoclast activity in vitro. In clinical trials, calcitonin has had modest effects on BMD, with values in the hip and spine increasing by 1% to 3% after 3 to 5 years of treatment. Originally given by subcutaneous injection, calcitonin is now most often administered as the nasal spray, and this formulation is approved for treatment of postmenopausal osteoporosis in women at least 5 years past menopause. The drug is not approved for osteoporosis prevention since it failed to prevent bone loss in women in the first few years after menopause. Oral forms of calcitonin are in development.

In women with osteoporosis, nasal calcitonin therapy at 200 IU/day for 5 years reduced the risk of new vertebral fractures by 36%. No effect on spine fractures was seen with higher or lower doses, and no effect on nonvertebral fracture risk was observed at any dose.

Calcitonin has been shown to reduce bone pain from osteoporotic vertebral compression fractures more quickly than placebo immediately after a fracture; however, it has not been shown to decrease bone pain in other situations.

Calcitonin is typically dosed at 200 IU (1 spray) administered daily in alternating nostrils. Treatment with nasal calcitonin for 5 years has not been associated with unexpected side effects other than local nasal irritation with the nasal spray formulation. It is likely that the skeletal effect of therapy would disappear quickly when treatment is discontinued.

Due to its lower potency, calcitonin is reserved for women who cannot or choose not to take one of the other agents. Because efficacy of calcitonin has not been observed in early postmenopausal women, product labeling recommends its use only in women with osteoporosis who are at least 5 years beyond menopause.

Combining therapies. Combining potent agents for treating osteoporosis has not been widely studied, yet it is common in clinical practice. Prescribing combination alendronate plus HT has been shown to produce small but significantly greater gains in BMD than observed with either drug alone at the lumbar spine (8.1% vs 6%) and hip trochanter (3.5% vs 0.5%) in postmenopausal women with low BMD. In studies combining risedronate or cyclic etidronate with HT, BMD gains with combined therapy were slightly greater at the spine and 2% higher at the hip than gains made with HT alone. Similarly, combining raloxifene with alendronate or risedronate resulted in somewhat greater increase in BMD than was observed with raloxifene alone. One concern is that combining two antiresorptive therapies might oversuppress bone turnover, adversely affect bone quality, and thereby increase the likelihood of fracture. There are no fracture data or long-term safety data to suggest that combination therapy should be used.

Promising new therapies. Several new drugs show promise for the treatment and/or prevention of osteoporosis. Some are now available outside North America, while others are in clinical development. Currently, the only promising therapy that has demonstrated fracture efficacy in published trials is strontium ranelate (Protelos). This element is taken up by bone, and may have a dual action as an antiresorptive and as a stimulator of bone formation. It is approved in European countries and is taken orally (2 g/d). In large multicenter trials, strontium ranelate reduced vertebral fractures by 37%, nonvertebral fractures by 16%, and hip fractures by 36%. Its mechanism of action is not entirely clear. The most common side effect is diarrhea, and less commonly, vascular and central nervous effects.

Management of osteoporotic fractures. When osteoporotic fractures occur, pain management and rehabilitation are important clinical objectives. Healthcare providers should be alerted to the need for pain management, especially in those women who may attempt to "tough out" pain, and in those who may not exhibit usual pain behavior or are unable to express pain due to confusion or cognitive function decreased by dementia.

Chronic back pain, a common complication of osteoporotic vertebral fractures, can be reduced by improving muscle strength and posture. A back support is sometimes helpful. Because the pain is frequently related to strain on extensor muscles, exercises that improve extensor muscle strength and endurance can help, such as the use of a Posture Training Support. Some women achieve complete pain relief through an appropriately designed and monitored exercise program. Others achieve partial relief that enables them to resume many normal activities.

For women who have severe or intractable pain, drug therapy and site-specific analgesia are indicated. Multiple modalities, such as milder systemic pain medication in combination with site-specific analgesia, can help reduce the risk of side effects from any single pain therapy. They may provide alternatives to systemic narcotics and anticholinergics, which the elderly tolerate poorly. Trigger-point injections can decrease pain and improve the range of motion. If the woman's pain persists, referral to an anesthesiologist or pain management clinic may be warranted.

Open surgical management of vertebral fractures due to osteoporosis is rarely required. Vertebroplasty and kyphoplasty are invasive procedures in which bone cement is injected through a percutaneous needle into a fractured vertebra in an attempt to provide pain relief. Kyphoplasty may also partially reduce height loss. Serious adverse events include MI, CVD, and VTE from cement leakage. More studies are needed to evaluate the long-term outcome of these procedures on both symptoms and subsequent fracture risk.

Hip fractures are nearly always treated surgically, either by internal fixation or hip replacement. Appropriate management of the comorbidities frequently found in these women is essential, and adequate postoperative pain management is important. The mortality rate during the first 4 months after hip fracture is about 15% to 20%. Physical medicine and rehabilitation can help many women regain function after hip fracture and this is essential to avoid long-term nursing home care. Unfortunately, as the Surgeon General's report on osteoporisis showed, the great majority of hip fracture patients do not receive treatment for osteoporosis. All patients should receive bone-active agents in addition to adequate calcium and vitamin D (preferably vitamin D_3). Oral nutritional supplements containing protein have been shown to reduce further bone loss in elderly women who have sustained hip fracture. These supplements may also shorten the hospital stay after hip fracture and improve the clinical outcome.

Cardiovascular disease

Despite evidence-based gains in the treatment of cardiovascular disease (CVD), the disease remains the leading killer of women in the United States and Canada. Coronary heart disease (CHD) accounts for most CVD deaths in women. CHD is often fatal, and most women who die suddenly have no previously recognized symptoms. It is, therefore, important to implement management strategies to prevent CHD. Other types of CVD, including cerebrovascular disease and peripheral arterial disease (PAD), are also common in women as they age. However, it is beyond the scope of this textbook to present a complete discussion of the clinical management of CVD.

Risk factors. Risk factors associated with CVD in women include cigarette smoking, sedentary lifestyle, hypertension, diabetes mellitus (DM), abnormal plasma lipids, obesity, poor diet, family history of premature CVD, metabolic syndrome (see Box), poor exercise capacity on treadmill test and/or abnormal heart rate recovery after stopping exercise, and evidence of subclinical vascular disease (eg, coronary calcification). Whether a decline in estrogen levels is a risk factor, based on the association between increased risk of CVD and postmenopausal age, remains controversial.

Women should be stratified by risk. The 2007 guidelines from the American Heart Association (AHA) include the following definitions:

- *High risk:* defined as having established CHD, cerebrovascular disease, PAD, abdominal aortic aneurysm, DM, or chronic kidney disease.

- *At risk:* defined as having one or more major risk factors for CVD, including cigarette smoking, poor diet, physical inactivity, obesity (especially central adiposity), family history of premature CVD (<55 y in male relative and <65 y of age in female relative), hypertension, dyslipidemia, evidence of subclinical vascular disease (eg, coronary calcification), metabolic syndrome (see Box), and poor exercise capacity on treadmill test and/or abnormal heart rate recovery after stopping exercise.

- *Optimal risk:* defined as having optimal levels of risk factors and heart-healthy lifestyle and Framingham Risk Score (Framingham Heart Study) less than 10%.

The greater the risk, the more aggressive the prevention strategy should be. The guidelines note that a Framingham Risk Score greater than 20% could be used to identify a woman at high risk, but that a lower score is not sufficient to ensure low risk. They focus on the lifetime risk for CVD at age 50 being increased for women with even one single risk factor for CVD.

The *metabolic syndrome* is closely associated with the generalized metabolic disorder of insulin resistance. Although there are no universally accepted criteria for diagnosing the metabolic syndrome, many healthcare clinicians use criteria proposed in the third report of the Expert Panel on Detection, Evaluation, and Treatment of High Blood Cholesterol in Adults (Adult Treatment Panel III, or ATP III).

In women, the ATP III defines the metabolic syndrome as the presence of three or more of the following factors. (Note that the mmol/L value for HDL-C is from the Canadian guidelines, not directly converted from mg/dL.)

- Central obesity (≥35-inch or 88-cm waist measurement)
- Elevated serum triglycerides ≥150 mg/dL (1.70 mmol/L)
- Low serum HDL-C <50 mg/dL (1.3 mmol/L)
- Elevated blood pressure (≥130/85 mm Hg)
- Fasting plasma glucose level ≥100 mg/dL (5.6 mmol/L)

The ATP III did not find conclusive evidence to recommend routine measurement of insulin resistance, prothrombotic state, or proinflammatory state.

Underlying causes of this syndrome are overweight/obesity, physical inactivity, and genetic factors. Women with the metabolic syndrome are at increased risk of CHD, stroke, peripheral vascular disease, and type 2 DM.

Screening. Developing a standardized procedure for cardiovascular risk factor assessment and management is important for evaluating women at risk for CVD.

The ATP III recommends adopting the Framingham Risk Score method to estimate a woman's 10-year risk for developing cardiac events. Points are assigned to various levels of risk, which are then translated into the 10-year estimated risk for cardiovascular events. Risk factors included in the Framingham risk calculation include age, total cholesterol, HDL-C, systolic blood pressure (BP), ongoing treatment for hypertension, and active cigarette smoking. Framingham estimates are more robust for total cholesterol than for LDL-C, but LDL-C remains the primary target of therapy. The Framingham Risk Score gives estimates for myocardial infarction (MI) and coronary death. A risk assessment tool for estimating the 10-year CVD risk is available at: http://hin.nhlbi.nih.gov/atpiii/calculator.asp? usertype=prof

Blood pressure. It is important to identify and manage high BP. Elevated BP is strongly related to the risk of cardiovascular, cerebrovascular, and renal diseases. Treatment and control of elevated BP in the United States has contributed substantially to the reduction in stroke and heart disease mortality during the past 30 years, especially in women. For details on BP measurement, see Section F, page 194.

Hypertension is defined by the Joint National Committee on Prevention, Detection, Evaluation, and Treatment of High Blood Pressure (JNC 7) as BP greater than 140 mm Hg systolic or greater than 90 mm Hg diastolic. The JNC 7 guidelines also define normal BP as less than 120 mg Hg systolic and less than 80 mm Hg diastolic. Table 9 provides a classification of BP for adults aged 18 years or older.

Table 9. JNC 7 classification of blood pressure for adults aged 18 years or older

BP Classification	Systolic BP (mm Hg)		Diastolic BP (mm Hg)
Normal	<120	and	<80
Prehypertension	120-139	or	80-89
Stage 1 hypertension	140-159	or	90-99
Stage 2 hypertension	≥160	or	≥100

Source: Chobanian et al *JAMA* 2003.

Similarly, the 2006 AHA scientific statement on dietary approaches to prevent and treat hypertension states that less than 120/80 mm Hg is an optimal BP, calling for initial dietary intervention before pharmacotherapy in uncomplicated stage 1 hypertension levels established by JNC 7.

Referral for hypertension management does not require specialty consultation. An evaluation including history, physical examination, and laboratory testing (consisting of urinalysis, checking for albuminuria; complete blood count; blood chemistry, including electrolytes, creatinine, fasting glucose, and fasting lipids; and electrocardiogram [ECG]) should be performed initially to assess associated risks, target organ damage, and identify potential secondary causes (including sleep apnea). More extensive testing for secondary causes may be needed depending on initial screening results.

Lipid tests. Elevated serum cholesterol levels, particularly elevated LDL-C, are clearly established major risk factors for CVD. New guidelines have been established for the evaluation and management of hyperlipidemia that focus on the primacy of LDL-C as the target of evaluation and therapy. The ATP III recommends that a complete *fasting* lipoprotein profile be performed as the initial screening test for all adults. These tests should include a measurement of total cholesterol, LDL-C, HDL-C, and triglycerides. The classifications for cholesterol levels recommended by the ATP III are listed in Table 10.

Lifestyle modification. Women with any modifiable risk factors for CVD should be urged to initiate lifestyle changes to decrease their overall risk. The AHA guidelines stress the importance of lifestyle interventions, not only because of their potential to reduce clinical CVD, but also because heart-healthy lifestyles may prevent the development of major risk factors for CVD. Such prevention may minimize the need for more intensive future interventions.

Cigarette smoking. Use of tobacco is the single most important preventable risk factor for CVD in women. A woman who smokes is two to six times more likely to have a heart attack than a woman who does not smoke. The effect of smoking on risk of fatal CVD is dose related (ie, heavier smokers have a greater relative risk). However, if a woman stops smoking—no matter how long or how much she has smoked—her risk of heart disease drops rapidly. The 2007 AHA guidelines for smoking cessation include counseling, nicotine replacement, and other pharmacotherapy as indicated, in conjunction with a behavioral program or formal smoking cessation program. Women should also avoid environmental (ie, secondhand) smoke. Although oral contraceptive (OC) use does not increase CVD risk in nonsmokers, use of these drugs synergistically increases CVD risk in women who smoke.

Table 10. ATP III screening classifications for lipids (fasting)

Serum levels	In mg/dL	In mmol/L	Classification
LDL cholesterol	<100	<2.5	Optimal
	100-129	2.5-3.3	Near optimal/ above optimal
	130-159	3.4-4.0	Borderline high
	160-189	4.1-4.8	High
	≥190	≥4.9	Very high
Total cholesterol	<200	<5.1	Desirable
	200-239	5.1-6.1	Borderline high
	≥240	≥6.2	High
HDL cholesterol	<50	<1.3	Low
	≥60	≥1.5	High

Source: American Heart Association 2001.

Exercise. Physical inactivity is almost as great a risk factor as smoking. Studies have shown that middle-aged women who exercise regularly have lower weight, BP, and plasma glucose levels, as well as more favorable lipid profiles, than sedentary women. Regular physical activity, particularly aerobic exercise, promotes cardiovascular health. Adoption of a regular aerobic exercise program reduces the risk of coronary events in women. The AHA recommends that women accumulate a minimum of 30 minutes of moderate-intensity exercise (eg, brisk walking) on most, and preferably all, days of the week to maintain weight, and 60 to 90 minutes daily to lose weight.

Nutrition. The AHA guidelines suggest a heart-healthy diet that includes intake of a variety of fruits, vegetables, and whole-grain, high-fiber foods. The diet should include fish, especially oily fish, at least twice a week. The AHA recommends limiting intake of trans-fatty acids (<1% of energy), saturated fat (<10% of energy), and cholesterol (<300 mg/d). Sodium intake should be limited to less than 2.3 g/day (approximately 1 tsp salt). As an adjunct to diet, omega-3 fatty acid supplementation may be considered in high-risk women. See also Section J.

Additional nutrition-related approaches include:

- *Antioxidants.* Epidemiologic studies have shown a lower incidence of heart disease in those who eat more fruits and vegetables high in antioxidants and whole grains. To date, however, no large RCTs have established a benefit of taking antioxidant vitamin supplements, such as vitamin C, vitamin E, beta-carotene, lycopene, and folic acid. Some studies suggest that supplements may cause harm. See also Section H.

Eating less meat and taking supplements of the B vitamins folate, B_6, and B_{12} will lower homocysteine levels, although no studies document that lowering homocysteine prevents CVD.

The 2007 AHA guidelines indicate that antioxidant vitamin supplements should not be used to prevent CVD. Folic acid with or without B_6 and B_{12} supplementation should not be used for the primary or secondary prevention of CVD.

- *Plant sterols and stanols.* Naturally occuring plant sterols and stanols may help to reduce the risk of CHD by lowering blood cholesterol levels. These compounds chemically resemble cholesterol and inhibit cholesterol absorption in the small intestine. Sterols are present in small quantities in many fruits, vegetables, nuts, seeds, cereals, legumes, and other plant sources. Stanols occur in even smaller quantities in many of the same sources. For example, both plant sterols and stanols are found in vegetable oils.

Since everyday amounts are not great enough to have significant cholesterol-lowering effects, these compounds have been incorporated into low-fat foods, including bread, cereals, dressings, low-fat milk and yogurt, and fruit juice. New food products, such as spreads, have also been developed. Dietary supplements in softgel form are also available.

In 2000, the FDA authorized labeling health claims for sterol- or stanol-containing foods regarding their role in reducing risk of CHD if consumed as part of a diet low in saturated fat and cholesterol. Foods that carry the claim must also meet the requirements for low saturated fat and low cholesterol. Although the health claim recommends consuming these compounds with two meals, more recent research suggests that frequency may not matter so long as the daily amount is consumed.

In its 2006 Diet and Lifestyle Recommendations, the AHA recommended consumption of plant sterols and stanols from a variety of foods and beverages, just as they would use cholesterol-lowering medication, in order to maintain

LDL cholesterol reductions. The AHA also noted that maximum effects are achieved at intakes of about 2 g/day. This is consistent with the evidence statement made by the ATP III which stated that daily intakes of 2 to 3 g/day will reduce LDL cholesterol by 6% to 15%.

Patients on statin therapy (see page 132 for more about statins) may achieve further reductions in their blood cholesterol levels when consuming a diet rich in plant sterols/stanols. These compounds appear to be somewhat more effective than doubling the statin dose, which usually produces an additional lowering of LDL cholesterol levels by only 5% to 7%. A review suggested that long-term use of plant sterols/stanols resulted in a 20% reduction in the incidence of CHD.

A growing body of evidence also suggests other positive health outcomes that include the reduced risk of certain types of cancer.

- *Soy/isoflavones.* While not mentioned specifically in the AHA 2007 preventive guidelines, an AHA science advisory panel from 2006 reviewed the use of soy and isoflavones and their impact on cardiovascular health. This update looked at 22 RCTs of soy protein. The effect of isolated soy protein with isoflavones showed minimal LDL-C reductions in the range of 3%. No significant effects on HDL-C, triglycerides, lipoprotein(a), or BP were evident. Further review of 19 studies of soy isoflavones showed no effect on LDL-C and other lipid risk factors. Use of isoflavone supplements in food or pills was *not* recommended. The review does note, however, that many soy products should be beneficial to cardiovascular and overall health because of their high content of polyunsaturated fats, fiber, vitamins and minerals, and their low content of saturated fat.

Alcohol consumption. The 2007 AHA guidelines encourage limiting alcohol consumption to no more than one drink per day (a drink being equal to a 12-oz bottle of beer, a 5-oz glass of wine, or 1.5 oz of 80-proof spirit). Some evidence suggests that light to moderate use of alcohol lowers the cardiovascular mortality rate among women over age 50 who are at greater risk for CHD; however, higher levels (>7 drinks/wk) may increase risk of hypertension, stroke, and coronary disease.

Weight. Maintaining an ideal weight has been estimated to reduce the overall risk of CVD by 35% to 55%. Central obesity (ie, apple shape) is more dangerous for heart health. The AHA recommends weight maintenance or reduction through an appropriate balance of physical activity, caloric intake, and formal behavioral programs, when indicated, to maintain or achieve a BMI between 18.5 and 24.9 kg/m^2 and a waist circumference of less than 35 inches (88 cm). (See also Section J.)

For women who need to lose weight or sustain weight loss, the AHA guidelines recommend a minimum of 60 to 90 minutes of moderate-intensity exercise on most and preferably all days of the week. A combined approach of exercise and diet seems to be superior to diet only. Three 10-minute exercise sessions have been shown to be more effective than one 30-minute session. A reasonable goal is losing 10% of body weight over a 6-month period.

Psychosocial factors. Women with CVD should be evaluated for depression and treated appropriately, as necessary.

Aspirin. The benefit of aspirin use for individuals with heart disease remains unchallenged, and the use of daily low-dose aspirin (81 mg) to prevent recurrence of MI has become common practice. Dozens of studies conducted during the last 30 years have shown that aspirin impairs platelet function, which aids blood flow in those with atherosclerosis.

A meta-analysis of pooled data from five trials examining the effects of aspirin for the primary prevention of cardiovascular events over periods of 4 to 7 years showed that daily or every other day aspirin therapy reduced the risk for CHD by 28%, with no significant effects on mortality and stroke. Most participants were men older than age 50.

In the Nurses' Health Study (NHS), a large trial of healthy women aged 34 to 59 years who were monitored over 14 years, those who took aspirin (325 mg, 1-6 times/wk) had a lower risk of ischemic stroke, although women who took higher doses (>15 tablets/wk) were approximately twice as likely to suffer hemorrhagic strokes. This risk was increased further in older women with hypertension.

Data from the Massachusetts Women's Health Study published in 2005 evaluated the effects of low-dose aspirin (100 mg every other day) versus placebo in healthy women aged 45 years or older. Aspirin was shown to lower the risk of stroke without affecting the risk of MI or death from cardiovascular causes. While overall stroke risk decreased, there was a nonsignificant increase in hemorrhagic stroke. Aspirin did increase the risk of GI bleeding requiring transfusion compared with the placebo group. Subgroup analyses demonstrated that aspirin significantly reduced the risk of major cardiovascular events, ischemic stroke, and MI among women aged 65 years or older.

A meta-analysis published in 2006 reviewed aspirin for primary prevention of cardiovascular events in men and women. The conclusion was that, for both women and men, the risk of cardiovascular events was decreased due to a reduction in ischemic stroke in women and MI in men. Aspirin did increase the risk of bleeding to a similar effect in men and women.

A meta-analysis published in 2007 evaluated the dosing of aspirin for CVD prevention. Currently available clinical data do not support doses of aspirin greater than 75 to 81 mg/day in the setting of CVD prevention. Higher doses, which may be commonly prescribed, have not been found to be more effective at preventing events, but are associated with increased risks of GI bleeding.

The 2007 AHA guidelines recommend that women at high risk for CVD take aspirin (75-325 mg/d) unless contraindicated. If a high-risk woman is intolerant of aspirin therapy, clopidogrel (eg, Plavix) should be substituted.

Additionally, the 2007 AHA guidelines recommend that at-risk or healthy women aged 65 years or older consider aspirin therapy (81 mg/d or 100 mg every other day) if BP is controlled and benefit for ischemic stroke and MI prevention is likely to outweigh the risk of GI bleeding and hemorrhagic stroke. For women younger than 65 years, the same doses should be used when the benefit of ischemic stroke prevention is likely to outweigh the adverse effects of therapy. (See Section H, page 243, for precautions when using anticoagulant therapies.)

Aspirin use has been shown to significantly increase the rate of upper GI bleeding and is contraindicated for those who have an allergy to aspirin, tendency for bleeding, recent GI bleeding, or clinically active hepatic disease. Even enteric-coated or buffered aspirin may damage the intestinal lining. However, studies have shown that individuals who regularly take aspirin (and other anti-inflammatory drugs) have unusually low rates of digestive tract cancers. Data are not clear regarding an adverse association with cancers of the pancreas, prostate, and breast.

Pharmacologic interventions. For women with higher risks for CVD, prescription therapies may be necessary. If diet and exercise modifications for 6 weeks fail to obtain the desired levels for BP and cholesterol, appropriate drug intervention is recommended.

Prevention. Recommendations for primary prevention (based on the ATP III) focus on reducing risks through management of lipids, hypertension, and DM.

- *Lipids.* Increased serum levels of cholesterol can cause coronary artery atherosclerosis, limiting the blood flow to the heart. Atherosclerosis increases an individual's risk for MI. More than one third of women have abnormal cholesterol levels, which increases the risk for heart disease. It is estimated that a 25% reduction in total blood cholesterol can reduce heart disease risk by 50%. Reducing cholesterol to a normal range is a therapeutic goal.

  Triglycerides may be a more significant predictor of cardiovascular risk in women than in men. Attention should therefore be focused on the potential higher risk associated with women who have elevated triglyceride levels. In women who have levels of triglycerides of 128 mg/dL (1.4 mmol/L) or greater along with increased waist circumference of 35 inches (88 cm) or greater, risk for CVD is elevated. It is important to note that those women with abnormalities in the triglyceride/HDL-C axis often associated with increased waist circumference or metabolic syndrome may need aggressive triglyceride lowering along with reduction of LDL-C.

Guidelines for the management of hyperlipidemia now focus on LDL-C as the target of therapy. Optimal LDL-C levels are less than 100 mg/dL (2.5 mmol/L). High levels are set at 160 to 189 mg/dL (4.1-4.8 mmol/L). For women with known CVD or a CHD risk equivalent (ie, DM, 10-y risk ≥20%), the target LDL-C level is less than 100 mg/dL (2.5 mmol/L). For women with two or more major risk factors but no CHD risk equivalent (10-y risk ≤ 20%), the target is less than 130 mg/dL (3.3 mmol/L), and for those with one or no additional major risk factors, the target is less than 160 mg/dL (4.1 mmol/L). HDL-C goals are more than 50 mg/dL (1.3 mmol/L) in women and triglyceride goals are less than 150 mg/dL (1.7 mmol/L).

In 2004, the National Cholesterol Education Program released an update of the ATP III guidelines, based on available clinical trial evidence. Although the general goal of lipid-lowering remained the same, it recommended even lower LDL-C levels as reasonable clinical goals. Drug therapy for lowering LDL-C in high- or moderate-risk women should be aimed toward achieving a 30% to 40% reduction in LDL-C. Benefits of LDL-C–lowering therapy apply to older women. See Table 11.

Statin therapy is the best option for initial cholesterol control for older women. For example, lovastatin (eg, Mevacor) (20-40 mg/d), in addition to a diet that is low in saturated fat and cholesterol, has been shown to reduce the risk for the first acute major coronary event in women with average triglycerides and LDL-C levels and below-average levels of HDL-C. Women taking statin therapy should be monitored for adverse LDL-C effects (and other potential drug side effects).

- *Hypertension.* Hypertension is defined by JNC 7 and AHA as systolic BP greater than 140 mm Hg or diastolic BP greater than 90 mm Hg. Even mild elevations of BP can double the risk for stroke. The risk for hypertension increases with age. Postmenopausal women are at greater risk—with more than 50% affected beyond age 55—and black women are especially susceptible. Since hypertension rarely has symptoms, regular screening is important.

These guidelines also recommend aiming for an optimal BP of less than 120/80 mm Hg through lifestyle approaches. If BP is 140/90 mm Hg or greater, pharmacotherapy is indicated. For patients with DM or chronic kidney disease, the treatment goal is 130/80 mm Hg. A wide variety of antihypertensive agents can be

---

Table 11. Lipid-lowering guidelines in high- or moderate-risk women

Levels of lipids and lipoproteins recommended by the AHA through lifestyle approaches:

- LDL-C <100 mg/dL (2.5 mmol/L)
- HDL-C >50 mg/dL (1.3 mmol/L)
- Triglycerides <150 mg/dL (1.7 mmol/L)
- Non-HDL-C (total cholesterol minus HDL-C) <130 mg/dL (3.3 mmol/L)

If a woman is at high risk or has hypercholesterolemia:

- Intake of saturated fat should be <7% and cholesterol intake <200 mg/day
- LDL-C–lowering drug therapy should be used simultaneously with lifestyle therapy in high-risk women to achieve an LDL-C <100 mg/dL (2.5 mmol/L)

For at-risk women:

- If there are multiple risk factors, LDL-C–lowering drug therapy should be used if LDL-C is ≥130 mg/dL (3.3 mmol/L) with lifestyle therapy, even if the 10-year absolute risk is 10% to 20%
- LDL-C–lowering therapy should be used if LDL-C level is ≥160 mg/dL (4.1 mmol/L) with lifestyle therapy and multiple risk factors even if the 10-year absolute risk is <10%
- LDL-C–lowering therapy should be used if LDL-C is ≥190 mg/dL (4.9 mmol/L), regardless of the presence or absence of other risk factors or CVD on lifestyle therapy

For low HDL-C or elevated non-HDL-C in high-risk women:

- Niacin or fibrate therapy should be used after the LDL-C goal is reached

For women with multiple risk factors and a 10-year risk of 10% to 20%:

- Niacin or fibrates can be used when HDL-C is low or non-HDL-C is elevated after LDL-C goal is reached

Source: American Heart Association 2004.

---

prescribed, including diuretics. The AHA recommends including thiazide diuretics as part of the BP management plan for most women unless contraindicated or if there are compelling indications for other agents in specific CVD states. Initial treatment of high-risk women should be with beta-blockers, angiotensin-converting enzyme (ACE) inhibitors, or angiotensin II receptor blockers (ARBs), with addition of other drugs as needed, such as thiazides, to achieve goal BP.

- *Diabetes.* Another independent risk factor for CVD morbidity and mortality is DM. This disease is diagnosed in individuals with a fasting blood glucose of 126 mg/dL (7.0 mmol/L) or above. The disease accelerates atherosclerosis and increases the risk of acute coronary ischemia in women. It is usually associated with obesity, hypertension, and unfavorable plasma lipid profiles, which act synergistically to raise CVD risk. Programs aimed at reducing CVD risk in women with DM focus on controlling plasma glucose and insulin levels, controlling cholesterol, reducing obesity, and promoting exercise. The AHA recommends lifestyle and pharmacotherapy to achieve glycated hemoglobin (HbA1C) less than 7%, if this can be accomplished without significant hypoglycemia. (See page 135 for more about diabetes.)

- *Role of HT.* Oral estrogen alters the ratio of lipoproteins, raising HDL-C, lowering LDL-C, and raising triglycerides. Transdermal estrogen has been shown to increase HDL and lower LDL-C to a lesser degree than oral estrogen and does not affect triglycerides. Nonoral estrogens avoid the first-pass hepatic metabolism, which is partially responsible for diminished lipid effects.

The observed effects of estrogen differ markedly according to preparation, route of delivery, and dose. In the PEPI trial, oral CE alone or, for women with a uterus, in combination with a progestin, significantly increased HDL-C and decreased LDL-C. The addition of MPA slightly reduced the lipid benefits of using CE alone; progesterone had less of an adverse effect.

The beneficial effect of estrogen on endothelial function may occur via the promotion of nitric oxide release, which results in vasodilation, inhibition of adhesion molecule expression, and increased endothelial proliferation and migration to repair areas of injury. The improved lipid profile and endothelial cell function are thought to contribute to stabilization of atherosclerotic plaques. Estrogen increases the production of prostacyclin in the endothelium of blood vessels and decreases the production of thromboxane A_2 by platelets, thus reducing platelet adhesiveness. A 2007 WHI substudy by Manson et al found that among women 50 to 59 years old at enrollment, calcified plaque in the coronary arteries was less in women assigned to the estrogen arm than in those assigned to placebo.

Most observational studies support use of estrogen to prevent CVD in postmenopausal women. A meta-analysis of these data suggests 35% to 50% less risk for CVD. The effect seems to be independent of age, type of menopause (natural or surgical), or presence or absence of CVD. In the NHS, a survival benefit was observed in estrogen users with one or more cardiovascular risk factors; among women with no risk factors, a 30% lower relative risk was observed, although there was an increase in CVD events in the first years of HT use.

Recent RCTs have revealed a different risk-benefit ratio, moving from a presumption of benefit to evidence of harm. This highlights the complexity of HT use and underscores the value of RCTs to assess the safety and efficacy of therapeutic interventions. Despite new data, many questions regarding use of HT and CVD risk remain.

Data from the WHI suggest a reversed benefit-risk ratio. Initial reports from this trial indicated that a pattern of increased risk was emerging in the ET and EPT arms that resembled the pattern of early risk observed in the Heart and Estrogen/progestin Replacement Study (HERS). The WHI trial was allowed to continue because the risk was not statistically significant and because of the possibility that other noncoronary benefits might produce an overall net clinical benefit. Later, however, the EPT arm of the trial, using continuous-combined oral CE 0.625 mg/day plus MPA 2.5 mg/day, was stopped prematurely after a mean of 5.2 years of follow-up (original study design was for 8 y) due to significantly increased risk for CHD events and invasive breast cancer. These risks outweighed the statistically significant beneficial effects of EPT, including reduced hip fracture and colorectal cancer.

The unopposed ET arm of the WHI (all women had undergone a hysterectomy) was stopped prematurely after an average follow-up of 6.8 years, largely because of an increased risk of stroke and a lack of CHD benefits, the primary endpoint.

These WHI data and other findings contributed to the recommendations from NAMS (2007), AHA (2007), and other US and Canadian organizations that combined EPT not be initiated solely to prevent CVD in postmenopausal women. NAMS and AHA also advised that unopposed ET should not be initiated or continued to prevent CVD in postmenopausal women.

In its 2007 position statement on HT use, NAMS advised that data from studies, such as the WHI and HERS should be extrapolated only with caution to women younger than age 50 who initiate HT. WHI and HERS involved women aged 50 years and older (with mean ages of 63 and 67, respectively), and HERS was conducted solely in women with known coronary artery disease. The data should not be extrapolated to women experiencing premature menopause (<40 y) and initiating HT at that time. Likewise, data from these studies should not be extrapolated to the use of oral or other hormonal contraception by pre- or perimenopausal women.

Results from a substudy of the WHI (the Coronary-Artery Calcium Study), published in 2007 after the NAMS position statement, found that younger postmenopausal women who use unopposed estrogen have less calcified atheroma in the coronary artery than do similar women who do not use estrogen.

Premature menopause is associated with earlier onset of CHD, but there are no clear data as to whether ET or EPT will reduce morbidity or mortality from that condition.

The benefit-risk ratio for HT may be more favorable for younger women experiencing premature menopause.

The 2007 NAMS position statement notes that analysis of the time trend in the EPT arm of the WHI showed a significant interaction between CHD risk and the time since initiation of EPT, with an increased risk in the first year after initiation and decreased risk of CHD events in the later years of EPT use. A similar pattern was observed with EPT in the HERS secondary prevention trial in postmenopausal women with preexisting CHD. No increased risk of CHD soon after initiation of therapy was observed in the ET arm of the WHI or in any other ET-alone studies. The WHI and HERS studies enrolled women more than a decade after menopause on average, and most events occurred in older women. There was an insufficient number of younger, symptomatic, newly postmenopausal women to determine whether similar events apply to this cohort. NAMS points out that it remains unclear whether CHD risk is or is not increased soon after initiation of EPT in younger, newly postmenopausal women, and the results of these trials (WHI and HERS) should be applied to these women with caution.

Analysis of the data from WHI shows a trend toward reduction of CHD events in women who initiated HT less than 10 years since menopause and a significantly greater risk of CHD with initiation of HT more than 10 years after menopause. In women aged 50 to 59 years, there was a statistically significant reduction in the composite endpoint of MI, coronary artery revascularization, and CHD death randomized to ET in WHI.

In addition, analysis of the HERS data showed that the early increase of events was not seen in women taking statins.

Observational studies and RCTs have found a significant increase in the risk of VTE in postmenopausal women using systemic HT. There are limited observational data but no RCT data regarding the VTE risk differences between transdermal ET and oral therapies. The NAMS 2007 update suggests that lower doses of oral estrogens may be safer than higher doses.

Estrogen loss has been related to increased stroke rates in postmenopausal women. Randomized trials, however, show increased risk of stroke in women receiving HT. Longer lifetime exposure to ovarian estrogens may protect against noncardioembolic ischemic stroke. Very early age of exposure to ovarian estrogen may have negative effects.

The 2007 NAMS position statement notes that ET and EPT seem to increase the risk of ischemic stroke in postmenopausal women. The EPT and ET arms of WHI showed increased risk for ischemic stroke; however, other large trials did not. The absolute stroke risk in WHI is lower in women aged 50 to 59 years than in women further away from menopause. In secondary prevention (women with CHD or prior stroke), HT may not significantly increase stroke risk, but because these patients are at high baseline risk for a stroke, HT should be avoided. NAMS recommends that no HT regimen should be used for primary or secondary prevention of stroke.

The FDA now requires manufacturers of all HT products marketed in the United States to include in labeling a black box warning that all estrogens, with or without progestins, should not be used for the primary prevention of CVD. Health Canada has issued a similar advisory.

Treatment. Postmenopausal women have an extremely high risk for recurrent MI and CVD mortality. Therapies that result in even a small reduction in CVD risk can have a major impact on public health. In postmenopausal women with preexisting CVD, dietary and pharmacologic management of hypertension, hyperlipidemia, and DM should be initiated where appropriate, according to established guidelines from leading US and Canadian organizations, including the AHA.

- *Role of beta-blockers.* Beta-blocker agents should be prescribed indefinitely in all women after MI, acute coronary syndrome, or left ventricular dysfunction with or without heart failure symptoms, unless contraindicated.
- *Role of ACE inhibitors/ARBs.* ACE inhibitors should be used (unless contraindicated) in women after MI and in those with clinical evidence of heart failure, a left ventricular ejection function (LVEF) of 40% or less, or DM. In women after MI and in those with clinical evidence of heart failure or an LVEF of 40% or less, or those with DM who are intolerant of ACE inhibitors, ARBs should be used instead.
- *Aldosterone blockade.* Aldosterone blockade should be used after MI in women who do not have significant renal dysfunction or hyperkalemia, who are already receiving therapeutic doses of an ACE inhibitor and beta-blocker, and have an LVEF 40% or less with symptomatic heart failure.
- *Role of HT.* Several observational, secondary prevention studies had suggested that HT use could lower the risk of mortality and future cardiac events. However, based on RCTs that have found no effect of HT on clinical or anatomic progression of CVD, HT is not recommended by NAMS, AHA, or other US and Canadian organizations for the secondary prevention of CVD. For women with CVD, it would be prudent to emphasize cardiovascular risk reduction with established evidence-based treatments.

Diabetes mellitus

Type 1 diabetes mellitus (DM) is usually diagnosed in children and young adults. In type 1 DM, the body does not produce enough insulin, a hormone needed to convert glucose (sugar), starches, and other food into energy needed for daily life. Individuals with type 1 DM are treated with insulin. Type 1 DM is often called "insulin-dependent" DM.

As men and women age, they are more likely to develop "non-insulin-dependent" DM, often called "adult-onset" DM or "type 2" DM. Approximately 12.5% of US women aged 50 to 59 years have type 2 DM, with the prevalence increasing to about 17% at age 60 and older. Type 2 DM remains undiagnosed in approximately one third of women with the disease and is more prevalent in non-Caucasian women.

Risk factors. Women with or at high risk for type 2 DM have a substantially higher risk for developing CVD and this risk increases with age. A postmenopausal woman who has type 2 DM is three times more likely to develop CVD or stroke and is four times more likely to die from an MI than a woman without type 2 DM. Studies have shown the efficacy of reducing cardiovascular risk factors, such as hypertension, dyslipidemia, and smoking, in preventing or slowing CVD.

Patients with type 2 DM have an increased prevalence of lipid abnormalities, which contributes to higher rates of CVD. Lipid management aimed at lowering LDL-C, raising HDL-C, and lowering triglycerides has been shown to reduce macrovascular disease and mortality in those with DM.

Obesity and the loss of lean muscle mass, which amplify the type 2 DM risk, increase as the population ages. In women, the composition change typically presents as an increase in abdominal adipose tissue (central obesity). The presence of abdominal adipose tissue increases the propensity toward insulin resistance, which is often linked with dyslipidemia and coagulation abnormalities. A sedentary lifestyle may also contribute to obesity.

Skeletal muscle is the primary tissue responsible for insulin-mediated glucose uptake. A reduction in muscle mass can lead to insulin resistance, as observed in women of ideal body weight in early postmenopause. After menopause, pancreatic insulin secretion decreases and insulin resistance increases. These changes may be due to a combination of aging and estrogen deficiency.

Women with type 2 DM are at increased risk for other diseases as well. Their risk for developing endometrial cancer or gallstones is doubled. Many experience complications of uncontrolled type 2 DM that include vision loss, renal failure, neuropathy, or amputation.

The incidence of breast cancer, however, does not seem to be affected by type 2 DM, and the risk of osteoporosis may be lower. The role of obesity in both these conditions may outweigh any effect of type 2 DM, since it has been shown that obesity is protective for osteoporosis and is a risk factor for breast cancer after menopause.

Screening. The goal of glucose screening is to identify women who have or who are at risk for type 2 DM. Screening should be considered for all women over age 45, especially in those with a BMI of 25 kg/m^2 or more. Screening should also be considered in women younger than age 45 who are overweight. Other indications for DM testing include:

- Physical inactivity
- Having a first-degree relative with DM
- Being part of a high-risk ethnic population (eg, African American, Latino, American Indian, Asian American, Pacific Islander)
- Having delivered a baby weighing >9 lb (4 kg) or having been diagnosed with gestational DM
- BP ≥140/90 mm Hg
- HDL-C level <35 mg/dL (0.9 mmol/L) and/or a triglyceride level >250 mg/dL (6.4 mmol/L)
- Polycystic ovarian syndrome
- Impaired glucose tolerance on prior testing
- History of vascular disease.

Studies have shown that menopause does not lead to increases in impaired fasting glucose (IFG; or "prediabetes") levels. Repeat testing should be conducted every 3 years.

The US Preventive Services Task Force concluded in its 2003 clinical guidelines that the evidence is insufficient to recommend for or against routinely screening asymptomatic adults for type 2 DM, impaired glucose tolerance (IGT), or IFG. Type 2 DM is often not diagnosed until complications appear. Screening for type 2 DM should be conducted in a healthcare setting. A fasting plasma glucose (FPG) test or a 2-hour oral glucose tolerance test (OGTT), 75 g glucose load, is appropriate; however, the recommended screening method is the FPG. OGTT identifies persons with IGT who are at increased risk for the development of type 2 DM and CVD. An OGTT may be considered in those with IFG to better define the risk of type 2 DM.

Type 2 DM is diagnosed based on any one of the following criteria, provided the value can be confirmed on two or more occasions:
- Symptoms of type 2 DM and high casual plasma glucose concentration (≥200 mg/dL or 11.0 mmol/L)
- FPG is 126 mg/dL (7.0 mmol/L) or greater
- 2-hour postload glucose is 200 mg/dL (11.0 mmol/L) or greater

Management of DM consists of glycemic control and prevention of macrovascular and microvascular disease. According to the American Diabetes Association (ADA), the HbA1C should be less than 7%. Preprandial capillary glucose should be 90 mg/dL to 130 mg/dL (4.9-7.2 mmol/L) while peak postprandial glucose should be lower than 180 mg/day (9.9 mmol/L). The American Association of Clinical Endocrinologists guidelines proposed that the HbA1C should be less than 6.5% with a preprandial glucose lower than 110 mg/dL (6.0 mmol/L) and a postprandial glucose lower than 140 mg/dL (7.7 mmol/L).

Cholesterol screening should be performed annually, more often if needed, to achieve goals. According to the 2007 ADA guidelines, in women with DM, without CVD, the LDL-C target should be lower than 100 mg/dL (2.5 mmol/L). Triglycerides should be lower than 159 mg/dL (1.7 mmol/L) and HDL-C should be higher than 50 mg/dL (1.3 mmol/L).

Target BP in women with type 2 DM is less than 130/80 mm Hg.

Studies have shown a higher risk of morbidity and premature death from macrovascular complications among diabetic smokers. Smoking is also related to the premature development of microvascular complications of type 2 DM and may contribute to the development of type 2 DM. All patients with type 2 DM should be counseled on smoking cessation.

Diabetic nephropathy occurs in 20% to 40% of patients with type 2 DM and is the single leading cause of end-stage renal disease. Microalbuminuria (30-299 mg/24 h) has been shown to be the earliest stage of diabetic nephropathy in type 1 DM and a marker for development of nephropathy in type 2 DM. Microalbuminuria should be checked annually in type 1 diabetic patients with DM duration of 5 years or more and in all patients with type 2 DM, starting at diagnosis. Serum creatinine should be measured annually to estimate glomerular filtration rate (GFR). Optimal glucose control and BP control reduces the risk and may slow the progression of nephropathy.

Lifestyle modification. Many studies have shown that individuals at high risk for developing DM can be prescribed interventions that significantly delay, and sometimes prevent, the onset of type 2 DM. An intensive lifestyle modification program has been shown to be effective.

The Diabetes Prevention Program Research Group found that a 7% decrease in weight combined with at least 150 minutes of exercise per week decreased by 58% (vs placebo) the risk of type 2 DM in women at high risk. In other studies, exercise has been shown to reduce insulin resistance and improve control of glucose levels and lipids in individuals with type 2 DM. The ADA recommends at least 30 minutes of moderate physical activity on most days of the week. Weight reduction has been shown to also decrease insulin resistance, and weight loss programs that limit fat intake will improve the lipid profile.

Excessive alcohol consumption is associated with hyper- and hypoglycemia and should be avoided. Smoking should also be avoided, as smokers with type 2 DM have an increased risk of morbidity and premature death associated with development of macrovascular complications. Moreover, smoking is related to the premature development of microvascular complications of type 2 DM.

Aspirin. Use of low-dose aspirin (75-162 mg/d) should be recommended as a primary prevention strategy in those with type 2 DM at increased cardiovascular risk, including those who are older than 40 years or who have additional risk factors (family history of CVD, hypertension, smoking, dyslipidemia, or albuminuria). A meta-analysis of 145 prospective, controlled trials of antiplatelet therapy estimated that 38 vascular events per 1,000 patients with type 2 DM would be prevented if aspirin therapy were used for secondary prevention. This finding was further supported by the Early Treatment Diabetic Retinopathy Study.

Pharmacologic interventions. Various prescription therapies are available to manage the patient with diabetes.

Glycemic control. Management of glycemic control is outside the scope of this textbook.

Lipid control. For those over age 40, statin therapy is recommended to achieve an LDL-C reduction of 30% to 40%, regardless of baseline LDL-C levels. In those with overt CVD, all patients should be treated with a statin to achieve an LDL-C reduction of 30% to 40%. For high-risk patients, a lower LDL-C goal of lower than 70 mg/dL (1.8 mmol/L), using a high dose of a statin, is an option (Class B evidence).

BP control. In management of DM, BP control is important, as higher BP increases risks for renal dysfunction and CVD. Patients with hypertension should receive drug therapy as well as lifestyle and behavioral therapy. Initial drug therapy should begin with agents that have been shown to reduce CVD events in diabetics, such as ACE inhibitors, ARBs, beta-blockers, diuretics, and calcium channel blockers. Expert consensus opinion promotes use of an ACE or ARB in treating all diabetics with hypertension.

ACE inhibitors or ARBs should be used in the treatment of micro- and macroalbuminuria in diabetics with hypertension (Class A evidence). These agents have been shown to delay the progression of nephropathy in diabetics with hypertension and microalbuminuria (>300 mg/24 h) (Class A).

Role of hormones. Women with type 1 or type 2 DM present a clinical challenge when hormones are indicated as a contraceptive or as menopause therapy.

One comparative study in women with DM found that low-dose OC users (compared with copper T 380A intrauterine system users) had significantly higher triglycerides and HDL-C and lower LDL-C; DMPA users had significantly higher triglycerides and LDL-C and lower HDL-C. Partial thromboplastin time was prolonged in users of subdermal levonorgestrel (Norplant). The investigators concluded that, in women with DM, DMPA has an unfavorable metabolic outcome and low-dose OCs produce some metabolic alterations, whereas subdermal levonorgestrel has minimal metabolic alterations. In women aged 18 to 50 years at high risk for DM, DMPA was associated with a greater risk of DM compared with combination OCs. The 2006 guidelines from the American College of Obstetricians and Gynecologists (ACOG) indicate that use of combination OCs is not appropriate for women with DM who are over age 35, who smoke, and who show evidence of hypertension, nephropathy, retinopathy, or other vascular disease. Progestin-only contraceptive methods may be an option for older women with DM. See also Section G on oral contraceptives.

In postmenopausal women with type 2 DM, several short-term RCTs of ET or EPT and glycemic control have been conducted, involving fewer than 60 women per trial. In three trials that used oral estrogen, ET (17β-estradiol or CE) improved glycemic control. A trial that used oral CE plus MPA also found improved glycemic control. However, in other trials, no significant differences in glycemic control were observed for oral CE plus cyclic medrogestone or transdermal 17β-estradiol plus oral norethisterone. In all trials, only transdermal 17β-estradiol plus norethisterone did not worsen triglyceride levels.

The PEPI study, a 3-year RCT in women without type 2 DM, found that oral CE alone or combined with a progestogen (MPA or micronized progesterone) slightly decreased FPG levels, compared with placebo, while CE in combination with MPA increased 2-hour FPG levels.

In the large prospective NHS, after 12 years of follow-up, there was no evidence that the risk for type 2 DM was associated with the dose or duration of combined HT or with use of ET versus EPT. In the prospective Rancho Bernardo Study, the risk for DM was not significantly increased or decreased by HT in postmenopausal women followed for 11 years. Another prospective study of over 21,000 postmenopausal women found no association between HT use and risk of type 2 DM.

HERS demonstrated that the incidence of DM was 6.2% in those on daily combined EPT, compared with 9.5% in the placebo arm. In the randomized, double-blind WHI, which enrolled 15,641 postmenopausal women aged 50 to 79, the cumulative incidence of treated DM was 3.5% in the oral CE plus MPA group compared with 4.2% in the placebo arm after 5.6 y of follow-up. In the first year of follow-up, changes in fasting insulin and glucose levels indicated a decrease in insulin resistance in those on EPT. The WHI also looked at 10,739 postmenopausal women who had a hysterectomy and were placed on oral CE alone; the cumulative incidence of treated DM was 8.3% compared with 9.3% in the placebo group, although the difference was insignificant. HT, however, is not recommended for prevention of type 2 DM.

The Wisconsin Epidemiologic Study of Diabetic Retinopathy concluded that use of OCs or HT among women with type 1 or type 2 DM does not seem to affect the severity of diabetic retinopathy or incidence of macular edema.

In women with DM who need HT for menopausal symptom control, transdermal ET may offer advantages over the oral route. Serum triglyceride levels, often increased in women who have DM, are not increased further with transdermal ET. Low-dose and transdermal 17β-estradiol also seem to have less effect on DVT, gallbladder disease, and inflammatory markers; however, conclusive clinical trial evidence is lacking.

A daily dose equivalent to oral doses of 17β-estradiol (1 mg) or CE (≤0.625 mg) is recommended, even if vasomotor symptoms are still present at this dose. Higher doses have not been associated with increased benefit on the lipid profile but have been associated with decreased insulin sensitivity in a small study.

Observational studies have shown that ET has beneficial effects on plasma lipids, insulin sensitivity, vasodilation, atherosclerosis, and arterial response to injury. Research suggests that the progestogen component of EPT may attenuate the beneficial effects of estrogen on HDL-C, insulin sensitivity, and endothelial function. The 2000 NAMS consensus opinion on HT in women with DM concluded that, if EPT is required in a woman with DM, exposure to progestogen should be minimized. Selecting a metabolically neutral progestogen for EPT, such as micronized progesterone or norgestimate, is recommended to maintain higher plasma HDL-C. Progestins with a higher androgenic potency reduce more beneficial effects of estrogens on vasodilation; progesterone and 19-norpregnane derivatives have less of an adverse effect. For women with type 2 DM, continuous-sequential EPT regimens are recommended to minimize progestogen exposure; low-dose oral micronized progesterone is also recommended.

Postmenopausal women with type 2 DM are likely to be taking multiple medications to treat concomitant diseases, thereby increasing the likelihood of poor adherence to medication regimens. Counseling, therefore, is extremely important.

Most of the NAMS recommendations for postmenopausal women who have or are at risk for developing type 2 DM apply to women with type 1 DM. They include the following:

- Optimal glucose control (eg, glycated hemoglobin <7%) and controlling risk factors for cardiovascular events are primary goals of therapy for all women who have DM.

- Controlling CVD risk factors through pharmacologic and nonpharmacologic means can significantly decrease the risk for cardiovascular events.

- A broad-based recommendation for postmenopausal HT cannot be made; the benefits and risks must be weighed in the context of each woman's risk factors. HT cannot be recommended for primary or secondary prevention of CVD.

- If HT is recommended, the greatest benefits may be obtained through use of transdermal estrogen preparations and low doses of oral estrogens.
- If oral EPT is required, continuous-sequential therapy is recommended, rather than continuous-combined therapy, to minimize exposure to progestogen. The use of low-dose, oral micronized progesterone is recommended, although vaginal or intrauterine progesterone formulations may also minimize the potential for negative metabolic events.
- Counseling can maximize the woman's adherence to multiple medication regimens and increase her understanding of the potential benefits and risks of HT.

Cancers

Cancer is the second leading cause of death for women in the United States and Canada, surpassed only by heart disease. In the United States in 2007, 1,500 people die every day from cancer. Nearly 80% of all cancers are diagnosed at age 55 and older. Women have a one in three lifetime risk of developing cancer.

Menopause is not associated with increased cancer risk. However, since cancer rates increase with age, women in midlife and beyond should be evaluated for risk of cancer of the lung, breast, uterus, ovary, colon, rectum, and skin—the most common cancers that affect women.

The causes of various cancers are not known; however, risk factors have been identified. The top cancer risk factors are related to behavior, and include tobacco use, alcohol use, poor nutrition, and lack of exercise. Certain cancers related to viruses can be prevented through lifestyle change. Vaccines have been developed for hepatitis B (Hep B) and the human papillomavirus (HPV) and are being developed for the human immunodeficiency virus (HIV). Protecting the skin from direct sunlight can prevent most skin cancers.

In the United States and Canada, it is estimated that more than 85% of lung cancer deaths are attributed to smoking. The number of newly diagnosed cases is continuing to rise, which parallels the increasing number of women who smoke cigarettes.

Secondhand tobacco smoke (ie, environmental tobacco smoke) also poses health risks. One study showed that, among nonsmoking women, the risk of lung cancer is approximately 30% higher for wives of smokers than for wives of nonsmokers. Smoking is also related to an increased risk of cancer of the mouth and throat as well as cervical cancer. New screening techniques for lung cancer that are being evaluated include low-dose helical CT scans and molecular markers found in sputum samples.

It is estimated that about one third of all US cancer deaths are attributed to diet and obesity. Excessive alcohol consumption and physical inactivity also increase cancer risk. Healthy nutrition, increased physical activity, smoking cessation, and reduced alcohol intake may decrease cancer risk.

In US and Canadian women, breast cancer has the highest incidence, whereas lung cancer has the highest mortality (see Table 12). If all cancers were diagnosed at a localized stage, 5-year survival could reach 95%.

Table 12. Estimated new cancer cases and deaths in women in 2007

Site	United States		Canada	
	Estimated new cases	Estimated deaths	Estimated new cases	Estimated deaths
Lung and bronchus	98,620	70,880	10,900	8,900
Breast	178,480	40,460	22,300	5,300
Genital system:	78,290	28,020	7,850	2,830
Ovary	22,430	15,280	2,400	1,700
Endometrium	39,080	7,400	4,100	740
Uterine cervix	11,150	3,670	1,350	390
Vulva	3,490	880	NA	NA
Vagina	2,140	790	NA	NA
Colorectal:	74,630	26,180	9,400	4,000
Colon	57,050	26,180	NA	NA
Rectum	17,580	NA	NA	NA
Urinary bladder	17,120	4,120	1,700	520
Melanoma-Skin	26,030	2,890	2,100	340
Thyroid	25,480	880	2,900	110
Pancreas	18,340	16,530	1,850	1,850

NA, not available

Sources: American Cancer Society 2007; Canadian Cancer Society 2007.

Overall, African Americans are more likely to develop cancer than any other US racial or ethnic group. African Americans have the highest incidence of colon and rectal cancer, as well as lung and bronchial cancer, followed by Caucasians, Asian/Pacific Islanders, Hispanic Americans, and American Indians.

The Canadian Cancer Society publishes information about cancer incidence and mortality according to age, gender, and geographic location but not according to race/ethnicity. During their lifetimes, 39% of Canadian women will develop cancer, and cancer incidence is rising in women up to age 39, but deaths from cancer are declining for Canadian women under age 70. Generally, both cancer incidence and mortality rates are higher in eastern provinces and lower in western provinces.

This section provides overviews of the common cancers affecting women.

Breast cancer. For many women, breast cancer is their primary health concern.

Incidence. Breast cancer is the second major cause of cancer mortality in US and Canadian women. A woman's lifetime risk of developing breast cancer is approximately 1 in 8, and the risk increases with age; it is not specifically affected by menopause. Nearly one half of all breast cancer cases occur in women aged 65 years and older.

In the United States, less than 10% of cases occur in women under age 40 and approximately 15% occur in women under age 50. Current estimates are that by age 50, 2% of US women will have developed breast cancer. By age 60, between 4% and 5% will have the disease; by age 70, approximately 7%; and by age 80, between 9% and 10%. Contralateral breast cancer in women with a personal history of breast cancer is estimated to occur at a rate of 0.5% to 1% per year after the initial diagnosis.

Among racial/cultural groups in the United States, white non-Hispanic women have the highest incidence of breast cancer, although African-American women have the highest mortality from the disease, possibly related to later stages of diagnosis, more estrogen-receptor (ER) negative tumors, and more aggressive tumors. The 5-year survival rate for African Americans is 71% versus 86% for Caucasians.

Although the incidence of breast cancer has increased in recent years, mortality rates have decreased, perhaps due to earlier intervention. Smaller, less-advanced tumors that would have been missed without mammography can now be detected. According to US statistics, if breast cancer is detected while it is still localized, the 5-year survival rate is 95%, up from 72% in the 1940s. For regional metastases, however, the rate is 81%. For distant metastases, the rate is 26%. Survival at 10 years is also stage-dependent.

In Canada, the 5-year survival rate is 86%. After three decades of small annual increases, breast cancer incidence in women has leveled off since 1993 and the mortality rate has declined to the lowest it has been since 1950. These trends are attributed to screening programs and improved treatments.

Risk factors. Medical research has identified several potential cancer-causing genes, including *BRCA1* (linked to breast and ovarian cancers) and *BRCA2* (associated with breast cancer and postmenopausal ovarian cancer). Although the genes have been identified, more research is needed to identify which women to test, how to protect from gene discrimination, and what to do if the test results are positive.

Several potential risk factors for breast cancer have been identified (see Table 13). Data regarding the importance of a positive family history as a risk factor for breast cancer are not conclusive. However, most breast cancers occur in women without a positive family history.

Table 13. Potential risk factors for breast cancer

- Personal history of breast, endometrial, ovarian, or (possibly) colon carcinoma
- History of breast cancer in a mother, sister, or daughter, especially while premenopausal
- History of breast cancer in a father
- Menarche before age 12
- Late menopause (after age 55)
- Nulliparity or having the first child after age 30
- Obesity after menopause (≥20 kg [44 lb] weight gain)
- Alcohol consumption (>2 drinks/d)
- Lack of exercise (<4 hr/wk)
- Low levels of vitamin D
- Diet low in vegetables and fruits
- Exposure to intense radiation
- Long-term use (>5 y) of estrogen plus progestogen therapy

The National Cancer Institute has developed a breast cancer risk assessment tool, based on the Gail model. It assesses the 5-year risk based on five primary factors: a woman's age, age at first live birth, age at menarche, previous breast biopsy results, and personal or family (first-degree relatives) history of cancer.

Benign breast masses (eg, fibroadenomas, cysts) become much less common after menopause among women not using hormones. Any new growth observed after menopause is suggestive of breast cancer, and biopsy should be considered.

Role of hormone therapy. Menopausal HT may stimulate the growth of benign breast masses. Some recent studies report a greater increase in breast cancer risk with combined EPT than ET alone. Some data link greater occurrence of lobular breast cancers with progestogen use.

When making decisions regarding HT, it is important to note that some epidemiologic data suggest an association between the timing of menopause and breast cancer risk. The data have shown that early menopause is associated with decreased risk and delayed menopause is associated with an increased risk.

Recent large trials have provided conflicting data regarding the association between HT and breast cancer risk:

- *Women's Health Initiative (WHI)*. Data from the WHI found that oral daily EPT (CE plus MPA) increased the relative risk of invasive breast cancer by 26%, although this increase was not statistically significant (95% confidence interval [CI], 1.00-1.59). In absolute risk, EPT users had an additional eight cases of breast cancer per 10,000 person-years versus placebo. The EPT arm of the trial was discontinued prematurely after 5.2 years of a planned 8-year study, primarily because of the breast cancer findings. The increased risk began during year 3; EPT-treated patients had a lower risk during years 1 and 2. In April 2006, the WHI released findings that women (with prior hysterectomy) in the unopposed ET arm of the trial had no significant change in breast cancer risk after an average follow-up of 6.8 years.

- *Million Women Study (MWS)*. A large cohort study in Europe, the MWS confirmed the findings from the WHI EPT-arm of an increased risk for current EPT users. Although the ET-alone users in this study had significantly increased breast cancer risk, this risk was substantially less than with EPT. Breast cancer risk increased as duration of use increased. Past use did not increase the risk of incidence or mortality, and risk decreased with time since last use. Little variation was found between specific types of estrogen and progestogen, doses, their routes of administration, or whether the regimen was continuous or sequential. With estrogen only, increased risk was seen with oral, transdermal, and implant formulations, although vaginal estrogen did not increase the risk of breast cancer. Because this was an observational study, it has potential for error, but it does serve to confirm the WHI findings of a small increase in absolute risk of breast cancer with EPT.

Other recent observational studies from the United States and Sweden have found an increased risk with EPT but not ET. Data from the National Cancer Institute's Breast Cancer Detection Demonstration Project (BCDDP), a re-analysis of published data from 51 observational studies, as well as the NHS (published in abstract form only), found a positive association between HT use and increased breast cancer risk, especially in women using hormones for 5 to 15 years. Short-term or past users were not at significantly increased risk. The increased risk associated with hormone use disappeared within 5 years of its discontinuation.

A woman's BMI also may be a factor associated with breast cancer risk. The reports suggest an increased risk associated with use of ET alone in long-term users who had lean body mass. This effect, however, may be no greater than the effect associated with increased estrogen production in overweight women. One case-control study from Sweden found a significantly increased risk of breast cancer associated with 10 or more years of current HT use in women who were not overweight.

Most of the studies that have examined the breast cancer mortality rates in HT users have documented improved survival rates. Even those studies that found an increased risk of breast cancer in hormone users have reported better outcomes, perhaps because of earlier diagnosis. In the BCDDP reanalysis of the published data, the excess risk of breast cancer was confined to localized disease among current or recent users of HT. There is also evidence to suggest that HT users develop smaller, lower-grade tumors. However, these earlier findings are contraindicted by the findings of the WHI of slightly larger tumors with 10% more positive nodes in EPT users compared with placebo users.

In most studies that examined the relationship between HT and breast cancer, little attention was paid to the histologic type of breast cancer. In a recent case-control study of women aged 50 to 64 years, combined EPT use for at least 6 months was found to increase the risk of lobular, but not ductal, breast cancer. Lobular tumors represent 5% to 10% of all breast cancer cases; ductal tumors account for 80% to 85%. Lobular tumors are more difficult to palpate and are more likely to be missed by mammographic screening, but women with lobular cancer have a better prognosis than women with ductal cancer. The investigators concluded that, regarding absolute risk, even if combined EPT use is associated with an increased risk of lobular breast cancer, only a small percentage of EPT users are likely to be affected.

According to the NAMS 2007 position statement on HT, breast cancer risk is increased with use of EPT beyond 5 years (Table 14). In the WHI report, 4 to 6 additional invasive cancers per 10,000 person-years occurred in the group receiving EPT. There was no increase in breast cancer in the women in the ET arm of the WHI study after an average of 7.1 years of use. There are limited observational studies suggesting that using ET for more than 15 years may increase the risk of breast cancer. The effects of HT on risk for breast cancer in symptomatic *perimenopausal* women have not been established in RCTs.

Most women initiate HT for relief of vasomotor symptoms. They usually experience prompt symptom relief and can taper off HT long before the breast cancer risk increases. Evaluating whether to continue HT over the long term is more complicated. Use of ET or EPT should be consistent with treatment goals, benefits, and risks for the individual woman, taking into account cause of menopause, time since menopause, symptoms, and domains (eg, sexuality and sleep) that may have an impact on quality of life and the underlying risk of CVD, stroke, VTE, DM, and other conditions. It is especially important that each woman weigh known and probable risks and benefits. (See Section G.)

Table 14. NAMS position on breast cancer risk associated with menopausal hormone therapy

- Breast cancer risk is increased with EPT use beyond 5 years. Progestogen seems to contribute substantially to that adverse effect. EPT and, to a lesser extent, ET increase breast cell proliferation, breast pain, and mammographic density.

- EPT may impede the diagnostic interpretation of mammograms.

- The effects of HT on risk for breast cancer (and osteoporotic fracture) in symptomatic perimenopausal women have not been established in RCTs. The findings from trials in different populations (eg, WHI) should, therefore, be extrapolated with caution. There is, however, no evidence that symptomatic women differ from asymptomatic women in cancer (or bone) outcomes.

Source: NAMS *Menopause* 2007.

Lower-than-standard doses of ET and EPT should be considered (ie, daily doses of 0.3 mg oral CE, 0.25-0.5 mg oral micronized 17β-estradiol, 0.025 mg transdermal 17β-estradiol patch, or the equivalent). Many studies have demonstrated nearly equivalent vasomotor and vulvovaginal symptom relief. However, some women may require additional local therapy for persistent vaginal symptoms. Lower ET and EPT doses are better tolerated and may have a better risk-benefit ratio than standard doses. However, lower doses have not been tested in long-term trials. For younger perimenopausal women or women reaching menopause prematurely, the risks are likely to be lower.

All women should have a breast examination and mammogram before beginning HT (if they have not had one in the past 12 months) and at regular intervals thereafter.

Role of tibolone. Tibolone is a synthetic steroid prescribed as oral tablets in many countries (though not available in North America) for the treatment of vasomotor symptoms and the prevention of osteoporosis in postmenopausal women. Tibolone is inactive but is metabolically converted into three major metabolites, two of which are estrogens and one which is a progestogen with androgenic activity. Clinical studies have shown only minor changes in breast density during tibolone treatment. However, an excess of breast cancer was identified in women who used tibolone and participated in the MWS. The safety of tibolone in relation to breast cancer needs to be established through large-scale RCTs.

Women with a history of breast cancer. The number of women surviving breast cancer has increased as a result of earlier detection due to widespread application of mammographic screening and the efficacy of adjuvant systemic therapies. For women in remission, breast cancer recurrence is a possibility.

Premenopausal women receiving chemotherapy or radiation therapy have an increased risk of induced menopause (see Section D).

During peri- or postmenopause, if breast cancer survivors need relief from menopause-related symptoms, primarily vasomotor and vaginal atrophy symptoms, therapeutic choices must be weighed for their potential to cause breast cancer recurrence.

- *Systemic HT use in women with a history of breast cancer.* Breast cancer survivors and/or their healthcare providers generally do not choose systemic HT. The rationale is that avoiding hormones will reduce the risk of recurrence and of new contralateral tumors. Also, systemic HT increases mammographic density and could potentially decrease surveillance effectiveness for new breast cancer (although stopping HT for at least 2 weeks before a mammogram can resolve most of the breast density concerns). However, some breast cancer survivors may experience debilitating menopause-related symptoms, such as hot flashes and night sweats, which require the symptom relief that HT offers.

A number of studies, mostly uncontrolled, have evaluated the effects of HT in women with a history of breast cancer. Most, but not all, have enrolled women 10 or more years after the initial breast cancer diagnosis. The weight of evidence indicates that initiating HT at this point has no deleterious effects on tumor recurrence. No RCTs have demonstrated that HT increases the relapse rate. One randomized, open-label trial of HT in 424 breast cancer survivors (mean age, 55 y) was stopped prematurely after 2 years due to an increased rate of breast cancer.

A history of (or a high-risk profile for) breast cancer is not generally considered to be an absolute contraindication for HT use. In certain situations, the therapeutic benefits of HT may outweigh its risks. The decision must be made with the woman's full awareness that therapy may promote more rapid tumor growth, although observational studies have failed to show untoward effects of HT even in ER-positive breast cancer patients. However, caution is recommended in all cases, since there are no specific data from clinical trials regarding particular stages or histologic types of the disease to provide guidance regarding women at highest risk. Alternatives should be tried first.

- *Cognitive dysfunction.* Women who reach menopause as a result of adjuvant therapy for breast cancer often report complaints of difficulty with thinking and memory. These complaints could be the result of a direct neurotoxic effect of chemotherapy. Additional studies are needed to further define these effects. Similarly, little is known about the potential effects of tamoxifen on cognitive decline with aging.

- *Weight gain.* After breast cancer, menopause seems to be a significant factor in the development of weight gain, precipitated by adjuvant chemotherapy, decreased exercise during treatment, and/or to increased food intake related to depression. Obesity is an important health concern for postmenopausal breast cancer survivors (as it is for all postmenopausal women) because it increases the risk for CVD and DM. In some studies, weight gain has been associated with an increased risk of breast cancer recurrence, possibly due to higher levels of endogenous estrogen. Weight gain also affects body image and self-esteem, and it may be more of an issue for women than changes in the breast or mastectomy.

Women with benign breast disease. Women with premalignant breast disease are at increased risk for breast cancer. Compared with women with nonproliferative benign histology, those with proliferative, nonmalignant breast disease have an increased risk for developing breast cancer (relative risk, 3.6 and 1.8, respectively, with and without atypical hyperplasia). HT use has not been found to affect these risks. Women at risk for breast cancer because of family history can be referred for evaluation of genetic testing for *BRCA1* and *BRCA2*. Ductal lavage is sometimes performed as a diagnostic modality for high-risk women.

Screening. Monthly self-examination should be encouraged, as most breast cancers are detected by women themselves, although RCTs do not support this screening method. Mammography recommendations for peri- and postmenopausal women are presented in Table 15.

A clinical breast examination should be performed annually (close to the scheduled mammogram). The best time for a breast examination or mammogram is immediately after menses or EPT-induced uterine bleeding. From a practical perspective, however, most clinicians do not order mammography on a timed basis.

The following physical signs and symptoms should be investigated by mammography:

- Breast lump, thickening, swelling, distortion, or tenderness
- Skin irritation or dimpling
- Nipple pain, scaliness, or retraction

Mammography is a screening tool and does not provide an accurate diagnosis. The false-negative rate for screening mammography is approximately 10% to 15%.

Table 15. Recommendations for mammograms in peri- and postmenopausal women

- *The American Cancer Society:* Annual mammograms beginning at age 40, in the absence of unusual findings.
- *The Canadian Cancer Society:* Mammogram every 2 years between the ages 50 and 69, with more frequent mammograms or more detailed testing when abnormalities are found.
- *The National Cancer Institute:* Mammograms every 1 or 2 years between ages 40 and 50, then annually thereafter.
- *The North American Menopause Society:* Annual mammograms beginning at age 40 (in the absence of unusual findings) and before initiating HT.
- *The US Preventive Services Task Force:* Screening mammography, with or without clinical breast examination, every 1 to 2 years for women age 40 and older.

Mammography sensitivity depends on a number of factors, including the size of the lesion, the woman's age, current use of any HT, and the extent of follow-up. In the 5-year BCDDP, the estimated sensitivity of the combined clinical examination and mammography was 75%; mammography alone was 71%. The specificity was 94% to 99%.

The appearance of breast tissue on a mammogram changes according to its composition. Fat is radiolucent and appears dark on a mammogram, while stromal and epithelial tissues have greater optical density and appear light.

Several studies confirm that mammographic density is a strong predictor of breast cancer risk. In a review of studies looking at more than 2,200 Canadian women, those with denser breasts were three to five times more likely to be diagnosed with breast cancer during the study period.

Factors that are associated with a reduction in breast density include increasing age, menopause, an elevated BMI, pregnancy at an early age, and tamoxifen treatment. Factors associated with an increase in breast density include an increased age at first birth and postmenopausal use of ET or EPT. Women with breast implants and those older than age 40 with fibrocystic changes have denser breasts, but they are not necessarily at greater risk for breast cancer.

The mammographic appearance of the breasts becomes increasingly radiolucent after menopause, in response to decreased estrogen and progesterone levels. For example, 76% of women aged 75 to 79 years and not using HT have radiolucent breasts, compared with 38% of women aged 25 to 29 years.

Use of HT increases breast density. Sensitivity of mammography may be reduced by 15% in women using HT. Former HT users have the same mammographic sensitivity as never users. Because of this hormonal effect, some clinicians discontinue HT for 2 weeks before a mammogram to allow breast density to decrease.

In the PEPI trial, almost all increases in breast density occurred within the first year of HT. In other trials, women who use estrogen plus progestin, especially continuous-combined EPT, have shown the greatest increase in breast density. ET and cyclic EPT have not produced as much of an effect. HT use may also contribute to more homogeneous breast tissue, which may result in breast enlargement.

Ultrasound is being used more frequently to evaluate developing focal asymmetric densities and any palpable masses of the breast. New methods for detection include digital mammography, which is similar to regular mammography except that images are digitized and can be stored on film. This may improve the sensitivity of mammography in women with dense breasts, although clinical trials are needed to confirm this. Ductal lavage is a recently approved minimally invasive technique in which a small flexible catheter is inserted into a periareolar duct to collect cells for examination. Prospective randomized trials from Europe support the use of magnetic resonance imaging (MRI) in the routine evaluation of women of reproductive age who have an inherited susceptibility to breast cancer.

The American Cancer Society (ACS) has issued new guidelines for women at increased risk for breast cancer that employ MRI as an adjunct to mammography. MRI is more sensitive in identifying mammographically occult disease in this targeted population, identified as women who meet at least one of the following conditions:

- Have a *BRCA1* or *BRCA2* mutation
- Have a first-degree relative (parent, sibling, child) with a *BRCA1* or *BRCA2* mutation, even if they have yet to be tested themselves
- Their lifetime risk of breast cancer has been scored at 20%-25% or greater, based on one of several accepted risk assessment tools that look at family history and other factors
- Had radiation to the chest between the ages of 10 and 30
- Have Li-Fraumeni syndrome, Cowden syndrome, or Bannayan-Riley-Ruvalcaba syndrome, or may have one of these syndromes based on a history in a first-degree relative

However, it must be noted that all studies to date have reported that the specificity for MRI in detecting breast cancer is significantly lower than that of mammography. This may be acceptable to women at very high risk for breast cancer, such as women with an inherited pre-disposition to develop breast cancer. MRI screening for women at low risk for breast cancer is inappropriate as the technique will lead to an excessive number of recalls and biopsies for benign disease.

Lifestyle modification. All women should be assisted in modifying unhealthy lifestyle habits, with some having a significant effect on breast cancer risk.

- *Recreational physical activity* and risk of postmenopausal breast cancer was evaluated in the Iowa Women's Health Study, a prospective cohort of 41,836 postmenopausal women followed for 18 years. Compared with low physical activity, high physical activity was associated with a significant (14%) reduction in breast cancer, and a significant reduction in ER-positive/PR-negative breast cancer, a clinically more aggressive tumor phenotype. This study gave similar risk reductions for breast cancer compared with that reported by the WHI—a 14% reduction in breast cancer among 74,171 women engaged in regular strenuous physical activity at age 35 and an 8% reduction for women engaged in regular physical activity at age 50. Physical activity seems to reduce the risk of breast cancer, but more research is needed to determine the level of activity necessary. A lifetime of physical activity may be the key.

- *Diet* also affects breast cancer risk. Consumption of well-done meats and exposure to heterocyclic amines (or other compounds) formed during high-temperature cooking may increase breast cancer risk. The evidence linking dietary fat intake to breast cancer risk has been conflicting. The Women's Intervention Nutrition Study evaluated the effects of a low-fat diet on recurrence rates of 2,400 women with early stage, resected breast cancer. Participants were prospectively randomized to continue with a normal diet (control group) or a diet in which 20% or fewer calories were from fat. Relapse-free and overall survivals were significantly improved in women on a low-fat diet compared with controls. Interestingly, no improvement in survival was seen in ER-positive breast cancer patients on the low-fat diet. The benefits accrued to patients whose cancers were estrogen- and progestin-receptor negative. Nevertheless, even after a diagnosis of breast cancer, it is important to use dietary discretion and follow a low-fat diet.

Alcohol consumption has been associated with breast cancer in many studies, including a 2006 meta-analysis by Key et al, although there is some evidence that excess risk from alcohol consumption may be reduced by adequate folate intake. The role of phytoestrogens on breast cancer risk is being explored, but with mixed results. Tomatoes and tomato-based products contain lycopenes that may play a protective role in breast and cervical cancer.

Levels of 25-hydroxyvitamin D below 20 ng/mL (74.88 nmol/L) are associated with a 30% to 50% increased risk of incident colon, prostate, and breast cancer, along with higher mortality from these cancers, according to both prospective and retrospective epidemiologic studies. For instance, pooled data for 980 women showed that the highest vitamin D intake, as compared with the lowest, correlated with a 50% lower risk of breast cancer. And, participants in the WHI who at baseline had a 25-hydroxyvitamin D concentration of less than 12 ng/mL (30 nmol/L) had a 253% increase in the risk of colorectal cancer over a follow-up period of 8 years.

- *Weight management* is also important. One report found that avoiding adult weight gain may contribute to the prevention of breast cancer after menopause, particularly among women who do not use HT. A positive association between adiposity and breast cancer risk has been documented.

Pharmacologic interventions. Various prescription options are available.

- *Prevention.* Selective estrogen-receptor modulators (SERMs) have now moved into the clinical realm for the primary prevention of breast cancer. (Note that the FDA now disallows the term "selective estrogen-receptor modulator" [SERM], preferring "estrogen agonist/antagonist.")

Tamoxifen, the first clinically significant SERM, was noted in the 1960s to prevent the initiation and promotion of rat mammary carcinogenesis. It was subsequently shown to decrease the incidence of contralateral breast cancer in postmenopausal women with ER-positive breast cancers. However, tamoxifen stimulated the growth of endometrial cancer.

The National Surgical Adjuvant Breast and Bowel Project (NSABP) P-1 trial, a prospective, randomized, placebo-controlled trial, demonstrated that tamoxifen (20 mg/d) reduced the risk of breast cancer by 50% in women at high risk for breast cancer based on a Gail model score of 1.6 or higher. Additionally, hyperplasia of the breast was reduced by 80% and ductal carcinoma in situ by 50%. However, tamoxifen was associated with a 2.5-fold increased risk of endometrial cancer and a significant increase in DVT and pulmonary emboli (PE).

Two recent European trials support the long-term chemopreventive effect of tamoxifen on breast cancer reduction once it is discontinued. The first International Breast Cancer Intervention Study randomized 7,145 women aged 35 to 70 years at an increased risk for breast cancer to receive tamoxifen (20 mg/d) or placebo for 5 years. Significantly fewer breast cancers (n = 42) were identified in the tamoxifen group compared with the placebo (n = 195) group. No diminution of the tamoxifen effect was observed for up to 10 years after randomization. Tamoxifen significantly reduced the number of ER-positive breast cancers compared with placebo (87 vs 132 cases) but had no impact on the incidence of ER-negative cancers (35 in each arm). DVT/PE were significantly more likely to occur in the tamoxifen arm of this trial (52 vs 23 cases).

The Royal Marsden Trial randomized 2,494 healthy women aged 30 to 70 years to tamoxifen (20 mg/d) or placebo for 8 years. At a 20-year follow-up, a significant reduction in breast cancer was identified in the tamoxifen treated group (n = 82) compared with the placebo group (n = 104). A statistically significant reduction in ER-positive breast cancer (23 vs 47 cases) was seen in the posttreatment period, supporting the value of tamoxifen in the long-term prevention of estrogen-dependent breast cancer.

Tamoxifen (marketed as Nolvadex oral tablets) was FDA approved in 1978 for reduction of breast cancer incidence in high-risk women and, in 2000, for reduction of risk of invasive cancer in ductal carcinoma. In 2002, labeling was revised to include a black box warning for uterine malignancies, stroke, and pulmonary embolism. Use of the drug has been limited, as reports indicate that many high-risk women have not been willing to accept the side effects of therapy. Generic tamoxifen, not Nolvadex, is now available in the United States and Canada.

Raloxifene, another clinically effective SERM (marketed as Evista oral tablets), is approved in the United States and Canada for the prevention and treatment of osteoporosis (for more about osteoporosis, see page 113). The MORE trial and its extension through 8 years, the Continuing Outcomes Relative to Evista (CORE) trial, found that raloxifene significantly reduces the incidence of postmenopausal breast cancer compared with placebo in osteoporotic women (1.4 vs 4.2 cancers/1,000 person-years of treatment).

The results of the NSABP Study of Tamoxifen STAR P-2 trial revealed that raloxifene is equivalent to tamoxifen in reducing the incidence of invasive breast cancer in postmenopausal women at high risk for the disease. However, at 2 years of treatment, raloxifene failed to completely control the development of noninvasive breast cancer (2.1 vs 1.5/1,000 person-years of treatment) compared with tamoxifen. Raloxifene significantly reduced the incidence of endometrial cancer, endometrial hyperplasia, hysterectomies, cataracts, cataract surgery, and DVT/PE, compared with tamoxifen. It should be noted that there was no placebo control arm in the STAR trial.

Raloxifene also significantly reduced the incidence of breast cancer in the RUTH trial, a prospective randomized, placebo-controlled trial in which 5,044 patients received raloxifene (60 mg/d), and 5,075 patients received placebo. The incidence of breast cancer was 2.7/1,000 person-years of placebo versus 1.5/1,000 person-years of raloxifene, a 44% reduction in breast cancer. In the RUTH trial, raloxifene had no impact on coronary events (death, MI, hospitalization for acute coronary syndrome), but it was associated with an increase in deaths from cerebral vascular accidents (59 deaths for raloxifene vs 39 for the control group).

In mid-2007, raloxifene was approved by the FDA to reduce invasive breast cancer risk in postmenopausal women with osteoporosis and in postmenopausal women at high risk for breast cancer. It does not treat existing breast cancer, reduce the risk of recurrent breast cancer, or reduce the risk of all forms of breast cancer.

A black box warning in the raloxifene labeling emphasizes that the drug is contraindicated in women with an active or past history of VTE and that women at risk for stroke should use raloxifene only after evaluating the risk-benefit ratio. This drug should not be prescribed to women experiencing periods of prolonged immobilization or to those with a history of clotting disorders.

The most commonly reported side effects are hot flashes, leg cramps, peripheral edema, athralgia, flu syndrome, and sweating.

Aromatase inhibitors are now being evaluated as chemopreventive agents for women at high risk for breast cancer. These agents (anastrozole, letrozole, exemestane) lower the amount of estrogen produced outside the ovaries by inhibiting the enzyme aromatase from turning androgen intro estrogen. With less estrogen in the bloodstream and reaching estrogen receptors, there is less cancer cell growth. Aromatase inhibitors have been shown to be superior to tamoxifen in clinical trials for reducing contralateral breast cancer in postmenopausal women with ER-positive breast cancer. However, patients treated with aromatase inhibitors are more likely to develop osteoporosis, bone fractures, arthralgia, low-grade hypercholesterolemia, and cardiovascular events other than ischemia and cardiac failure. Zoledronic acid (4 mg) intravenously every 6 months has been shown to be effective in preventing osteoporosis when initiated with an aromatase inhibitor in premenopausal and postmenopausal breast cancer patients.

In selecting a therapy for the primary prevention of breast cancer, it is important to note that raloxifene is not approved for use in premenopausal women and aromatase inhibitors are not effective in premenopausal women with an intact hypothalamic-pituitary-ovarian axis. Raloxifene would be the choice therapy for postmenopausal women with or without osteoporosis. Tamoxifen would be the choice therapy for premenopausal women at very high risk for breast cancer, including those with atypical ductal hyperplasia and lobular carcinoma in situ.

For women with *BRCA1* and *BRCA2* gene mutations, risk-reduction bilateral salpingo-oophorectomy (ie, the prophylactic removal of both ovaries and fallopian tubes) has been associated with a significant reduction (up to 53%) in their risk for breast cancer.

- *Treatment.* Because many breast cancer risk factors are nonmodifiable and some risks are unknown, early detection is the best strategy. Treatment of breast cancer is outside the scope of this textbook.

Endometrial cancer. Endometrial cancer affects cells that line the inside of the uterus (the endometrium). Endometrial cancer may sometimes be referred to as "uterine cancer." However, different cancers may develop from other tissues of the uterus, including cervical cancer, sarcoma of the myometrium, and trophoblastic disease.

There are many microscopic subtypes of endometrial cancer, including the common *endometrioid* type, in which the cancer cells grow in patterns reminiscent of normal endometrium, and the far more aggressive *papillary serous* and *clear cell* endometrial cancers. All forms of endometrial cancer almost always present with abnormal uterine bleeding or spotting. Some authorities have proposed that endometrial cancers be classified into two pathogenetic groups:

- *Type 1.* These cancers occur in pre- and perimenopausal women, often with a history of unopposed estrogen exposure and/or endometrial hyperplasia. They are often minimally invasive into the underlying uterine wall, are of the *low-grade endometrioid* type, and carry a good prognosis. They represent approximately 90% of all endometrial cancers.

- *Type 2.* These cancers occur in older, postmenopausal women, are more common in African Americans than Caucasians, and are not associated with increased exposure to estrogen. They are typically of the *high-grade endometrioid*, *papillary serous*, or *clear cell* types, and carry a generally poor prognosis. They represent approximately 10% of endometrial cancers and represent approximately 50% of all endometrial cancer relapses.

Incidence. Fewer than 3 in 100 US women who live to age 50 will develop cancer of the endometrium in their remaining lifetime, and far fewer will die from the disease. Endometrial cancer is the sixth leading cause of cancer death in US and Canadian women. Approximately 25% of uterine cancers occur in premenopausal women.

The 1-year relative survival rate for type 1 endometrial cancer is 93%. The high survival rate is related to the finding of the cancer being confined to the uterus in approximately 75% of cases. The 5-year relative survival rate is 95%, if diagnosed at an early stage, but 64% if diagnosed at a regional metastasized stage. At every stage, relative survival rates for Caucasians exceed those for African Americans by at least 18%. Recent data suggest that African Americans are more likely to have type 2 endometrial cancers.

Risk factors. A woman's lifetime risk of developing endometrial cancer is small and unrelated to menopause. Various risk factors for endometrial cancer have been identified (see Table 16). These factors are most often associated with hyperestrogenism.

Table 16. Risk factors for developing endometrial cancer
• >50 years of age
• Family history
• Obesity
• Diet high in fat
• Diabetes mellitus
• Hypertension
• Hereditary colon cancer
• Endometrial hyperplasia
• Early menarche
• Late menopause
• Nulliparity
• History of anovulation
• Use of unopposed estrogen
• Use of tamoxifen, tibolone (?)

Role of hormone therapy. For the postmenopausal woman, use of unopposed systemic ET is associated with increased risk related to the dose and duration of the ET. Unopposed ET, when used for more than 3 years, is associated with a fivefold increased risk of endometrial cancer; if used for 10 years, the risk increases tenfold. This increased risk persists for several years after discontinuation of estrogen. Because abnormal uterine bleeding usually bring the disease to medical attention early in its course, most cases do not reduce life expectancy.

Role of tamoxifen and tibolone. Two other prescription therapies commonly used by postmenopausal women are associated with an increased risk of endometrial cancer.

• *Tamoxifen* is a common therapy for breast cancer (see page 145 for more). It is now well established that women who have completed tamoxifen therapy for breast cancer are at a subsequent increased risk for developing endometrial cancer (particularly type 2). Although adding progestogen to ET reduces the risk of endometrial cancer, the effect of adding progestogen to tamoxifen is undetermined. ACOG recommends that women using tamoxifen be educated about its effects on the endometrium and be monitored closely. Tamoxifen use should be limited to 5 years. ACOG further advises that tamoxifen use may be considered after hysterectomy for endometrial cancer, provided that the woman makes an informed decision. Aromatase inhibitors and raloxifene do not increase the risk of endometrial cancer.

• *Tibolone*, a synthetic steroid that, when metabolized, has estrogenic, progestogenic and androgenic activity, has been used for the control of vasomotor symptoms and the prevention of osteoporosis in postmenopausal women (see page 113 for more about osteoporosis). This compound was not thought to stimulate endometrial growth. However, the Million Women Study (an observational study) reported an unexpected increase in the incidence of endometrial cancer in women who had

taken tibolone. In contrast, a prospective randomized trial involving 3,240 women, the Tibolone Histology of the Endometrium and Breast Endpoints Study (THEBES), demonstrated that tibolone did not induce endometrial hyperplasia or carcinoma. Tibolone is not currently available in North America.

Women with a history of endometrial cancer. HT has traditionally been withheld from women with a history of endometrial cancer, based on the belief that HT might increase the risk of recurrence. Despite epidemiologic studies linking prolonged use of unopposed ET with the development of endometrial cancer, two recent retrospective studies in women who received HT after their treatment for endometrial cancer did not seem to show an excessive increased risk for recurrence.

In 2006, the Gynecologic Oncology Group (GOG) published the results of a prospective, double-blind, randomized trial by Barakat et al that tested the hypothesis that ET had a deleterious effect on the risks of recurrence in endometrial cancer patients. Participants were all stage I and II endometrial cancer patients within 20 weeks of completing initial cancer treatment. Estrogen was to be given for 3 years. The study was closed prematurely because of the publication of the WHI data revealing that the risks of EPT exceeded the benefits. The study accrued 1,236 of the planned 2,108 patients. Of those participating, 87.2% had stage IA (37.7%) or stage IB (49.5%) disease. Only 7.3% had histologic grade 3 lesions. In the ET group, 14 patients (2.3%) experienced disease recurrence, compared with 12 patients (1.9%) in the placebo group. Only one (0.2%) patient developed breast cancer, compared with three patients (0.5%) in the placebo group. Three patients in the ET group died of MIs or coronary artery disease, compared with four patients in the placebo group. The progression-free survival for the entire group at 3 years was 94.8%. All patients participating in the study were required to have an indication for treatment with EPT, including hot flashes, vaginal atrophy, increased risk for CVD, or an increased risk for osteoporosis. This incomplete study was not able to refute or support the safety of exogenous estrogen for symptomatic women recently treated for endometrial cancer. Nevertheless, the low recurrence rate (2.1%) in women receiving ET is noteworthy.

ACOG has advised that, in the absence of well-designed studies, the decision to recommend HT for women after endometrial cancer should be based on prognostic indicators, including depth of invasion, degree of differentiation, and cell type. The Society of Obstetricians and Gynaecologists of Canada (SOGC) similarly advises that HT may be recommended to women who have been treated for endometrial cancer and who fall in a low-risk group (eg, with stage I disease, grade 1 or 2 histology, and less than 50% depth of myometrial invasion). Careful counseling regarding perceived benefits and risks should be conducted to assist each woman in making an informed decision. The need for adding progestogen therapy is undetermined, although progestogen supplementation has not been found to affect the recurrence rate.

Screening. Endometrial cancer screening parameters for women using HT are found in Table 17.

Table 17. NAMS screening parameters for endometrial cancer for women using ET and EPT

- Women using continuous-sequential EPT (estrogen every day plus cycled progestogen) should undergo a baseline pelvic examination. Endometrial evaluation should be considered if uterine bleeding occurs at any time other than the expected time of withdrawal uterine bleeding, or when heavier or more prolonged withdrawal uterine bleeding occurs.

- Women using continuous-combined EPT (estrogen and progestogen every day) should undergo a baseline pelvic examination. Endometrial evaluation must be considered when irregular uterine bleeding persists more than 6 months after beginning therapy. Early evaluation can be considered based on individual circumstances.

- Women with a uterus generally should not use unopposed ET. When the regimen is used despite this recommendation, women should undergo routine pelvic examinations and endometrial evaluations at baseline and annually thereafter. Endometrial evaluation should be performed after any episode of uterine bleeding; reevaluation is necessary when uterine bleeding is persistent.

The ACS and NAMS recommend that all women over age 40 should have an annual pelvic examination. Although a pelvic examination does not uncover uterine cancers, the examination is valuable for detecting other cancers, as well as other adverse health conditions.

Lifestyle modification. As with almost all medical conditions, lifestyle modification can reduce risk. Obesity is one of the most common risk factors associated with the development of type 1 endometrial cancers, histologically the most common form of the disease. A healthy diet and exercise are imperative to avoid development of these cancers. There are no etiologic factors for type 2 cancers.

Obesity is associated with a decreased life expectancy even in women who do not have cancer. In a study of early-stage endometrial cancer patients, designed to determine rates of disease recurrence and survival differences between obese (BMI 30-39.9 kg/m²), morbidly obese (BMI ≥40 kg/m²), and nonobese women, obesity was associated with a higher mortality from causes other than endometrial cancer, but not from disease recurrence. Thus, the impact of obesity on the overall survival of endometrial cancer patients is different than its impact in breast cancer. In the latter disease, obesity is associated with recurrence and

morbidity rates secondary to the cancer. A prospective study reported that the relative risk of death for morbidly obese women (BMI ≥40 kg/m²) with endometrial cancer was 6.25 compared with those of a normal weight. These studies did not evaluate weight reduction efforts to possibly improve survival.

Pharmacologic interventions. Well-studied options are available.

- *Prevention.* The simplest way for a woman to reduce her risk for developing endometrial cancer is to use combination oral contraceptives (OCs) for a prolonged period of time during her reproductive years. It is estimated that women who have used OCs have a 50% reduction in risk for developing endometrial cancer compared with those who have never used them. Longer duration of use (≥6 y in one study and ≥10 y in another) was associated with substantially greater risk reduction compared with never-users. The protective effect continues for up to 20 years after use is discontinued. Use of nonoral estrogen-progestin contraceptives may have a similar benefit.

For the postmenopausal woman using systemic ET, adding progestogen therapy to ET reduces the risk of endometrial cancer induced by ET to the level found in women not taking hormones. Data from the PEPI trial showed that women who took unopposed ET during the 3-year trial had a significantly increased risk of hyperplasia (34%) whereas those taking EPT had a risk of only 1%. Progestogen does not eliminate endometrial cancer risk completely because there is a risk independent of hormone use.

In the WHI, postmenopausal women taking oral CE, 0.625 mg/day, plus MPA, 2.5 mg/day, did not experience a significant increase in endometrial cancer (27 cases vs 31 with placebo). Compared with placebo, the hazard ratio for EPT recipients was 0.81 (95% CI, 0.48-1.36). No appreciable differences were found in the distribution of tumor histology, stage, or grade. However, significantly more women using EPT required endometrial biopsies.

The primary menopause-related indication for progestogen use is endometrial protection from unopposed ET. For all women with an intact uterus who are using ET, clinicians are advised to also prescribe adequate progestogen. With some women and some dose schedules of progestogen, the endometrial lining sheds and passes from the uterus as bleeding, similar to a menstrual period. This progestogen-induced bleeding is not associated with menstrual cramps, and ovulation does not occur.

Some women regard this progestogen-induced bleeding as an unacceptable nuisance. For many women, it is difficult to decide whether to tolerate the uterine bleeding in exchange for the EPT reductions in short-term menopausal symptoms, such as hot flashes, and lowering the risk of other diseases later in life.

With an oral progestin used in a cyclic regimen with a standard estrogen dose (eg, 0.625 mg CE, 1 mg oral estradiol, or 0.05 mg patch), the minimum effective dose for endometrial protection is 5 mg/day of MPA, or the equivalent, for 12 to 14 days each month. With oral micronized progesterone, the minimum effective dose is 200 mg/day for 12 to 14 days each month. Progestogen-containing intrauterine devices or vaginal gels offer another possibility for endometrial protection, although long-term efficacy data are lacking regarding their endometrial cancer protection. (See Section G for more about progestogen.)

The newer continuous-combined EPT dose schedules, in which a smaller amount of progestogen is taken daily along with estrogen, usually result in amenorrhea over time. However, many women (particularly those who are recently postmenopausal) have uterine spotting and bleeding during the first year or so of this regimen. With continuous-combined EPT, the minimum effective dose of oral progestogen for endometrial protection against standard doses of estrogen is 2.5 mg/day of MPA (or the equivalent) or 100 mg/day of oral micronized progesterone. The continuous-combined regimen is the most popular regimen in the United States. (See Section G for more about EPT.)

Other alternatives to reduce uterine bleeding include dosing progestogen every few months or not at all. However, ET without a progestogen is rarely advisable for a woman with an intact uterus. If either of these options is chosen, some uterine evaluation (transvaginal ultrasound or endometrial biopsy) must be performed every year to monitor for adverse changes. Uterine bleeding can also occur when ET is taken alone and may be associated with endometrial hyperplasia or carcinoma.

Women who use a cyclic progestogen regimen universally experience uterine bleeding when the progestogen is withdrawn. These women should be encouraged to report any uterine bleeding that occurs at unusual times.

- *Treatment.* The most effective management of endometrial cancer is to promptly evaluate the endometrium at the first indication of abnormal uterine spotting or bleeding. The overwhelming majority of women with endometrial cancer will present with postmenopausal spotting or bleeding. An office endometrial biopsy or an ultrasound-based approach will often identify the disease and lead to definitive treatment, which involves a complete hysterectomy, removal of the fallopian tubes and ovaries, removal of pelvic and paraaortic lymph nodes, and peritoneal cytology evaluation. Treatment of uterine cancer is extremely successful, because at least 70% of patients are diagnosed with stage I disease, which is associated with an excellent prognosis.

Cervical cancer. In North America, the mortality rate from cervical cancer has dropped sharply over the years but remains a serious concern. As screening with the Pap test has become more prevalent, preinvasive lesions are detected more frequently than invasive cancer.

Incidence. From 2000 to 2004, 15.1% of new cancer cases and more than 19% of cancer deaths from cervical cancer occurred in US women between ages 55 and 64. In Canada, figures are similar. The 1-year survival rate for cervical cancer is 89%, with a 5-year survival rate of 70%. When detected at an early stage, the 5-year survival rate improves to 91%. Survival with preinvasive lesions is nearly 100%. However, many women who develop invasive cervical cancer have never had a Pap test.

Incident rates are higher in African Americans; however, Caucasian-American women are more likely than African Americans to have cancers detected at an early stage.

Risk factors. Several risk factors for cervical cancer have been identified (see Table 18).

Table 18. Risk factors for cervical cancer
• HPV
• Sexual intercourse at an early age
• Multiple sexual partners
• Sexual partners who have had multiple partners
• HIV-positive status
• Smoking

Studies have found that virtually all cervical cancers are related to infection by the sexually transmitted, high-risk (oncogenic) types of HPV. An HPV infection is characterized by benign growths in the genital area (genital warts) for men and women, but it can be asymptomatic. A recent study of HPV infection in US women aged 15 to 59 years suggested that 24.9 million women in this age range have prevalent HPV infections. There was a statistically significant trend for increasing HPV prevalence with each year of age from 14 to 24 years, followed by a significant gradual decline in HPV prevalence through age 59. Multivariate analysis demonstrated that being a single woman younger than age 25 and having increasing numbers of recent or lifetime sex partners were factors independently associated with HPV infection.

No epidemiological studies have linked HT use with squamous cell cancers of the cervix. One small epidemiologic study demonstrated a statistically increased risk for cervical cancer among unopposed ET users. It should be noted that, in the same study, women using a progestogen had no statistically increased risk for the development of adenocarcinoma of the cervix. In the WHI, women taking EPT had no significant increase in cervical cancer versus those taking placebo; eight and five cases were reported, respectively.

Screening. A pelvic examination and Pap test are key elements of a comprehensive physical examination for women older than age 40. However, approximately one half of US women diagnosed with cervical cancer have never had a Pap test. In addition, many women stop having pelvic examinations and Pap tests when they reach menopause.

The Pap test is used primarily for diagnosis of precancerous and cancerous conditions of the cervix and vagina. Most deaths from cervical cancer could be prevented by having routine Pap tests and by adhering to safer sex practices.

The Pap test is a simple office procedure in which samples for cytologic evaluation are obtained from the cervix and endocervix. Cells obtained from the lateral vaginal wall can be evaluated for hormonal effect and microorganisms.

Pap tests are especially important in women who do the following:

- Smoke cigarettes
- Have unprotected sexual intercourse
- Have had HPV detected in their Pap test or have had genital warts
- Have HIV infection (or AIDS)

New tests and methods have been developed that increase the accuracy of the Pap test analysis. A computer-based evaluation technique is available in which a computer screens and identifies the most abnormal cells to be reviewed. Liquid-based thin-layer cytology (ThinPrep, AutoCyte Prep) Pap testing is a technique in which cells are washed into a fluid, allowing abnormal cells to be more easily detected by reducing preparation variables and decreasing ambiguous atypical cells. These techniques may improve Pap test accuracy in the detection of precancerous changes by as much as 30%. Currently, there is no "best" method. Liquid-based Pap tests also can be used to detect HPV and other viruses.

Because cervical cancer is slow growing, considerable uncertainty surrounds the issue of the optimal screening interval. An annual pelvic examination is recommended for all peri- and postmenopausal women. However, recommendations regarding annual Pap tests are inconsistent. A large study that included data from the National Breast Cancer and Cervical Cancer Early Detection Program together with modeling found little further mortality reduction from cervical cancer for screening every year, compared with screening every 3 years. The ACS recommends annual screening with the regular Pap test or every 2 years with the liquid-based Pap test. However, the guidelines indicate that another reasonable option for women over age 30 is screening every 3 years with the conventional or liquid-based Pap test, plus the HPV DNA test.

The general consensus is that women who do not have any risk factors for developing cervical cancer and who have had three consecutive normal Pap tests may be screened every 2 to 3 years with the conventional or liquid-based Pap test (although these women should continue to have an annual pelvic examination).

The ACS recommends that women age 70 or older who have had at least three consecutive normal Pap tests and no abnormal Pap test results in the last 10 years may choose to stop having cervical cancer screening.

Included among those who many need to continue screening are women with abnormal Pap test results; those with a history of cervical cancer, diethylstilbestrol (DES) exposure before birth, HIV infection, or a weakened immune system; as well as women who were young at first intercourse, have more than one sexual partner, or smoke cigarettes. Some of these women may need more frequent screening or additional testing, such as colposcopy (magnified visual examination of the cervix) and biopsy.

Women who have had a hysterectomy with removal of the cervix for benign disease rarely have important abnormalities found on Pap testing. Several studies have shown that the rate of high-grade vaginal lesions or vaginal cancer is fewer than 1 in 1,000 tests. No study has shown that screening for vaginal cancer reduces mortality from this rare condition. Women who have had a hysterectomy without removal of the cervix should continue to follow the ACS guidelines.

Lifestyle modification. The risk factors provided in Table 18 indicate that early age of first intercourse, multiple sexual partners, sexual partners who have had multiple partners, being HIV positive, and cigarette smoking are all associated with increasing a woman's chances for developing cervical cancer. Smoking cessation, changes in sexual behavior, and use of condoms may reduce these risks for cervical cancer.

Pharmacologic interventions. At least one option is available to lower cervical cancer risk.

- *Prevention.* The single most important clinical development in gynecologic oncology in recent times has been the introduction of vaccines to prevent cervical cancer. The FDA and Health Canada have approved the use of Gardasil, a quadravalent vaccine prepared from the major capsid proteins of HPV 6, 11, 16 and 18. Worldwide, approximately 70% of invasive cervical cancers are caused by HPV types 16 and 18. Additionally, about 500,000 cases of precancerous lesions (cervical intraepithelial neoplasm [CIN] grade 2 and 3) are diagnosed annually in the United States. Approximately 50% to 60% of CIN 2 and CIN 3 are attributable to HPV 16 and 18. The ACS has developed recommendations for the use of this vaccine; currently, it is not currently recommended for women over age 26. Spread of HPV can be reduced considerably through the use of condoms.

Even if a woman has been vaccinated against HPV 16 and 18, she still is at risk for cervical cancer caused by other high oncogenic risk HPV types. Pap smear screening remains important for all women, even those who have been immunized against HPV 16 and 18.

- *Treatment.* Symptoms of cervical cancer include abnormal uterine bleeding and spotting as well as abnormal vaginal discharge. These symptoms do not necessarily indicate that the cancer is at an advanced stage. Prompt medical evaluation is necessary when these symptoms occur. Treatment of cervical cancer is outside the scope of this textbook.

Ovarian cancer. Cancer of the ovaries causes more deaths than any other cancer of the reproductive system, primarily because it usually is detected in an advanced stage.

Incidence. In the United States, the 1-year and 5-year survival rates are 79% and 53%, respectively. If ovarian cancer is detected and treated early, 95% of women survive at least 5 years; however, only 25% of cases are detected at the earliest, localized stage. Ovarian cancer accounts for 4% of all malignancies among US women and is the fifth leading cause of cancer deaths among US and Canadian women.

Risk factors. In 2007, new recommendations for early symptom warnings for ovarian cancer were released by the ACS and the Gynecological Cancer Foundation. The risk for ovarian cancer increases with age, particularly in nulliparous women, and peaks during the eighth decade. Women with a family or personal history of breast or ovarian cancer, including those with *BRCA1* and *BRCA2* gene mutations, are among those at increased risk for the disease. An association has been found between the hereditary nonpolyposis colorectal cancer syndrome and endometrial and ovarian cancer. Obesity is another risk factor.

Some epidemiologic studies have reported an association between genital area talc exposure and ovarian cancer; however, this association remains controversial. The NHS provided little support for any substantial association, although the investigators reported that talc use in the genital area may modestly increase the risk of ovarian cancer. A review of the epidemiologic literature revealed that the genital application of powder containing only cornstarch is not a risk factor for ovarian cancer.

A history of pregnancy, breastfeeding, past use of OCs, or bilateral tubal ligation has been associated with lower ovarian cancer risk.

Role of hormone therapy. Published data on the role of HT and risk of ovarian cancer are conflicting. Most epidemiologic studies have shown no association or a modest increase.

There is a relatively large volume of observational trial data that points to an association between HT use and increased ovarian cancer risk. In a cohort of 44,241 postmenopausal women who participated in the Breast Cancer Detection Demonstration Project (BCDDP), use of unopposed ET, especially for more than 10 years, increased the risk for ovarian cancer. Overall, ever-use of unopposed ET was associated with a 60% greater risk of developing ovarian cancer, compared with never-use. The risk increased with duration of use; those who used ET for 10 to 19 years had an RR of 1.8 and those with 20 or more years had an RR of 3.2. Women who used combined EPT did not have a significantly increased risk of developing ovarian cancer in BCDDP.

Similar findings were reported previously. A large, prospective, epidemiologic observational study by Rodriguez et al following 211,581 postmenopausal women from 1982 to 1996 found that ever-users of HT (either ET or EPT) had a significantly increased risk for death from ovarian cancer. Duration of use also was associated with a higher risk of ovarian cancer mortality. Women who used HT for 10 or more years had a statistically increased risk for ovarian cancer mortality compared with never users. Women using HT for less than 10 years did not have an increased risk.

In this study, risk decreased with time since last HT use. Women who had not used hormones for at least 15 years did not have a significantly increased risk, whereas women who had stopped hormone use within 15 years had a significantly increased risk. This series is limited by the relatively small number of ovarian cancer deaths in women who were HT users at the time of study entry (n = 31) and those who were former users (n = 35). The impact of progestin therapy was unknown.

A European study that updated a collaborative analysis of European case-control ovarian cancer studies found a similar trend. Women who had stopped HT (either ET or EPT) within the past 10 years had an increased risk for ovarian cancer that reached statistical significance. If the time since the last hormone use was 10 years or more, there was no increased risk for ovarian cancer.

A meta-analysis of 15 case-control studies of HT use and the risk of epithelial ovarian cancer failed to demonstrate that HT had an important effect on risk of epithelial ovarian cancer.

In the WHI (the only RCT to date), postmenopausal women taking daily continuous-combined CE (0.625 mg) and MPA (2.5 mg) for an average follow-up of 5.6 years did not exhibit a statistically significant increase in ovarian cancer. There were 20 cases of invasive ovarian cancer among EPT recipients (n = 8,506) and 12 cases among those taking placebo (n = 8,102).

Role of tamoxifen. Use of tamoxifen may result in the development of benign ovarian cysts, but an increase in ovarian cancer risk has not been found.

Screening. No satisfactory screening tests are available for ovarian cancer. Ovarian cancer is a deadly disease because it lacks obvious early warning symptoms and there are few commercially available tests that allow early detection.

The most common sign of ovarian cancer is enlargement of the abdomen, caused by accumulation of fluid or a large ovarian mass. However, many women have bloating or weight gain in the abdominal area, making this sign nonspecific. In women over age 40, digestive disturbances (eg, stomach discomfort, gas, distention) that persist and cannot be explained by any other cause indicate the need for a thorough evaluation for ovarian cancer, including a carefully performed pelvic examination and ultrasound. Abnormal uterine bleeding is rarely associated with ovarian cancer.

Ovarian cancer symptoms are often subtle. A study of 1,725 US and Canadian women who had been diagnosed with ovarian cancer revealed that the overwhelming majority experienced symptoms for 3 to 6 months before the disease was identified. A second study reported that the most common symptoms associated with ovarian cancer were bloating, increased abdominal size, fatigue, urinary tract symptoms, and pelvic or abdominal pain. These symptoms were more frequent and more severe in ovarian cancer patients than in women presenting to a general health clinic. Compared with women with irritable bowel syndrome (IBS), bloating and urinary tract symptoms were more severe in ovarian cancer patients, whereas diarrhea was more severe in the IBS patients.

Based on these observations, the ACS, the Gynecologic Cancer Foundation, and the Society for Gynecolgic Oncologists recommended in 2007 that women who have the symptoms of abdominal bloating, abdominal or pelvic pain, early satiety, and/or urinary urgency or frequency that occurs almost daily for a few weeks see their healthcare provider, preferably a gynecologist, to rule out ovarian cancer. Prompt medical evaluation may lead to the early detection of ovarian cancer, which is asssociated with an excellent prognosis.

Currently, serum CA 125 levels and endovaginal ultrasound examinations have been used to identify ovarian cancer in women at high risk for the disease based on family and personal medical histories and in those with known or suspected gene mutations associated with ovarian cancer. However, serum CA 125 is neither specific nor sensitive enough for the early detection of ovarian cancer. The CA 125 test is slightly more accurate after menopause, although its cost-effectiveness has been questioned. The addition of pelvic ultrasound as a second screen increases the specificity.

Proteomic technology has been employed in the diagnosis of ovarian cancer. The study of protein expression in ovarian cancer patients continues at many institutions. This may lead to practical screening techniques for the early detection of the disease.

Lifestyle modification. Ovarian cancer, like many other cancers, is more likely to develop in overweight women. Dietary discretion is one approach designed to reduce risk. Breastfeeding also seems to reduce risk, extending the time period for postpartum anovulation. Pregnant women should be encouraged to breastfeed postpartum, not only for the salubrious benefits to their child, but also for the health benefit they themselves might experience regarding reduced risk of ovarian cancer.

Pharmacologic interventions.

- *Prevention.* It is now well recognized that factors suppressing ovulation—including pregnancy, post-partum breastfeeding, and OC use—are associated with a reduced incidence of ovarian cancer. The simplest pharmacologic intervention to suppress ovulation is the use of OCs. Multiple observational studies have supported this approach. The Royal College of General Practitioners' study of 47,000 women with a 25-year follow-up confirmed a significant reduction of ovarian cancer among women who had ever used OCs compared with never users. As with many other studies, long-term use was associated with greater protection and this protection lasted for 20 years or more after stopping OCs. Similar observations were made in the Oxford Family Planning Association Study of 17,032 women and the Norwegian-Swedish Women's Lifestyle and Health Cohort Study of 103,551 women.

  Case-control studies have generally supported the finding that OC use is also effective in preventing ovarian cancer in women at highest risk for the disease—women who have inherited a mutation in the *BRCA1* or *BRCA2* genes. Longer duration of use was associated with a reduced incidence of ovarian cancer.

  Long-term use of OCs (>10 y) is associated with a 50% reduction in the incidence of ovarian cancer. Ever use of OCs is associated with a 30% reduction in the disease. There is a decrease in the RR of ovarian cancer of 5% per year of use. There is no particular type of OC that is especially likely to confer the cancer-sparing advantages. Other estrogen-progestin contraceptives may provide the same benefit.

- *Treatment.* Treatment of ovarian cancer is outside the scope of this textbook.

Colorectal cancer. Although fewer North American women are being diagnosed with cancer of the colon or rectum than in the recent past, this type of cancer is still a significant threat.

Incidence. Colorectal cancer is the third leading cause of cancer death in US and Canadian women. More than 31,000 North American women were expected to die from this disease during 2006. The decline in incident rates is attributed to increased screening and removal of adenomatous polyps, which prevents progression to invasive cancer.

The overall 1-year survival rate is 82%, with a 5-year survival rate of 61% (but 8% for distant metastasized carcinoma). If detected in an early, localized stage, the 5-year survival rate increases to 90%; however, only 37% of colorectal cancers are discovered early.

Risk factors. Various risk factors for colorectal cancer have been identified (see Table 19).

Table 19. Risk factors for colorectal cancer
• Age (risk increases markedly after age 50)
• Family or personal history of colorectal cancer
• Adenomatous polyps
• Inflammatory bowel disease
• Diabetes mellitus
• Diet mostly from animal sources (low in fruits and vegetables)
• Physical inactivity
• Obesity
• Smoking
• Heavy alcohol use
• Low levels of vitamin D
Source: American Cancer Society 2007.

A particular inherited form of colorectal cancer is known as the hereditary nonpolyposis colorectal cancer (HNPCC) or Lynch syndrome. It is characterized by an autosomal dominant inheritance pattern of early-onset colorectal cancer and an increased risk of other cancers, such as those of the endometrium, ovary, stomach, urinary tract, hepatobiliary tract, pancreas, and small bowel. HNPCC is caused by a germline mutation in DNA mismatch repair genes.

Levels of 25-hydroxyvitamin D below 74.88 nmol/L (20 ng/mL) are associated with a 30% to 50% increased risk of incident colon, prostate, and breast cancer, along with higher mortality from these cancers, according to both prospective and retrospective epidemiologic studies. For instance, pooled data for 980 women showed that the highest vitamin D intake, as compared with the lowest, correlated with a 50% lower risk of breast cancer. And, participants in the WHI who at baseline had a 25-hydroxyvitamin D concentration of less than 30 nmol/L (12 ng/mL) had a 253% increase in the risk of colorectal cancer over a follow-up period of 8 years.

Screening. Rectal bleeding, blood in the stool, and a change in bowel habits may be a sign of colon or rectal malignant tumors. These symptoms require prompt medical evaluation. Other causes of these symptoms can include diverticulitis, ileitis, colitis, and polyps.

The principal screening tests for detecting colorectal cancer are fecal occult blood testing, digital rectal examination, sigmoidoscopy, colonoscopy, and barium enema.

- *Fecal occult blood testing* is the standard of care for annual screening. The most common fecal occult blood test is the guaiac-impregnated card. The positive predictive value for cancer is only approximately 5% to 10%, however, which can result in discomfort, cost, and occasional complications from unnecessary follow-up tests. The best way to conduct this test is to have the woman obtain a stool sample on three consecutive days. Improved methods of fecal occult blood testing and genetic-based fecal screening are also being developed.

- *Digital rectal examination* is of limited value as a screening test for colorectal cancer as it can evaluate only 7 to 8 cm of the 11-cm rectal mucosa. Nevertheless, it should be performed before sigmoidoscopy, colonoscopy, or double-contrast barium enema and during the annual pelvic examination.

- *Sigmoidoscopy* uses a flexible proctosigmoidoscope to examine up to 50 cm of the rectum and sigmoid colon. Its primary use is to detect cancers and other abnormalities of the GI tract, such as hemorrhoids, polyps, or ulcers that could cause blood in the stool, because it evaluates only the lower colon. If there is a polyp or tumor present, colonoscopy is indicated. Combining sigmoidoscopy with fecal occult blood testing increases the identification of cancer to 76% relative to colonoscopy. The perforation risk with sigmoidoscopy is 1:10,000 compared with 1:500 to 1:4,000 with colonoscopy.

- *Colonoscopy* is the examination of the large intestine with a flexible fiber optic colonoscope. Air introduced through the colonoscope distends the intestinal walls to enhance visualization. Colonoscopy is also used to evaluate polypoid lesions that are beyond the reach of a sigmoidoscope. During colonoscopy, polyps are removed for biopsy, and photographs of visualized lesions can be taken. Colonoscopy can be used to follow women with previous polyps, colon cancer, or high-risk factors. Colonoscopy is considered the gold standard for screening because of its ability to visualize, sample, and/or remove lesions from the entire colon.

Colonoscopy and polypectomy have been shown to decrease the morbidity and mortality of patients with the HNPCC syndrome. Colonoscopy should start at 2-year intervals beginning at age 25 for HNPCC individuals. For family members on non-HNPCC-associated colorectal cancer patients, screening should start at least 10 years before the earliest age of onset in the family and continue at intervals of 2 to 5 year.

- *Barium enema* with air contrast increases the contrast and quality of x-rays of the rectum.

- *Other screening tests* include virtual colonoscopy, a method of using a CT scan to examine the colon. A three-dimensional approach, as opposed to a two-dimensional approach, provides sensitivity ratings of 93% for polyps at least 10 mm in diameter to 89% for polyps at least 6 mm in diameter. Specificity for adenomatous polyps ranged from 80% (>6 mm in diameter) to 96% (>10 mm in diameter). The two-dimensional approach has a false-positive rate of 17% for lesions larger than 10 mm in diameter.

Screening recommendations from the ACS are presented in Table 20.

Table 20. Colorectal screening recommendations for women age 50 and older

For women at least age 50 and with average risks for colorectal cancer, the American Cancer Society recommends selecting one of the following five screening options:

- Annual fecal occult blood test (FOBT)
- Flexible sigmoidoscopy every 5 years
- Annual FOBT plus flexible sigmoidoscopy every 5 years (preferred by ACS)
- Double-contrast barium enema every 5 years
- Colonoscopy every 10 years

Source: American Cancer Society 2007.

Women at high risk for colorectal cancer should be considered for a more frequent and possibly earlier testing schedule. Having any one of the following risk factors places a woman in the high-risk category:

- A strong family history of colorectal cancer or polyps in a first-degree relative (parent, sibling, or child) occurring before age 60 or in two first-degree relatives at any age
- Families with hereditary colorectal cancer syndromes, defined as familial adenomatous polyposis and hereditary nonpolyposis colon cancer
- A personal history of colorectal cancer or adenomatous polyps
- A personal history of chronic inflammatory bowel disease

Lifestyle modification. Colorectal cancer risk may be lowered by exercise, healthy eating habits, and not smoking. It is well recognized that countries with significantly lower fat intake than the US population had one third the risk of colorectal cancer compared with the US population. However, the WHI Dietary Modification Trial, an RCT involving 48,835 postmenopausal women, demonstrated

that reducing fat ingestion and increasing intake of fruits, vegetables, and grains did not reduce the incidence of colorectal cancer. In the trial, intervention group participants reduced fat as a percentage of energy intake by 10.7% more than the control group at 1 year and mostly maintained this difference (8.1%) at 6 years. There was no evidence that this intervention reduced colorectal cancer incidence in the following years. The study group did tend to have more women taking aspirin, HT, and calcium and vitamin D supplementation, which may have influenced the findings. These findings were consistent with those of the Polyp Prevention Trial, which showed no reduction in polyp formation in 2,079 participants followed for 4 years. The results were also consistent with a polled analysis of prospective cohort studies evaluating dietary fiber intake and the risk of colorectal cancer.

Pharmacologic interventions.

- *Prevention.* Observational studies suggest colorectal cancer risk may be reduced with calcium or with aspirin or other nonsteroidal anti-inflammatory drugs. However, the Massachusetts Women's Health Study, a prospective RCT in which 19,934 women received aspirin (100 mg every other day) and 19,942 women received placebo for an average treatment period of 10 years, failed to show a reduction in risk of development of colorectal or breast cancer. These results were consistent with the other RCTs assessing colorectal cancer risks and use of aspirin.

  RCTs, including the WHI, have shown that EPT use is associated with an overall decreased risk of colorectal cancer. However, colorectal tumors diagnosed in EPT users are more advanced, possibly because rectal bleeding might not be evaluated as early in such women. Data are insufficient to support a global recommendation for EPT use to reduce the risk of colorectal cancer in postmenopausal women.

- *Treatment.* Treatment of colorectal cancer is outside the scope of this textbook.

Pancreatic cancer. Pancreatic cancer is more common in men than in women, yet it is of particular interest to menopause practitioners since ERs are present in the exocrine pancreas from which 95% of pancreatic cancers arise.

Incidence. Pancreatic cancer is the fourth leading cause of cancer death in US and Canadian women. Pancreatic cancer is more likely to occur in postmenopausal than in premenopausal women. A prospective cohort study of 89,835 Canadian women who were followed at a mean of 16.4 years failed to show an association between pancreatic cancer risk and age at first live birth, parity, age at menarche, the use of OCs, or use of HT.

Pancreatic cancer is a rapidly fatal disease. The 1-year survival rate is 20% and 5-year survival is 4%. Average survival is 6 months or less from date of diagnosis.

Risk factors. Cigarette smoking is the only well-established risk factor for pancreatic cancer. Risk of pancreatic cancer seems to increase with age, diet high in fat, and, possibly, alcohol intake. Recent studies also suggest a causal role for type 2 DM (adult onset), chronic pancreatitis, and obesity.

Screening. There are no effective methods for the early detection of pancreatic cancer. Cancer of the pancreas is generally asymptomatic until advanced stages. Jaundice may be the first symptom if the cancer develops near the common bile duct. Pancreatic cancer frequently presents with lower extremity DVT, thrombophlebitis migrans, and pulmonary emboli. Portal vein thrombosis in pancreatic cancer patients is more frequently being recognized on routine CT scans in the absence of symptoms. A patient presenting with manifestations of thromboembolic disease must be evaluated promptly for the possibility of pancreatic cancer.

Lifestyle modification. Cigarette smoking and dietary indiscretion should be avoided. Several studies have reported adverse effects on survival in patients diagnosed to have pancreatic cancer associated with high levels of tobacco use.

Vitamin D may lower pancreatic cancer risk. An analysis of two large prospective cohort studies (the NHS and the Health Professional Follow-up Study) observed a 41% lower risk for pancreatic cancer in participants consuming 600 IU/day or more of vitamin D compared with those consuming less than 150 IU/day. Increasing vitamin D consumption may serve as primary prevention. However, a recent prospective case-control study involving 29,133 male smokers gave conflicting results.

Pharmacologic interventions. No prescription therapies are known to reduce the risk of pancreatic cancer. Treatment of pancreatic cancer is outside the scope of this textbook.

Skin cancer. It is estimated that more than 1 million Americans will be diagnosed with skin cancer each year. Despite public health efforts to warn about this cancer and its association with skin exposure, the public tends to trivialize the disease. Cancers of the skin can be divided into melanomas and nonmelanomas.

Melanoma. The most deadly form of skin cancer is the melanoma. Its incidence has increased more than 500% in the last 50 years. Melanoma is a cancer that begins in the melanocytes. Because most melanoma cells still produce melanin, melanoma tumors are usually brown or black. Some melanomas do not contain pigment and are difficult to diagnose. Although melanoma is much less common than basal cell and squamous cell cancers, it is much more likely to metastasize. The 5-year survival rate for malignant melanoma is 88%. If diagnosed at a localized stage, the 5-year survival rate is 96%.

Melanoma is predominantly a cutaneous disease, but may in rare instances occur at other sites, including the mucous membrane (vulva, vagina, perianal region, lip, throat, and esophagus), as well the eye (uvea and retina). Melanomas in these sites have a worse prognosis than cutaneous melanomas.

Although fair-skinned individuals are at highest risk, those with darkly pigmented skin are not risk free. Risk factors for melanoma include excessive exposure to ultraviolet (UVA) radiation, coal tar, pitch, creosote, arsenic, or radon. Having severe sunburns during childhood greatly increases the risk for melanoma later in life. Additional risk factors include a family history of melanoma, and multiple nevi or atypical nevi.

Nonmelanomas. The most common cancers of the skin are nonmelanomas—usually basal cell and squamous cell cancers. Because they rarely metastasize, they are less worrisome than melanomas.

Benign tumors that develop from other types of skin cells include:

- Actinic keratoses—Sun-induced growths that are sometimes burning and tender. Wrinkles and telangiectasia (skin lesions related to vascular dilation) are associated with increased risks of actinic keratoses, which are strongly associated with an increased risk of squamous cell cancer.
- Seborrheic keratoses—Benign tan, brown, or black raised spots with a waxy texture or rough surface.
- Hemangiomas—Benign blood vessel growths often called strawberry spots or port wine stains.
- Warts—Rough-surfaced benign growths caused by a virus.
- Lipomas—Soft growths of benign fat cells.

Cumulative exposure to sunlight and exposure within the past 10 years are strongly associated with the risk of actinic keratoses and, thus, squamous cell cancer. Recent exposure is not associated with the risk of basal cell cancer. Risk factors for photoaging and skin cancer include fair skin, difficulty tanning, ease of sunburning, sunburns before age 20, and advancing age. Smoking is an independent risk factor for wrinkling, telangiectasia, and squamous cell cancer.

Screening. All women, but particularly those who are fair-skinned, should be undergoing total body skin examinations periodically for skin cancers and precursors to skin cancer.

Moles should be evaluated for asymmetry, border irregularities, variability in color, diameter greater than 6 mm, or a sudden or progressive increase in size. The typical presenting sign of melanoma is any change in appearance of a mole or other dark pigmented growths or spots. Other signs and symptoms of melanoma include a change in appearance of a skin bump or nodule, spread of pigmentation beyond the border, scaliness, oozing, bleeding, change in sensation, itchiness, tenderness, or pain.

Basal cell carcinoma may present with a persistant, nonhealing sore on the skin; a reddish or irritated patch of skin; a shiny bump or nodule that may be mistaken for a mole; a pink, elevated growth; or a scar-like area on the skin.

Squamous cell tumors appear thick, rough, horny and shallow on the skin. They may ulcerate, meaning that the epidermis above the cancer is not intact.

Lifestyle modification. It is well established that prolonged exposure to solar ultraviolet radiation (particularly UVB) is the major cause of photoaging and skin cancers. The following strategies can be employed to reduce the risk of developing skin cancer:

- Avoid the sun during midday hours (10 am to 4 pm)
- When in the sun, wear clothing (including hats) and sunglasses, to avoid excessive ultraviolet radiation.
- Apply adequate amounts of sunscreen with a sun protective factor (SPF) of at least 15 (if one cannot avoid sun exposure). Self-tanning lotions containing dihydroxyacetome may be used to achieve a darker appearance.
- Avoid tanning salons because exposure to UVA radiation may induce photoaging and photo-allergic responses. Tanning outdoors should also be avoided. Patients can be reminded that there is no such thing as a "healthy tan"—tanned skin means that skin is damaged.
- Do not smoke.

Pharmacologic interventions. These therapies are outside the scope of this textbook.

Sexually transmitted infections

Although postmenopausal women cannot get pregnant, they are not protected against sexually transmitted infections (STIs), which are often called sexually transmitted diseases, or STDs. The risk of STIs—including syphilis, gonorrhea, genital herpes, HPV (genital warts), hepatitis B, and HIV—is a lifelong concern for women not in long-term, mutually monogamous relationships.

Most STIs are more easily transmitted man-to-woman than woman-to-man. Women are twice as likely as men to contract gonorrhea, hepatitis B, and HIV, if exposed. Moreover, STIs are less likely to produce symptoms in women and are, therefore, more difficult to diagnose until serious complications develop.

Sexually active postmenopausal women with genital atrophy may be at increased risk for STIs because the delicate genital tissue is prone to small tears and cuts that can act as pathways for infection.

Safer sex guidelines. Avoidance of STIs is an important behavior to reinforce (see Table 21).

Table 21. Safer sex guidelines for all women

- Choose sex partners selectively.
- Discuss sexual history with a partner; do not let embarrassment compromise health.
- Always insist that male partners use a latex condom for genital, oral, and anal sex, unless in a longstanding, mutually monogamous relationship. Never use petroleum-based oils as lubrication for condoms because they can damage the condom, potentially causing a leak.
- Have an annual physical examination, including (when indicated) a Pap test, as well as tests to identify STIs. Ensure that vaccinations are up to date (eg, hepatitis B vaccine).
- If exposed to an STI, or after a confirmed diagnosis, urge any partner(s) to be examined and treated.

Lesbians tend to have fewer STIs than heterosexual women, but STIs can still be passed from woman to woman. Lesbians and bisexual women not in long-term, mutually monogamous relationships are at an increased risk. Clinicians can provide counseling to lower this risk (see Tables 21 and 22).

Table 22. Preventing STIs in a woman-to-woman sexual relationship

- Prevent transfer of any body fluids, including menstrual blood and vaginal fluids, to cuts or other openings.
- During oral sex, cover the partner's vaginal area with a barrier impermeable to fluid to avoid contact with vaginal secretions.
- Use a latex barrier between vaginas during vulva-to-vulva sex.
- Avoid sharing sex toys. Either clean them in hot, soapy water or use a new condom before switching users.

Screening. Clinicians should not assume that older women are not at risk for STIs. Vaginal atrophy increases the risk for contracting an STI. In addition, older women may not be as knowledgeable about infection risks or willing to take steps to minimize these risks as are younger women who have lived with the threat of AIDS their entire sexually active lives.

STI testing could include screening for the following pathogens (listed alphabetically).

Bacterial vaginosis. The most common abnormal vaginal flora in women of childbearing age is bacterial vaginosis (BV). Peri- and postmenopausal women are also susceptible. Although the cause is not fully understood, BV is associated with an imbalance in the normal vaginal bacterial flora. The risk for BV increases by having a new sex partner or multiple sex partners and using an intrauterine contraceptive device.

Symptoms of BV include a white or gray vaginal discharge with a high pH and a strong fishy odor, but some women have no signs or symptoms. Complications for peri- and postmenopausal women include an increased susceptibility to other STIs and pelvic inflammatory disease. BV is diagnosed through microscopic examination of the vaginal fluid, pH determination, and KOH (10% K hydroxide) use for "whiff" testing.

Chlamydia. Most chlamydial infections occur in women under age 25. In peri- and postmenopausal women, testing is recommended only for those at high risk for STIs. These include women with multiple sex partners, a sex partner who has had multiple sexual contacts, or a sex partner with a chlamydial infection. In addition, all women with purulent cervical discharge should be screened.

Antigen-detection and direct nucleic-acid probe assays provide sensitivity, availability, and lower cost than cell culture. Urine-based screening, as well as the traditional cervical swab approach, may be used.

Genital herpes. From 1999 to 2004, the overall seroprevalence of genital herpes infection was 17%, compared with 21% from 1988 to 1994 (constituting a relative decrease of 19% between surveys). Almost 20% of all US adults have been infected. Genital herpes is caused by the herpes simplex viruses type 1 (HSV-1) and type 2 (HSV-2). HSV-2 is more common in women (1 in 4) than in men (1 in 5), possibly due to male-to-female transmission being more efficient than female-to-male. Also, most persons infected with HSV-2 have not been diagnosed.

Most genital herpes is caused by HSV-2, and infection typically occurs during sexual contact. HSV-1 can cause genital herpes, but it more commonly causes infections of the mouth and lips ("fever blisters"). HSV-1 infection of the genitals can be caused by oral-genital contact. Although HSV-1 is less likely to result in severe recurrent outbreaks, it is possible to genitally transmit HSV-1 as well as HSV-2. Anyone with a history of either type should be aware of the transmissibility of the infection through genital, oral, and anal contact.

Most individuals have no or only minimal signs or symptoms from HSV-1 or HSV-2 infection. When signs do occur, they typically appear as one or more blisters on or around the genitals or rectum. The blisters break, leaving tender ulcers that may require 2 to 4 weeks to heal the first time they occur. Typically, another outbreak can appear weeks or months after the first, although it is almost always less severe and of shorter duration. Other signs and symptoms during the primary episode may include a second crop of sores and flu-like symptoms, including fever and swollen glands. Complications include an increased susceptibility to other STIs, including HIV.

The clinical diagnosis of genital herpes is insensitive and nonspecific. Up to 30% of first-episode cases of genital herpes are caused by HSV-1, but recurrences are much less frequent for genital HSV-1 infection than genital HSV-2 infection. Therefore, the distinction between HSV serotypes influences prognosis and counseling. For these reasons, some experts believe that the clinical diagnosis of genital herpes should be confirmed by laboratory testing. Virologic tests and type-specific serologic tests for HSV are often used, as the sensitivity of the culture methods decline rapidly as lesions begin to heal.

Gonorrhea. Caused by the bacterium *Neisseria gonorrhoeae* that multiplies easily in warm, moist areas, gonorrhea infection can be found in the reproductive tract, anus, urethra, mouth, throat, and eyes. Gonorrhea is easily transmitted, primarily through sexual contact.

In women, symptoms are often mild and so nonspecific as to be mistaken for a bladder or vaginal infection. Initial symptoms may include a painful or burning sensation when urinating, increased vaginal discharge, or vaginal bleeding between periods. Many women who are infected have no symptoms, but are still at risk of developing serious complications. Symptoms of rectal infection may include discharge, anal itching, soreness, bleeding, or painful bowel movements. Untreated gonorrhea can cause pelvic inflammatory disease and serious sequelae, including long-lasting pelvic pain. Gonorrhea can spread to the blood or joints, and can become life-threatening.

Several laboratory tests are available to confirm the diagnosis. A positive Gram's stain is highly suggestive for diagnosing gonorrhea that is present in the cervix or urethra.

Hepatitis B virus (HBV). HBV is transmitted via percutaneous or mucous membrane exposure to infectious body fluids. Most HBV infections in the United States result from sexual transmission, with heterosexual transmission accounting for 40% of the cases. HBV is concentrated primarily in the blood, but is also present to a lesser extent in semen, vaginal secretions, and wound exudates.

HBV infection is diagnosed through serologic testing. Acute HBV infection is diagnosed by the presence of IgM antibody to hepatitis B core antigen (IgM anti-HBc). Chronic HBV infection is identified by the presence of HBsAg (hepatitis B surface antigen) with a negative test for IgM anti-HBc. Postmenopausal women may not have received the HBV vaccination since its introduction in 1982, and therefore may be at increased risk for infection.

Human immunodeficiency virus (HIV). For peri- and postmenopausal women, routine screening for HIV (the AIDS virus) is recommended only in women seeking treatment for sexually transmitted disease; past or present intravenous drug users; women with multiple sex partners;

women having sexual contact with partners who were HIV-infected, bisexual, or intravenous drug users; women born or living in an area with a high prevalence of HIV infection; and women who received a blood transfusion between 1978 and 1985. Little is known about HIV risk and older women.

The initial screening test to detect antibodies to HIV is the ELISA test. This test has high sensitivity and specificity; however, false-negative results can occur in the first 6 to 12 weeks after infection, before antibodies develop. Some immunologic disorders may cause a false-positive test result; thus, a second test is warranted in women with a positive HIV result on an ELISA test.

Other tests to validate positive ELISA results for HIV include the Western blot test, radioimmunoprecipitation assays, and indirect immunofluorescence assays. The Western blot test is the most accurate test and has a false-positive rate of less than 0.001%.

Human papillomavirus (HPV). By age 50, at least 80% of US women will have acquired genital HPV infection, a group of viruses that includes more than 100 different strains or types. More than 30 of these viruses are sexually transmitted, living in the skin or mucous membranes of the reproductive tract, vulva, and rectum. Most people with HPV will not have any symptoms and will clear the infection on their own. Some of these viruses are termed high-risk, and may cause abnormal Pap test results; persistent infection may lead to cancer of the cervix, vulva, vagina, or anus. The low-risk HPV viruses may cause mild Pap test abnormalities or genital warts.

There is a substantial body of evidence indicating that almost all cervical cancers are related to HPV infection. Most women are diagnosed with HPV on the basis of abnormal Pap test findings. Almost all women who are past menopause still require regular Pap tests. The 2007 guidelines from the American Society for Colposcopy and Cervical Pathology include recommendations for HPV testing in the evaluation of atypical squamous cells of undetermined significance (ASC-US). Women with ASC-US should be managed using a program of two repeat cytology tests, immediate colposcopy, or DNA testing for high-risk types of HPV.

Syphilis. This STI, caused by the bacterium *Treponema pallidum*, is often called the "great imitator" because so many of its signs and symptoms are indistinguishable from those of other diseases. Many people infected with syphilis have no symptoms for years, yet remain at risk for complications. The primary stage is usually marked by a single or multiple chancre, which heals within 3 to 6 weeks. Skin rash and mucous membrane lesions characterize the second stage, followed by the latent stage when symptoms disappear. Untreated, death can result from progressive syphilitic infection.

Syphilis should be diagnosed by examining the exudate from a chancre with dark-field microscopy. Syphilis screening tests (RPR, VDRL) and serum antibody tests (MHATP, FTAbs) are more reliable, but results are not often positive early in the lesions' presence.

Routine screening of women is not recommended, based on the low incidence of syphilis in the general population. However, screening is justified in women who engage in sex with multiple partners, have another STI, live in areas where syphilis is prevalent, or who had sexual contact with persons with syphilis.

Trichomoniasis. This is the most common curable STI in sexually active women. Caused by the single-cell protozoan parasite, *Trichomonas vaginalis*, trichomoniasis is most often found in women in the vagina. Only about 20% of women are asymptomatic. When women have symptoms, they usually appear within 5 to 28 days of exposure. Many infected women exhibit a heavy, yellow-green or gray vaginal discharge with a strong unpleasant odor, possibly with discomfort during intercourse and urination, as well as genital irritation and itching. On rare occasions, lower abdominal pain can be present. In about two thirds of infected women, there is edema, inflammation, cell hypertrophy, and metaplasia. Diagnosis is confirmed with wet mount, culture, or nucleic acid testing.

Management. Treating these diseases is outside the scope of this textbook.

Thyroid disease

Thyroid disorders are common in women, increasing in prevalence with age. In a subset of more than 3,000 multiethnic women aged 42 to 52 years participating in the Study of Women's Health Across the Nation (SWAN), approximately 1 in 10 women had evidence of thyroid dysfunction—a thyroid-stimulating hormone (TSH) level outside of the normal range (two thirds were higher than normal and one third were below normal). Symptoms of thyroid dysfunction (eg, altered cycle length, change in amount of bleeding, sleep disruption, fatigue, mood swings, forgetfulness, heat intolerance, palpitations) can be confused with symptoms common to the menopause transition.

The primary function of the thyroid is to regulate metabolism. Thyroid hormone is synthesized when the thyroid gland extracts iodine from the circulation, combines it with the amino acid tyrosine, and converts it to the thyroid hormones triiodothyronine (T_3) and thyroxine (T_4). The thyroid gland stores thyroid hormone until it is released into the bloodstream. Most thyroid hormones circulate bound to proteins. Thyroid hormones affect the liver, muscle, heart, bone, and central nervous system. TSH secreted by the pituitary gland reflects circulating thyroid hormone concentration and via a negative feedback loop, regulates thyroid hormone release.

Hypothyroidism. Hypothyroidism is the most common thyroid disorder in women; by age 60, up to 17% of women have an underactive thyroid. A hypothyroid woman may complain of fatigue, dry skin, leg cramps, and heavier, longer menstrual cycles. If a woman has a family history of thyroid disorders, experienced postpartum thyroiditis, received radioactive iodine treatment for Graves' disease, or reports a history of DM, polycystic ovarian syndrome, or other endocrine disorders, her risk of hypothyroidism increases. Another clue to the diagnosis of an underactive thyroid gland may be an elevated triglyceride level on a lipid panel.

The serum TSH determination is the current gold standard to detect hypothyroidism. The normal range is defined as 0.45 to 4.5 mIU/L. Elevated TSH and FT_4 (free T_4) should be measured to confirm the diagnosis. A high TSH value with an *elevated* FT_4 may be suggestive of a rare TSH-producing pituitary adenoma, but more likely may confirm that a patient may have taken extra thyroid hormone before her appointment. If the patient has symptoms of hypothyroidism and a low FT_4, and the TSH level is also low, an evaluation of the pituitary and hypothalamus is indicated.

Recommendations for screening for hypothyroidism vary. Contrary to recommendations by the American Thyroid Association (ATA) (ie, screen all adults beginning at age 35 and every 5 years thereafter), the US Preventive Services Task Force concluded that the evidence is insufficient to recommend for or against routine screening for thyroid disease in adults. The Canadian Task Force on the Periodic Health Examination recommends maintaining a high index of clinical suspicion for nonspecific symptoms consistent with hypothyroidism when examining perimenopausal and postmenopausal women. NAMS recommends that all perimenopausal women have TSH testing, as vasomotor symptoms and irregular menses may have their origin in thyroid dysfunction.

Management. Recent guidelines recommend treatment for women with TSH levels higher than 10 mIU/L. An asymptomatic woman with no history of thyroid disease who has a TSH value of 4.5 to 10 mIU/L with FT_4 in the normal range would qualify for a diagnosis of mild thyroid failure, also referred to as "subclinical hypothyroidism," and would merit close monitoring of her thyroid function at annual intervals, particularly if her antithyroperoxidase antibodies were positive. Positive antibodies predict a higher likelihood of developing overt hypothyroidism.

The usual replacement dose of synthetic thioxine (levothyroxine) averages 1.6 µg/kg body weight/day. Therapy should be initiated at 50 to 100 µg/day and titrated at 6-week intervals by 25 to 50 µg depending on the TSH levels (more gingerly if your patient is older or at substantial risk for CHD). In treated patients, the target range for TSH is 0.5 to 2.0 mIU/L. At this level of TSH, the FT_4 should fall in the upper third of the normal range.

Once the replacement dose is established, monitor TSH values every 6 to 12 months or, if the patient changes thyroid hormone preparations (eg, insurance or pharmacy change), recheck the TSH after 6 weeks. Because concurrent administration of thyroxine with food, vitamins, calcium, and iron may significantly interfere with absorption, patients should take thyroxine separately. Case reports suggest that an increase in the dose of thyroxine might be necessary when raloxifene or soy supplements are initiated in hypothyroid women.

The effects of thyroid hormone on BMD and fracture risk are of interest. In the Study of Osteoporotic Fractures, use of thyroid hormone itself did not increase risk of fracture if the TSH was maintained in the normal range. However, suppressed TSH levels (<0.1 mIU/L)—either as a result of excess endogenous thyroid hormone production or exogenous thyroid hormone use—were associated with a threefold increase in hip fractures and a fourfold increase in vertebral fractures in women older than age 65. As assessed by TSH measurements, approximately 20% of patients receiving thyroxine therapy may be overtreated. BMD should be measured, preferably at a cortical site, such as the hip, in women with a long history of thyroxine therapy, particularly since doses used in the past were often higher than currently recommended.

Role of hormone therapy. If the patient receiving thyroid hormone starts HT to alleviate menopause-related symptoms, monitor TSH levels 6 weeks later. Anticipate that the dose of thyroxine may need to be increased. Oral estrogens, in particular, increase thyroid-binding globulin which, in turn, reduces the FT_4 values. A normal functioning thyroid gland compensates by increasing thyroid hormone production to maintain FT_4, but a hypothyroid gland with compromised thyroid reserve cannot do this. Conversely, when HT is discontinued, monitor thyroid function again 6 weeks later. The dose of thyroxine may be reduced.

Hyperthyroidism. Symptoms of hyperthyroidism—including anxiety, palpitations, lighter and less frequent menses, and heat intolerance—may also mimic menopausal symptoms.

The initial diagnostic test of choice for hyperthyroidism remains the TSH level:

- If the TSH value is suppressed to less than 0.1 mIU/L, FT_4 should be measured to assess the degree of thyroid hormone excess.
- If FT_4 is normal, total T_3 should also be measured and, if elevated, might point to the presence of an autonomously functioning thyroid nodule.
- When FT_4 is above the normal range, a radioactive iodine uptake scan can be used to confirm the diagnosis of hyperthyroidism and define thyroid anatomy.

Markedly increased uptake in a homogenous distribution is consistent with Graves' disease, while a heterogenous distribution is consistent with multinodular goiter. A lack of uptake points to the diagnosis of thyroiditis, either Hashimoto's autoimmune thyroiditis or glandular destruction due to a viral infection.

Management. Most hyperthyroid women should be referred to an endocrinologist for consultation and therapy. Therapy often includes beta-blockers for symptomatic relief and, if the diagnosis is Graves' disease or multinodular goiter, concurrent antithyroid drugs (propylthiouracil or methimazole). A radioactive iodine uptake scan is the most definitive therapy for Graves' disease and toxic multinodular goiter. Patients with TSH levels of 0.1 to 0.45 mIU/L and normal FT_4 meet the criteria for "subclinical hyperthyroidism," for which the potential risks (eg, atrial fibrillation) and benefits of treatment are less certain.

Thyroid nodules. Ultrasound examination of asymptomatic patients suggests that nodules occur in as many as 19% to 67% of the US population. The vast majority of nodules are benign, but 5% to 10% harbor thyroid cancers. The risk of thyroid cancer increases with age, a history of radiation, a family history of radiation, rapid growth of the nodule, and hoarseness. The ATA issued guidelines in 2006 for evaluation and management of thyroid nodules and thyroid cancers. If a thyroid nodule is suspected on physical examination, the next step is a thyroid ultrasound to define the anatomy of the gland and accurately measure the nodule—an important parameter for management decisions and long-term follow-up. If the patient's TSH level is low, a radioactive iodine uptake scan should be performed to see if the nodule is functioning autonomously. Because "hot nodules" are rarely malignant, therapy for hyperthyroidism can be considered. If the TSH value is normal or elevated and the nodule is greater than 1 to 1.5 cm in diameter, the patient should be referred to an endocrinologist for fine-needle aspiration.

Management. The cytology of the cellular aspirate will dictate further management. Most benign nodules can be monitored with annual serial ultrasounds, and, depending on whether the nodule has grown, a repeat of the fine-needle aspiration may be indicated.

Epilepsy

Epilepsy is a chronic neurologic disease characterized by recurrent seizures. In most women with epilepsy, seizures do not occur randomly. Instead, in more than 50% of cases, they tend to cluster. Seizure clusters, in turn, may occur with temporal rhythmicity in a significant proportion of both women (35%) and men (29%).

Role of ovarian hormones. In women, seizures may cluster in relation to the menstrual cycle, commonly known as "catamenial epilepsy". This is attributable to the neuro-active properties of reproductive hormones and the cyclic variation of their serum levels.

Estrogen generally has neuroexcitatory properties and can promote seizure occurrence. Progesterone, in contrast, has metabolites with potent antiseizure effects. Mid-cycle elevations in estrogen and premenstrual withdrawal of progesterone are triggers for seizures in about one third of women with epilepsy.

Statistical evidence supports the concept of catamenial epilepsy and the existence of at least three distinct patterns of seizure exacerbation in relation to the menstrual cycle: (1) perimenstrual, (2) preovulatory patterns in women with ovulatory cycles, and (3) entire luteal and perimenstrual phase pattern in women with anovulatory or inadequate luteal phase cycles. These inadequate luteal phase cycles are more common among women with epilepsy than in the general population. This may result from epilepsy-related disruption of ovulation and luteal progesterone production.

Menopause occurs earlier in women with epilepsy than in the general population, especially in women with a high lifetime seizure frequency and with polytherapy using enzyme-inducing antiepileptic drugs. Perimenopause is sometimes associated with increased seizure frequency, which is more pronounced in women who have shown previous evidence of hormonal sensitivity in the form of catamenial seizure exacerbation. Perimenopausal seizure exacerbation may relate to unopposed estrogen effects that accompany the greater frequency of anovulatory cycles during this transition.

Role of hormone therapy. Progesterone therapy may benefit some women with catamenial epilepsy. Two open-label trials have shown that cyclic, oral progesterone supplementation at physiologic range levels during the luteal phase of each cycle may be associated with substantially and significantly lower seizure frequencies than optimal antiepileptic drug therapy alone. In contrast, oral progestins, administered cyclically or continuously, have not proven to be an effective therapy. An NIH-sponsored, multicenter investigation is under way to evaluate the efficacy of progesterone as a supplemental treatment for epilepsy.

The effects of menopausal HT on epilepsy have not been rigorously assessed, although ET has demonstrated epileptogenic effects in women with epilepsy who do not have an intact uterus. A small randomized, double-blind, placebo-controlled multicenter NIH investigation by Harden et al in 2006 did show that treatment of postmenopausal women with epilepsy using CE and MPA was associated with a significant increase in seizure frequency of the most severe seizure type during the 3-month treatment phase as compared to the 3-month baseline phase. The increase in seizure frequency correlated with the dosage of EPT.

Antiepileptic drug interaction effects with HT have not been established, but they may be similar to the effects on oral contraceptives. Enzyme-inducing antiepileptic drugs (eg, carbamazepine, oxcarbazepine, phenobarbital, phenytoin, primidone, topiramate) can make OCs less effective, reducing steroid concentrations in OC users by up to 50%. Antiepileptic medications that do not seem to interfere, or interfere minimally, with the effectiveness of OCs include gabapentin, lamotrigine, levetiracetam, tiagabine, and the infrequently used felbamate. Lamotrigine, and possibly valproate levels, however, do drop markedly by as much as 40% to 50% on active pill and recover within days on inactive pill. A comparable effect of HT needs to be considered but has not yet been reported.

Management. Epilepsy management, including screening and treatment, is outside the scope of this textbook. However, in addition to the relationship between hormones and epilepsy described above, it is important for the menopause practitioner to realize that antiepileptic drug therapy results in a significant increase in the risk of osteoporosis and fracture. Enzyme-inducing antiepileptic drugs induce the hydrolase enzymes in the hepatic microsomal system to accelerate the conversion of vitamin D sterols to inactive polar metabolites. They also reduce levels of 1,25-dihydroxycholecalciferol, the vitamin D metabolite needed for transport of calcium from the intestine into the bloodstream and for bone formation. The precise magnitude of osteoporosis risk, however, is difficult to establish because of the frequent coexistence of other risk factors, such as lack of ambulation, falls, and inadequate sunlight exposure. The use of vitamin D and calcium supplements, as well as bone absorption inhibitors, may be particularly important in women with epilepsy, especially those that take or have taken enzyme-inducing antiepileptic drugs.

Some studies have found that one antiseizure medication, gabapentin, is effective in managing mild hot flashes (see Section C, page 39 for more).

Asthma

The relationship between sex hormones and asthma is complex. Compared with men, women have more hospital admissions as a result of the disease. Studies are inconsistent regarding which phase of the menstrual cycle (premenstrual or preovulatory) is more strongly associated with asthma flares. It is possible that sharp decreases in serum estradiol levels are associated with increased risk of asthma flare.

The relationship between estrogen therapy (either in hormonal contraceptives or menopausal HT) and asthma is also inadequately characterized. During the reproductive years, women experience an increased incidence and severity of asthma. Some clinicians have postulated that HT may increase susceptibility to this disease in midlife.

The NHS's epidemiologic study of HT and asthma found that current HT use was associated with increased asthma severity and that longer use was associated with an increased incidence of asthma. Women who used HT for 10 or more years had twice the age-adjusted risk of asthma as nonusers. Previous use of OCs did not affect the results. In contrast, a 2003 review of literature published from 1966 to 2001 found HT to be associated with improved pulmonary function and a decrease in the risk of asthma exacerbation.

A small (N = 20) prospective, crossover study of asthmatic women who were at least 2 years postmenopausal found that neither discontinuation nor reinitiation of HT had any effect on objective measures of airway function. However, women with corticosteroid-dependent asthma, those older than age 70, and smokers were not included in the study. The authors concluded that, until data to the contrary are available, HT should not be withheld from postmenopausal women due to concerns about detrimental effects on asthma.

In a nonrandomized study of asthmatic and healthy postmenopausal women aged 48 to 60 years, measurement of endocrine and spirometric parameters before and after 6 months of transdermal 17β-estradiol and cyclic oral MPA treatment led to the conclusion that EPT use in postmenopausal asthmatic women has a favorable influence on the course of asthma. EPT was found to reduce daily use of glucocorticoids and frequency of asthma exacerbations. Preliminary epidemiologic research suggests that EPT may relax the bronchial smooth muscle and may be associated with higher levels of forced expiratory volume in 1 second (FEV1), an indicator of pulmonary function. Adequately sized RCTs are needed to verify these proposed favorable consequences of EPT on the course of asthma and resolve the contradictions in the literature.

Treatment of asthma is outside the scope of this textbook.

Gallbladder disease

The incidence of gallstones in the US population has been estimated at 8% to 10%. Women are more likely than men to have gallstones. A woman's risk of gallstones increases with obesity, parity, and hormone use. Ovarian hormones, whether OCs or menopausal HT, increase biliary cholesterol saturation, a prerequisite for cholesterol gallstone formation.

A 2005 review of the epidemiologic literature, which included the NHS and two RCTs (PEPI and HERS), concluded that HT increases risk of gallbladder disease and cholecystectomy. Furthermore, the HERS trial found that HT use among postmenopausal women with known coronary disease resulted in a marginally significant increase in the risk of biliary tract surgery. The increased risk was expressed as one additional woman undergoing surgery for every 185 women treated with CE 0.625 mg/ MPA 2.5 mg.

One RCT compared the impact of transdermal and oral estrogens on gallstone formation and focused on biliary markers of gallstone formation, an intermediate outcome, as opposed to clinical gallstone formation. The study found that both estrogen formulations altered bile comparably in ways that would be expected to form gallstones. A small, nonrandomized study suggested that the degree of elevation of circulating estrone levels manifested during oral, but not transdermal, estradiol therapy may predict the level of lithogenic bile during oral estrogen therapy use.

HT should be administered with caution to postmenopausal women who have gallstones or a history of gallbladder disease, although no RCTs have directly compared the impact of HT on gallstones in women with or without a history of gallstones.

Treatment of gallbladder disease is outside the scope of this textbook.

Suggested reading

Osteoporosis

American Association of Oral and Maxillofacial Surgeons. American Association of Oral and Maxillofacial Surgeons position paper on bisphosphonate-related osteonecrosis of the jaws. Available at: http://www.aaoms.org/docs/position_papers/osteonecrosis.pdf. Accessed July 16, 2007.

Anderson GL, Limacher M, Assaf AR, et al, for the Women's Health Initiative Steering Committee. Effects of conjugated equine estrogen in postmenopausal women with hysterectomy: the Women's Health Initiative randomized controlled trial. *JAMA* 2004;291:1701-1712.

Atkinson C, Compston JE, Day NE, Dowsett M, Bingham SA. The effects of phytoestrogen isoflavones on bone density in women: a double-blind, randomized, placebo-controlled trial. *Am J Clin Nutr* 2004;79:326-333.

Bagger YZ, Tanko LB, Alexandersen P, et al. Two to three years of hormone replacement treatment in healthy women have long-term preventive effects on bone mass and osteoporotic fractures: the PERF study. *Bone* 2004; 34:728-735.

Banks E, Beral V, Reeves G, Balkwill A, Barnes I, for the Million Women Study Collaborators. Fracture incidence in relation to the pattern of use of hormone therapy in postmenopausal women. *JAMA* 2004;291:2212-2220.

Barad D, Kooperberg C, Wactawski-Wende J, Liu J, Hendrix SL, Watts NB. Prior oral contraception and postmenopausal fracture: a Women's Health Initiative observational cohort study. *Fertil Steril* 2005;84:374-383.

Baron JA, Farahmand BY, Weiderpass E, et al. Cigarette smoking, alcohol consumption, and risk for hip fracture in women. *Arch Intern Med* 2001; 161:983-988.

Barrett-Connor E, Grady D, Sashegvi A, et al, for the MORE Investigators (Multiple Outcomes of Raloxifene Evaluation). Raloxifene and cardiovascular events in osteoporotic postmenopausal women: four-year results from the MORE (Multiple Outcomes of Raloxifene Evaluation) randomized trial. *JAMA* 2002;287:847-857.

Barrett-Connor E, Wehren LE, Siris ES, et al. Recency and duration of postmenopausal hormone therapy: effects on bone mineral density and fracture risk in the National Osteoporosis Risk Assessment (NORA) study. *Menopause* 2003;10:412-419.

Bassey EJ, Ramsdale SJ. Increase in femoral bone density in young women following high-impact exercise. *Osteoporos Int* 1994;4:72-75.

Bauer DC, Browner WS, Cauley JA, et al. Factors associated with appendicular bone mass in older women: the Study of Osteoporotic Fractures Research Group. *Ann Intern Med* 1993;118:657-665.

Bilezikian JP. Osteonecrosis of the jaw—do bisphosphonates pose a risk? *N Engl J Med* 2006;355:2278-2281.

Bischoff-Ferrari HA, Willett WC, Wong JB, Giovannucci E, Dietrich T, Dawson-Hughes B. Fracture prevention with vitamin D supplementation: a meta-analysis of randomized controlled trials. *JAMA* 2005;293:2257-2264.

Black DM, Bilezikian JP, Ensrud KE, et al, for the PaTH Study Investigators. One year of alendronate after one year of parathyroid hormone (1-84) for osteoporosis. *N Engl J Med* 2005;353:555-565.

Black DM, Cummings SR, Karpf DB, et al. Randomised trial of effect of alendronate on risk of fracture in women with existing vertebral fractures: Fracture Intervention Trial Research Group. *Lancet* 1996;348:1531-1541.

Black DM, Delmas PD, Eastell R, et al, for the HORIZON Pivotal Fracture Trial. Once yearly zoledronic acid for treatment of postmenopausal osteoporosis. *N Engl J Med* 2007;356:1809-1822.

Black DM, Schwartz AV, Ensrud KE, et al, for the FLEX Research Group. Effects of continuing or stopping alendronate after 5 years of treatment: the Fracture Intervention Trial Long-Term Extension (FLEX): a randomized trial. *JAMA* 2006;296:2927-2938.

Black DM, Thomson DE, Bauer DC, et al, for the FIT Research Group. Fracture risk reduction with alendronate in women with osteoporosis: the Fracture Intervention Trial. *J Clin Endocrinol Metab* 2000;85:4118-4124.

Blau LA, Hoehns JD. Analgesic efficacy of calcitonin for vertebral pain. *Ann Pharmacother* 2003;37:564-570.

Bolland M, Hay D, Grey A, Reid I, Cundy T. Osteonecrosis of the jaw and bisphosphonates—putting the risk in perspective. *N Z Med J* 2006;119:U2339.

Bone HG, Greenspan SL, McKeever C, et al, for the Alendronate/Estrogen Study Group. Alendronate and estrogen effect in postmenopausal women with low bone mineral density. *J Clin Endocrinol Metab* 2000;85:720-726.

Bone HG, Hosking D, Devogelaer JP, et al, for the Alendronate Phase III Osteoporosis Treatment Study Group. Ten years' experience with alendronate for osteoporosis in postmenopausal women. *N Engl J Med* 2004; 350:1189-1199.

Boniva [package insert]. Roche Laboratories Inc, 2006.

Briot K, Tremollieres F, Thomas T, Roux C, for the Comité scientifique du GRIO. How long should patients take medications for postmenopausal osteoporosis? *Joint Bone Spine* 2007;74:24-31.

Brown JP, Kendler DL, McClung MR, et al. The efficacy and tolerability of risedronate once a week for the treatment of postmenopausal osteoporosis. *Calcif Tissue Int* 2002;71:103-111.

Brown JP, Olszynski WP, Hodsman A, et al. Positive effect of etidronate therapy is maintained after drug is terminated in patients using corticosteroids. *J Clin Densitom* 2001;4:363-371.

Campbell AJ, Robertson MC, Gardner MM, Norton RN, Buchner DM. Psychotropic medication withdrawal and a home-based exercise program to prevent falls: a randomized, controlled trial. *J Am Geriatr Soc* 1999; 47:850-853.

Cauley JA, Lui LY, Ensrud KE, et al. Bone mineral density and the risk of incident nonspinal fractures in black and white women. *JAMA* 2005; 293:2012-2108.

Cauley JA, Robbins J, Chen Z, et al, for the Women's Health Initiative investigators. Effects of estrogen plus progestin on risk of fracture and bone mineral density: the Women's Health Initiative randomized trial. *JAMA* 2003;290:1729-1738.

Chapuy MC, Arlot ME, Duboeuf F, et al. Vitamin D_3 and calcium to prevent hip fractures in elderly women. *N Engl J Med* 1992;327:1637-1642.

Chapurlat RD, Delmas PD. Drug insight: bisphosphonates for postmenopausal osteoporosis. *Nat Clin Pract Endocrinol Metab* 2006;2:211-219.

Chesnut CH, Silverman S, Andriano K, et al. A randomized trial of nasal spray calcitonin in postmenopausal women with established osteoporosis: the Prevent Recurrence of Osteoporotic Fracture Study. PROOF Study Group. *Am J Med* 2000;109:267-276.

Chestnut CH, Skag A, Christiansen C, et al. Effects of oral ibandronate administered daily or intermittently on fracture risk in postmenopausal osteoporosis. *J Bone Miner Res* 2004;19:1241-1249.

Clark MK, Sowers MR, Nichols S, Levy B. Bone mineral density changes over two years in first-time users of depot medroxyprogesterone acetate. *Fertil Steril* 2004;82:1580-1586.

Cosman F, Nieves J, Woelfert L, et al. Parathyroid hormone added to established hormone therapy: effects on vertebral fracture and maintenance of bone mass after parathyroid hormone withdrawal. *J Bone Miner Res* 2001;16:925-931.

Cosman F, Nieves J, Zion M, Woelfert L, Luckey M, Lindsay R. Daily and cyclic parathyroid hormone in women receiving alendronate. *N Engl J Med* 2005;353:566-575.

Cranney A, Guyatt G, Griffith L, Wells G, Tugwell P, Rosen C, for the Osteoporosis Methodology Group and The Osteoporosis Research Advisory Group. Meta-analyses of therapies for postmenopausal osteoporosis. IX: Summary of meta-analyses of therapies for postmenopausal osteoporosis. *Endocr Rev* 2002;23:570-578.

Cranney A, Guyatt G, Krolicki N, et al. A meta-analysis of etidronate for the treatment of postmenopausal osteoporosis. Osteoporosis Research Advisory Group. *Osteoporos Int* 2001;12:140-151.

Cummings SR, Black DM, Nevitt MC, et al. Bone density at various sites for prediction of hip fractures: the Study of Osteoporotic Fractures Research Group. *Lancet* 1993;341:72-75.

Cummings SR, Black DM, Thompson DE, et al. Effect of alendronate on risk of fracture in women with low bone density but without vertebral fractures: results from the Fracture Intervention Trial. *JAMA* 1998;280:2077-2082.

Cummings SR, Eckert S, Krueger KA, et al, for the Multiple Outcomes of Raloxifene Evaluation. The effect of raloxifene on risk of breast cancer in postmenopausal women: results from the MORE randomized trial. *JAMA* 1999;281:2189-2197.

Cummings SR, Melton LJ. Epidemiology and outcomes of osteoporotic fractures. *Lancet* 2002;359:1761-1767.

Cummings SR, Nevitt MC, Browner WS, et al. Risk factors for hip fracture in white women: Study of Osteoporotic Fractures Research Group. *N Engl J Med* 1995;332:767-773.

Cummings SR, Palermo L, Browner W, et al. Monitoring osteoporosis therapy with bone densitometry: misleading changes and regression to the mean. Fracture Intervention Trial Research Group. *JAMA* 2000;283:1318-1321.

Dawson-Hughes B, Dallal GE, Krall EA, et al. A controlled trial of the effect of calcium supplementation on bone density in postmenopausal women. *N Engl J Med* 1990;323:878-883.

Dawson-Hughes B, Harris SS, Krall EA, Dallal GE. Effect of calcium and vitamin D supplementation on bone density in men and women 65 years of age and older. *N Engl J Med* 1997;337:670-676.

De Laet C, Kanis JA, Oden A, et al. Body mass index as a predictor of fracture risk: a meta-analysis. *Osteoporos Int* 2005;16:1330-1338.

Delmas PD. Treatment of osteoporosis. *Lancet* 2002;359:2018-2026.

Delmas PD, Bjarnason NH, Mitlak BH, et al. Effects of raloxifene on bone mineral density, serum cholesterol concentrations, and uterine endometrium in postmenopausal women. *N Engl J Med* 1997;337:1641-1647.

Delmas PD, Eastell R, Garnero P, Seibel MJ, Stepan J, for the Committee of Scientific Advisors of the International Osteoporosis Foundation. The use of biochemical markers of bone turnover in osteoporosis. Committee of Scientific Advisors of the International Osteoporosis Foundation. *Osteoporos Int* 2000;11(Suppl 6):S2-S17.

Delmas PD, Ensrud KE, Adachi JD, et al, for the Multiple Outcomes of Raloxifene Evaluation Investigators. *J Clin Endocrinol Metab* 2002; 87:3609-3617.

Delmas PD, Recker RR, Chestnut CH, et al. Daily and intermittent oral ibandronate normalize bone turnover and provide significant reduction in vertebral fracture risk: results from the BONE study. *Osteoporos Int* 2004;15:792-798.

Delmas PD, Seeman E. Changes in bone mineral density explain little of the reduction in vertebral or nonvertebral fracture risk with anti-resorptive therapy. *Bone* 2004;34:599-604.

Dempster DW, Cosman F, Kurland ES, et al. Effects of daily treatment with parathyroid hormone on bone microarchitecture and turnover in patients with osteoporosis: a paired biopsy study. *J Bone Miner Res* 2001;16:1846-1853.

Devine A, Dick IM, Dhaliwal SS, Naheed R, Beilby J, Prince RL. Prediction of incident osteoporotic fractures in elderly women using the free estradiol index. *Osteoporos Int* 2005;16:216-221.

Diem SJ, Blackwell TL, Stone KL, et al. Use of antidepressants and rates of hip bone loss in older women: the Study of Osteoporotic Fractures. *Arch Intern Med* 2007;167:1240-1245.

Dodin S, Lemay A, Jacques H, Legare F, Forest JC, Basse B. The effects of flaxseed dietary supplement on lipid profiles, bone mineral density, and symptoms in menopausal women: a randomized, double-blind, wheat germ placebo-controlled clinical trial. *J Clin Endocrinol Metab* 2005;90:1390-1397.

Durlach J, Bac P, Durlach V, Rayssiguier Y, Bara M, Guiet-Bara A. Magnesium status and ageing: an update. *Magnes Res* 1998;11:25-42.

Ensrud KE, Barrett-Connor EL, Schwartz A, et al, for the Fracture Intervention Trial Long-Term Extension Research Group. Randomized trial of effect of alendronate continuation versus discontinuation in women with low BMD: results from the Fracture Intervention Trial long-term extension. *J Bone Miner Res* 2004;19:1259-1269.

Ensrud KE, Ewing SK, Stone KL, Cauley JA, Bowman PJ, Cummings SR, for the Study of Osteoporotic Fractures Research Group. Intentional and unintentional weight loss increase bone loss and hip fracture risk in older women. *J Am Geriatr Soc* 2003;51:1740-1747.

Ettinger B, Black DM, Mitlak BH, et al. Reduction of vertebral fracture risk in postmenopausal women with osteoporosis treated with raloxifene. *JAMA* 1999;282:637-645.

Ettinger B, Ensrud KE, Wallace R, et al. Effects of ultralow-dose transdermal estradiol on bone mineral density: a randomized clinical trial. *Obstet Gynecol* 2004;104:443-451.

Evans RA, Marel GM, Lancaster EK, et al. Bone mass is low in relatives of osteoporotic patients. *Ann Intern Med* 1988;109:870-873.

Felson DT, Kiel DP, Anderson JJ, Kannel WB. Alcohol consumption and hip fractures: the Framingham Study. *Am J Epidemiol* 1988;128:1102-1110.

Felson DT, Zhang Y, Hannan MT, Kannel WB, Kiel DP. Alcohol intake and bone mineral density in elderly men and women: the Framingham Study. *Am J Epidemiol* 1995;142:485-492.

Ferrar L, Jiang G, Barrington NA, Eastell R. Identification of vertebral deformities in women: comparison of radiological assessment and quantitative morphometry using morphometric radiography and morphometric x-ray absorptiometry. *J Bone Miner Res* 2000;15:575-585.

Ferreira E, Brown TER. Pharmacotherapy: Canadian consensus on menopause and osteoporosis. *J Obstet Gynaecol Can* 2001;23:1105-1114.

Folgelman I, Herd RJ, Blake GM, Balena R. Cyclical etidronate therapy for prevention of postmenopausal bone loss: a 1-year open-label follow-up study. *Calcif Tissue Int* 2000;66:348-354.

Food and Drug Administration. FDA Talk Paper. Black box warning added concerning long-term use of Depo-Provera contraceptive injection. Available at: http://www.fda.gov/bbs/topics/answers/2004/ans01325.html. Accessed September 14, 2007.

Forteo [package insert]. Eli Lilly and Company, 2004.

Fujita K, Kasayama S, Hashimoto J, et al. Inhaled corticosteroids reduce bone mineral density in early postmenopausal but not premenopausal asthmatic women. *J Bone Miner Res* 2001;16:782-787.

Gallagher JC, Baylink DJ, Freeman R, McClung M. Prevention of bone loss with tibolone in postmenopausal women: results of two randomized, double-blind, placebo-controlled, dose-finding studies. *J Clin Endocrinol Metab* 2001;86:4717-4726.

Gallagher JC, Rapuri PB, Haynatzki G, Detter JR. Effect of discontinuation of estrogen, calcitriol, and the combination of both on bone density and bone markers. *J Clin Endocrinol Metab* 2002;87:4914-4923.

Gallagher JC, Satpathy R, Rafferty K, Haynatzka V. The effect of soy protein isolate on bone metabolism. *Menopause* 2004;11:290-298.

Genant HK, Jergas M, Palermo L, et al. Comparison of semiquantitative visual and quantitative morphometric assessment of prevalent and incident vertebral fractures in osteoporosis: the Study of Osteoporotic Fractures Research Group. *J Bone Miner Res* 1996;11:984-996.

Genant HK, Wu CY, van Kuijk C, Nevitt MC. Vertebral fracture assessment using a semiquantitative technique. *J Bone Miner Res* 1993;8:1137-1148.

Gerdhem P, Obrant KJ. Bone mineral density in old age: the influence of age at menarche and menopause. *J Bone Miner Metab* 2004;22:372-375.

Gillespie LD, Gillespie WJ, Robertson MC, Lamb SE, Cumming RG, Rowe BH. Interventions for preventing falls in elderly people. *Cochrane Database Syst Rev* 2003;4:CD000340.

Globus RK, Bikle DD, Morey-Holton E. The temporal response of bone to unloading. *Endocrinology* 1986;118:733-742.

Gordon S, Walsh BW, Ciaccia AV, Siddhanti S, Rosen AS, Plouffe L. Transition from estrogen-progestin to raloxifene in postmenopausal women: effect on vasomotor symptoms. *Obstet Gynecol* 2004;103:267-273.

Grady D, Ettinger B, Moscarelli E, et al, for the Multiple Outcomes of Raloxifene Evaluation Investigators. Safety and adverse effects associated with raloxifene: multiple outcomes of raloxifene evaluation. *Obstet Gynecol* 2004;104:837-844.

Grady D, Rubin SM, Petitti DB, et al. Hormone therapy to prevent disease and prolong life in postmenopausal women. *Ann Intern Med* 1992;117:1016-1037.

Grant AM, Avenell A, Campbell MK, et al, for the RECORD Trial Group. Oral vitamin D3 and calcium for secondary prevention of low-trauma fractures in elderly people (Randomised Evaluation of Calcium Or vitamin D, RECORD): a randomised placebo-controlled trial. *Lancet* 2005;365:1621-1628.

Greendale GA, Espeland M, Slone S, Marcus R, Barrett-Connor E, for the PEPI Safety Follow-up Study. Bone mass response to discontinuation of long-term hormone replacement therapy: results from the Postmenopausal Estrogen/Progestin Interventions (PEPI) Safety Follow-up Study. *Arch Intern Med* 2002;162:665-672.

Greenspan SL, Bone HG, Ettinger MP, et al, for the Treatment of Osteoporosis with Parathyroid Hormone Study Group. Effect of recombinant human parathyroid hormone (1-84) on vertebral fracture and bone mineral density in postmenopausal women with osteoporosis: a randomized trial. *Ann Intern Med* 2007;146:326-339.

Greenspan SL, Emkey RD, Bone HG, et al. Significant differential effects of alendronate, estrogen, or combination therapy on the rate of bone loss after discontinuation of treatment of postmenopausal osteoporosis: a randomized, double-blind, placebo-controlled trial. *Ann Intern Med* 2002;137:875-883.

Greenspan SL, von Stetten E, Emond SK, Jones L, Parker RA. Instant vertebral assessment: a noninvasive dual x-ray absorptiometry technique to avoid misclassification and clinical mismanagement of osteoporosis. *J Clin Densitom* 2001;4:373-380.

Gutin B, Kasper JM. Can vigorous exercise play a role in osteoporosis prevention? A review. *Osteoporos Int* 1992;2:55-69.

Harris ST, Eriksen EF, Davidson M, et al. Effect of combined risedronate and hormone replacement therapies on bone mineral density in postmenopausal women. *J Clin Endocrinol Metab* 2001;86:1890-1897.

Harris ST, Watts NB, Genant HK, et al. Effects of risedronate treatment on vertebral and nonvertebral fractures in women with postmenopausal osteoporosis: a randomized controlled trial. *JAMA* 1999;282:1344-1352.

Harris ST, Watts NB, Jackson RD, et al. Four-year study of intermittent cyclic etidronate treatment of postmenopausal osteoporosis: three years of blinded therapy followed by one year of open therapy. *Am J Med* 1993;95:557-567.

Hedlund LR, Gallagher JC, Meeger C, Stoner S. Change in vertebral shape in spinal osteoporosis. *Calcif Tissue Int* 1989;44:168-172.

Hochberg MC, Ross PD, Black D, et al. Larger increases in bone mineral density during alendronate therapy are associated with a lower risk of new vertebral fractures in women with postmenopausal osteoporosis: Fracture Intervention Trial Research Group. *Arthritis Rheum* 1999;42:1246-1254.

Hodgson SF, Watts NB, Bilezikian JP, et al, for the American Association of Clinical Endocrinologists. American Association of Clinical Endocrinologists 2001 medical guidelines for clinical practice for the prevention and management of postmenopausal osteoporosis. *Endocr Pract* 2001;7:293-312.

Hodsman A, Adachi J, Olszynski W. Use of bisphosphonates in the treatment of osteoporosis: prevention and management of osteoporosis: consensus statements from the scientific advisory board of the Osteoporosis Society of Canada. *Can Med Assoc J* 1996;155(Suppl):S945-S948.

Holbrook TL, Barrett-Connor E, Wingard DL. Dietary calcium and risk of hip fracture: 14-year prospective population study. *Lancet* 1988;2:1046-1049.

Holick MF. Vitamin D deficiency. *N Engl J Med* 2007;357:266-281.

Jackson RD, Wactawski-Wende J, LaCroix AZ, et al. Effects of conjugated equine estrogen on risk of fractures and BMD in postmenopausal women with hysterectomy: results from the Women's Health Initiative randomized trial. *J Bone Miner Res* 2006;21:817-828.

Jensen J, Christiansen C, Rodbro P. Cigarette smoking, serum estrogens and bone loss during hormone-replacement therapy early after menopause. *N Engl J Med* 1985;313:973-975.

Johnell O, Gullberg B, Kanis JA, et al. Risk factors for hip fracture in European women: the MEDOS Study. Mediterranean Osteoporosis Study. *J Bone Miner Res* 1995;10:1802-1815.

Johnell O, Pauwels R, Lofdahl CG, et al. Bone mineral density in patients with chronic obstructive pulmonary disease treated with budesonide Turbuhaler. *Eur Resp J* 2002;19:1058-1063.

Kanis JA, Borgstrom F, De Laet C, et al. Assessment of fracture risk. *Osteoporos Int* 2005;16:581-589.

Kanis JA, De Laet C, Delmas P, et al. A meta-analysis of previous fracture and fracture risk. *Bone* 2004;35:375-382.

Kanis JA, Glüer CC, for the Committee of Scientific Advisors, International Osteoporosis Foundation: an update on the diagnosis and assessment of osteoporosis with densitometry. *Osteoporos Int* 2000;11:192-202.

Kanis JA, Johansson H, Johnell O, et al. Alcohol intake as a risk factor for fracture. *Osteoporos Int* 2005;16:737-742.

Kanis JA, Johansson H, Oden A, et al. A family history of fracture and fracture risk: a meta-analysis. *Bone* 2004;35:1029-1037.

Kanis JA, Johansson H, Oden A, et al. A meta-analysis of prior corticosteroid use and fracture risk. *J Bone Miner Res* 2004;19:893-899.

Kanis JA, Johnell O, Oden A, et al. Smoking and fracture risk: a meta-analysis. *Osteoporos Int* 2005;16:155-162.

Kanis JA, Johnell O, Oden A, Dawson A, De Laet C, Jonsson B. Ten-year probabilities of osteoporotic fractures according to BMD and diagnostic thresholds. *Osteoporos Int* 2001;12:989-995.

Kato I, Toniolo P, Akhmedkhanov A, et al. Prospective study of factors influencing the onset of natural menopause. *J Clin Epidemiol* 1998;51:1271-1276.

Kelley GA, Kelley KS, Tran ZV. Exercise and lumbar spine bone mineral density in postmenopausal women: a meta-analysis of individual patient data. *J Gerontol A Biol Sci Med Sci* 2002;57:599-604.

Kemp JP, Osur S, Shrewsbury SB, et al. Potential effects of fluticasone propionate on bone mineral density in patients with asthma: a 2-year randomized, double-blind, placebo-controlled trial. *Mayo Clin Proc* 2004;79:459-466.

Kerlikowske K, Shepherd J, Creasman J, et al. Are breast density and bone mineral density independent risk factors for breast cancer? *J Natl Cancer Inst* 2005;97:368-374.

Klotzbuecher CM, Ros PD, Landsman PB, Abbott TA, Berger M. Patients with prior fractures have an increased risk of future fractures: a summary of the literature and statistical synthesis. *J Bone Miner Res* 2000;15:721-739.

Knoke JD, Barrett-Connor E. Weight loss: a determinant of hip bone loss in older men and women. The Rancho Bernardo Study. *Am J Epidemiol* 2003;158:1132-1138.

Krall EA, Dawson-Hughes B. Smoking and bone loss among postmenopausal women. *J Bone Miner Res* 1991;6:331-338.

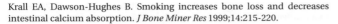

Krall EA, Dawson-Hughes B. Smoking increases bone loss and decreases intestinal calcium absorption. *J Bone Miner Res* 1999;14:215-220.

Kreijkamp-Kaspers S, Kok L, Grobbee DE, et al. Effect of soy protein containing isoflavones on cognitive function, bone mineral density, and plasma lipids in postmenopausal women: a randomized controlled trial. *JAMA* 2004;292:65-74.

Leipzig RM, Cumming RG, Tinetti ME. Drugs and falls in older people: a systematic review and meta-analysis. *J Am Geriatr Soc* 1999;47:30-50.

Leslie WD, Lix LM, Tsang JF, Caetano PA, for the Manitoba Bone Density Program. Single-site vs multisite bone density measurement for fracture prediction. *Arch Intern Med* 2007;167:1641-1647.

Liberman UA, Weiss SR, Broll J, et al. Effect of oral alendronate on bone mineral density and the incidence of fractures in postmenopausal osteoporosis. The Alendronate Phase III Osteoporosis Treatment Study Group. *N Engl J Med* 1995;333:1437-1443.

Lindsay R, Gallagher JC, Kleerekoper M, Pickar JH. Effect of lower doses of conjugated equine estrogens with and without medroxyprogesterone acetate on bone in early postmenopausal women. *JAMA* 2002;287:2668-2676.

Lindsay R, Nieves J, Formica C, et al. Randomised controlled study of effect of parathyroid hormone on vertebral-bone mass and fracture incidence among postmenopausal women on oestrogen with osteoporosis. *Lancet* 1997;350:550-555.

Lindsay R, Pack S, Li Z. Longitudinal progression of fracture prevalence through a population of postmenopausal women with osteoporosis. *Osteoporos Int* 2005;16:306-312.

Lindsay R, Silverman SL, Cooper C, et al. Risk of new vertebral fracture in the year following a fracture. *JAMA* 2001;285:320-323.

Lips P. Vitamin D deficiency and secondary hyperparathyroidism in the elderly: consequences for bone loss and fractures and therapeutic implications. *Endocr Rev* 2001;22:477-501.

Liu JH, Muse KN. The effects of progestins on bone density and bone metabolism in postmenopausal women: a randomized controlled trial. *Am J Obstet Gynecol* 2005;192:1216-1324.

Lyles KW, Colon-Emeric CS, Magaziner JS, et al, for the HORIZON Recurrent Fracture Trial. Zoledronic acid and clinical fractures and mortality after hip fracture. *N Engl J Med* 2007 Sep 17:[Epub ahead of print].

Lyritis GP, Ioannidis GV, Karachalios T, et al. Analgesic effect of salmon calcitonin suppositories in patients with acute pain due to recent osteoporotic vertebral crush fractures: a prospective double-blind, randomized, placebo-controlled clinical study. *Clin J Pain* 1999;15:284-289.

Majumdar SR, Kim N, Colman I, et al. Incidental vertebral fractures discovered with chest radiography in the emergency department: prevalence, recognition, and osteoporosis management in a cohort of elderly patients. *Arch Intern Med* 2005;165:905-909.

Marcus R, Holloway L, Wells B, et al. The relationship of biochemical markers of bone turnover to bone density changes in postmenopausal women: results from the Postmenopausal Estrogen/Progestin Interventions (PEPI) trial. *J Bone Miner Res* 1999;14:1583-1595.

Maricic M, Adachi JD, Sarkar S, Wu W, Wong M, Harper KD. Early effects of raloxifene on clinical vertebral fractures at 12 months in postmenopausal women with osteoporosis. *Arch Intern Med* 2002;162:1140-1143.

Marshall D, Johnell O, Wedel H. Meta-analysis of how well measures of bone mineral density predict occurrence of osteoporotic fractures. *BMJ* 1996;312:1254-1259.

Marx RE, Sawatari Y, Fortin M, Broumand V. Bisphosphonate-induced exposed bone (osteonecrosis/osteopetrosis) of the jaws: risk factors, recognition, prevention, and treatment. *J Oral Maxillofac Surg* 2005;63:1567-1575.

McClung M. Bisphosphonates. *Endocrinol Metab Clin North Am* 2003;32:253-271.

McClung M, Clemmesen B, Daifotis A, et al. Alendronate prevents postmenopausal bone loss in women without osteoporosis: a double-blind, randomized, controlled trial. *Ann Intern Med* 1998;128:253-261.

McClung MR, Geusens P, Miller PD, et al. Effect of risedronate on the risk of hip fracture in elderly women. *N Engl J Med* 2001;344:333-340.

McClung MR, Lewiecki EM, Cohen SB, et al, for the AMG 162 Bone Loss Study Group. Denosumab in postmenopausal women with low bone mineral density. *N Engl J Med* 2006;354:821-831.

McClung MR, San Martin J, Miller PD, et al. Opposite bone remodeling effects of teriparatide and alendronate in increasing bone mass. *Arch Intern Med* 2005;165:1762-1768.

McClung MR, Wasnich RD, Hosking DJ, et al, for the Early Postmenopausal Intervention Cohort Study. Prevention of postmenopausal bone loss: six-year results from the Early Postmenopausal Intervention Cohort Study. *J Clin Endocrinol Metab* 2004;89:4879-4885.

McClung MR, Wasnich RD, Recker R, et al, for the Oral Ibandronate Study Group. Oral daily ibandronate prevents bone loss in early postmenopausal women without osteoporosis. *J Bone Miner Res* 2004;19:11-18.

McCombs JS, Thiebaud P, McLaughlin-Miley C, Shi J. Compliance with drug therapies for the treatment and prevention of osteoporosis. *Maturitas* 2004;48:271-287.

McLean RR, Jacques PF, Selhub J, et al. Homocysteine as a predictive factor for hip fracture in older persons. *N Engl J Med* 2004;350:2042-2049.

Mellstrom DD, Sorensen OH, Goemaere S, Roux C, Johnson TD, Chines AA. Seven years of treatment with risedronate in women with postmenopausal osteoporosis. *Calcif Tissue Int* 2004;75:462-468.

Melton LJ III, Thamer M, Ray NF, et al. Fractures attributable to osteoporosis: report from the National Osteoporosis Foundation. *J Bone Miner Res* 1997;12:16-23.

Meunier PJ, Roux C, Seeman E, et al. The effects of strontium ranelate on the risk of vertebral fracture in women with postmenopausal osteoporosis. *N Engl J Med* 2004;350:459-468.

Michaelsson K, Baron JA, Farahmand BY, et al. Hormone replacement therapy and risk of hip fracture: population based case-control study. The Swedish Hip Fracture Study Group. *BMJ* 1998;316:1858-1863.

Migliorati CA, Casiglia J, Epstein J, Jacobsen PL, Siegel MA, Woo S-B. Managing the care of patients with bisphosphonate-associated osteonecrosis: an American Academy of Oral Medicine position paper. *J Am Dent Assoc* 2005;136:1658-1668.

Migliorati CA, Schubert MM, Peterson DE, Seneda LM. Bisphosphonate-associated osteonecrosis of mandibular and maxillary bone: an emerging oral complication of supportive cancer therapy. *Cancer* 2005;104:83-93.

Miller PD, Baran DT, Bilezikian JT, et al. Practical clinical applications of biochemical markers of bone turnover: consensus of an expert panel. *J Clin Densitom* 1999;2:323-342.

Miller PD, Barlas S, Brenneman SK, et al. An approach to identifying osteopenic women at increased short-term risk of fracture. *Arch Intern Med* 2004;164:1113-1120.

Miller PD, Hochberg MC, Wehren LE, Ross PD, Wasnich RD. How useful are measures of BMD and bone turnover? *Curr Med Res Opin* 2005;21:545-554.

Miller PD, McClung MR, Macovei L, et al. Monthly oral ibandronate therapy in postmenopausal osteoporosis: 1-year results from the MOBILE study. *J Bone Miner Res* 2005;20:1315-1322.

Miller PD, Watts NB, Licata AA, et al. Cyclical etidronate in the treatment of postmenopausal osteoporosis: efficacy and safety after seven years of treatment [erratum in: *Am J Med* 1998;104:608]. *Am J Med* 1997;103:468-476.

Mortensen L, Charles P, Bekker PJ, et al. Risedronate increases bone mass in an early postmenopausal population: two years of treatment plus one year of follow-up. *J Clin Endocrinol Metab* 1998;83:396-402.

National Osteoporosis Foundation. National Osteoporosis Foundation's Updated recommendations for calcium and vitamin D3 intake. 2007. Available at: http://www.nof.org/prevention/calcium_and_VitaminD.htm. Accessed July 16, 2007.

National Osteoporosis Foundation. *Osteoporosis: Physician's Guide to Prevention and Treatment of Osteoporosis.* Washington, DC: National Osteoporosis Foundation, 2003.

Neele SJ, Evertz R, De Valk-De Roo G, Roos JC, Netelenbos JC. Effect of 1 year of discontinuation of raloxifene or estrogen therapy on bone mineral density after 5 years of treatment in healthy postmenopausal women. *Bone* 2002;30:599-603.

Neer RM, Arnaud CD, Zanchetta JR, et al. Effect of parathyroid hormone (1-34) on fractures and bone mineral density in postmenopausal women with osteoporosis. *N Engl J Med* 2001;344:1434-1441.

Nieves JW, Golden AL, Siris E, Kelsey JL, Lindsay R. Teenage and current calcium intake are related to bone mineral density of the hip and forearm in women aged 30-39 years. *Am J Epidemiol* 1995;141:342-351.

NIH Consensus Development Panel on Osteoporosis Prevention, Diagnosis, and Therapy. Osteoporosis prevention, diagnosis, and therapy. *JAMA* 2001;85:785-795.

The North American Menopause Society. Estrogen and progestogen use in peri- and postmenopausal women: March 2007 position statement of The North American Menopause Society. *Menopause* 2007;14:168-182.

The North American Menopause Society. Management of osteoporosis in postmenopausal women: 2006 position statement of The North American Menopause Society. *Menopause* 2006;13:340-367.

The North American Menopause Society. The role of calcium in peri-and postmenopausal women: 2006 position statement of The North American Menopause Society. *Menopause* 2006;13:862-877.

The North American Menopause Society. The role of isoflavones in menopausal health: consensus opinion of The North American Menopause Society. *Menopause* 2000;7:215-229.

Notelovitz M, Martin D, Tesar R, et al. Estrogen therapy and variable-resistance weight training increase bone mineral in surgically menopausal women. *J Bone Miner Res* 1991;6:583-590.

Ohta H, Sugimoto I, Masuda A, et al. Decreased bone mineral density associated with early menopause progresses for at least ten years: cross-sectional comparisons between early and normal menopausal women. *Bone* 1996;18:227-231.

O'Loughlin JL, Robitaille Y, Boivin JF, Suissa S. Incidence of and risk factors for falls and injurious falls among the community-dwelling elderly. *Am J Epidemiol* 1993;137:342-354.

Overgaard K, Hansen MA, Jensen SB, Christiansen C. Effect of salcatonin given intranasally on bone mass and fracture rates in established osteoporosis: a dose-response study. *BMJ* 1992;305:556-561.

Perrien DS, Achenbach SJ, Bledsoe SE, et al. Bone turnover across the menopause transition: correlations with inhibins and follicle-stimulating hormone. *J Clin Endocrinol Metab* 2006;91:1848-1854.

Pocock NA, Eisman JA, Hopper JL, et al. Genetic determinants of bone mass in adults: a twin study. *J Clin Invest* 1987;80:706-710.

Porthouse J, Cockayne S, King C, et al. Randomised controlled trial of calcium and supplementation with cholecalciferol (vitamin D_3) for prevention of fractures in primary care. *BMJ* 2005;330:1003-1009.

Pouilles JM, Tremollieres F, Bonneu M, Ribot C. Influence of early age at menopause on vertebral bone mass. *J Bone Miner Res* 1994;9:311-315.

Pouilles JM, Tremollieres F, Ribot C. Vertebral bone loss in perimenopause: results of a 7-year longitudinal study. *Presse Med* 1996;25:277-280.

Prestwood KM, Kenny AM, Kleppinger A, Kulldorff M. Ultralow-dose micronized 17beta-estradiol and bone density and bone metabolism in older women: a randomized controlled trial. *JAMA* 2003;290:1042-1048.

Prince RL, Devine A, Dhaliwal SS, Dick IM. Effects of calcium supplementation on clinical fracture and bone structure: results of a 5-year, double-blind, placebo-controlled trial in elderly women. *Arch Intern Med* 2006;166:869-875.

Prince RL, Price RI, Ho S. Forearm bone loss in hemiplegia: a model for the study of immobilization osteoporosis. *J Bone Miner Res* 1988;3:305-310.

Pun KK, Chan LW. Analgesic effect of intranasal salmon calcitonin in the treatment of osteoporotic vertebral fractures. *Clin Ther* 1989;11:205-209.

Raisz LG, Wiita B, Artis A, et al. Comparison of the effects of estrogen alone and estrogen plus androgen on biochemical markers of bone formation and resorption in postmenopausal women. *J Clin Endocrinol Metab* 1996; 81:37-43.

Rapuri PB, Gallagher JC, Balhorn KE, Ryschon KL. Alcohol intake and bone metabolism in elderly women. *Am J Clin Nutr* 2000;72:1206-1213.

Rapuri PB, Gallagher JC, Balhorn KE, Ryschon KL. Smoking and bone metabolism in elderly women. *Bone* 2000;27:429-436.

Ravn P, Christensen JO, Baumann M, Clemmesen B. Changes in biochemical markers and bone mass after withdrawal of ibandronate treatment: prediction of bone mass changes during treatment. *Bone* 1998;22:559-564.

Recker RR, Davies KM, Dowd RM, Heaney RP. The effect of low-dose continuous estrogen and progesterone therapy with calcium and vitamin D on bone in elderly women: a randomized, controlled trial. *Ann Intern Med* 1999;130:897-904.

Recker RR, Lappe J, Davies K, Heaney R. Characterization of perimenopausal bone loss: a prospective study. *J Bone Miner Res* 2000;15:1965-1973.

Reclast [package insert]. Novartis Pharmaceuticals Corporation, 2007.

Reginster J, Minne HW, Sorensen OH, et al. Randomized trial of the effects of risedronate on vertebral fractures in women with established postmenopausal osteoporosis. Vertebral Efficacy with Risedronate Therapy (VERT) Study Group. *Osteoporos Int* 2000;11:83-91.

Reginster JY, Adami S, Lakatos P, et al. Efficacy and tolerability of once-monthly oral ibandronate in postmenopausal osteoporosis: 2 year results from the MOBILE study. *Ann Rheum Dis* 2006;65:654-661.

Reginster JY, Seeman E, De Vernejoul MC, et al. Strontium ranelate reduces the risk of nonvertebral fractures in postmenopausal women with osteoporosis: treatment of peripheral osteoporosis (TROPOS) study. *J Clin Endocrinol Metab* 2005;90:2816-2822.

Rejnmark L, Vestergaard P, Tofteng CL, et al. Response rates to oestrogen treatment in perimenopausal women: 5-year data from the Danish Osteoporosis Prevention Study (DOPS). *Maturitas* 2004;48:307-320.

Richards JB, Papaioannou A, Adachi JD, et al, for the Canadian Multicentre Osteoporosis Study Research Group. Effect of selective serotonin reuptake inhibitors on the risk of fracture. *Arch Intern Med* 2007;167:188-194.

Robertson MC, Campbell AJ, Gardner MM, Devlin N. Preventing injuries in older people by preventing falls: a meta-analysis of individual-level data. *J Am Geriatr Soc* 2002;50:905-911.

Rosen CJ, Hochberg MC, Bonnick SL, et al, for the Fosamax Actonel Comparison Trial investigators. *J Bone Miner Res* 2000;20:141-151.

Rossouw JE, Anderson GL, Prentice RL, et al, for the Writing Group for the Women's Health Initiative Investigators. Risks and benefits of estrogen plus progestin in healthy postmenopausal women: principal results from the Women's Health Initiative randomized controlled trial. *JAMA* 2002; 288:321-333.

Roux C, Seeman E, Eastell R, et al. Efficacy of risedronate on clinical vertebral fractures within six months. *Curr Med Res Opin* 2004;20:433-439.

Rude RK, Olerich M. Magnesium deficiency: possible role in osteoporosis associated with gluten-sensitive enteropathy. *Osteoporos Int* 1996;6:453-461.

Ruggiero SL, Mehrotra B, Rosenberg TJ, Engroff SL. Osteonecrosis of the jaws associated with the use of bisphosphonates: a review of 63 cases. *J Oral Maxillofac Surg* 2004;62:527-534.

Sagsveen M, Farmer JE, Prentice A, Breeze A. Gonadotrophin-releasing hormone analogues for endometriosis: bone mineral density. *Cochrane Database Syst Rev* 2003;4:CD001297.

Schneider DL, von Muhlen D, Barrett-Connor E, Sartoris DJ. Kyphosis does not equal vertebral fractures: the Rancho Bernardo study. *J Rheumatol* 2004; 31:747-752.

Schnitzer T, Bone HG, Crepaldi G, et al. Therapeutic equivalence of alendronate 70 mg once-weekly and alendronate 10 mg daily in the treatment of osteoporosis. Alendronate Once-Weekly Study Group. *Aging* (Milano) 2000;12:1-12.

Scholes D, LaCroix AZ, Ichikawa LE, Barlow WE, Ott SM. Injectable hormone contraception and bone density: results from a prospective study. *Epidemiology* 2002;13:581-587.

Seeman E, Hopper JL, Bach LA, et al. Reduced bone mass in daughters of women with osteoporosis. *N Engl J Med* 1989;320:554-558.

Segal E, Tamir A, Ish-Shalom S. Compliance of osteoporotic patients with different treatment regimens. *Isr Med Assoc J* 2003;5:859-862.

Shane E, Goldring S, Christakos S, et al. Osteonecrosis of the jaw: more research needed. *J Bone Miner Res* 2006;21:1503-1505.

Sherwin BB. Hormones and the brain: Canadian consensus on menopause and osteoporosis. *J SOGC* 2001;23:1102-1104.

Sikon A, Thacker HL, Deal C, Carey J, Licata A. Secondary Osteoporosis: are we recognizing it? *J Womens Health* 2006;15:1174-1183.

Silverman SL, Greenwald M, Klein RA, Drinkwater BL. Effect of bone density information on decisions about hormone replacement therapy: a randomized trial. *Obstet Gynecol* 1997;89:321-325.

Silverman SL, Watts NB, Delmas PD, Lange JL, Lindsay R. Effectiveness of bisphosphonates on nonvertebral and hip fractures in the first year of therapy: the risedronate and alendronate (REAL) cohort study. *Osteoporos Int* 2007;18:25-34.

Siminoski K, Jiang G, Adachi JD, et al. Accuracy of height loss during prospective monitoring for detection of incident vertebral fractures. *Osteoporos Int* 2005;16:403-410.

Siris ES, Harris ST, Eastell R, et al, for the Continuing Outcomes Relevant to Evista (CORE) Investigators. Skeletal effects of raloxifene after 8 years: results from the continuing outcomes relevant to Evista (CORE) study. *J Bone Miner Res* 2005;20:1514-1524.

Siris ES, Miller PD, Barrett-Connor E, et al. Identification and fracture outcomes of undiagnosed low bone mineral density in postmenopausal women: results from the National Osteoporosis Risk Assessment. *JAMA* 2001;286:2815-2822.

Slemenda CW, Christian JC, Williams CJ, et al. Genetic determinants of bone mass in adult women: a reevaluation of the twin model and the potential importance of gene interaction on heritability estimates. *J Bone Miner Res* 1991;6:561-567.

Slemenda CW, Hui SL, Longcope C, et al. Cigarette smoking, obesity, and bone mass. *J Bone Miner Res* 1989;4:737-741.

Snow-Harter C, Bouxsein ML, Lewis BT, Carter DR, Marcus R. Effects of resistance and endurance exercise on bone mineral status of young women: a randomized exercise intervention trial. *J Bone Miner Res* 1992;18:761-769.

Sorensen OH, Crawford GM, Mulder H, et al. Long-term efficacy of risedronate: a 5-year placebo-controlled clinical experience. *Bone* 2003; 32:120-126.

Spencer H, Fuller H, Norris C, Williams D. Effect of magnesium on the intestinal absorption of calcium in man. *J Am Coll Nutr* 1994;13:485-492.

Speroff L, Rowan J, Symons J, Genant H, Wilborn W, for the CHART Study Group. The comparative effect on bone density, endometrium, and lipids of continuous hormones as replacement therapy (CHART Study): a randomized controlled trial. *JAMA* 1996;276:1397-1403.

Standing Committee on the Scientific Evaluation of Dietary Reference Intakes. Institute of Medicine. *Dietary Reference Intakes: Calcium, Phosphorus, Magnesium, Vitamin D, and Fluoride.* Washington, DC: National Academy Press, 1997.

Storm T, Thamsborg G, Steiniche T, et al. Effect of intermittent cyclical etidronate therapy on bone mass and fracture rate in women with postmenopausal osteoporosis. *N Engl J Med* 1990;322:1265-1271.

Taaffe DR, Robinson TL, Snow CM, Marcus R. High-impact exercise promotes bone gain in well-trained female athletes. *J Bone Miner Res* 1997;12:255-260.

Tinetti ME, Speechley M, Ginter SF. Risk factors for falls among elderly persons living in the community. *N Engl J Med* 1988;319:1701-1707.

Torgerson DJ, Bell-Syer SE. Hormone replacement therapy and prevention of nonvertebral fractures: a meta-analysis of randomized trials. *JAMA* 2001;285:2891-2897.

Tosteson ANA, Grove MR, Hammond CS, et al. Early discontinuation of treatment for osteoporosis. *Am J Med* 2003;115:209-216.

Tremollieres FA, Pouilles JM, Ribot C. Withdrawal of hormone replacement therapy is associated with significant vertebral bone loss in postmenopausal women. *Osteoporos Int* 2001;12:385-390.

Trivedi DP, Doll R, Khaw KT. Effect of four monthly oral vitamin D3 (cholecalciferol) supplementation on fractures and mortality in men and women living in the community: randomised double blind controlled trial. *BMJ* 2003;326:469-475.

US Department of Health and Human Services. *Bone Health and Osteoporosis: A Report of the Surgeon General.* Rockville, MD: US Department of Health and Human Services; 2004.

van der Voort DJ, Geusens PP, Dinant GJ. Risk factors for osteoporosis related to their outcome: fractures. *Osteoporos Int* 2001;12:630-638.

van Staa TP, Leufkens HG, Cooper C. Use of inhaled corticosteroids and risk of fractures. *J Bone Miner Res* 2001;16:581-588.

Vestergaard P, Rejnmark L, Mosekilde L. Fracture reducing potential of hormone replacement therapy on a population level. *Maturitas* 2006; 54:285-293.

Wactawski-Wende J, Morley Kotchen J, Anderson GL, et al, for the Women's Health Initiative Investigators. Calcium plus vitamin D supplementation and the risk of colorectal cancer. *N Engl J Med* 2006;354:684-696.

Wasnich RD. Vertebral fracture epidemiology. *Bone* 1996;18(Suppl):179S-183S.

Wasnich RD, Bagger YZ, Hosking DJ, et al, for the Early Postmenopausal Intervention Cohort Study Group. Changes in bone density and turnover after alendronate or estrogen withdrawal. *Menopause* 2004;11:622-630.

Watts NB, Cooper C, Lindsay R, et al. Relationship between changes in bone mineral density and vertebral fracture risk associated with risedronate: greater increases in bone mineral density do not relate to greater decreases in fracture risk. *J Clin Densitom* 2004;7:255-261.

Weiss SR, Ellman H, Dolker M. A randomized controlled trial of four doses of transdermal estradiol for preventing postmenopausal bone loss: Transdermal Estradiol Investigator Group. *Obstet Gynecol* 1999;94:330-336.

Wells G, Tugwell P, Shea B, et al, for the Osteoporosis Methodology Group and the Osteoporosis Research Advisory Group. Meta-analyses of therapies for postmenopausal osteoporosis. V. Meta-analysis of the efficacy of hormone replacement therapy in treating and preventing osteoporosis in postmenopausal women. *Endocr Rev* 2002;23:529-539.

Welsh L, Rutherford OM. Hip bone mineral density is improved by high-impact aerobic exercise in postmenopausal women and men over 50 years. *Eur J Appl Physiol Occup Physiol* 1996;74:511-517.

Wolff I, van Croonenberg JJ, Kemper HC, Kostense PJ, Twisk JW. The effect of exercise training programs on bone mass: a meta-analysis of published controlled trials in pre- and postmenopausal women. *Osteoporos Int* 1999;9:1-12.

Woo SB, Hellstein JW, Kalmar JR. Narrative review: bisphosphonates and osteonecrosis of the jaws. *Ann Intern Med* 2006;144:753-761.

World Health Organization. Assessment of fracture risk and its application to screening for postmenopausal osteoporosis. Report of a WHO Study Group. *World Health Organ Tech Rep Ser* 1994;843:1-129.

The Writing Group for the Postmenopausal Estrogen/Progestin Interventions (PEPI) trial. Effects of hormone therapy on bone mineral density: results from the PEPI trial. *JAMA* 1996;276:1389-1396.

The Writing Group for the Women's Health Initiative Investigators. Risks and benefits of estrogen plus progestin in healthy postmenopausal women: principal results from the Women's Health Initiative randomized controlled trial. *JAMA* 2002;288:321-333.

Wu CY, Li J, Jergas M, Genant HK. Comparison of semiquantitative and quantitative techniques for the assessment of prevalent and incident vertebral fractures. *Osteoporos Int* 1995;5:354-370.

Yates J, Barrett-Connor E, Barlas S, Chen YT, Miller PD, Siris ES. Rapid loss of hip fracture protection after estrogen cessation: evidence from the National Osteoporosis Risk Assessment. *Obstet Gynecol* 2004;103:440-446.

Cardiovascular disease

Abramson B, Derzko C, Lalonde A, Reid R, Turek M, Wielgosz A. Hormone replacement therapy and cardiovascular disease: position statement of the Canadian Cardiovascular Society. Ottawa, ON, Canada: Canadian Cardiovascular Society 2002. Available at: http://www.ccs.ca/download/position_statements/2002_10_HRT_Statement_2.pdf. Accessed August 13, 2007.

Akhrass F, Evans AT, Wang Y, et al. Hormone replacement therapy is associated with less coronary atherosclerosis in postmenopausal women. *J Clin Endocrinol Metab* 2003;88:5611-5614.

Albers GW, Hart RG, Lutsep HL, Newell DW, Sacco R. Supplement to the guidelines for the management of transient ischemic attacks: a statement from the Ad Hoc Committee on Guidelines for the Management of Transient Ischemic Attacks, Stroke Council, American Heart Association. *Stroke* 1999;30:2502-2511.

American Heart Association. Third Report of the National Cholesterol Education Program (NCEP) Expert Panel on Detection, Evaluation, and Treatment of High Blood Cholesterol in Adults (Adult Treatment Panel III, or ATP III). 2001. Available at: http://www.americanheart.org/presenter.jhtml?identifier=11206. Accessed September 10, 2007.

Angerer P, Stork S, Kothny W, Schmitt P, van Schacky C. Effect of oral postmenopausal hormone replacement on progression of atherosclerosis: a randomized, controlled trial. *Arterioscler Thromb Vasc Biol* 2001;21:262-268.

Antiplatelet Trialists' Collaboration. Collaborative overview of randomised trials of antiplatelet therapy. I. Prevention of death, myocardial infarction, and stroke by prolonged antiplatelet therapy in various categories of patients. *BMJ* 1994;308:81-106.

Appel LJ, Brands MW, Daniels SR, Karanja N, Elmer PJ, Sacks FM. Dietary approaches to prevent and treat hypertension: a scientific statement from the American Heart Association. *Hypertension* 2006;47:296-308.

Appel LJ, Sacks FM, Carey VJ, et al, for the OmniHeart Collaborative Research Group. Effects of protein, monounsaturated fat, and carbohydrate intake on blood pressure and serum lipids. Results of the OmniHeart randomized trial. *JAMA* 2005;294:2455-2464.

Arana A, Varas C, González-Pérez A, Gutiérrez L, Bjerrum L, García Rodgríguez LA. Hormone therapy and cerebrovascular events: a population-based nested case-control study. *Menopause* 2006;13:730-735.

Bairey Merz CN, Johnson BD, Berga S, Braunstein G, Reis SE, Bittner V, for the WISE Study Group. Past oral contraceptive use and angiographic coronary artery disease in postmenopausal women: data from the National Heart, Lung and Blood Institute-sponsored Women's Ischemia Syndrome Evaluation. *Fertil Steril* 2006;85:1425-1431.

Bairey Merz CN, Johnson BD, Sharaf BL, et al, for the WISE Study Group. Hypoestrogenemia of hypothalamic origin and coronary artery disease in premenopausal women: a report from the NHLB-sponsored WISE Study. *J Am Coll Cardiol* 2003;41:413-419.

Bazzano LA, Reynolds K, Holder KN, He J. Effect of folic acid supplementation on risk of cardiovascular diseases: a meta-analysis of randomized controlled trials. *JAMA* 2006;296:2720-2726.

Berger JS, Roncaglioni MC, Avanzini F, Pangrazzi I, Tognoni G, Brown DL. Aspirin for the primary prevention of cardiovascular events in women and men: a sex-specific meta-analysis of randomized controlled trials. *JAMA* 2006;295:306-313.

Best PJM, Berger PB, Miller VM, Lerman A. The effects of estrogen replacement therapy on plasma nitric oxide and endothelin-1 levels in postmenopausal women. *Ann Intern Med* 1998;128:285-288.

Campbell CL, Smyth S, Montalescot G, Steinhubl SR. Aspirin dose for the prevention of cardiovascular disease: a systematic review. *JAMA* 2007; 297:2018-2024.

Canonico M, Oger E, Plu-Bureau G, et al, for the Estrogen and Thromboembolism Risk (ESTHER) Study Group. Hormone therapy and venous thromboembolism among postmenopausal women: impact of the route of estrogen administration and progestogens—the ESTHER Study. *Circulation* 2007;115:840-845.

Chan AT, Manson JE, Feskanich D, Stampfer MJ, Colditz GA, Fuchs CS. Long-term aspirin use and mortality in women. *Arch Intern Med* 2007; 167:562-572.

Chobanian AV, Bakris GL, Black HR, et al, for the National High Blood Pressure Education Program Coordinating Committee. The seventh report of the Joint National Committee on Prevention, Detection, Evaluation, and Treatment of High Blood Pressure: the JNC 7 report. *JAMA* 2003;289:2560-2572.

Clearfield M. Coronary heart disease risk reduction in postmenopausal women: the role of statin therapy and hormone replacement therapy. *Prev Cardiol* 2004;7:131-136.

Collaborative Group of the Primary Prevention Project (PPP). Low-dose aspirin and vitamin E in people at cardiovascular risk: a randomized trial in general practice. *Lancet* 2001;357:89-95.

Curb JD, Prentice RL, Bray PF, et al, for the Women's Health Initiative Investigators. Venous thrombosis and conjugated equine estrogen in women without a uterus: data from the Women's Health Initiative. *Arch Int Med* 2006;166:772-780.

Cushman M, Kuller LH, Prentice R, et al, for the Women's Health Initiative Investigators. Estrogen plus progestin and risk of venous thrombosis. *JAMA* 2004;292:1573-1580.

Dayspring T, Pokrywka G. Pharmacotherapeutic decisions in menopausal women with cardiovascular risk. *Future Lipidology* 2007;2:197-210.

de Lecinana MA, Egido JA, Fernandez C, et al; PIVE Study Investigators of the Stroke Project of the Spanish Cerebrovascular Diseases Study Group. *Neurology* 2007;68:33-38.

Despres JP, Lamarche B, Mauriege P, et al. Hyperinsulinemia as an independent risk factor for ischemic heart disease. *N Engl J Med* 1996;334:952-957.

Devaraj S, Jialal I, Vega-Lopez S. Plant sterol-fortified orange juice effectively lowers cholesterol levels in mildly hypercholesterolemic healthy individuals. *Arterioscler Thromb Vasc Biol* 2004;24:e25-e28.

Downs JR, Clearfield M, Weis S, et al. Primary prevention of acute coronary events with lovastatin in men and women with average cholesterol levels: results of AFCAPS/TexCAPS, Air Force/Texas Coronary Atherosclerosis Prevention Study. *JAMA* 1998;279:1615-1622.

Feng Y, Hong X, Wilker E, et al. Effects of age at menarche, reproductive years, and menopause on metabolic risk factors for cardiovascular diseases. *Atherosclerosis* 2007 Aug 3; [Epub ahead of print].

Folsom AR, Mink PJ, Sellers TA, Hong CP, Zheng W, Potter JD. Hormonal replacement therapy and morbidity and mortality in a prospective study of postmenopausal women. *Am J Public Health* 1995;85:1128-1132.

Food and Drug Administration. FDA authorizes new coronary heart disease health claim for plant sterol and plant stanol esters. *FDA Talk Paper*, 2000. Available at: http://www.cfsan.fda.gov/~lrd/tpsterol.html. Accessed September 21, 2007.

Galie N, Ghofrani HA, Torbicki A, et al, for the Sildenafil Use in Pulmonary Artery Hypertension (SUPER) Study Group. Sildenafil citrate therapy for pulmonary arterial hypertension. *N Engl J Med* 2005;353:2148-2157.

Gorodeski EZ, Gorodeski GI. Epidemiology and risk factors of cardiovascular disease in postmenopausal women. In: Lobo RA, ed. *Treatment of the Postmenopausal Woman: Basic and Clinical Aspects*, 3rd ed. San Diego, CA: Academic Press, 2007:405-452.

Grady D, Herrington D, Bittner V, et al, for the HERS Research Group. Heart and Estrogen/progestin Replacement Study follow-up (HERS II). Part 1: Cardiovascular outcomes during 6.8 years of hormone therapy. *JAMA* 2002;288:49-57.

Greiser C, Greiser EM, Dören M. Menopausal hormone therapy and risk of breast cancer: a meta-analysis of epidemiological studies and randomized controlled trials. *Hum Reprod Update* 2005;11:561-573.

Grodstein F, Manson JE, Stampfer MJ. Hormone therapy and coronary heart disease: the role of time since menopause and age at hormone initiation. *J Womens Health* 2006;15:35-44.

Grodstein F, Stampfer MJ. The epidemiology of coronary heart disease and estrogen replacement in postmenopausal women. *Prog Cardiovasc Dis* 1995; 38:199-210.

Grodstein F, Stampfer MJ, Colditz GA, et al. Postmenopausal hormone therapy and mortality. *N Engl J Med* 1997;336:1769-1775.

Grodstein F, Stampfer MJ, Goldhaber SZ, et al. Prospective study of exogenous hormones and risk of pulmonary embolism in women. *Lancet* 1996;348:983-987.

Grodstein F, Stampfer MJ, Manson JE, et al. Postmenopausal estrogen and progestin use and the risk of cardiovascular disease. *N Engl J Med* 1996;335:453-461.

Guetta V, Cannon RO III. Cardiovascular effects of estrogen and lipid-lowering therapies in postmenopausal women. *Circulation* 1996;93:1928-1937.

Gutthann SP, Rodriguez LAG, Castellsague J, et al. Hormone replacement therapy and risk of venous thromboembolism: population based case-control study. *BMJ* 1997;314:796-800.

Grundy SM, Cleeman JI, Bairey Merz N, et al, for the Coordinating Committee of the National Cholesterol Education Program. Implications of recent clinical trials for the National Cholesterol Education Program Adult Treatment Panel III guidelines. *Circulation* 2004;110:227-239.

Hayden M, Pignone M, Phillips C, Mulrow C. Aspirin for the primary prevention of cardiovascular events: a summary of the evidence for the US Preventive Services Task Force. *Ann Intern Med* 2002;136:161-172.

He J, Whelton PK, Vu B, Klag MJ. Aspirin and risk of hemorrhagic stroke: a meta-analysis of randomized controlled trials. *JAMA* 1998;280:1930-1935.

Hendrix SL, Wassertheil-Smoller S, Johnson KC, et al, for the WHI Investigators. Effects of conjugated equine estrogen on stroke in the WHI. *Circulation* 2006;113:2425-2434.

Herrington DM, Reboussin DM, Brosnihan KB, et al. Effects of estrogen replacement on the progression of coronary-artery atherosclerosis. *N Engl J Med* 2000;343:522-529.

Herrington DM, Vittinghoff E, Lin F, et al, for the HERS Study Group. Statin therapy, cardiovascular events, and total mortality in the Heart and Estrogen/progestin Replacement Study (HERS). *Circulation* 2002;105:2962–2967.

Hiroyasu I, Hennekens CH, Stampfer MJ, et al. Prospective study of aspirin use and risk of stroke in women. *Stroke* 1999;30:1764-1771.

Hodis HN, Mack WJ, Lobo RA, et al, for the Estrogen in Prevention of Atherosclerosis Trial (EPAT) research group. Estrogen in the prevention of atherosclerosis: a randomized, double-blind, placebo-controlled trial. *Ann Intern Med* 2001;135:939-953.

Hsia J, Langer RD, Manson JE, et al, for the Women's Health Initiative Investigators. Conjugated equine estrogens and coronary heart disease: the Women's Health Initiative. *Arch Intern Med* 2006;166:357-365.

Hu FB, Grodstein F, Hennekens CH, et al. Age at natural menopause and risk of cardiovascular disease. *Arch Intern Med* 1999;159:1061-1066.

Hulley S, Furberg C, Barrett-Connor E, et al, for the HERS Research Group. Heart and Estrogen/progestin Replacement Study follow-up (HERS II). Part 2: Non-cardiovascular outcomes during 6.8 years of hormone therapy. *JAMA* 2002;288:58-66.

Hulley S, Grady D, Bush T, et al, for the Heart and Estrogen/progestin Replacement Study (HERS) Research Group. Randomized trial of estrogen plus progestin for secondary prevention of coronary heart disease in postmenopausal women. *JAMA* 1998;280:605-613.

Iso H, Hennekens CH, Stampfer MJ, et al. Prospective study of aspirin use and risk of stroke in women. *Stroke* 1999;30:1764-1771.

Jick H, Darvy LE, Myers MW, et al. Risk of hospital admission for idiopathic venous thromboembolism among users of postmenopausal estrogens. *Lancet* 1996;348:981-983.

Kannel WB, Hjortland MC, McNamara PM, Gordon T. Menopause and risk of cardiovascular disease: the Framingham study. *Ann Intern Med* 1976; 85:447-452.

Katan MB, Grundy SM, Jones P, Law M, Miettinen T, Paoletti R; Stresa Workshop Participants. Efficacy and safety of plant stanols and sterols in the management of blood cholesterol levels. *Mayo Clin Proc* 2003;78:965-978.

Kurth T, Everett BM, Buring JE, Kase CS, Ridker PM, Gaziano JM. Lipid levels and the risk of ischemic stroke in women. *Neurology* 2007;68:556-562.

Lemaitre RN, Weiss NS, Smith NL, et al. Esterified estrogen and conjugated equine estrogen and the risk of incident of myocardial infarction and stroke. *Arch Intern Med* 2006;166:399-404.

Lichtenstein AH, Appel LJ, Brands M, et al. Diet and lifestyle recommendations revision 2006: a scientific statement from the American Heart Association Nutrition Committee. *Circulation* 2006;114:82-96.

Lloyd-Jones DM, Leip EP, Larson MG, et al. Prediction of lifetime risk for cardiovascular disease by risk factor burden at 50 years of age. *Circulation* 2006;113:791-798.

Manson JE, Allison MA, Rossouw JE, et al, for the WHI and WHI-CACS Investigators. Estrogen therapy and coronary artery calcification. *N Engl J Med* 2007;356:2591-2602.

Manson JE, Colditz GA, Stampfer MJ, et al. A prospective study of obesity and risk of coronary heart disease in women. *N Engl J Med* 1990;322:882-889.

Manson JE, Tosteson H, Ridker PM, et al. The primary prevention of myocardial infarction. *N Engl J Med* 1992;326:1406-1416.

Miettenen TA, Gylling H. Plant stanol and sterol esters in prevention of cardiovascular diseases: A review. *Int J Clin Pharmacol Ther* 2006;44:247-250.

Mikkola TS, Clarkson TB. Coronary heart disease and postmenopausal HT: conundrum explained by timing? *J Womens Health* 2006;15:51-53.

Moriusi KG, Oosthuizen W, Opperman AM. Phytosterols/stanols lower cholesterol concentrations in familial hypercholesterolemic subjects: A systematic review with meta-analysis. *J Am Coll Nutr* 2006;25:41-48.

Mosca L, Banka CL, Benjamin EJ, Berra K, et al, for the Expert Panel/Writing Group. Evidence-based guidelines for cardiovascular disease prevention in women: 2007 update. *Circulation* 2007;115:1481-1501.

Mosca L, Jones WK, King KB, Ouyang P, Redberg RF, Hill MN, for the American Heart Association Women's Heart Disease and Stroke Campaign Task Force. Awareness, perception, and knowledge of heart disease risk and prevention among women in the United States. *Arch Fam Med* 2000;9:506-515.

Mosca L, Linfante AH, Benjamin EJ, et al. National study of physician awareness and adherence to cardiovascular disease prevention guidelines. *Circulation* 2005;111:499-510.

Mosca L, Merz NB, Blumenthal RS, et al. Opportunity for intervention to achieve American Heart Association guidelines for optimal lipid levels in high risk women in a managed care setting. *Circulation* 2005;111:488-493.

Murabito JM, Yang Q, Fox C, Wilson PWF, Cuples LA. Heritability of age at natural menopause in the Framingham Heart Study. *J Clin Endocrinol Metab* 2005;90:3247-3430.

National Institutes of Health, National Heart, Lung, and Blood Institute. Clinical guidelines on the identification, evaluation, and treatment of overweight and obesity in adults: executive summary. *Am J Clin Nutr* 1998; 68:899-917.

Nissen SE, Tuzcu EM, Schoenhagen P, et al, for the Reversal of Atherosclerosis with Aggressive Lipid Lowering (REVERSAL) Investigators. Statin therapy, LDL cholesterol, C-reactive protein, and coronary artery disease. *N Engl J Med* 2005;352:29-38.

National Cholesterol Education Program (NCEP) Expert Panel on Detection, Evaluation, and Treatment of High Blood Cholesterol in Adults (Adult Treatment Panel III). Final Report. NIH Publication No. 02-5215. September 2002.

The North American Menopause Society. Estrogen and progestogen use in peri- and postmenopausal women: March 2007 position statement of The North American Menopause Society *Menopause* 2007;14:168-182.

The North American Menopause Society. The role of isoflavones in menopausal health: consensus opinion of The North American Menopause Society. *Menopause* 2000;7:215-229.

Patrono C, Garcia Rodriguez LA, Landolfi R, Baigent C. Low-dose aspirin for the prevention of atherothrombosis. *N Engl J Med* 2005;353:2373-2383.

Pedersen TR, Faergeman O, Kastelein JJP, et al, for the Incremental Decrease in End Points Through Aggressive Lipid Lowering (IDEAL) Study Group. High-dose atorvastatin vs usual-dose simvastatin for secondary prevention after myocardial infarction. The IDEAL Study: a randomized controlled trial. *JAMA* 2005;294:2347-2445.

Pepine CJ. Ischemic heart disease in women. *J Am Coll Cardiol* 2006;47:S1-S3.

Pepine CJ, von Mering GO, Kerensky RA, et al, for the WISE Study Group. Phytoestrogens and coronary macrovascular function in women with suspected myocardial ischemia: a report from the Women's Ischemia Syndrome Evaluation (WISE) Study. *J Womens Health* 2007;16:481-488.

Prentice RL, Langer RD, Stefanick ML, et al, for the Women's Health Initiative Investigators. Combined analysis of Women's Health Initiative observational and clinical trial data on postmenopausal hormone treatment and cardiovascular disease. *Am J Epidemiol* 2006;163:589-599.

Ridker P, Cook N, Lee IM, et al. A randomized trial of low-dose aspirin in the primary prevention of cardiovascular disease in women. *N Engl J Med* 2005;352:1293-1304.

Ridker PM, Buring JE, Rifai N, Cook NR, Development and validation of improved algorithms for the assessment of global cardiovascular risk in women: The Reynolds Risk Score. *JAMA* 2007;297:611-619.

Ridker PM, Rifai N, Cook NR, Bradwin G, Buring JE. Non-HDL cholesterol, apolipoproteins A-I and B100, standard lipid measures, lipid ratios, and CRP as risk factors for cardiovascular disease in women. *JAMA* 2005;294:326-333.

Roderick PJ, Wilkes HC, Meade TW. The gastrointestinal toxicity of aspirin: an overview of randomized controlled trials. *Br J Clin Pharmacol* 1993; 35:219-226.

Rosenberg L, Hennekens CH, Rosner B, Belanger C, Rothman KJ, Speizer FE. Early menopause and the risk of myocardial infarction. *Am J Obstet Gynecol* 1981;139:47-51.

Rossouw JE, Prentice RL, Manson, JE, et al. Post-menopausal hormone therapy and risk of cardiovascular disease by age and years since menopause. *JAMA* 2007;297:1465-1477.

Sacks FM, Lichtenstein A, Van Horn L, Harris W, Kris-Etherton P, Winston M, for the American Heart Association Nutrition Committee. Soy, isoflavones, and cardiovascular health: an American Heart Association A Science Advisory for professionals from the Nutrition Committee. *Circulation* 2006;113:1034-1044.

Salpeter SR, Walsh JM, Greyber E, Salpeter EE. Brief report: coronary heart disease events associated with hormone therapy in younger and older women: a meta-analysis. *J Gen Intern Med* 2006;21:363-366.

Sambrook PN, Geusens P, Ribot C, et al. Alendronate produces greater effects than raloxifene on bone density and bone turnover in postmenopausal women with low bone density: results of EFFECT (EFficacy of Fosamax versus Evista Comparison Trial) international. *J Intern Med* 2004;255:503-511.

Scarabin PY, Oger E, Plu-Bureau G, for the EStrogen and THromboEmbolism Risk (ESTHER) Study Group. Differential association of oral and transdermal oestrogen-replacement therapy with venous thromboembolism risk. *Lancet* 2003;362:428-432.

Schernhammer ES, Kang JH, Chan AT, et al. A prospective study of aspirin use and the risk of pancreatic cancer in women. *J Natl Cancer Inst* 2004;96:22-28.

Shaw LJ, Bairy Merz CN, Pepine CJ, et al. Insights from the NHLBI-sponsored Women's Ischemia Syndrome Evaluation (WISE) Study: Part I: gender differences in traditional and novel risk factors, symptom evaluation, and gender-optimized diagnostic strategies. *J Am Coll Cardiol* 2006;47(suppl): S4-S20.

Sidelmann JJ, Jespersen J, Andersen LF, Skouby SO. Hormone replacement therapy and hypercoagulability: results from the prospective Danish Climacteric Study. *Br J Obstet Gynecol* 2003;110:541-547.

Siris ES, Chen YT, Abbott TA, et al. Bone mineral density thresholds for pharmacological intervention to prevent fractures. *Arch Intern Med* 2004; 164:1108-1112.

Smith NL, Heckbert SR, Lemaitre RN, et al. Esterified estrogen and conjugated equine estrogens and the risk of venous thrombosis. *JAMA* 2004; 292:1581-1587.

Sowers MR, Symons JP, Jannausch ML, Chu J, Kardia SR. Sex steroid hormone polymorphisms, high-density lipoprotein cholesterol, and apolipoprotein A-1 from the Study of Women's Health Across the Nation (SWAN). *Am J Med* 2006;119(Suppl 1):S61-S68.

Speroff L, Rowan J, Symons J, Genant H, Wilborn W, for the CHART Study Group. The comparative effect on bone density, endometrium, and lipids of continuous hormones as replacement therapy (CHART Study): a randomized controlled trial. *JAMA* 1996;276:1397-1403.

Stampfer MJ, Willett WC, Colditz GA, Rosner B, Speizer FE, Hennekens CH. A prospective study of postmenopausal estrogen therapy and coronary heart disease. *N Engl J Med* 1985;313:1044-1049.

Steiner AZ, Hodis HN, Lobo RA, Shoupe D, Xiang M, Mack WJ. Postmenopausal oral estrogen therapy and blood pressure in normotensive and hypertensive subjects: the Estrogen in the Prevention of Atherosclerosis Trial. *Menopause* 2005;12:728-733.

Steingrimsdottir L, Gunnarsson O, Indridason OS, Franzson L, Sigurdsson G. Relationship between serum parathyroid hormone levels, vitamin D sufficiency, and calcium intake. *JAMA* 2005;294:2336-2341.

Stenson WF, Newberry R, Lorenz R, Baldus C, Civitelli R. Increased prevalence of celiac disease and need for routine screening among patients with osteoporosis. *Arch Intern Med* 2005;165:393-399.

Stephens NG, Parsons A, Schofield PM, Kelly F, Cheeseman K, Mitchinson MJ. Randomised controlled trial of vitamin E in patients with coronary disease: Cambridge Heart Antioxidant Study. *Lancet* 1996;347:781-786.

Suk Danik J, Rifai N, Buring JE, Ridker PM. Lipo-protein(a), measured with an assay independent of apolipoprotein(a) isoform size, and risk of future cardiovascular events among initially healthy women. *JAMA* 2006; 296:1363-1370.

Sullivan JM, VanderSwag R, Hughes JP, et al. Estrogen replacement and coronary artery disease: effect on survival in postmenopausal women. *Arch Intern Med* 1990;150:2557-2562.

Tankó LB, Bagger YZ, Qin G, Alexandersen P, Larsen PJ, Christiansen C. Enlarged waist combined with elevated triglycerides is a strong predictor of accelerated atherogenesis and related cardiovascular mortality in postmenopausal women. *Circulation* 2005;111:1883-1890.

Tsimikas S, Brilakis ES, Miller ER, et al. Oxidized phospholipids, Lp(a) lipoprotein, and coronary artery disease. *N Engl J Med* 2005;353:46-57.

US Preventive Services Task Force. Aspirin for the primary prevention of cardiovascular events. *Ann Intern Med* 2002;136:157-160.

Vasilakis C, Jick H, del Mar Melero-Montes M. Risk of idiopathic venous thromboembolism in users of progestagens alone. *Lancet* 1999;354:1610-1611.

Verhoef P, Stampfer MJ, Buring JE, et al. Homocysteine metabolism and risk of myocardial infarction: relation with vitamins B6, B12, and folate. *Am J Epidemiol* 1996;143:845-859.

Viscoli CM, Brass LM, Kernan WN, Sarrel PM, Suissa S, Horwitz RI. A clinical trial of estrogen-replacement therapy after ischemic stroke. *N Engl J Med* 2001;345:1243-1249.

Wadden TA, Berkowitz RI, Womble LG, et al. Randomized trial of lifestyle modification and pharmacotherapy for obesity. *N Engl J Med* 2005; 353:2111-2120.

Walsh BW, Kuller LH, Wild RA, et al. Effects of raloxifene on serum lipids and coagulation factors in healthy postmenopausal women. *JAMA* 1998; 279:1445-1451.

Wassertheil-Smoller S, Hendrix SL, Limacher M. Effect of estrogen plus progestin on stroke in postmenopausal women: the Women's Health Initiative: a randomized trial. *JAMA* 2003;289:2673-2684.

Whelton PK, He J, Appel LJ, et al, for the National High Blood Pressure Education Program Coordinating Committee. Primary prevention of hypertension: clinical and public health advisory from the National High Blood Pressure Education Program. *JAMA* 2002;288:1882-1888.

Wolf PA, Clagett GP, Easton JD, et al. Preventing ischemic stroke in patients with prior stroke and transient ischemic attack: a statement for healthcare professionals from the Stroke Council of the American Heart Association. *Stroke* 1999;30:1991-1994.

The Women's Health Initiative Steering Committee. Effects of conjugated equine estrogen in postmenopausal women with hysterectomy: the Women's Health Initiative randomized controlled trial. *JAMA* 2004;291:1701-1712.

The Writing Group for the American Heart Association Statistics Committee and Stroke Statistics Subcommittee. Heart Disease and Stroke Statistics—2007 Update: a report from the American Heart Association Statistics Committee and Stroke Statistics Subcommittee. Available at: http://circ.ahajournals.org/cgi/content/full/circulationaha.106.179918. Accessed July 2, 2007.

The Writing Group for the PEPI Trial. Effects of estrogen or estrogen/progestin regimens on heart disease risk factors in postmenopausal women. *JAMA* 1995;273:199-208.

The Writing Group for the Women's Health Initiative Investigators. Risks and benefits of estrogen plus progestin in healthy postmenopausal women: principal results from the Women's Health Initiative randomized controlled trial. *JAMA* 2002;288:321-333.

Yaffe K, Kanaya A, Lindquist K, et al. The metabolic syndrome, inflammation, and risk of cognitive decline. *JAMA* 2004;292:2237-2242.

Yeboah J, Reboussin DM, Waters D, Kowalchuk G, Herrington DM. Effects of estrogen replacement with and without medroxyprogesterone acetate on brachial flow-mediated vasodilator responses in postmenopausal women with coronary artery disease. *Am Heart J* 2007;153:439-444.

Diabetes

ACOG Committee on Practice Bulletins-Gynecology. Use of hormonal contraception in women with coexisting medical conditions. ACOG practice bulletin. No. 73: *Obstet Gynecol* 2006;107:1453-1472.

American Association of Clinical Endocrinologists, American College of Endocrinology. Medical guidelines for the management of diabetes mellitus: the AACE system of intensive diabetes self-management—2002 update. *Endocr Pract* 2002;8(Suppl 1):40-82.

American Diabetes Association. Standards of medical care in diabetes—2007. *Diabetes Care* 2007;30(Suppl):S4-S41.

Andersson B, Mattsson LA, Hahn L, et al. Estrogen replacement therapy decreases hyperandrogenicity and improves glucose homeostasis and plasma lipids in postmenopausal women with noninsulin-dependent diabetes mellitus. *J Clin Endocrinol Metab* 1997;82:638-643.

Antiplatelet Trialists' Collaboration. Collaborative overview of randomised trials of antiplatelet therapy. I: Prevention of death, myocardial infarction, and stroke by prolonged antiplatelet therapy in various categories of patients. *BMJ* 1994;308:81-106.

Barnard RJ, Jung T, Inkeles SB. Diet and exercise in the treatment of NIDDM: the need for early emphasis. *Diabetes Care* 1994;17:1469-1472.

Barrett-Connor E, Grady D. Hormone replacement therapy, heart disease, and other considerations. *Annu Rev Public Health* 1998;19:55-72.

Bonds DE, Larson JC, Schwartz AV, et al. Risk of fracture in women with type 2 diabetes: the Women's Health Initiative Observational Study. *J Clin Endocrinol Metab* 2006;91:3404-3410.

Bonds DE, Lasser N, Qi L, et al. The effect of conjugated equine estrogens on diabetes incidence: the Women's Health Initiative randomised trial. *Diabetologia* 2006;49:459-468.

Brussaard HE, Gevers Leuven JA, Frolich M, Kluft C, Krans HM. Short-term oestrogen replacement therapy improves insulin resistance, lipids and fibrinolysis in postmenopausal women with NID diabetes. *Diabetologia* 1997;40:843-849.

Buse J, Ginsberg HN, Bakris GL, et al, for the American Heart Association, American Diabetes Association. Primary prevention of cardiovascular disease in people with diabetes mellitus: a scientific statement from the American Heart Association and the American Diabetes Association. *Circulation* 2007;115:114-126.

Chobanian AV, Bakris GL, Black HR, et al, for the National High Blood Pressure Education Program Coordinating Committee. The seventh report of the Joint National Committee on Prevention, Detection, Evaluation, and Treatment of High Blood Pressure: the JNC 7 report. *JAMA* 2003;289:2560-2572.

Cowie CC, Rust KF, Byrd-Holt DD, et al. Prevalence of diabetes and impaired fasting glucose in adults in the US population: National Health And Nutrition Examination Survey 1999-2002. *Diabetes Care* 2006;21:1263-1268.

Diab KM, Zaki MM. Contraception in diabetic women: comparative metabolic study of Norplant, depot medroxyprogesterone, low dose oral contraceptive pill and CuT380A. *J Obstet Gynaecol Res* 2000;26:17-26.

Diabetes Prevention Program Research Group. Reduction in the incidence of type 2 diabetes with lifestyle intervention or metformin. *N Engl J Med* 2002;346:393-403.

Early Treatment Diabetic Retinopathy Study investigators. Aspirin effects on mortality and morbidity in patients with diabetes mellitus. *JAMA* 1992;268:1292-1300.

Expert Panel on Detection, Evaluation, and Treatment of High Blood Cholesterol in Adults. Executive summary of the Third Report of the National Cholesterol Education Program (NCEP) Expert Panel on Detection, Evaluation, and Treatment of High Blood Cholesterol in Adults (Adult Treatment Panel III). *JAMA* 2001;285:2486-2497.

Friday KE, Dong C, Fontenot RU. Conjugated equine estrogen improves glycemic control and blood lipoproteins in postmenopausal women with type 2 diabetes. *J Clin Endocrinol Metab* 2001;86:48-52.

Gabal LL, Goodman-Gruen D, Barrett-Connor E. The effect of postmenopausal estrogen therapy on the risk of non-insulin-dependent diabetes mellitus. *Am J Public Health* 1997;87:443-445.

Goldberg RB, Mellies MJ, Sacks FM, et al. Cardiovascular events and their reduction with pravastatin in diabetic and glucose-intolerant and myocardial infarction survivors with average cholesterol levels: subgroup analyses in the cholesterol and recurrent events (CARE) trial. *Circulation* 1998;98:2513-2519.

Goldberg RJ, Larson M, Levy D. Factors associated with survival to 75 years of age in middle-aged men and women. The Framingham Study. *Arch Intern Med* 1996;156:505-509.

Grady D, Herrington D, Bittner V, et al, for the HERS Research Group. Heart and Estrogen/progestin Replacement Study follow-up (HERS II). Part 1: Cardiovascular outcomes during 6.8 years of hormone therapy. *JAMA* 2002;288:49-57.

Grundy SM, Cleeman JI, Bairey Merz N, et al, for the Coordinating Committee of the National Cholesterol Education Program. Implications of recent clinical trials for the National Cholesterol Education Program Adult Treatment Panel III Guidelines. *Circulation* 2004;110:227-239.

Haffner SM, Diehl AK, Mitchell DB, Stern MP, Hazuda HP. Increased prevalence of clinical gallbladder disease in subjects with noninsulin-dependent diabetes mellitus. *Am J Epidemiol* 1990;132:327-335.

Harris MI, Flegal KM, Cowie CC, et al. Prevalence of diabetes, impaired fasting glucose, and impaired glucose tolerance in US adults. The Third National Health and Nutrition Examination Survey, 1988-1994. *Diabetes Care* 1998;21:518-524.

Herrington DM, Reboussin DM, Brosnihan KB, et al. Effects of estrogen replacement on the progression of coronary-artery atherosclerosis. *N Engl J Med* 2000;343:522-529.

Hoogeveen EK, Kostense PJ, Jakobs C, et al. Hyperhomocysteinemia increases risk of death, especially in type 2 diabetes: 5-year follow-up of the Hoorn Study. *Circulation* 2000;101:1506-1511.

Hu FB, Manson JE, Stampfer MJ, et al. Diet, lifestyle, and the risk of type 2 diabetes mellitus in women. *N Engl J Med* 2001;345:790-797.

Inzucchi SE. *Yale Diabetes Center Facts and Guidelines*. New Haven, CT: Yale Diabetes Center, 2001:10.

Kalish GM, Barrett-Connor E, Laughlin GA, Gulanski BI. Association of endogenous sex hormones and insulin resistance among postmenopausal women: results from the Postmenopausal Estrogen/Progestin Intervention Trial. *J Clin Endocrinol Metab* 2003;88:1646-1652.

Kanaya AM, Herrington D, Vittinghoff E, et al. Glycemic effects of postmenopausal hormone therapy: the Heart and Estrogen/progestin Replacement Study. *Ann Intern Med* 2003;128:1-9.

Kaplan RC, Heckbert SR, Weiss NS, et al. Postmenopausal estrogens and risk of myocardial infarction in diabetic women. *Diabetes Care* 1998;21:1117-1121.

Khoo CL, Perera M. Diabetes and the menopause. *J Br Menopause Soc* 2005; 11:6-11.

Kim C, Seidel KW, Begier EA, Kwok YS. Diabetes and depot medroxyproges-terone contraception in Navajo women. *Arch Intern Med* 2001;161:1766-1771.

Klein BE, Klein R, Moss SE. Exogenous estrogen exposures and changes in diabetic retinopathy. The Wisconsin Epidemiologic Study of Diabetic Retinopathy. *Diabetes Care* 1999;22:1984-1987.

Lindstrom J, Louheranta A, Mannelin M, et al, for the Finnish Diabetes Prevention Study Group. The Finnish Diabetes Prevention Study (DPS): lifestyle intervention and 3-year results on diet and physical activity. *Diabetes Care* 2003;26:3230-3236.

Liu S, Tinker L, Song Y, et al. A prospective study of inflammatory cytokines and diabetes mellitus in a multiethnic cohort of postmenopausal women. *Arch Intern Med* 2007;167:1676-1685.

Lo JC, Zhao X, Scuteri A, Brockwell S, Sowers MR. The association of genetic polymorphisms in sex hormone biosynthesis and action with insulin sensitivity and diabetes mellitus in midlife women. *Am J Med* 2006;119(9 Suppl 1):S69-S78.

Manning PJ, Allum A, Jones S, Sutherland WH, Williams SM. The effect of hormone replacement therapy on cardiovascular risk factors in type 2 diabetes: a randomized controlled trial. *Arch Intern Med* 2001;161:1772-1776.

Manson JE, Colditz GA, Stampfer MJ, et al. A prospective study of maturity-onset diabetes mellitus and risk of coronary heart disease and stroke in women. *Arch Intern Med* 1991;151:1141-1147.

Manson JE, Rimm EB, Colditz GA, et al. A prospective study of postmeno-pausal estrogen therapy and subsequent incidence of non-insulin-dependent diabetes mellitus. *Ann Epidemiol* 1992;2:665-673.

Margolis KL, Bonds DE, Rodabough RJ, et al, for the Women's Health Initiative Investigators. Effect of oestrogen plus progestin on the incidence of diabetes in postmenopausal women: results from the Women's Health Initiative Hormone Trial. *Diabetologia* 2004;47:1175-1187.

McKenzie J, Jaap AJ, Gallacher S, et al. Metabolic, inflammatory and haemostatic effects of a low-dose continuous combined HRT in women with type 2 diabetes: potentially safer with respect to vascular risk? *Clin Endocrinol* 2003;59:682-689.

Mosca L, Appel LJ, Benjamin EJ, for the Expert Panel/Writing Group. Evidence-based guidelines for cardiovascular disease prevention in women. American Heart Association scientific statement. *Circulation* 2004;109:672-693.

Mosca L, Collins P, Herrington DM, et al. Hormone replacement therapy and cardiovascular disease: a statement for healthcare professionals from the American Heart Association. *Circulation* 2001;104:499-503.

The North American Menopause Society. Effects of menopause and estrogen replacement therapy or hormone replacement therapy in women with diabetes mellitus: consensus opinion of The North American Menopause Society. *Menopause* 2000;7:87-95.

Pan XR, Li GW, Hu YH, et al. Effects of diet and exercise in preventing NIDDM in people with impaired glucose tolerance: the Da Qing IGT and Diabetes Study. *Diabetes Care* 1997;20:537-544.

Perera M, Sattar N, Petrie JR, et al. The effects of transdermal estradiol in combination with oral norethisterone on lipoproteins, coagulation, and endothelial markers in postmenopausal women with type 2 diabetes: a randomized, placebo-controlled study. *J Clin Endocrinol Metab* 2001; 86:1140-1143.

Petitti DB. Combination estrogen-progestin oral contraceptives. *N Engl J Med* 2003;349:1443-1450.

Sacks FM, Pfeffer MA, Moye LA, et al. The effects of pravastatin on coronary events after myocardial infarction in patients with average cholesterol levels. *N Engl J Med* 1996;335:1001-1009.

The Sixth Report of the Joint National Committee on prevention, detection, evaluation, and treatment of high blood pressure. *Arch Intern Med* 1997; 157:2413-2446.

Sowers JR. Diabetes mellitus and cardiovascular disease in women. *Arch Intern Med* 1998;158:617-621.

Tuomilehto J, Lindstrom J, Eriksson JG, et al, for the Finnish Diabetes Prevention Group. Prevention of type 2 diabetes mellitus by changes in lifestyle among subjects with impaired glucose tolerance. *N Engl J Med* 2001;344:1343-1350.

US Preventive Services Task Force. Screening for type 2 diabetes mellitus in adults: recommendations and rationale. *Ann Intern Med* 2003;138:212-214.

van Daele PL, Stolk RP, Burger H, et al. Bone density in non-insulin-dependent diabetes mellitus. The Rotterdam Study. *Ann Intern Med* 1995;122:409-414.

Weiderpass E, Gridley G, Persson I, et al. Risk of endometrial and breast cancer in patients with diabetes mellitus. *Int J Cancer* 1997;71:360-363.

Wilson PWF, Meigs JB, Sullivan L, Fox CS, Nathan DM, D'Agostino RB Sr. Prediction of incident diabetes mellitus in middle-aged adults: the Framingham Offspring Study. *Arch Intern Med* 2007;167:1068-1074.

Wingard DL, Barrett-Connor E. Heart disease and diabetes. In: Harris MI, Courie CC, Beiber G, Boyko E, Stern M, Bennet P, eds. *Diabetes in America*, 2nd ed. (NIH Publication No. 95-1468). Washington, DC: US Government Printing Office, 1995.

The Writing Group for the PEPI Trial. Effects of estrogen or estrogen/progestin regimens on heart disease risk factors in postmenopausal women. *JAMA* 1995;273:199-208.

The Writing Group for the Women's Health Initiative Investigators. Risks and benefits of estrogen plus progestin in healthy postmenopausal women: principal results from the Women's Health Initiative randomized controlled trial. *JAMA* 2002;288:321-333.

Cancers

American Cancer Society. *Cancer Facts & Figures 2007*. Available at: http://www.cancer.org/docroot/STT/content/STT_1x_Cancer_Facts__Figures_2007.asp. Accessed September 15, 2007.

Canadian Cancer Society. *Canadian Cancer Statistics 2006*. Available at: http://www.cancer.ca/vgn/images/portal/cit_86751114/31/21/935505792c w_2006stats_en.pdf. Accessed September 15, 2007.

Cook NR, Lee IM, Gaziano M, et al. Low-dose aspirin in the primary prevention of cancer. *JAMA* 2005;294:47-55.

Gotay CC. Behavior and cancer prevention. *J Clin Oncol* 2005;23:301-310.

National Cancer Institute of Canada. *Canadian Cancer Statistics 2007*. Available at: http://www.ncic.cancer.ca/vgn/images/portal/cit_86751114/2 1/40/1835950430cw_2007stats_en.pdf. Accessed September 20, 2007.

Breast cancer

The American College of Obstetricians and Gynecologists. Hormone replacement therapy in women with previously treated breast cancer: ACOG Committee Opinion Number 226. Washington, DC: The American College of Obstetricians and Gynecologists, November 1999.

Anderson GL, Judd HL, Kaunitz AM, et al, for the Women's Health Initiative investigators. Effects of estrogen plus progestin on gynecologic cancers and associated diagnostic procedures: the Women's Health Initiative randomized trial. *JAMA* 2003;290:1739-1748.

Armstrong K, Eisen A, Weber B. Assessing the risk of breast cancer. *N Engl J Med* 2000;342:564-571.

Baines CJ, McFarlane DV, Miller AB. Sensitivity and specificity of first screen mammography in 15 NBSS centres. *Can Assoc Radiol J* 1988;39:273-276.

Bardia A, Hartmann LC, Vachon CM, et al. Recreational physical activity and risk of postmenopausal breast cancer based on hormone receptor status. *Arch Intern Med* 2006;166:2478-2483.

Barrett-Connor E, Grady D, Sashegyi A, et al. Raloxifene and cardiovascular events in osteoporotic postmenopausal women: four-year results from the MORE (Multiple Outcomes of Raloxifene Evaluation) randomized trial. *JAMA* 2002;287:847-857.

Barrett-Connor E, Mosca L, Collins P, et al. Effects of ralixofene on cardio-vascular events and breast cancer in postmenopausal women. *N Engl J Med* 2006;355:125-137.

Belisle S, Derzko C. Hormone replacement therapy and cancer: Canadian consensus on menopause and osteoporosis. *J SOGC* 2001;23:1198-1203.

Bentrem DJ, Jordan VC. Targeted antiestrogens for the prevention of breast cancer. *Oncol Res* 1999;11:401-409.

Beral V, for the Million Women Study collaborators. Breast cancer and hormone-replacement therapy in the Million Women Study. *Lancet* 2003; 362:419-427.

Berry DA, Cronin KA, Pleviritis SK, et al, for the Cancer Intervention and Surveillance Modeling Network (CISNET) Collaborators. Effect of screening and adjuvant therapy on mortality from breast cancer. *N Engl J Med* 2005;353:1784-1792.

Bertelli G, Venturini M, Del Mastro L, et al. Tamoxifen and the endometrium: findings of pelvic examination and endometrial biopsy in asymptomatic breast cancer patients. *Breast Cancer Res Treat* 1998;47:41-46.

Boyd NF, Byng JW, Jong RA, et al. Quantitative classification of mammographic densities and breast cancer risk: results from the Canadian National Breast Cancer Screening Study. *J Natl Cancer Inst* 1995;87:670-675.

Boyd NF, Dite GS, Stone J, et al. Heritability of mammographic density, a risk factor for breast cancer. *N Engl J Med* 2002;12:886-894.

Boyd NF, Guo H, Martin LJ, et al. Mammographic density and the risk and detection of breast cancer. *N Engl J Med* 2007;356:227-236.

Breast Cancer in Canada (April 1999). Population and Public Health Branch. Available at: http://www.phac-aspc.gc.ca/publicat/updates/breast-99_e.html. Accessed June 26, 2007.

Breast International Group (BIG) 1-98 Collaborative Group; Thurlimann B, Keshaviah A, Coates AS, et al. A comparison of letrozole and tamoxifen in postmenopausal women with early breast cancer. *N Engl J Med* 2005; 353:2747-2757.

Brezden CB, Phillips KA, Abdolell M, Bunston T, Tannock IF. Cognitive function in breast cancer patients receiving adjuvant chemotherapy. *J Clin Oncol* 2000;18:2695-2701.

Brufsky A, Harker WG, Beck JT, et al. Zoledronic acid inhibits adjuvant letrozole-induced bone loss in postmenopausal women with early breast cancer. *J Clin Oncol* 2007;25:829-836.

Burstein HJ, Winer EP. Primary care for survivors of breast cancer. *N Engl J Med* 2000;343:1086-1094.

Byrne C, Connolly JL, Colditz GA, Schnitt SJ. Biopsy confirmed benign breast disease, postmenopausal use of exogenous female hormones, and breast carcinoma risk. *Cancer* 2000;89:2046-2052.

Byrne C, Schairer C, Wolfe J, et al. Mammographic features and breast cancer risk: effects with time, age, and menopause status. *J Natl Cancer Inst* 1995;87:1622-1629.

Cauley JA, Norton L, Lippman ME, et al. Continued breast cancer risk reduction in postmenopausal women treated with raloxifene: 4-year results from the MORE trial. Multiple Outcomes of Raloxifene Evaluation (MORE) Investigators. *Breast Cancer Res Treat* 2001;65:125-134.

Cecchini S, Ciatto S, Bonardi R, et al. Screening by ultrasonography for endometrial carcinoma in postmenopausal breast cancer patients under adjuvant tamoxifen. *Gynecol Oncol* 1996;60:409-411.

Chang-Claude J, Andrieu N, Rookus M, et al, for the Epidemiological Study of Familial Breast Cancer (EMBRACE), Gene Etude Prospective Sein Ovaire (GENEPSO), Genen Omgeving studie van de werkgroep Hereditiair Borstkanker Onderzoek Nederland (GEO-HEBON), the International *BRCA1/2* Carrier Cohort Study (IBCCS) collaborators group. Age at menarche and menopause and breast cancer risk in the International *BRCA1/2* Carrier Cohort Study. *Cancer Epidemiol Biomarkers Prev* 2007;16:740-746.

Chen CL, Weiss NS, Newcomb P, Barlow W, White E. Hormone replacement therapy in relation to breast cancer. *JAMA* 2002;287:734-741.

Chen WY, Manson JE, Hankinson SE, et al. Unopposed estrogen therapy and the risk of invasive breast cancer. *Arch Intern Med* 2006;166:1027-1032.

Chez Z, Maricic M, Bassford TL, et al. Fracture risk among breast cancer survivors: results from the Women's Health Initiative Study. *Arch Intern Med* 2005;165:552-558.

Chlebowski RT, Chen Z, Anderson GL, et al. Ethnicity and breast cancer: factors influencing differences in incidence and outcome. *J Natl Cancer Inst* 2005;97:439-448.

Chlebowski RT, Hendrix SL, Langer RD, et al, for the WHI investigators. Influence of estrogen plus progestin on breast cancer and mammography in healthy postmenopausal women: the Women's Health Initiative Randomized Trial. *JAMA* 2003;289:3243-3253.

Coates AS, Keshaviah A, Thurlimann B, et al. Five years of letrozole compared with tamoxifen as initial adjuvant therapy for postmenopausal women with endocrine-responsive early breast cancer: Update of study BIG 1-98. *J Clin Oncol* 2007;25:486-492.

Colditz GA, Hankinson SE, Hunter DJ, et al. Estrogen replacement therapy and progestins and the risk of breast cancer in postmenopausal women. *N Engl J Med* 1995;332:1589-1593.

Colditz GA, Rosner B. Cumulative risk of breast cancer to age 70 years according to risk factor status: data from the Nurses' Health Study. *Am J Epidemiol* 2000;152:950-964.

Collaborative Group on Hormone Factors in Breast Cancer. Breast cancer and hormone replacement therapy: collaborative re-analysis of data from 51 epidemiological studies of 52,705 women with breast cancer and 108,411 women without breast cancer [erratum in: *Lancet* 1997;350:1484]. *Lancet* 1997;350:1047-1059.

Committee on Gynelogical Practice. Risk of breast cancer with estrogen-progestin replacement therapy. ACOG committee opinion (no. 262). *Obstet Gynecol* 2001;98:1181-1184.

Committee on Gynecological Practice. Tamoxifen and endometrial cancer. ACOG committee opinion. *Int J Gynaecol Obstet* 2001;73:77-79.

Conner P. Breast response to menopausal hormone therapy—aspects on proliferation apoptosis, and mammographic density. *Ann Med* 2007;39:28-41.

Conner P, Svane G, Azavedo E, et al. Mammographic breast density, hormones, and growth factors during continuous combined hormone therapy. *Fertil Steril* 2004;81:1617-1623.

Coombes RC, Hall E, Gibson JL, et al. A randomized trial of exemestane after two to three years of tamoxifen therapy in postmenopausal women with primary breast cancer. *N Engl J Med* 2004;350:1081-1092.

Costantino JP, Kuller LH, Ives DG, Fisher B, Dignam J. Coronary heart disease mortality and adjuvant tamoxifen therapy. *J Natl Cancer Inst* 1997;89:776-782.

Cummings SR, Eckert S, Krueger KA, et al. The effect of raloxifene on risk of breast cancer in postmenopausal women: results from the MORE randomized trial. Multiple Outcomes of Raloxifene Evaluation [erratum in: *JAMA* 1999;282:2124]. *JAMA* 1999;281:2189-2197.

Cuzick J, Forbes JF, Sestak I, et al, for the International Breast Cancer Intervention Study I Investigators. Long-term results of tamoxifen prophylaxis for breast cancer–96 month follow-up of the IBIS-I trial. *J Natl Cancer Inst* 2007;99:272-282.

Day R, Ganz PA, Costantino JP, Cronin WM, Wickerham DL, Fisher B. Health-related quality of life and tamoxifen in breast cancer prevention: a report from the National Surgical Adjuvant Breast and Bowel Project P-1 study. *J Clin Oncol* 1999;17:2659-2669.

Delmas PD, Bjarnason NH, Mitlak BH, et al. Effects of raloxifene on bone mineral density, serum cholesterol concentrations, and uterine endometrium in postmenopausal women. *N Engl J Med* 1997;337:1641-1647.

DiSaia PJ, Brewster WR, Ziogas A, Anton-Culver H. Breast cancer survival and hormone replacement therapy: a cohort analysis. *Am J Clin Oncol* 2000;23:541-545.

Dupont WD, Page DL, Parl FF, et al. Estrogen replacement therapy in women with a history of proliferative breast disease. *Cancer* 1999;85:1279-1283.

Erel CT, Senturk LM, Kaleli S. Tibolone and breast cancer. *Postgrad Med* 2006;82:658-662.

Evista [package insert]. Eli Lilly and Company, 2007.

Fabian CJ, Kimler BF, Zalles CM, et al. Short-term breast cancer prediction by random periareolar fine-needle aspiration cytology and the Gail risk model. *J Natl Cancer Inst* 2000;92:1217-1227.

Fisher B, Costantino J, Wickerham D, et al. Tamoxifen for the prevention of breast cancer: report of the NSABP Project P-1. *J Natl Cancer Inst* 1998; 90:1371-1388.

Fisher B, Dignam J, Bryant J, et al. Five versus more than five years of tamoxifen therapy for breast cancer patients with negative lymph nodes and estrogen receptor-positive tumors. *J Natl Cancer Inst* 1996;88:1529-1542.

Fletcher AS, Erbas B, Kavanagh AM, Hart S, Rodger A, Gertig DM. Use of hormone replacement therapy (HRT) and survival following breast cancer diagnosis. *Breast* 2005;14:192-200.

Fournier A, Berrino F, Riboli E, Avenel V, Clavel-Chapelon F. Breast cancer risk in relation to different types of hormone replacement therapy in the E3N-EPIC cohort. *Intl J Cancer* 2004;114:448-454.

Friedenreich CM, Bryant HE, Courneya KS. Case-control study of lifetime physical activity and breast cancer. *Am J Epidemiol* 2001;154:336-347.

Friedenreich CM, Rohan TE. A review of physical activity and breast cancer. *Epidemiology* 1995;6:311-317.

Gail MH, Brinton LA, Byar DP, et al. Projecting individualized probabilities of developing breast cancer for white females examined annually. *J Natl Cancer Inst* 1989;81:1879-1886.

Ganz PA, Desmond KA, Belin TR, Meyerowitz BE, Rowland JH. Predictors of sexual health in women after a breast cancer diagnosis. *J Clin Oncol* 1999;17:2371-2380.

Ganz PA, Greendale GA, Kahn B, et al. Are older breast carcinoma survivors willing to take hormone replacement therapy? *Cancer* 1999;86:814-820.

Ganz PA, Greendale GA, Petersen L, et al. Managing menopausal symptoms in breast cancer survivors: results of a randomized controlled trial. *J Natl Cancer Inst* 2000;92:1054-1064.

Ganz PA, Rowland JH, Desmond K, Meyerowitz BE, Wyatt GE. Life after breast cancer: understanding women's health-related quality of life and sexual functioning. *J Clin Oncol* 1998;16:501-514.

Gapster SM, Morrow M, Sellars TA. Hormone replacement therapy and risk of breast cancer with a favorable histology: results of the Iowa Women's Health Study. *JAMA* 1999;281:2091-2097.

Garland CF, Garland FC, Gorham ED, et al. The role of vitamin D in cancer prevention. *Am J Public Health* 2006;96:252-261.

Gnant MFX, Mlineritsch B, Luschin-Ebengreuth, et al. Zoledronic acid prevents cancer treatment-induced bone loss in premenopausal women receiving adjuvant endocrine therapy for hormone-responsive breast cancer: A report from the Austrian breast and colorectal cancer study group. *J Clin Oncol* 2007;25:820-828.

Goldberg RM, Loprinzi CL, O'Fallon JR, et al. Transdermal clonidine for ameliorating tamoxifen-induced hot flashes [erratum in: *J Clin Oncol* 1996;14:2411]. *J Clin Oncol* 1994;12:155-158.

Goodwin PJ, Ennis M, Pritchard KI, et al. Adjuvant treatment and onset of menopause predict weight gain after breast cancer diagnosis. *J Clin Oncol* 1999;17:120-129.

Goodwin PJ, Ennis M, Pritchard KI, Trudeau M, Hood N. Risk of menopause during the first year after breast cancer diagnosis. *J Clin Oncol* 1999; 17:2365-2370.

Goss PE, Ingle JN, Martino S, et al. Randomized trial of letrozole following tamoxifen as extended adjuvant therapy in receptor-positive breast cancer; updated findings from NCIC CTG MA.17. *J Natl Cancer Inst* 2005; 97:1262-1271.

Greendale GA, Reboussin BA, Sie A, et al, for the Postmenopausal Estrogen/Progestin Interventions (PEPI) Investigators. Effects of estrogen and estrogen-progestin on mammographic parenchymal density. *Ann Intern Med* 1999;130:262-269.

Hartmann LC, Sellers TA, Frost MH, et al. Benign breast disease and the risk of breast cancer. *N Engl J Med* 2005;353:229-237.

Harvey J, Scheuerer C, Kawakami FT, Quebe-Fehling E, de Palacios PI, Ragavan VV. Hormone replacement therapy and breast density changes. *Climacteric* 2005;8:185-192.

Hershman D, Sundararajan V, Jacobson JS, et al. Outcomes of tamoxifen chemoprevention for breast cancer in very high-risk women: A cost-effectiveness analysis. *J Clin Oncol* 2002;20:9-16.

Holmberg L, Anderson H, for the HABITS steering and data monitoring committees. HABITS (hormonal replacement therapy after breast cancer—is it safe?), a randomised comparison: trial stopped. *Lancet* 2004;363:453-455.

Holmgren PA, Lindskog M, von Schoultz B. Vaginal rings for continuous low-dose release of oestradiol in the treatment of urogenital atrophy. *Maturitas* 1989;11:55-63.

Howell A, Cuzick J, Baum M, et al. Results of the ATAC (Arimidex, Tamoxifen, Alone or in Combination) trial after completion of 5 years' adjuvant treatment for breast cancer. *Lancet* 2005;365:60-62.

Huang Z, Hankinson SE, Colditz GA, et al. Dual effects of weight and weight gain on breast cancer risk. *JAMA* 1997;278:1407-1411.

Hughes KS, Schnaper LA, Berry D, et al, for the Cancer and Leukemia Group B, Radiation Therapy Oncology Group, and Eastern Cooperative Oncology Group. Lumpectomy plus tamoxifen with or without irradiation in women 70 years of age or older with early breast cancer. *N Engl J Med* 2004;351:971-977.

Hulley S, Furberg C, Barrett-Connor E, et al, for the HERS Research Group. Noncardiovascular disease outcomes during 6.8 years of hormone therapy: Heart and Estrogen/progestin Replacement Study follow-up (HERS II). *JAMA* 2002;288:58-66.

Jordan V. Optimising endocrine approaches for the chemoprevention of breast cancer beyond the Study of Tamoxifen and Raloxifene (STAR) trial. *Eur J Cancer* 2006;42:2909-2913.

Kanis JA, McCloskey EV, Powles T, et al. A high incidence of vertebral fracture in women with breast cancer. *Br J Cancer* 1999;79:1179-1181.

Kauff ND, Satagopan JM, Robson ME, et al. Risk-reducing salpingo-oophorectomy in women with a *BRCA1* or *BRCA2* mutation. *N Engl J Med* 2002;346:1609-1615.

Kavanagh AM, Mitchell H, Giles GG. Hormone replacement therapy and accuracy of mammographic screening. *Lancet* 2000;355:270-274.

Kedar RP, Bourne TH, Powles TJ, et al. Effects of tamoxifen on uterus and ovaries of postmenopausal women in a randomised breast cancer prevention trial. *Lancet* 1994;343:1318-1321.

Kerlikowske K, Ichikawa L, Miglioretti DL, et al, for the National Institutes of Health Breast Cancer Surveillance Consortium. Longitudinal measurement of clinical mammographic breast density to improve estimation of breast cancer risk. *J Natl Cancer Inst* 2007;99:386-395.

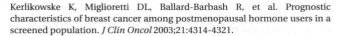

Kerlikowske K, Miglioretti DL, Ballard-Barbash R, et al. Prognostic characteristics of breast cancer among postmenopausal hormone users in a screened population. *J Clin Oncol* 2003;21:4314-4321.

Key J, Hodgson S, Omar RZ, et al. Meta-analysis of studies of alcohol and breast cancer with consideration of the methodological issues. *Cancer Causes Control* 2006;17:759-770.

Knekt P, Jarvinen R, Seppanen R, Pukkala E, Aromaa A. Intake of dairy products and the risk of breast cancer. *Br J Cancer* 1996;73:687-691.

Knight JA, Martin LJ, Greenberg CV, et al. Macronutrient intake and change in mammographic density at menopause: results from a randomized trial. *Cancer Epidemiol Biomarkers Prev* 1999;8:123-128.

Kriege M, Brekelmans CTM, Boetes C, et al, for the Magnetic Resonance Imaging Screening Study Guide. Efficacy of MRI and mammography for breast-cancer screening in women with a familial or genetic predisposition. *N Engl J Med* 2004;351:427-437.

Land SR, Wickerham DL, Costantino JP, et al. Patient-reported symptoms and quality of life during treatment with tamoxifen or raloxifene for breast cancer prevention: the NSABP Study of Tamoxifen and Raloxifene (STAR) P-2 trial. *JAMA* 2006;295:2742-2751.

Larsson SC, Giovannucci E, Wolk A. Folate and risk of breast cancer: a meta-analysis. *J Natl Cancer Inst* 2007;99:64-76.

Laya MB, Larson EB, Taplin SH, White E. Effect of estrogen replacement therapy on the specificity and sensitivity of screening mammography. *J Natl Cancer Inst* 1996;88:643-649.

Lehman CD, Gatsonis C, Kuhl CK, et al. MRI evaluation of the contralateral breast in women with recently diagnosed breast cancer. *N Engl J Med* 2007; 356:1295-1303.

Li CI, Malone KE, Porter PL, et al. Relationship between long durations and different regimens of hormone therapy and risk of breast cancer. *JAMA* 2003; 289:3254-3263.

Li CI, Weiss NS, Stanford JL, Daling JR. Hormone replacement therapy in relation to risk of lobular and ductal breast carcinoma in middle-aged women. *Cancer* 2000;88:2570-2577.

Lippman ME, Krueger KA, Eckert S, et al. Indicators of lifetime estrogen exposure: effect on breast cancer incidence and interaction with raloxifene therapy in the multiple outcomes of raloxifene evaluation study participants. *J Clin Oncol* 2001;19:3111-3116.

Lochner DM, Brubaker KL. Incidence of malignancy in hormone therapy users with indeterminate calcifications on mammogram. *Am J Obstet Gynecol* 2006;194:82-85.

Longnecker MP, Newcomb PA, Mittendorf R, et al. Risk of breast cancer in relation to lifetime alcohol consumption. *J Natl Cancer Inst* 1995;87:923-929.

Loprinzi CL, Abu-Ghazaleh S, Sloan JA, et al. Phase III randomized double-blind study to evaluate the efficacy of a polycarbophil-based vaginal moisturizer in women with breast cancer. *J Clin Oncol* 1997;15:969-973.

Loprinzi CL, Kugler JW, Sloan JA, et al. Venlafaxine in management of hot flashes in survivors of breast cancer: a randomised controlled trial. *Lancet* 2000;356:2059-2063.

Loprinzi CL, Michalak JC, Quella SK, et al. Megestrol acetate for the prevention of hot flashes. *N Engl J Med* 1994;331:347-352.

Lyytinen H, Pukkala E, Ylikorkala. Breast cancer risk in postmenopausal women using estrogen-only therapy. *Obstet Gynecol* 2006;108:1354-1360.

Magnusson C, Baron JA, Correia N, Bergström R, Adami HO, Persson I. Breast cancer risk following long-term oestrogen- and oestrogen-progestin-replacement therapy. *Int J Cancer* 1999;81:339-344.

Martino S, Cauley JA, Barrett-Connor E, et al, for the CORE investigators. Continuing outcomes relevant to EVISTA: Breast cancer incidence in postmenopausal osteoporotic women in a randomized trial of raloxifene. *J Natl Cancer Inst* 2004;96:1751-1761.

McTiernan A, Kooperberg C, White E, et al, for the Women's Health Initiative Cohort Study. Recreational physical activity and the risk of breast cancer in postmenopausal women: the Women's Health Initiative Cohort Study. *JAMA* 2003;290:1331-1336.

Meyerowitz BE, Desmond KA, Rowland JH, et al. Sexuality following breast cancer. *J Sex Marital Ther* 1999;25:237-250.

Million Women Study Collaborators. Breast cancer and hormone-replacement therapy in the Million Women Study. *Lancet* 2003;362:419-427.

Naessen T, Rodriguez-Macias K. Menopausal estrogen therapy counteracts normal aging effects on intima thickness, media thickness and intima/media ratio in carotid and femoral arteries. *Atherosclerosis* 2006;189:387-392.

National Cancer Institute. Breast cancer risk assessment tool. Available at: http://bcra.nci.nih.gov/brc. Accessed August 16, 2007.

National Cancer Institute. Screening for breast cancer (Last date modified 02/20/2004). Available at: http://www.cancer.gov/cancerinfo/pdq/screening/breast/healthprofessional. Accessed June 26, 2007.

National Cancer Institute of Canada. *Canadian Cancer Statistics 2002.* Toronto, ON, Canada: National Cancer Institute of Canada, 2002.

Natrajan PK, Soumakis K, Gambrell RD Jr. Estrogen replacement therapy in women with previous breast cancer. *Obstet Gynecol* 1999;181:288-295.

Negri E, Tzonou A, Beral V, et al. Hormonal therapy for menopause and ovarian cancer in a collaborative re-analysis of European studies. *Int J Cancer* 1999;80:848-851.

Newcomb PA, Longnecker MP, Storer BE, et al. Long-term hormone replacement therapy and risk of breast cancer in postmenopausal women. *Am J Epidemiol* 1995;142:788-795.

The North American Menopause Society. Estrogen and progestogen use in peri- and postmenopausal women: March 2007 position statement of The North American Menopause Society. *Menopause* 2007;14:168-182.

The North American Menopause Society. Role of progestogen in hormone therapy for postmenopausal women: position statement of The North American Menopause Society. *Menopause* 2003;10:113-132.

The North American Menopause Society. Treatment of menopause-associated vasomotor symptoms: position statement of The North American Menopause Society. *Menopause* 2004;11:11-33.

Olsen O, Gøtzsche PC. Cochrane review on screening for breast cancer with mammography. *Lancet* 2001;358:1340-1342.

Olsson HL, Ingvar C, Bladstrom A. Hormone replacement therapy containing progestins and given continuously increases breast carcinoma risk in Sweden. *Cancer* 2003;97:1387-1392.

Persson I, Yuen J, Bergkvist L, Shairer C. Cancer incidence and mortality in women receiving estrogen and estrogen-progestin replacement therapy: long-term follow-up of a Swedish cohort. *Int J Cancer* 1996;67:327-332.

Powles TJ, Ashley S, Tidy A, Smith IE, Dowsett M. Twenty-year follow-up of the Royal Marsden randomized, double-blinded tamoxifen breast cancer prevention trial. *J Natl Cancer Inst* 2007;99:283-290.

Powles TJ, Hickish T, Kanis JA, et al. Effect of tamoxifen on bone mineral density measured by dual-energy x-ray absorptiometry in healthy premenopausal and postmenopausal women. *J Clin Oncol* 1996;14:78-84.

Prentice RL, Caan B, Chlebowski RT, et al, for the Women's Health Initiative Investigators. Low-fat dietary pattern and risk of invasive breast cancer: the Women's Health Initiative randomized controlled Dietary Modification Trial. *JAMA* 2006;295:629-642.

Ravdin PM, Cronin KA, Howlader N, et al. The decrease in breast-cancer incidence in 2003 in the United States. *N Engl J Med* 2007;356:1670-1674.

Rebbeck TR, Friebel T, Wagner T, et al, for the Prose Study Group. Effect of short-term hormone replacement therapy on breast cancer risk reduction after bilateral prophylactic oophorectomy in *BRCA1* and *BRCA2* mutation carriers. *J Clin Oncol* 2005;23:7804-7810.

Rebbeck TR, Lynch HT, Neuhausen SL, et al, for the Prevention and Observation of Surgical End Points Study Group. Prophylactic oophorectomy in carriers of *BRCA1* or *BRCA2* mutations. *N Engl J Med* 2002;346:1616-1622.

Rosenberg L, Palmer JR, Wise LA, Adams-Campbell LL. A prospective study of female hormone use and breast cancer among black women. *Arch Intern Med* 2006;166:760-765.

Rosenberg RD, Hunt WC, Williamson MR, et al. Effects of age, breast density, ethnicity, and estrogen replacement therapy on screening mammographic sensitivity and cancer stage at diagnosis: review of 183,134 screening mammograms in Albuquerque, New Mexico. *Radiology* 1998;209:511-518.

Ross RK, Paganini-Hill A, Wan PC, Pike MC. Effect of hormone replacement therapy on breast cancer risk: estrogen versus estrogen plus progestogen. *J Natl Cancer Inst* 2000;92:328-332.

Roubidoux MA, Wilson TE, Orange RJ, Fitzgerald JT, Helvie MA, Packer SA. Breast cancer in women who undergo screening mammography: relationship of hormone replacement therapy to stage and detection method. *Radiology* 1998;208:725-728.

Saslow D, Boetes C, Burke W, et al. American Cancer Society guidelines for breast screening with MRI as an adjunct to mammography. *CA Cancer J Clin* 2007;57:75-89.

Schagen SB, van Dam FS, Muller MJ, et al. Cognitive deficits after postoperative adjuvant chemotherapy for breast carcinoma. *Cancer* 1999;85:640-650.

Schairer C, Gail M, Byrne C, et al. Estrogen replacement therapy and breast cancer survival in a large screening study. *J Natl Cancer Inst* 1999;91:264-270.

Schairer C, Lubin J, Troisi R, Sturgeon S, Brinton L, Hoover R. Menopausal estrogen and estrogen-progestin replacement therapy and breast cancer risk. *JAMA* 2000;283:485-491.

Sellers TA, Mink PJ, Cerhan JR, et al. The role of hormone replacement therapy in the risk for breast cancer and total mortality in women with a family history of breast cancer. *Ann Intern Med* 1997;127:973-980.

Shantakumar S, Terry MB, Paykin A, et al. Age and menopausal effects of hormonal birth control and hormone replacement therapy in relation to breast cancer risks. *Am J Epidemiol* 2007;165:1187-1198.

Singletary KW, Gapstur SM. Alcohol and breast cancer: review of epidemiologic and experimental evidence and potential mechanisms. *JAMA* 2001;286:2143-2151.

Smith RA, Saslow D, Sawyer KA, et al, for the Breast Cancer Advisory Group. American Cancer Society guidelines for breast cancer screening: update 2003. *CA Cancer J Clin* 2003;54:141-169.

Speroff L. Endometrial cancer—surprising reports. *Maturitas* 2005; 51:329-333.

Speroff L. Postmenopausal estrogen-progestin therapy and breast cancer: a clinical response to epidemiological reports. *Climacteric* 2000;3:3-12.

Stanford JL, Weiss NS, Voigt LF, Daling JR, Habel LA, Rossing MA. Combined estrogen and progestin hormone replacement therapy in relation to risk of breast cancer in middle-aged women. *JAMA* 1995;274:137-142.

Stefanick ML, Anderson GL, Margolis KL et al, for the Women's Health Initiative Investigators. Effects of conjugated equine estrogens on breast cancer and mammography screening in postmenopausal women with hysterectomy: the Women's Health Initiative. *JAMA* 2006;295:1647-1657.

Tamimi RM, Hankinson SE, Chen WY, Rosner B, Colditz GA. Combined estrogen and testosterone use and risk of breast cancer in postmenopausal women. *Arch Intern Med* 2006;166:1483-1489.

Tilanus-Linthorst MM, Obdeijn IM, Bartels KC, de Koning HJ, Oudkirk M. First experiences in screening women at high risk for breast cancer with MR imaging. *Breast Cancer Res Treat* 2000;63:53-60.

Ursin G, Ma H, Wu AH, et al. Mammographic density and breast cancer in three ethnic groups. *Cancer Epidemiol Biomarkers Prev* 2003;12:332-338.

US Preventive Services Task Force. Screening for breast cancer: recommendations and rationale. *Ann Intern Med* 2002;137:344-346.

van Dam FS, Schagen SB, Muller MJ, et al. Impairment of cognitive function in women receiving adjuvant treatment for high-risk breast cancer: high-dose versus standard-dose chemotherapy. *J Natl Cancer Inst* 1998;90:210-218.

Van Duijnhoven FJB, Peeters PHM, Warren RML, et al. Postmenopausal hormone therapy and changes in mammographic density. *J Clin Oncol* 2007;25:1323-1328.

Van Leeuwen FE, Klokman WJ, Stovall M, et al. Roles of radiation dose, chemotherapy, and hormonal factors in breast cancer following Hodgkin's disease. *J Natl Cancer Inst* 2003;95:971-980.

Vogel VG, Costantino JP, Wickerham DL, et al, for the National Surgical Adjuvant Breast and Bowel Project (NSABP). Effects of tamoxifen vs raloxifene on the risk of developing invasive breast cancer and other disease outcomes. The NSABP Study of Tamoxifen and Raloxifene (STAR) P-2 trial. *JAMA* 2006;295:2727-2741.

von Schoultz E, Rutqvist LE, for the Stockholm Breast Cancer Study Group. Menopausal hormone therapy after breast cancer: the Stockholm Randomized Trial. *J Natl Cancer Inst* 2005;97:533-535.

Wagner TM, Moslinger RA, Muhr D, et al. *BRCA1*-related breast cancer in Austrian breast and ovarian cancer families: specific *BRCA1* mutations and pathological characteristics. *Int J Cancer* 1998;77:354-360.

Walsh T, Casadei S, Coats KH, Swisher E, et al. Spectrum of mutations in *BRCA1, BRCA2, CHEK2,* and *TP53* in families at high risk of breast cancer. *JAMA* 2006;295:1379-1388.

Weiss LK, Burkman RT, Cushing-Haugen KL, et al. Hormone replacement therapy regimens and breast cancer risk. *Obstet Gynecol* 2002;100:1148-1158.

Wile AG, Opfell RW, Margileth DA. Hormone replacement therapy in previously treated breast cancer patients. *Am J Surg* 1993;165:372-375.

Writing Group for the Women's Health Initiative Investigators. Risks and benefits of estrogen plus progestin in healthy postmenopausal women: principal results from the Women's Health Initiative randomized controlled trial. *JAMA* 2002;288:321-333.

Zhang S, Hunter DJ, Hankinson SE, et al. A prospective study of folate intake and the risk of breast cancer. *JAMA* 1999;281:1632-1637.

Zheng W, Gustafson DR, Sinha R, et al. Well-done meat intake and the risk of breast cancer. *J Natl Cancer Inst* 1998;90:1724-1729.

Endometrial cancer

Acharya S, Hensley ML, Montag AC, et al. Rare uterine tumors. *Lancet Oncol* 2005;6:961-971.

Anderson GL, Judd HL, Kaunitz AM, et al, for the Women's Health Initiative Investigators. Effects of estrogen plus progestin on gynecologic cancers and associated diagnostic procedures: the Women's Health Initiative Randomized Trial. *JAMA* 2003;290:1739-1748.

Archer DF, Hendrix S, Gallagher JC, et al. Endometrial effects of tibolone. *J Clin Endocrinol Metab* 2007;92:911-918.

Barakat RR, Bundy BN, Spirtos NM, Bell J, Mannel RS, for the Gynecologic Oncology Group Study. Randomized double-blind trial of estrogen replacement therapy versus placebo in stage I or II endometrial cancer: a Gynecologic Oncology Group study. *J Clin Oncol* 2006;24:587-592.

Belisle S, Derzko C. Hormone replacement therapy and cancer: Canadian consensus on menopause and osteoporosis. *J SOGC* 2001;23:1198-1203.

Beral V, Bull D, Reeves G, for the Million Women Study Collaborators. Endometrial cancer and hormone-replacement therapy in the Million Women Study. *Lancet* 2005;365:1543-1551.

Beresford SA, Weiss NS, Voigt LF, McKnight B. Risk of endometrial cancer in relation to use of oestrogen combined with cyclic progestogen therapy in postmenopausal women. *Lancet* 1997;349:458-461.

Bernstein L. The risk of breast, endometrial and ovarian cancer in users of hormonal preparations. *Basic Clin Pharmacol Toxic* 2006;98:288-296.

Bertelli G, Venturini M, Del Mastro L, et al. Tamoxifen and the endometrium: findings of pelvic examination and endometrial biopsy in asymptomatic breast cancer patients. *Breast Cancer Res Treat* 1998;47:41-46.

Calle EE, Rodriguez C, Walker-Thurmond K, et al. Overweight, obesity, mortality from cancer in a prospectively studied cohort of US adults. *N Engl J Med* 2003;348;1625-1638.

Cecchini S, Ciatto S, Bonardi R, et al. Screening by ultrasonography for endometrial carcinoma in postmenopausal breast cancer patients under adjuvant tamoxifen. *Gynecol Oncol* 1996;60:409-411.

Cicinelli E, de Ziegler D, Galantino P, et al. Twice-weekly transdermal estradiol and vaginal progesterone as continuous combined hormone replacement therapy in postmenopausal women: a 1-year prospective study. *Am J Obstet Gynecol* 2002;187:556-560.

Clark TJ, Barton PM, Coomarasamy A, Gupta JK, Khan KS. Investigating postmenopausal bleeding for endometrial cancer: cost-effectiveness of initial diagnostic strategies. *BJOG* 2006;113:502-510.

Clevenger-Hoeft M, Syrop CH, Stovall DW, et al. Sonohysterography in premenopausal women with and without abnormal bleeding. *Obstet Gynecol* 1999;94:516-520.

Committee on Gynecologic Practice. Hormone replacement therapy in women treated for endometrial cancer. ACOG committee opinion (no. 234). *Int J Gynaecol Obstet* 2001;73:283-284.

Committee on Gynecologic Practice. Tamoxifen and endometrial cancer. ACOG committee opinion (no. 232). *Int J Gynaecol Obstet* 2001;73:77-79.

Creasman WT, Henderson D, Hinshaw W, Clarke-Pearson DL. Estrogen replacement therapy in the patient treated for endometrial cancer. *Obstet Gynecol* 1986;67:326-330.

Daly E, Vessey MP, Hawkins MM, Carson JL, Gough P, Marsh S. Risk of venous thromboembolism in users of hormone replacement therapy. *Lancet* 1996;348:977-980.

de Lignieres B. Endometrial hyperplasia: risks, recognition and the search for a safe hormone replacement regimen. *J Reprod Med* 1999;44:191-196.

Dijkhuizen FP, Mol BW, Brolmann HA, Heinz AP. The accuracy of endometrial sampling in the diagnosis of patients with endometrial carcinoma and hyperplasia: a meta-analysis. *Cancer* 2000;89:1765-1772.

Doherty JA, Cushing-Haugen KL, Saltzman BS, et al. Long-term use of postmenopausal estrogen and progestin hormone therapies and the risk of endometrial cancer. *Am J Obstet Gynecol* 2007;197:139.e1-e7.

Ferguson SE, Soslow RA, Amsterdam A, et al. Comparison of uterine malignancies that develop during and following tamoxifen therapy. *Gynecol Oncol* 2006;101:322-326.

Goldstein RB, Bree RL, Benson CB, et al. Evaluation of the woman with postmenopausal bleeding. *J Ultrasound Med* 2001;20:1025-1036.

Henderson BE, Casagrande JT, Pike MC, Mack T, Rosario I, Duke A. The epidemiology of endometrial cancer in young women. *Br J Cancer* 1983;47:749-756.

Hill DA, Weiss NA, Beresford SA, et al. Continuous combined hormone replacement therapy and risk of endometrial cancer. *Am J Obstet Gynecol* 2000;183:1456-1461.

Huang GS, Gebb JS, Einstein MH, et al. Accuracy of preoperative endometrial sampling for the detection of high-grade endometrial tumors. *Am J Obstet Gynecol* 2007;196:243-244.

Jirecek S, Lee A, Pavo I, Crans G, Eppel W, Wenzl R. Raloxifene prevents the growth of uterine leiomyomas in premenopausal women. *Fertil Steril* 2004;81:132-136.

Judd HL, Lucas WE, Yen SS. Effect of oophorectomy on circulating testosterone and androstenedione levels in patients with endometrial cancer. *Am J Obstet Gynecol* 1974;118:793-798.

Kaunitz AM, Masciello A, Ostrowski M, et al. Comparison of endometrial biopsy with the endometrial Pipelle and Vabra aspirator. *J Reprod Med* 1988;33:427-431.

Kurman RJ, Kaminski PF, Norris HJ. The behavior of endometrial hyperplasia. A long-term study of "untreated" hyperplasia in 170 patients. *Cancer* 1985;56:403-412.

Langer RD, Pierce JJ, O'Hanlon KA, et al. Transvaginal ultrasonography compared with endometrial biopsy for the detection of endometrial disease. *N Engl J Med* 1997;337:1792-1798.

Lethaby A, Farquhar C, Sarkis A, Roberts H, Jepson R, Barlow D. Hormone replacement therapy in postmenopausal women: endometrial hyperplasia and irregular bleeding. *Cochrane Database Syst Rev* 2004;3:CD000402.

Magriples U, Naftolin F, Schwartz PE, Carcangiu ML. High-grade endometrial carcinoma in tamoxifen-treated breast cancer patients. *J Clin Oncol* 1993; 11:485-490.

Marchetti M, Vasile C, Chiarelli S. Endometrial cancer: asymptomatic endometrial findings. Characteristics of postmenopausal endometrial cancer. *Eur J Gynaecol Oncol* 2005;26:479-484.

Parsons AK, Londono JL. Detection and surveillance of endometrial hyperplasia and carcinoma. In: Lobo RA, ed. *Treatment of the Postmenopausal Woman: Basic and Clinical Aspects.* Philadelphia, PA: Lippincott Williams & Wilkins, 1999:513-538.

Reid RL. Progestins in hormone replacement therapy: impact on endometrial and breast cancer. *J SOGC* 2000;22:677-681.

Schlesselman J. Risk of endometrial cancer in relation to use of combined oral contraceptives. A practioner's guide to meta-analysis. *Hum Reprod* 1997;12:1851-1863.

Schwartz PE. The management of serous papillary uterine cancer. *Curr Opin Oncol* 2006;18:494-499.

Smith-Bindman R, Kerlikowske K, Feldstein VA, et al. Endovaginal ultrasound to exclude endometrial cancer and other endometrial abnormalities. *JAMA* 1998;280:1510-1517.

Soerjomataram I, deVries E, Pukkala E, Coebergh JW. Excess of cancers in Europe: a study of eleven major cancers amenable to lifestyle change. *Int J Cancer* 2007;120:1336-1343.

Spencer CP, Whitehead MI. Endometrial assessment re-visited. *Br J Obstet Gynaecol* 1999;106:623-632.

Speroff L. Endometrial cancer—surprising reports. *Maturitas* 2005; 51:329-333.

Stanford JL, Brinton LA, Berman ML, et al. Oral contraceptives and endometrial cancer: do other risk factors modify the association? *Int J Cancer* 1993;54:243-248.

Sturdee DW, Barlow DH, Ulrich LG, et al. Is the timing of withdrawal bleeding a guide to endometrial safety during sequential oestrogen-progestogen replacement therapy? UK Continuous Combined EPT Study Investigators. *Lancet* 1994;344:979-982.

von Gruenigen VE, Tian C, Frasure H, Waggoner S, Keys H, Barakat RR. Treatment effects, disease recurrence, and survival in obese women with early endometrial cancer. A Gyneocologic Oncology Group study. *Cancer* 2006;107:2786-2791.

Weber AM, Belinson JL, Piedmonte MR. Risk factors for endometrial hyperplasia and cancer among women with abnormal bleeding. *Obstet Gynecol* 1999;93:594-598.

The Women's Health Initiative Steering Committee. Effects of conjugated equine estrogen in postmenopausal women with hysterectomy: the Women's Health Initiative randomized controlled trial. *JAMA* 2004;291:1701-1712.

The Writing Group for the PEPI Trial. Effects of hormone replacement therapy on endometrial biopsy in postmenopausal women. *JAMA* 1996;275:370-375.

Cervical cancer

Anderson GL, Judd HL, Kaunitz AM, et al, for the Women's Health Initiative Investigators. Effects of estrogen plus progestin on gynecologic cancers and associated diagnostic procedures: the Women's Health Initiative randomized trial. *JAMA* 2003;290:1739-1748.

Day SJ, Deszo EL, Freund GG. Dual sampling of the endocervix and its impact on AutoCyte Prep endocervical adequacy. *Am J Clin Pathol* 2002;118:41-46.

Dunne EF, Unger ER, Sternberg M, et al. Prevalence of HPV infection among females in the United States. *JAMA* 2007;297:813-819.

Fox J, Remington P, Layde P, et al. The effect of hysterectomy on the risk of an abnormal screening Papanicolaou test result. *Am J Obstet Gynecol* 1999;180:1104-1109.

Lacey JV Jr, Brinton LA, Barnes WA, et al. Use of hormone replacement therapy and adenocarcinomas and squamous cell carcinomas of the uterine cervix. *Gynecol Oncol* 2000;77:149-154.

Papillo JL, Zarka MA, St. John TL. Evaluation of the ThinPrep Pap test in clinical practice. A seven-month, 16,314-case experience in northern Vermont. *Acta Cytol* 1998;42:203-208.

Pearce KF, Haefner HK, Sarwar SF, et al. Cytopathological findings on vaginal Papanicolaou smears after hysterectomy for benign gynecologic disease. *N Engl J Med* 1996;335:1559-1562.

Saslow D, Castle PE, Cox JT, et al, for the Gynecologic Cancer Advisory Group. American Cancer Society guideline for human papillomavirus (HPV) vaccine use to prevent cervical cancer and its precursors. *Ca Cancer J Clin* 2007; 57:7-28.

Sawaya GF, Grady D, Kerlikowske K, et al. The positive predictive value of cervical smears in previously screened postmenopausal women: the Heart and Estrogen/progestin Replacement Study (HERS). *Ann Intern Med* 2000;133:942-950.

Sawaya GF, McConnell KJ, Kulasingam SL, et al. Risk of cervical cancer associated with extending the interval between cervical-cancer screenings. *N Engl J Med* 2003;349:1501-1509.

Schiffman M, Solomon D. Findings to date from the ASCUS-LSIL Triage Study (ALTS). *Arch Pathol Lab Med* 2003;127:946-949.

Shi L, Sings HG, Bryan JT, et al. Gardasil®: Prophylactic human papilloma-virus vaccine development—from bench top to bed-side. *Discovery* 2007; 81:259-264.

Smith EM, Johnson SR, Ritchie JM, et al. Persistent HPV infection in postmenopausal age women. *Int J Gynecol Obstet* 2004;87:131-137.

Smith JS, Green J, Berrington de Gonzalez A, et al. Cervical cancer and use of hormonal contraceptives: a systematic review. *Lancet* 2003;361:1159-1167.

Stratton J, Pharoah P, Smith S, Easton D, Ponder B. A systematic review and meta-analysis of family history and risk of ovarian cancer. *Br J Obstet Gynaecol* 1998;105:493-499.

Villa LL, Costa RLR, Petta CA, et al. Prophylactic quadrivalent human papillomavirus (types 6, 11, 16, and 18) L1 virus-like particle vaccine in young women: a randomised double-blind placebo-controlled multicentre phase II efficacy trial. *Lancet Oncol* 2005;6:271-278.

Villa LL, Costa RLR, Petta CA, et al. High sustained efficacy of a prophylactic quadrivalent human papillomavirus type 6/11/16/18 L1 virus-like particle vaccine through 5 years of follow-up. *Br J Cancer* 2006;95:1459-1466.

Ovarian cancer

Ahmed N, Barker G, Oliva KT, et al. Proteomic-based identification of haptoglobin-1 precursor as a novel circulating biomarker of ovarian cancer. *Br J Cancer* 2004;91:129-140.

Beral V, for the Million Women Study Collaborators. Ovarian cancer and hormone replacement therapy in the Million Women Study. *Lancet* 2007;369:1703-1710.

Beral V, Hermon C, Kay C, Hannaford P, Darby S, Reeves G. Mortality associated with oral contraceptive use: 25 year follow up of cohort of 46,000 women from Royal College of General Practitioners' oral contraception study. *BMJ* 1999;318:96-100.

Bernstein L. The risk of breast, endometrial and ovarian cancer in users of hormonal preparations. *Basic Clin Pharmacol Toxicol* 2006;98:288-296.

Coughlin SS, Giustozzi A, Smith SJ, Lee NC. A meta-analysis of estrogen replacement therapy and risk of epithelial ovarian cancer. *J Clin Epidemiol* 2000;53:367-375.

Diamandis EP. Analysis of serum proteomic patterns for early cancer diagnosis: drawing attention to potential problems. *J Natl Cancer Inst* 2004;94:353-356.

Fathalla MF. Incessant ovulation—a factor in ovarian neoplasia? *Lancet* 1971;2:163.

Gertig DM, Hunter DJ, Cramer DW, et al. Prospective study of talc use and ovarian cancer. *J Natl Cancer Inst* 2000;92:249-252.

Godard B, Foulkes WD, Provencher D, et al. Risk factors for familial and sporadic ovarian cancer among French Canadians: a case-control study. *Am J Obstet Gynecol* 1998;179:403-410.

Goff BA, Mandel L, Melancon CH, et al. Frequency of symptoms of ovarian cancer in women presenting to primary care clinics. *JAMA* 2004;291:2705-2712.

Goff BA, Mandel L, Muntz HG, Melancon CH. Ovarian cancer diagnosis. *Cancer* 2000;89:2068-2075.

Greer JB, Modugno F, Allen GO, Ness RB. Androgenic progestins in oral contraceptives and the risk of epithelial ovarian cancer. *Obstet Gynecol* 2005;105:731-740.

Huddleston HG, Wong K-K, Welch WR, Berkowitz RS, Mok SC. Clinical applications of microarray technology: creatine kinase B is an up-regulated gene in epithelial ovarian cancer and shows promise as a tumor marker. *Gynecol Oncol* 2005;96:77-83.

Kotsopoulos J, Lubinski J, Neuhausen SL, et al. Hormone replacement therapy and the risk of ovarian cancer in *BRCA1* and *BRCA2* mutation carriers. *Gynecol Oncol* 2006;100:83-88.

Kumle M, Weiderpass E, Braaten T, Adami HO, Lund ME, Norwegian-Swedish Women's Lifestyle and Health Cohort study. Risk for invasive and borderline epithelial ovarian neoplasias following use of hormonal contraceptives: the Norwegian-Swedish Women's Lifestyle and Health Cohort study. *Br J Cancer* 2004;90:1386-1391.

Lacey JV Jr, Mink PJ, Lubin JH, et al. Menopausal hormone replacement therapy and risk of ovarian cancer. *JAMA* 2002;288:334-341.

La Vecchia C. Oral contraceptives and ovarian cancer: an update, 1998-2004. *Eur J Cancer Prev* 2006;15:117-124.

McGuire V, Felberg A, Mills M, et al. Relation of contraceptive and reproductive history to ovarian cancer risk in carriers and noncarriers of *BRCA1* gene mutations. *Am J Epidemiol* 2004;160:613-618.

Mor G, Visintin I, Lai V, et al. Serum protein markers for early detection of ovarian cancer. *Proc Natl Acad Sci USA* 2005;102:7677-7682.

Narod SA, Risch H, Moslehi R, et al. Oral contraceptives and the risk of hereditary ovarian cancer. *N Engl J Med* 1998;339:424-428.

Ness RB, Grisso JA, Klapper J, et al. Risk of ovarian cancer in relation to estrogen and progestin dose and use characteristics. *Am J Epidemiol* 2000;152:233-241.

Ness RB, Grisso JA, Vergona R, et al. Oral contraceptive, other methods of contraception and risk reduction for ovarian cancer. *Epidemiology* 2001; 12:307-312.

Petricoin EF, Ardekani AM, Hitt BA, et al. Use of proteomic patterns in serum to identify ovarian cancer. *Lancet* 2002;395:572-577.

Purdie DM, Siskind V, Bain CJ, Webb PM, Green AC. Reproduction-related risk factors for mucinous and nonmucinous epithelial ovarian cancer. *Am J Epidemiol* 2001;153:860-864.

Riman T, Persson I, Nilsson S. Hormonal aspects of epithelial ovarian cancer: review of epidemiologic evidence. *Clin Endocrinol* 1998;49:695-707.

Risch HA, Marrett LD, Jain M, Howe GR. Differences in risk factors for epithelial ovarian cancer by histologic type: results of a case-control study. *Am J Epidemiol* 1996;144:363-372.

Rodriguez C, Calle EE, Coates RJ, Miracle-McMahill HL, Thun MJ, Heath CW Jr. Hormone replacement therapy and fatal ovarian cancer. *Am J Epidemiol* 1995;141:828-835.

Rodriguez C, Patel AV, Calle EE, Jacob EJ, Thun MJ. Estrogen replacement therapy and ovarian cancer mortality in a large prospective study of US women. *JAMA* 2001;285:1460-1465.

Salazar-Martinez E, Lazcano-Ponce EC, Gonzalez Lira-Lira G, Escudero-De los Rios P, Salmeron-Castro J, Hernandez-Avila M. Reproductive factors of ovarian and endometrial cancer risk in a high fertility population in Mexico. *Cancer Res* 1999;59:3658-3662.

Tung KH, Goodman MT, Wu AH, et al. Reproductive factors and epithelial ovarian cancer risk by histologic type: a multiethnic case-control study. *Am J Epidemiol* 2003;158:629-638.

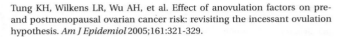

Tung KH, Wilkens LR, Wu AH, et al. Effect of anovulation factors on pre- and postmenopausal ovarian cancer risk: revisiting the incessant ovulation hypothesis. *Am J Epidemiol* 2005;161:321-329.

Vessey M, Painter R, Yeates D, et al. Mortality in relation to oral contraceptive use and cigarette smoking. *Lancet* 2003;362:185-191.

von Schoultz E, Rutqvist LE, for the Stockholm Breast Cancer Study Group. Menopausal hormone therapy after breast cancer: the Stockholm Randomized Trial. *J Natl Cancer Inst* 2005;97:533-535.

Wagner TM, Moslinger RA, Muhr D, et al. *BRCA1*-related breast cancer in Austrian breast and ovarian cancer families: specific *BRCA1* mutations and pathological characteristics. *Int J Cancer* 1998;77:354-360.

Whysner J, Mohan M. Perineal application of talc and cornstarch powders: evaluation of ovarian cancer risk. *Am J Obstet Gynecol* 2000;182:720-724.

Wong C, Hempling RE, Piver MS, Natarajan N, Mettlin CJ. Perineal talc exposure and subsequent epithelial ovarian cancer: a case-control study. *Obstet Gynecol* 1999;93:372-376.

Ye B, Cramer DW, Skates SJ, et al. Haptoglobin-alpha subunit as potential serum biomarker in ovarian cancer: identification and characterization using proteomic profiling and mass spectrometry. *Clin Cancer Res* 2003; 9:2904-2911.

Zhang Z, Bast RC Jr, Yu Y, et al. Three biomarkers identified from serum proteomic analysis for the detection of early stage ovarian cancer. *Cancer Res* 2004;64:5882-5890.

Colorectal cancer

Baron JA, Cole BF, Sandler RS, et al. A randomized trial to prevent colorectal adenomas. *N Engl J Med* 2003;348:891-899.

Beresford SAA, Johnson KC, Ritenbaugh NL, et al. Low-fat dietary pattern and risk of colorectal cancer. The Women's Health Initiative randomized controlled dietary modification trial. *JAMA* 2006;295:643-654.

Chan JA, Meyerhardt JA, Chan AT, Giovannucci EL, Colditz GA, Fuchs CS. Hormone replacement therapy and survival after colorectal cancer diagnosis. *J Clin Oncol* 2006;24:5680-5686.

Chlebowski RT, Wactawski-Wende J, Ritenbaugh C, et al, for the Women's Health Initiative Investigators. Estrogen plus progestin and colorectal cancer in postmenopausal women. *N Engl J Med* 2004;350:991-1004.

Cook NR, Lee IM, Gaziano JM, et al. Low-dose aspirin in the primary prevention of cancer. The Women's Health Study: a randomized controlled trial. *JAMA* 2005;294:47-55.

Gann PH, Manson JAE, Glynn RJ, Buring JE, Hennekens CH. Low-dose aspirin and incidence of colorectal tumors in a randomized trial. *J Natl Cancer Inst* 1993;85:1220-1224.

Gonzalez-Perez A, Rodriguez LAG, Lupez-Ridaura R. Effects of non-steroidal anti-inflammatory drugs on cancer sites other than the colon and rectum: a meta-analysis. *Cancer* 2003;3:28-40.

Imperiale TF, Wagner DR, Lin CY, Larkin GN, Rogge JD, Ransohoff DF. Risk of advanced proximal neoplasms in asymptomatic adults according to the distal colorectal findings. *N Engl J Med* 2000;343:169-174.

Lanza E, Schatzkin A, Daston C, et al. Implementation of a 4-y, high-fiber, high-fruit-and-vegetable, low-fat dietary intervention: results of dietary changes in the Polyp Prevention Trial. *Am J Clin Nutr* 2001;74:387-401.

Levin B, Brooks D, Smith RA, Stone A. Emerging technologies in screening for colorectal cancer: CT colonography, immunochemical fecal occult blood tests, and stool screening using molecular markers. *CA Cancer J Clin* 2003;53:44-55.

Lieberman DA, Weiss DG, Bond JH, Ahnen DJ, Garewal H, Chejfec G. Use of colonoscopy to screen asymptomatic adults for colorectal cancer. Veterans Affairs Cooperative Study Group 380. *N Engl J Med* 2000;343:162-168.

Park Y, Hunter DJ, Spiegelman D, et al. Dietary fiber intake and risk of colorectal cancer: a pooled analysis of prospective cohort studies. *JAMA* 2005;294:2849-2857.

Pickhardt PJ, Choi R, Hwang I, et al. Computed tomographic virtual colonoscopy to screen for colorectal neoplasia in asymptomatic adults. *N Engl J Med* 2003;349:2191-2200.

Robinson KL, Liu T, Vandrovcova J, et al. Lynch syndrome (hereditary non-polyposis colorectal cancer) diagnostics. *J Natl Cancer Inst* 2007;99:291-299.

Smith RA, Cokkinides V, Eyre HJ. American Cancer Society Guidelines for the early detection of cancer, 2006. *CA Cancer J Clin* 2006;56:11-25.

Wang WH, Huang JQ, Zheng GF, Lam SK, Karlberg J, Wong BC-Y. Non-steroidal anti-inflammatory drug use and the risk of gastric cancer: a systematic review and meta-analysis. *J Natl Cancer Inst* 2003;95:1784-1791.

Pancreatic cancer

Chan JM, Wang F, Holly EA. Vegetable and fruit intake and pancreatic cancer in a population-based case-control study in the San Francisco Bay area. *Cancer Epidemiol Biomarkers Prev* 2005;14:2093-2097.

Coughlin SS, Calle EE, Patel AV, Thun MJ. Predictors of pancreatic cancer mortality among a large cohort of United States adults. *Cancer Causes Control* 2000;11:915-923.

Khorana AA, Fine RL. Pancreatic cancer and thromboembolic disease. *Lancet Oncol* 2004;5:655-663.

Larsson SC, Permert J, Hakansson N, et al. Overall obesity, abdominal adiposity, diabetes, and cigarette smoking in relation to the risk of pancreatic cancer in two Swedish population-based cohorts. *Br J Cancer* 2005;93:1310-1315.

Lin YS, Tamakoshi A, Kawamura T, et al, for the JACC Study Group, Japan Collaborative Cohort. A prospective cohort study of cigarette smoking and pancreatic cancer in Japan. *Cancer Causes Control* 2002;13:249-254.

Michaud DS. Vitamin D and pancreatic cancer risk in the alpha-tocopherol, beta-carotene cancer prevention cohort. *Cancer Res* 2006;66:9802-9803.

Navarro Silvera SA, Miller AB, Rohan TE. Hormonal and reproductive factors and pancreatic cancer risk. *Pancreas* 2005;30:369-374.

Prizment AE, Anderson KE, Hong CP, Folsom AR. Pancreatic cancer incidence in relation to female reproductive factors: Iowa Women's Health Study. *JOP* 2007;8:16-27.

Rapp K, Schroeder J, Klenk J, et al. Obesity and the incidence of cancer: a large cohort study of over 145,000 adults in Austria. *Br J Cancer* 2005;93:1062-1067.

Skinner HG, Michaud DS, Giovannucci E, Willett WC, Colditz GA, Fuchs CS. Vitamin D intake and the risk for pancreatic cancer in two cohort studies. *Cancer Epidemiol Biomarkers Prev* 2006;15:1688-1695.

Stolzenberg-Solomon RZ, Vieth R, Azad A, et al. A prospective nested case-control study of vitamin D status and pancreatic cancer risk in male smokers. *Cancer Res* 2006;66:10213-10219.

Teras LR, Patel AV, Rodriguez C, Thun MJ, Calle EE. Parity, other reproductive factors, and risk of pancreatic cancer mortality in a large cohort of US women. *Cancer Causes Control* 2005;16:1035-1040.

Zell JA, Rhee JM, Ziogas A, Lipkin SM, Anton-Culver H. Race, socioeconomic status, treatment, and survival time among pancreatic cancer cases in California. *Cancer Epidemiol Biomarkers Prev* 2007;16:546-552.

Skin cancer

Dennis LK. Analysis of the melanoma epidemic, both apparent and real: data from the 1973 through 1994 Surveillance, Epidemiology, and End Results program registry. *Arch Dermatol* 1999;135:275-280.

Eide MJ, Weinstock MA. Public health challenges in sun protection. *Dermatol Clin* 2006;24:119-124.

Lowe NJ. An overview of ultraviolet radiation, sunscreens, and photo-induced dermatoses. *Dermatol Clin* 2006;24:9-17.

Poocharoen VN, Cockerell CJ. The war against skin cancer: the time for action is now. *Arch Dermatol* 2005;141:499-501.

Stanton WR, Janda M, Baade PD, Anderson P. Primary prevention of skin cancer: a review of sun protection in Australia and internationally. *Health Promot Int* 2004;19:369-378.

Weiss M, Loprinzi CL, Creagan ET, Dalton RJ, Novotny P, O'Fallon JR. Utility of follow-up tests for detecting recurrent disease in patients with malignant melanomas. *JAMA* 1995;274:1703-1705.

Sexually transmitted infections

Brook MG. Sexual transmission and prevention of the hepatitis viruses A-E and G. *Sex Transm Infect* 1998;74:395-398.

Centers for Disease Control and Prevention. *Chlamydia in the United States; April 2006.* Available at: http://www.cdc.gov/std/chlamydia/STDFact-Chlamydia.htm#Common. Accessed August 16, 2007.

Centers for Disease Control and Prevention. Update to CDC's sexually transmitted diseases treatment guidelines, 2006: fluoroquinolones no longer recommended for treatment of gonococcal infections. *Morb Mortal Wkly Rep (MMWR)* 2007;56:332-336.

Cohen MS. HIV and sexually transmitted diseases: the physician's role in prevention. *Postgrad Med* 1995;98:52-58.

Department of Health, United Kingdom. Cervical screening: launch of test for human papilloma virus (HPV) status; Jan 30, 1998. Available at: http://www.info.doh.gov.uk/doh/embroadcast.nsf/. Accessed August 16, 2007.

Elias C, Coggins C. Acceptability research on female-controlled barrier methods to prevent heterosexual transmission of HIV: Where have we been? Where are we going? *J Womens Health Gend Based Med* 2001;10:163-173.

Elias CJ, Coggins C. Female-controlled methods to prevent sexual transmission of HIV. *AIDS* 1996;10(Suppl):S43-S51.

Frame PT. HIV disease in primary care. *Prim Care* 2003;30:205-237.

Gilson RJ, Mindel A. Recent advances: sexually transmitted infections. *BMJ* 2001;322:1160-1164.

Holmes KK, Levine R, Weaver M. Effectiveness of condoms in preventing sexually transmitted infections. *Bull World Health Organ* 2004;82:454-461.

Holtgrave DR. The President's Fiscal Year 2007 Initiative for Human Immunodeficiency Virus Counseling and Testing Expansion in the United States: A Scenario Analysis of Its Coverage, Impact, and Cost-effectiveness. *J Public Health Manag Pract* 2007;13:239-243.

Holtgrave DR, Qualls NL, Curran JW, Valdiserri RO, Guinan ME, Parra WC. An overview of the effectiveness and efficacy of HIV prevention programs. *Public Health Rep* 1995;110:134-146.

Piper JM, Shain RN, Korte JE, Holden AEC. Behavioral interventions for prevention of sexually transmitted diseases in women: a physician's perspective. *Obstet Gynecol Clin North Am* 2003;30:659-669.

Pope V. Use of treponemal tests to screen for syphilis. *Infect Med* 2004; 21:399-402.

Reyes EM, Legg JJ. Prevention of HIV transmission. *Prim Care* 1997; 24:469-477.

Scoular A, Gillespie G, Carman WF. Polymerase chain reaction for diagnosis of genital herpes in genitourinal medicine clinic. *Sex Transmit Infect* 2002;78:21-25.

Shain RN, Perdue ST, Piper JM, et al. Behaviors changed by intervention are associated with reduced STD recurrence: the importance of context in measurement. *Sex Transm Dis* 2002;29:530-532.

Shepard CW, Simard EP, Finelli AE, Bell BP. Hepatitis B virus infection: epidemiology and vaccination. *Epidemiol Rev* 2006;28:112-125.

Stratton P, Alexander NJ. Prevention of sexually transmitted infections: physical and chemical barrier methods. *Infect Dis Clin North Am* 1993; 7:841-859.

US Preventive Services Task Force. Screening for chlamydial infection: recommendations and rationale. *Am J Prev Med* 2001;20:90-94.

Workowski KA, Berman SM. Centers for Disease Control and Prevention sexually transmitted diseases treatment guidelines. *Clin Infect Dis* 2007; 44(suppl 3):S73-76.

Wright TC Jr, Cox JT, Massad LS, Twiggs LB, Wilkinson EJ, for the ASCCP-sponsored consensus conference. 2001 consensus guidelines for the management of women with cervical cytological abnormalities. *JAMA* 2002;287:2120-2129.

Xu F, Sternberg MR, Kottiri BJ, et al. Trends in herpes simplex virus type 1 and 2 seroprevalence in the United States. *JAMA* 2006;296:964-973.

Yeni PG, Hammer SM, Hirsch MS, et al. Treatment for adult HIV infection: 2004 recommendations of the International AIDS Society-USA Panel. *JAMA* 2004;292:251-265.

Thyroid disease

American Association of Clinical Endocrinologists. Thyroid Fact Sheet. Available at: http://www.aace.com/public/awareness/tam/2006/pdfs/ThyroidFactSheet.pdf. Accessed August 16, 2007.

American Thyroid Association Guidelines Taskforce. Management guidelines for patients with thyroid nodules and differentiated thyroid cancer. *Thyroid* 2006;16:1-33.

Arafah BM. Increased need for thyroxine in women with hypothyroidism during estrogen therapy. *N Engl J Med* 2001;344:1743-1749.

Bauer DC, Ettinger B, Nevitt MC, Stone KL, for the Study of Osteoporotic Fractures Research Group. Risk for fracture in women with low serum levels of thyroid-stimulating hormone. *Ann Intern Med* 2001;134:561-568.

Canadian Task Force on the Periodic Health Examination. Canadian Guide to Clinical Preventive Health Care. Ottawa, ON, Canada: Canada Communication Group. 1994:611-618.

Cappola AR, Fried LP, Arnold AM, et al. Thyroid status, cardiovascular risk, and mortality in older adults. *JAMA* 2006;295:1033-1041.

Col NF, Surks MI, Daniels GH. Subclinical thyroid disease: clinical applications. *JAMA* 2004;291:239-243.

Demers LM, Spencer CA. NACB: Laboratory support for the diagnosis and monitoring of thyroid disease. In: NACB Laboratory Medicine Practice Guidelines. Available at: http://www.nacb.org/lmpg/thyroid_lmpg_pub.stm. Accessed August 16, 2007.

Greenspan SL, Greenspan FS. The effect of thyroid hormone on skeletal integrity. *Ann Intern Med* 1999;130:750-758.

Ladenson PW, Singer PA, Ain KB, et al. American Thyroid Association guidelines for detection of thyroid dysfunction. *Arch Intern Med* 2000; 160:1573-1575.

The North American Menopause Society. Clinical challenges of perimenopause: consensus opinion of The North American Menopause Society. *Menopause* 2000;7:5-13.

Sowers M, Luborsky J, Perdue C, et al. SWAN. Thyroid stimulating hormone (TSH) concentrations and menopausal status in women at the mid-life: SWAN. *Clin Endocrinol* 2003;58:340-347.

Surks MI, Ortiz E, Daniels GH, et al. Subclinical thyroid disease: scientific review and guidelines for diagnosis and management. *JAMA* 2004; 291:228-238.

US Preventive Services Task Force. Screening for thyroid disease: recommendation statement. *Ann Intern Med* 2004;140:125-127.

Epilepsy

Abbasi F, Krumholz A, Kittner SJ, Langenberg P. Effects of menopause on seizures in women with epilepsy. *Epilepsia* 1999;40:205-210.

Backstrom T. Epileptic seizures in women related to plasma estrogen and progesterone during the menstrual cycle. *Acta Neurol Scand* 1976;54:321-347.

Epilepsy Foundation. Epilepsy Answer Place. Available at: http://www.efa.org/answerplace. Accessed August 16, 2007.

Feldkamp J, Becker A, Witte OW, Scharff D, Scherbaum WA. Long-term anticonvulsant therapy leads to low bone mineral density: evidence for direct drug effects of phenytoin and carbamazepine on human osteoblast-like cells. *Exp Clin Endocrinol Diabetes* 2000;108:37-43.

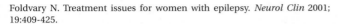

Foldvary N. Treatment issues for women with epilepsy. *Neurol Clin* 2001; 19:409-425.

Harden CL. Menopause and bone density issues for women with epilepsy. *Neurol* 2003;61(Suppl):S16-S22.

Harden CL, Koppel BS, Herzog AG, et al. Hormone replacement therapy in women with epilepsy. *Epilepsia* 2006;47:1447-1451.

Harden CL, Koppel BS, Herzog AG, Nikolov BG, Hauser WA. Seizure frequency is associated with age of menopause in women with epilepsy. *Neurology* 2003;61:451-455.

Harden CL, Pulver MC, Ravdin L, Jacobs AR. The effect of menopause and perimenopause on the course of epilepsy. *Epilepsia* 1999;40:1402-1407.

Herzog AG. Progesterone therapy in women with epilepsy: a 3-year follow up. *Neurology* 1999;52:1917-1918.

Herzog AG, Coleman AE, Jacobs AR, et al. Interictal EEG discharges, reproductive hormones, and menstrual disorders in epilepsy. *Ann Neurol* 2003;54:625-637.

Herzog AG, Farina EL, Blum AS. Fluctuation in serum valproate levels with oral contraceptive use. *Epilepsia* 2005;46:970-971.

Herzog AG, Klein P, Ransil BJ. Three patterns of catamenial epilepsy. *Epilepsia* 1997;38:1082-1088.

Klein P, Serje A, Pezzullo JC. Premature ovarian failure in women with epilepsy. *Epilepsia* 2001;42:1584-1589.

Mattson RH, Cramer JA, Caldwell BV, Siconolfi BC. Treatment of seizures with medroxyprogesterone acetate: preliminary report. *Neurology* 1984; 34:1255-1258.

Pedrera JD, Canal ML, Carvajal J, et al. Influence of vitamin D administration on bone ultrasound measurements in patients on anticonvulsant therapy. *Eur J Clin Invest* 2000;30:895-899.

Sabers A, Ohman I, Christensen J, Tomson T. Oral contraceptives reduce lamotrigine plasma levels. *Neurology* 2003;61:570-571.

Shorvon SD, Tallis RC, Wallace HK. Antiepileptic drugs: coprescription of proconvulsant drugs and oral contraceptives: a national study of antiepileptic drug prescribing practice. *J Neurol Neurosurg Psychiatry* 2001;72:114-115.

Asthma

Barr RG, Camargo CA Jr. Hormone replacement therapy and obstructive airway disease. *Treat Respir Med* 2004;3:1-7.

Barr RG, Wentowski CC, Grodstein F, et al. Prospective study of postmenopausal hormone use and newly diagnosed asthma and chronic obstructive pulmonary disease. *Arch Intern Med* 2004;164:379-386.

Barrett-Connor E. Postmenopausal estrogen therapy and selected (less-often-considered) disease outcomes. *Menopause* 1999;6:14-20.

Cohen PG. Estradiol induced inhibition of 11beta-hydroxysteroid dehydrogenase 1: an explanation for the postmenopausal hormone replacement therapy effects. *Med Hypotheses* 2005;64:989-991.

Gomez Real F, Svanes C, Bjornsson EH, et al. Hormone replacement therapy, body mass index and asthma in perimenopausal women: a cross sectional survey. *Thorax* 2006;61:34-40.

Haggerty CL, Ness RB, Kelsey S, Waterer GW. The impact of estrogen and progesterone on asthma. *Ann Allergy Asthma Immunol* 2003;90:284-291.

Hepburn MJ, Dooley DP, Morris MJ. The effects of estrogen replacement therapy on airway function in postmenopausal, asthmatic women. *Arch Intern Med* 2001;161:2717-2721.

Kasayama S, Fujita M, Goya K, et al. Effects of alendronate on bone mineral density and bone metabolic markers in postmenopausal asthmatic women treated with inhaled corticosteroids. *Metabolism* 2005;54:85-90.

Kos-Kudla B, Ostrowska Z, Marek B, et al. Circadian rhythm of androstene-dione and free testosterone in asthmatic women with postmenopausal hormone therapy. *Endocr Regul* 2004;38:111-118.

Kos-Kudla B, Ostrowska Z, Marek B, et al. Effects of hormone replacement therapy on endocrine and spirometric parameters in asthmatic postmenopausal women. *Gynecol Endocrinol* 2001;15:304-311.

Kos-Kudla B, Ostrowska Z, Marek B, et al. Hormone replacement therapy in postmenopausal asthmatic women. *J Clin Pharmacol Ther* 2000;25:461-466.

Mueller JE, Frye C, Brasche S, Heinrich J. Association of hormone replacement therapy with bronchial hyper-responsiveness. *Respir Med* 2003;97:990-992.

Siroux V, Curt F, Oryszczyn MP, Maccario J, Kauffmann F. Role of gender and hormone-related events on IgE, atopy, and eosinophils in the Epidemiological Study on the Genetics and Environment of Asthma, bronchial hyperresponsiveness and atopy. *J Allergy Clin Immunol* 2004;114:491-498.

Troisi RJ, Speizer FE, Willett WC, Trichopoulos D, Rosner B. Menopause, postmenopausal estrogen preparations, and the risk of adult-onset asthma: a prospective cohort study. *Am J Respir Crit Care Med* 1995;152:1183-1188.

Gallbladder disease

Barrett-Connor E. Postmenopausal estrogen therapy and selected (less-often-considered) disease outcomes. *Menopause* 1999;6:14-20.

Cirillo DJ, Wallace RB, Rodabough RJ, et al. Effect of estrogen therapy on gallbladder disease. *JAMA* 2005;293:330-339.

Everson GT, McKinley C, Kern F Jr. Mechanisms of gallstone formation in women. Effects of exogenous estrogen (Premarin) and dietary cholesterol on hepatic lipid metabolism. *J Clin Invest* 1991;87:237-246.

Farquhar CM, Marjoribanks J, Lethaby A, Lamberts Q, Suckling JA, for the Cochrane HT Study Group. Long term hormone therapy for perimenopausal and postmenopausal women. *Cochrane Database System Rev* 2005;CD004143.

Haffner SM, Diehl AK, Mitchell DB, Stern MP, Hazuda HP. Increased prevalence of clinical gallbladder disease in subjects with noninsulin-dependent diabetes mellitus. *Am J Epidemiol* 1990;132:327-335.

Hulley S, Grady D, Bush T, et al, for the Heart and Estrogen/progestin Replacement Study (HERS) Research Group. Randomized trial of estrogen plus progestin for secondary prevention of coronary heart disease in postmenopausal women. *JAMA* 1998;280:605-613.

Morimoto LM, Newcomb PA, Hamptom JM, Trentham-Dietz A. Cholecystectomy and endometrial cancer: a marker of long-term elevated estrogen exposure? *Int J Gynecol Cancer* 2006;16:1348-1353.

Simon JA, Grady D, Snabes MC, et al. Ascorbic acid supplement use and the prevalence of gallbladder disease. *J Clin Epidemiol* 1998;5:257-265.

Uhler ML, Marks JW, Judd HL. Estrogen replacement therapy and gallbladder disease in postmenopausal women. *Menopause* 2000;7:162-167.

Uhler ML, Marks JW, Voigt BJ, Judd HL. Comparison of the impact of transdermal versus oral estrogen on biliary markers of gallstone formation in postmenopausal women. *J Clin Endocrinol Metab* 1998;83:410-414.

Van Erpecum KJ, Van Berge Henegouwen GP, Verschoor L, Stoelwinder B, Willekens FL. Different hepatobiliary effects of oral and transdermal estradiol in postmenopausal women. *Gastroenterology* 1991;100:482-488.

The goals of a health evaluation of a woman around menopause are similar to those throughout her life span, tailored to her not only as an individual but also to the known physical and psychological consequences of menopause. Such an evaluation presents an opportunity to identify specific menopause-related issues and provide appropriate anticipatory guidance, plan preventive care, diagnose early disease, and determine the need for treatment, if any.

As women move through the menopause transition, regular health examinations are the standard of care. Although some experts have questioned the value of the periodic health examination, a recent systematic review concluded it was justified.

In general, the clinical evaluation includes the following:

- Detailed medical, psychological, and social history of the woman, including family history
- Complete physical examination, including vital signs, height and weight, as well as thyroid, breast, pelvic, and rectovaginal examinations
- Laboratory testing when indicated, such as fasting serum cholesterol (total, high-density lipoprotein cholesterol [HDL-C], and low-density lipoprotein cholesterol) [LDL-C], triglycerides, glucose, Papanicolaou (Pap) test, thyroid testing, urine screens, screens for sexually transmitted infections (STIs), and stool for occult blood
- Appropriate testing to evaluate problems (eg, abnormal uterine bleeding)
- Other age- and risk-appropriate screening tests (eg, bone density, mammogram, skin, colon cancer screening, glaucoma screening, and hearing test (see diagnostic and screening tests on page 189).

This discussion is general, so clinicians will want to consider the appropriate approach for each individual patient. Because this section of the textbook focuses on specific menopause-related issues, it does not include all the possible elements of a comprehensive physical examination.

History gathering

The comprehensive, nine-page Menopause Health Questionnaire developed by The North American Menopause Society (NAMS) can assist practitioners in gathering a menopause-focused history. This is available on the NAMS Web site (www.menopause.org/edumaterials/questionnaire.pdf).

Medical history. A complete medical history of a menopausal woman will include information from the following areas.

Symptom history. Ask detailed questions about symptoms that could be related to menopause and rate them according to frequency, severity, and duration. Although the 2005 State-of-the-Science Conference Statement on Management of

Menopause-Related Symptoms from the National Institutes of Health definitively attributes only vasomotor symptoms, painful intercourse, and possibly sleep disturbance to menopause, women often experience many additional physical and psychological symptoms around menopause. Whether these concerns are related to menopause or aging, potential areas of discussion include hot flashes, night sweats, difficulty sleeping, vaginal dryness, dyspareunia, moodiness, anxiety, depression, urinary symptoms, sexual issues (desire, arousal, orgasm), hair and skin changes, weight gain, joint pain, and memory.

Numerous symptom inventories can be used to evaluate menopausal women. The most widely used is the 21-question Greene Climacteric Scale, which is easily administered and scored.

Gynecologic history. Review a woman's menstrual history, including age at menarche and description of menses since her premenopausal years. Note all gynecologic problems, including ovarian cysts, polycystic ovarian syndrome, fibroids, infertility, endometriosis, STIs, abnormal Pap smears, diethylstilbestrol exposure in pregnancy, and gynecologic surgery.

It is important to establish the date and results of the patient's last clinical breast and pelvic examinations as well as laboratory and radiologic examinations and screening tests, such as Pap smear, mammogram, and tests for cholesterol and bone density.

Obstetric history. Establish the number of pregnancies, full-term births, premature births, abortions, and living children; the woman's age at time of first birth; and significant complications during pregnancy or delivery.

History of serious illness. Exploring a woman's self-perceived health status provides a context to address her response and her own approach to menopause. Put special emphasis on cardiovascular disease (CVD), diabetes mellitus (DM), cancer, and osteoporosis, although any serious medical condition is relevant (see identification of modifiable health risk factors on page 184). Review her hospitalizations.

Surgical history. Get a full history of all the patient's surgeries.

Medication history. In addition to current medication use (prescription, nonprescription, complementary and alternative therapies) and allergies to any of them, ask about current and past hormone use (eg, hormonal contraceptives and menopausal hormone therapy [HT]). It is often revealing to ask specifically about prior strategies to deal with symptoms attributed to menopause. For all medications—especially those used for menopause-related symptoms—ask about duration of use, effectiveness, and reasons for stopping if they are no longer used.

Psychological history. It is important to elicit a woman's history of psychotherapy, depression, and other mental health issues, especially hormone-related mood issues, such as premenstrual syndrome (PMS), premenstrual dysphoric disorder (PMDD), and postpartum depression.

Most women present to their primary care clinicians with symptoms of psychological problems before they consult a mental health professional. Thus, it is the responsibility of the primary care clinician to conduct an initial assessment of psychological health.

Social history. Marital status, sexual history, occupation, and living situation all affect a woman's health. Her financial status and access to care are relevant issues to explore. Ask her if she feels safe at home.

A sexual history (eg, sexual function) requires confidentiality and a nonjudgmental attitude. Be sensitive to the woman's specific conditions, including her sexual orientation; do not assume that all women are heterosexual. (See Section C, page 59, for more about evaluation of sexual function and Section J, page 279, about lesbian health.)

Quality of life. Maintaining optimal quality of life (QOL) is a priority for women through menopause and beyond. A woman's perception of her QOL is not limited to menopause-related symptoms, but involves a more global sense of well-being across the physical, behavioral, cognitive, and emotional functioning domains. QOL is a state of mind beyond the presence or absence of symptoms. The comprehensive clinical evaluation ideally incorporates the use of validated questionnaires that consider both the symptom profile and a scale of well-being.

There are two types of QOL: health-related QOL (HRQOL) and global QOL (GQOL). The former concentrates on symptoms and essentially relates symptom relief to sense of improvement in general life quality. The latter relates directly to sense of well-being, whether symptoms or handicaps are present or absent.

The only validated instrument for measuring GQOL in peri- and postmenopausal women is the Utian Quality of Life (UQOL) Scale. The World Health Organization QOL is possibly another, but it is designed for multiple populations and requires several hours for completion.

The validated HRQOL instruments include the Greene Climacteric Scale, Menopause-Specific QOL, Short Form-36 Health Survey, and the Schneider QOL. The Kupperman Index has never been validated and there is a vast literature explaining why it should be dropped from contemporary discussions.

In both research and clinical care, a global measure such as the UQOL should be combined with a symptom-profile index like the Greene to obtain a more complete picture.

There is currently no satisfactory validated instrument that properly measures both components.

Family history. In taking the family history, be especially attentive to breast and ovarian cancer, colon cancer, CVD, thromboembolic disease, DM, and osteoporosis (including fracture) as well as the age when each disease was diagnosed. The age when a woman's first-degree female relatives reached menopause is of interest because it can predict her own age at menopause.

Identification of modifiable health risk factors. Menopause can be either a difficult or simple transition for any woman, but it is an identifiable milestone for all. As such, this milestone provides an opportunity for a woman and her healthcare providers to review her overall health and her personal risk for disease. An important element of a menopause-related therapeutic plan is lifestyle modification. Information about a woman's lifestyle—including physical activity, weight changes, diet, stress management, physical activity, use of caffeine, alcohol, tobacco, and "recreational" drugs, wearing seat belts when traveling in a vehicle, and participating in safer sex practices during sexual encounters when both partners are not monogamous—is critical in helping to manage her present and future well-being. (See Section J, page 280, for information about lifestyle risk factors and their management.)

Weight changes. Weight is a concern for most women in the United States; over 70% of women aged 55 to 75 years and 65% of women aged 45 to 55 years are overweight (body mass index [BMI] >25). More than 40% are obese (BMI ≥30). More than 40% of Canadian women are overweight or obese. Higher weight and level of body fat are associated with adverse health consequences including type 2 DM, CVD, stroke, hypertension, some cancers, osteoarthritis, and premature mortality.

Longitudinal studies show that midlife women gain weight, although the factors contributing to this are not fully understood. Sedentary women, women who quit smoking, and those who are already overweight have been shown to be particularly at risk in one Australian study. Conversely, overweight women who lose just 10% of their body weight can reap many health benefits including a significant lowering of blood pressure (BP).

Plotting a woman's weight over time provides an opportunity to identify and discuss trends. Since women typically gain weight quite slowly at midlife, it is often beneficial for weight management goals to remind them that gaining "only a couple of pounds" every year can add up over a decade. (For more about weight, see Section C, page 68, and Section J, page 287.)

Substance use. Smoking, abuse of caffeine, alcohol, and prescription drugs, and use of recreational drugs are important habits to uncover in taking the history.

- *Smoking.* Cigarette smoking is the single greatest preventable cause of illness and premature death. Smoking causes more than 178,000 deaths annually of women in the United States and 15,000 deaths in Canadian women. Therefore, smoking cessation is the most important change a woman can make to guard her health. Smokers on average reach menopause up to 2 years earlier than nonsmokers, placing them at increased risk for the associated diseases. Altered endogenous levels of estradiol and estrone have not been associated with smoking in either pre- or postmenopausal women; however, among postmenopausal women who use oral HT, smokers have lower serum estrone and estradiol levels than nonsmokers. Use of snuff and chewing tobacco is also associated with adverse health outcomes.

  The role healthcare providers can play in helping women to quit smoking is well documented. This often requires repeated discussions. Identifying a woman's stage in the process of change as well as her history of tobacco use and prior attempts to quit will guide the clinician to appropriate support strategies for this process. (See Section J, page 282, for more about the effects of smoking and strategies to quit.)

- *Caffeine.* Caffeine-containing drinks (coffee, tea, colas, soft drinks) may have a negative effect on health. Caffeine ingestion may trigger hot flashes and can contribute to insomnia, even when consumed hours before bedtime. Caffeine is a natural diuretic, which increases dehydration. Caffeine has been proposed as a risk factor for bone loss in postmenopausal women; however, many of the studies linking caffeine to bone loss were confounded by covariates. A few studies have found a benefit from caffeine consumption, including a positive effect on Parkinson's disease and some cancers. Women are often unaware of the effects of caffeine or its sources. Clinicians are advised to include a discussion about caffeine in the evaluation.

- *Alcohol.* Drinking alcohol has been associated with both risks and benefits, depending on the amount consumed. In peri- and postmenopausal women, the effect of alcohol on endogenous estrogen levels remains unclear. Although some studies have suggested that alcohol consumption may lower estrogen levels, one study in postmenopausal women using HT found that acute alcohol consumption was associated with significant, sustained elevations in circulating estradiol up to levels 300% higher than those used clinically. Moderate alcohol consumption seems to lower the risk of hip fractures in women age 65 and above, possibly because it increases estradiol concentrations and calcitonin excretion, which may inhibit bone resorption. In addition, there is some evidence that light to moderate alcohol use is associated with reduced cardiovascular risk, better cognitive function, and perhaps reduced risk of dementia.

Women are more affected by alcohol than men because of many factors, including having less water in their bodies to dilute the alcohol, fewer enzymes to digest the alcohol, typically smaller body size, and hormonal differences that may affect absorption. Death rates from alcohol abuse are 50% to 100% higher for women than for men. Both women and men who drink have a higher risk of many forms of cancer. Women who consume one or two drinks daily may be at increased risk for breast cancer.

Risks often associated with excessive alcohol use include cirrhosis, cardiac failure secondary to cardiomyopathy, accidents, and victimization by physical, sexual, and emotional abuse.

Physical markers for recognizing alcohol abuse include frequent gastrointestinal disturbances, difficulty controlling health problems such as hypertension or DM, and unexplained seizures. Abnormal laboratory results that are consistent with alcoholism are an elevated γ-glutamyltransferase level or elevated mean corpuscular volume.

Drinking moderate amounts of alcohol can cause hair and skin to appear dull and can worsen acne and dandruff. Alcohol can lead to weight gain through its caloric content, primarily low-nutritional calories. Those who abuse alcohol may suffer from malnutrition. Moderate alcohol consumption is also associated with insomnia, even when consumed a long time before bed.

Traditional markers for alcoholism include tolerance, withdrawal symptoms, loss of control over drinking, social decline, and impaired working skills. Some of these symptoms may be confused with menopause-related symptoms. Be highly on guard for addictive disorders.

One method for determining if a woman is abusing alcohol is to use the "TACE" questions (see Table 1). Total score of 2 or more from the four questions suggests alcohol abuse.

Table 1. TACE questions for determining alcohol abuse

T (tolerance)
How many drinks does it take to make you feel high?
(If the answer is more than two drinks, give a score of 2)

A (annoyed)
Have people annoyed you by criticizing your drinking?
(Score 1 for yes)

C (cut down)
Have you felt you ought to cut down on your drinking?
(Score 1 for yes)

E (eye opener)
Have you ever had a drink first thing in the morning to steady your nerves or get rid of a hangover? (Score 1 for yes)

Because of the health risks associated with heavy alcohol consumption, it is important to counsel women who drink to limit themselves to one drink per day and a maximum of seven per week (one drink equals 12 oz beer, 4 oz wine, or 1 oz liquor). For women who do not drink, the potential benefits of moderate drinking do not outweigh the potential risks. (See Section J, page 284, for counseling techniques for those who abuse alcohol.)

- *Prescription and recreational drugs.* Abuse of legal and illegal drugs is a growing problem for aging women. Although the general perception is that illegal drug use is a problem of youth, it is estimated that up to 11% of older women misuse prescription drugs. Although methods to diagnose this problem are limited, be alert to this possibility, especially in women with the risk factors of social isolation, a history of substance use or mental illness, and access to prescription drugs with abuse potential. (See Section J, page 284, for counseling suggestions regarding drug abuse.)

Lack of exercise. Physical inactivity is a risk factor for many diseases, including CVD and DM. Women who exercise sleep better, are less depressed, and are more able to maintain a healthy weight. Nevertheless, national surveys report that more than one third of US women aged 45 years and older do not participate in leisure-time physical activity and fewer than 20% participate in regular, sustained physical activity of at least 30 minutes five or more times per week.

Reports in Canada are similar, with only 15% of Canadian women aged 40 to 54 years classified as sufficiently active. Another 54% reported regular participation in physical activity, 18% were occasionally active, and 23% were inactive. Physical inactivity increases as Canadian women age; 72% of women over age 70 are inactive.

Questions to elicit the level of activity are an important component of the evaluation. (For more about counseling strategies to increase physical activity, see Section J, page 285.)

Stress. Midlife is a stressful time for many women. Stress negatively affects QOL, produces a variety of symptoms, and can aggravate some medical conditions. Sometimes just asking a woman if there are any particular stresses in her life can provide an opening to hear about her specific concerns and allow discussion of stress-reducing strategies. (Stress-reducing strategies can be found in Section J, page 285.)

Nutrition. A complete nutrition history requires keeping a food diary; however, this exercise may provide more information than is needed. Asking women if they get five to seven fruits and vegetables a day reveals helpful information about diet. Determine what vitamins, minerals, and other "nutritional" supplements are used. Be sure to inquire about dietary restrictions.

Counseling about nutrition is found in Section J, page 286.

Abuse of women. Abuse can be physical, sexual, or mental. Older adults and female spouses or intimate partners are among the primary victims of abuse.

Several leading women's health organizations, including NAMS, the American Medical Association, the American College of Obstetricians and Gynecologists (ACOG), the Society of Obstetricians and Gynaecologists of Canada, and the Registered Nurses' Association of Ontario, recommend that healthcare providers look for signs of abuse through incorporation of universal screening during all health examinations. Detecting abuse can be challenging. For guidance, including suggested questions to pose to patients, see Section J, page 288.

If abuse is suspected, document the incident and physical findings as well as any treatments. In many US states, physicians are required to report elder abuse and intimate partner violence to government authorities.

Dental, eye care, skin care, hearing function, and injury prevention. These are parts of comprehensive lifestyle history counseling that, time permitting, the menopause clinician should address. A standard questionnaire can help make gathering this information time-efficient.

Physical examination

This section addresses height and weight measurements as well as pelvic, breast, and BP examinations.

Height. Current height and the maximal adult height are important components of the clinical evaluation. Height loss greater than 1.5 inches (3.8 cm) may be associated with vertebral compression fractures and indicate osteoporosis. The preferred method for height measurement is a stadiometer. Height should be measured (without shoes) during each visit, and, ideally, at approximately the same time of day. Women lose up to 0.24 inch (6 mm) of height over the course of a day.

Weight and body mass index. Recording a woman's weight is another essential component of clinical evaluation. Clinicians should be aware that weight is a sensitive matter for many women, and weight measurement should be performed discreetly.

BMI provides a measure of adiposity that is relatively independent of height. The formula for calculating BMI is as follows:

$$\text{BMI (in kg/m}^2) = \frac{\text{weight in kg}}{(\text{height in meters})^2}$$

Sometimes BMI is expressed simply as the number (without kg/m^2). Table 2 provides a chart to convert weight in pounds

Table 2. Determining body mass index									
BMI	18	20	22	24	26	28	30	32	34
Height (inches [cm])	Body weight (pounds)								
58 (147)	91	96	105	115	124	134	143	153	162
60 (152)	92	102	112	123	133	143	153	163	174
62 (157)	99	109	120	131	142	153	164	175	186
64 (163)	105	116	128	140	151	163	174	186	197
66 (168)	113	124	136	148	161	173	186	198	210
68 (173)	119	131	144	158	171	184	197	210	223
70 (178)	127	139	153	167	181	195	209	222	236
72 (183)	135	147	162	177	191	206	221	235	250
74 (188)	143	155	171	186	202	218	233	249	264
76 (193)	151	164	180	197	213	230	246	263	279

and height in inches to BMI. Web-based calculators are also available (eg, www.cdc.gov/nccdphp/dnpa/bmi).

Once the BMI has been calculated, the woman's weight status can be determined (eg, normal, underweight, obese). The National Institutes of Health has established definitions to classify BMI (see Table 3).

Table 3. Body mass index classification for women	
Classification	*BMI (kg/m²)*
Underweight	<18.5
Normal weight	18.5-24.9
Overweight	25.0-29.9
Obese	30.0-39.9
Morbidly obese	≥40.0
Source: National Library of Medicine 2006.	

In addition to BMI, the presence of central obesity out of proportion to total body fat is an independent predictor of DM, CVD, and total mortality. The accuracy of waist circumference (measured parallel to the ground, just above the iliac crest, while a woman is standing and after exhaling) should be measured for the initial assessment of obesity and also to monitor the efficacy of weight loss treatment. A waist circumference equal to or greater than 35 inches (88 cm) for Caucasians is associated with increased risk for type 2 DM, dyslipidemia, hypertension, and CVD. For Asian Indians, 32 inches (80 cm) portends similar risk. Waist circumference measurement is more useful for women who fall in the normal or overweight category of BMI.

In some studies, central adiposity, visceral, and android (male-type) obesity have been shown to confer excess risk for CVD.

The waist-to-hip ratio (WHR) is an alternative measure to classify body fat distribution as android obesity (fat in the waist and stomach or "apple-shaped") or gynecoid obesity (fat in the hips or "pear-shaped"). The ratio estimates the amount of intra-abdominal fat (which is greater with android obesity). A WHR greater than 0.85 is indicative of android obesity, whereas a ratio of less than 0.75 is indicative of gynecoid obesity. Some clinicians include a WHR measurement as part of the physical examination. Measuring the waist alone is just as accurate. Most clinicians simply determine android or gynecoid obesity by observation.

Android obesity is more strongly associated with adverse health conditions than is gynecoid obesity, including insulin resistance, type 2 DM, hypertension, stroke, left ventricular hypertrophy, arrhythmias, congestive heart failure, myocardial infarction, angina pectoris, and peripheral vascular disease.

Data from the third National Health and Nutrition Examination Survey (NHANES III) indicated that risk for type 2 DM increases dramatically when the BMI exceeds 27 and as overweight (particularly android obesity) increases. The increase in obesity observed over the past decade in the United States has been accompanied by a 25% increase in the prevalence of type 2 DM. In NHANES III, higher body weight was also associated with a greater risk of gallstones and cholecystectomy.

The Nurses' Health Study (NHS) found that women with a WHR of 0.74 or higher had a twofold increase in heart disease risk. The investigators concluded that an ideal WHR is less than 0.72. In addition, waist circumference was found to be an independent factor associated with risk of coronary heart disease in women.

Increasing body weight elevates the risk for osteoarthritis. Individuals with a BMI of at least 30 have a markedly increased risk for knee osteoarthritis. Conversely, increased body weight seems to offer protection against the development of osteoporosis.

Obesity, in general, is associated with increased incidence and mortality from certain cancers. An estimated 34% to 56% of cases of endometrial cancer are associated with increased body weight (BMI >29). Almost one half of breast cancer cases among postmenopausal women occur in those with a BMI greater than 29. In the NHS, women gaining more than 20 lb (9 kg) from 18 years of age to midlife doubled their risk for breast cancer compared with women who maintained stable weight. Compared with women of normal weight, obese women have a higher mortality rate from cancers of the endometrium, cervix, gallbladder, colon, ovary, and breast (in postmenopausal women).

For information about obesity management, see Section C, page 68.

Blood pressure. Hypertension is an important parameter in determining cardiovascular and stroke risk for women. BP increases with age, and the incidence of hypertension is 50% for individuals between the ages of 60 and 69, increasing to 75% in the 70-and-over age group. BP must be measured during every visit. The cutoff for treatment is 140/90 mg Hg. The designation "prehypertension"—BP in the range of 120-139/80-90—identifies women who probably need nonmedication interventions to reduce their BP and who must be followed closely. (See Section E, page 129, for more about BP measurement and cardiovascular effects.)

Manual breast examination. The clinical breast examination is a time-honored ritual in women's health. The American Cancer Society (ACS) and ACOG recommend yearly examinations for women over age 40. However, both the Cochrane Collaboration and the US Preventive Services Task Force (USPSTF) state that there is a lack of evidence to support this practice. One study that evaluated women who died from breast cancer showed a discouraging low pick-up rate of 21% in their community-based retrospective data. In contrast, a pick-up rate of 69% was found in the Canadian National Breast Cancer Screening study, during which the systematized breast examinations lasted 5 to 10 minutes. Other studies have shown that the duration of a typical clinical breast examination correlates with its effectiveness, and that breast examinations often last under 2 minutes whereas as much as 5 minutes or more is recommended. Therefore, a yearly systematic clinical breast examination is prudent and supportable in perimenopausal and postmenopausal women, especially in light of the burden of disease of breast cancer in North America and the fact that mammograms can miss breast cancers.

See Section E, page 140, for a comprehensive discussion of breast cancer, including screening.

Pelvic examination. NAMS and ACOG recommend that all women have an annual pelvic examination after they become sexually active. The ACS and NAMS recommend that all women over 40 have an annual pelvic examination regardless of whether they are sexually active. A thorough and sensitive pelvic examination of the peri- and postmenopausal woman provides an opportunity to screen for disease and to assess one of the most noticeable effects of estrogen loss.

Start this examination with a disciplined look at the external genitalia. The distribution of pubic hair suggests different levels of androgen. Pale, thin tissue at the introitus extending into the vagina suggests the absence of estrogen. A cotton-tipped applicator can be used to evaluate the sensitivity of the introitus just distal to the hymen. If a woman experiences any pain from a gentle touch, vulvovaginal pathology should be suspected. A visible clitoris and normal labia minora help rule out the vulvar dystrophies. Vulvar vestibulitis is characterized by entry dyspareunia, discomfort at the opening of the vagina, a positive swab test, tenderness localized within the vulvar vestibulum, and focal or diffuse vestibular erythema.

A wide spectrum of benign, premalignant, and malignant lesions may involve the vulva. The challenge to the clinician is to differentiate between normal variants, benign findings, and potentially serious disease. Most vulvar intraepithelial neoplasia lesions are multifocal and located in the hairless part of the vulva. The lesions are often raised and/or verrucose (warty) and white, but the color may be pink, gray, or brown. Macular lesions mostly occur on adjacent mucosal surfaces. Vulvar cancer presents with a unifocal vulvar plaque, ulcer, or mass (fleshy, nodular, or warty) on the labia majora. In Paget's disease, the lesions appear to have an eczematous or velvet-like surface.

Lichen sclerosus should be ruled out. With an unknown etiology, it appears as a white, usually symmetric lesion with a wrinkled, parchment-like surface, causing atrophy of the labia minora pudendi. Pathologic examination shows thinning of squamous epithelium, loss of rete pegs, and deep dermal inflammatory cells. Because of loss of elastic fibers in layers beneath the epithelium, the lesion can appear thickened. Over time, the introitus becomes narrowed and appears fibrotic. Diagnosis is based on the histologic finding of thinning of the epithelium.

Pelvic supports can be evaluated, and the presence of bladder, uterine, or rectal descensus should be recorded and correlated with symptoms.

Using a warm and small speculum minimizes the discomfort of the examination. Examination of the cervix allows identification of polyps and the opportunity to obtain a Pap smear, with the frequency indicated for the individual patient (see Section E, page 149, for more about cervical cancer). A vaginal pH obtained with a cotton-tipped applicator from the vaginal sidewall gives valuable information about the health of the vagina. A high vaginal pH suggests atrophy or vaginitis.

The bimanual pelvic examination is the clinician's window to the female reproductive organs. For women with lower abdominal and genital complaints, it provides especially useful information. Conditions that can be identified include dyspareunia, sexual inactivity, or vaginal stenosis. Unfortunately, the pelvic examination is not an effective screening test for ovarian cancer.

Rectal examination. The rectal examination is considered by many gynecologists as an extension of the pelvic examination—an opportunity to further evaluate the pelvic organs, especially when a woman's uterus is retroverted. It has also been part of some colorectal cancer screening strategies. If a fecal occult blood test (FOBT) is required, obtain stool samples from home in case there was tearing during the digital examination that would invalidate an office sample. With the more widespread use of colonoscopy, the value of this uncomfortable examination has come into question. (For more about colorectal cancer, see Section E, page 152.)

Other examinations. There are several other potential examinations that may be appropriate at menopause and beyond. Menopause clinicians must know what they can diagnose and treat, as well as when to refer.

Skin examination. A skin examination requires time and expertise. On the other hand, a clinician performing a physical examination of any sort has the opportunity to observe the skin. This is important because the median age at diagnosis of malignant melanoma is 53 years, although the USPSTF states there is insufficient evidence to recommend for or against routine screening for skin cancer by primary care providers. (See Section E, page 155, for more about skin cancer and Section C, page 74, for skin conditions and their relationship to menopause.)

Menopausal women often have concerns about changes in their hair (including facial hair). (For more about hair conditions, see Section C, page 76.)

Eye examination. An eye examination is not in the repertoire of most menopause clinicians. However, they should encourage their patients to see an expert and, in particular, to be screened for glaucoma at least every 3 years. (See Section C, page 78, for more about ocular issues.)

Dental/oral examination. The oral cavity is the source of health issues for the aging woman, and the menopause clinician can easily do a superficial assessment of dental hygiene and encourage appropriate dental care. (See Section C, page 73, for more about conditions of the oral cavity.)

Auditory examination. The prevalence of hearing impairment increases beyond age 50. Audiometric testing should be performed on all individuals with evidence of hearing impairment by patient inquiry. Simply whispering a question out of the sight of the patient should be a part of every postmenopausal woman's annual physical examination. Referral to a specialist for more specific testing and use of hearing aids may need to be considered.

Diagnostic and screening tests

Laboratory testing, such as standard blood screens, serum cholesterol (total, HDL and LDL cholesterol, and triglycerides), fasting glucose, thyroid testing, Pap test, colon cancer screening, mammogram, and, when indicated, urine screens and screens for STIs are an integral part of the regular health examination of women at menopause.

Appropriate testing to evaluate problems (eg, abnormal uterine bleeding) and specific chronic conditions (eg, DM, osteoporosis) might also be ordered.

This section of the textbook focuses on menopause-related issues. It does not include all elements of a laboratory evaluation.

Blood chemistries. A chemistry screen tests the blood for albumin alkaline phosphatase, alanine aminotransferase, aspartate aminotransferase, bilirubin, glucose, calcium, carbon dioxide, chloride, cholesterol, creatinine, γ-glutamyl-transferase, iron, lactic acid, phosphate, potassium, serum protein, sodium, triglycerides, urea nitrogen, and uric acid. Values are compared with standards.

Urinalysis. A urinalysis can help identify potential medical causes for incontinence. For example, the presence of hematuria may suggest bladder pathology (eg, stones or bladder cancer) and should be investigated. A urinalysis may also be done to screen for early signs of disease, blood in the urine, or urinary tract infection. This test may also be suggested if the woman has signs of DM or kidney disease. Measuring a postvoid residual within 15 minutes of voiding is recommended to evaluate for urinary retention and overflow incontinence.

Breast health. The best time for a breast examination or mammogram is immediately after menses or HT-induced bleeding; however, most clinicians do not order mammography on a timed basis. Mammography is a screening tool and does not provide an accurate diagnosis. The false-negative rate for screening mammography is approximately 10% to 15%. All women should have a clinical breast examination and mammogram before beginning HT and at regular intervals thereafter.

Ultrasound is used more frequently to evaluate developing focal asymmetric densities and any palpable masses of the breast. There are also newer methods for detection, including digital mammography, which is similar to regular mammography but with images that are digitized and can be stored on film. This method is especially useful for women with dense breasts.

In 2006, the ACS issued new guidelines for women at increased risk for breast cancer that employ magnetic resonance imaging (MRI) as an adjunct to mammography for women at high risk for breast cancer; however, many believe that MRI is inappropriate because the technique will lead to an excessive number of recalls and biopsies for benign disease.

See Section E, page 140, for comprehensive information about breast cancer, including screening.

Vaginal evaluation. The pelvic examination should include an assessment for vaginal atrophy whether or not vaginal problems have been disclosed. Friability and pallor of the vaginal epithelium should be noted, along with any bleeding from low levels of trauma (eg, speculum insertion). Biopsy may be indicated for persistent symptoms to rule out vulvar dystrophy or vulvar neoplasia.

Vaginal fluid should also be examined, noting the amount, character, and pH. An increase in vaginal pH of 5 or above is one sign of estrogen loss and atrophic changes, provided presence of pathogens (eg, *Trichomonas*) has been ruled out. If concern is raised about an abnormal discharge, a wet smear may be considered. (See Section C, page 51, for more about vulvovaginal symptoms.)

Uterine evaluation. The following procedures are used to evaluate the endometrium in perimenopausal women with AUB as well as in postmenopausal women in whom endometrial evaluation is indicated. Patient preference, clinician's training and skill, as well as cost and access issues will determine their use in individual women. (See Section C, page 30, for more about uterine bleeding changes at menopause and beyond, and Section E, page 146, for comprehensive information about endometrial cancer.)

Endometrial biopsy. An endometrial biopsy provides an inexpensive, office-based endometrial evaluation with sensitivity ranging from 60% to 97% in diagnosing endometrial cancer.

Transvaginal ultrasound. A probe inserted into the vagina produces images to measure the thickness of the endometrium and evaluate the uterine and adnexal anatomy. For a postmenopausal woman experiencing uterine bleeding, transvaginal ultrasonography can be used to exclude malignancy, provided that the entire endometrium can be visualized and the endometrial-myometrial interface is distinct.

Hysteroscopy. This is a procedure in which a small flexible or rigid endoscope is inserted into the vagina and through the cervix to view the uterine lining directly. The uterus is distended with carbon dioxide or fluid for better visualization. Hysteroscopy may be useful in identifying and taking biopsies of (or removing) endometrial polyps and submucous fibroids.

Dilation and curettage (D&C). D&C is a surgical procedure in which the cervix is dilated and the uterine lining is blindly sampled by scraping, or by suction and scraping. An older name for the procedure is "dilatation" and curettage. This procedure is performed much less frequently than endometrial biopsy because it usually requires anesthesia. D&C is often performed with hysteroscopy.

Cervical evaluation. A small percentage of cases of abnormal uterine bleeding (AUB) are caused by cancer of the uterus or cervix. Regular pelvic examinations and Pap smears plus endometrial biopsy, ultrasound, hysteroscopy and/or saline hysterography, colposcopy, and cervical biopsy, when appropriate, are effective methods for the diagnosis of these serious diseases.

See Section E, page 149, for comprehensive information about cervical cancer, including screening.

Pelvic evaluation. In women, pelvic ultrasound is used to evaluate the ovaries, bladder, uterus, cervix, and the area of the fallopian tubes.

Using transvaginal ultrasound with saline infused transcervically to distend the uterus, a sonohysterography can better visualize the endometrial cavity and identify focal lesions such as endometrial polyps and submucous fibroids.

Ovarian evaluation. The bimanual pelvic examination has not been proven to be an effective screening test for ovarian cancer. Serum CA-125 levels and transvaginal ultrasound examinations are used to identify ovarian cancer in women at high risk for the disease. Unfortunately, due to both high false positive and negative results, a routine clinical role for these tests has not yet been confirmed. The addition of pelvic ultrasound as a second screen increases the specificity. (See Section E, page 151, for comprehensive information about ovarian cancer, including risk factors.)

Colorectal evaluation. For women aged 50 years and above and with average risks for colorectal cancer, the ACS recommends selecting one of the following five screening options: annual FOBT, flexible sigmoidoscopy every 5 years, annual FOBT plus flexible sigmoidoscopy every 5 years (preferred by ACS), double-contrast barium enema every 5 years, and colonoscopy every 10 years. (See Section E, page 152, for comprehensive information about colorectal cancer, including screening.)

Hormonal evaluation. At present, there is no single test of ovarian function that will predict or confirm menopause. Practitioners must rely on clinical signs and hormone testing to determine whether it has been reached. Usually, a woman's medical and menstrual history and symptoms are sufficient to confirm menopause. However, tests of nonovarian hormone levels (eg, thyroid-stimulating hormone [TSH]) may be necessary to rule out other causes of symptoms (eg, thyroid disease).

Tests of ovarian function—follicle-stimulating hormone (FSH), estradiol, luteinizing hormone (LH), total and free testosterone (or bioavailable testosterone), and prolactin—can be important for differentiating various causes of amenorrhea, such as premature ovarian failure (POF), hypothalamic hypogonadotropic amenorrhea, and anovulatory cycles. These tests are not routinely recommended for confirming menopause. They are also not recommended in premenopausal women for predicting the timing of menopause.

Pituitary hormones. Because natural menopause is a retrospective diagnosis (ie, 12 months of consecutive amenorrhea for which there is no other physiologic or pathologic cause), serum FSH levels have been evaluated as a laboratory marker that would potentially allow earlier diagnosis of menopause as well as impending menopause. Self-tests approved by the US Food and Drug Administration (FDA) measure two urine FSH levels. In laboratory tests, these tests compared favorably with serum FSH tests.

It is generally accepted that a woman has reached menopause if she has consistently elevated levels of FSH greater than 30 mIU/mL or IU/L. The difficulty in using FSH as a marker of menopause is that, in perimenopausal women, FSH levels in the postmenopausal range can return to premenopausal ranges a few days, weeks, or months later. In the Massachusetts Women's Health Study, 20% of midlife women who experienced 3 months of amenorrhea began menstruating again. A single measurement of FSH greater than 30 mIU/mL in a perimenopausal woman cannot always be considered a definitive diagnosis of menopause; several FSH measurements consistently greater than 30 mIU/mL may be necessary. Furthermore, FSH levels in perimenopausal women are frequently normal or can be elevated even while serum estradiol levels are still in a premenopausal range. This seeming paradox underscores the shortcomings of using FSH determination alone as a marker of menopause.

Hormonal contraceptives may lower FSH levels, making it difficult to diagnose menopause in women who use them. One option is to discontinue the contraceptive, use a nonhormonal method of contraception, and check the FSH level several weeks to months later. A study of perimenopausal women taking oral contraceptives concluded that measuring FSH on the seventh pill-free day was not a sensitive test for confirming menopause. A serum FSH-to-LH ratio greater than 1 or estradiol less than 20 pg/mL (73 pmol/L) on the seventh pill-free day was found to more accurately reflect menopause status.

Much of the recent research on ovarian function tests comes from efforts to assess fertility. FSH has been used as an indicator of "ovarian reserve," a term coined to reflect the remaining reproductive capacity of the ovary. Measuring FSH in the early follicular phase has been used to predict the likelihood of a successful response to infertility treatment and correlates better with treatment outcome than does age.

Changes in FSH levels seem to be preceded by a decline in ovarian production of inhibin B. A lower fertility rate was observed in women who had a normal FSH level on day 3 but a low inhibin B level when compared with women in whom both FSH and inhibin B levels were normal. As inhibin B levels decline, FSH levels rise. Inhibin B levels are normal in hypothalamic amenorrhea but very low in menopause. The average level of inhibin B in POF is only slightly higher than after menopause at the normal age. However, the measurement of inhibin B levels is not widely used in clinical practice. Production of inhibin A does not decrease until close to menopause.

Although tests of ovarian reserve were designed to predict the success of infertility treatment in the older woman at risk for infertility, this is likely associated with the onset of the menopause transition. The Stages of Reproductive Aging Workshop (STRAW) proposed a staging system for menopause and discussed the relation between FSH levels and perimenopausal stages (see Section A, page 10,

for more). An elevated early follicular FSH in one cycle is sufficient to place a woman in the late reproductive stage. However, FSH levels can be unreliable. Because of the variability during this phase of life, a normal FSH level would require a second normal FSH level before it could be assumed that the woman was not approaching menopause. Sporadic elevations of estradiol could suppress the FSH and be misleading. Thus, measuring FSH and estradiol together would be more informative. However, neither of these tests will predict menopause.

The elevation of LH associated with menopause is a late occurrence, much later than the increase in FSH. LH has limited value in confirming perimenopause or menopause when used as an isolated test.

Estrogen/progesterone/testosterone. Women often ask for baseline and continuous hormone testing based on their own research and/or the insistence of some compounding pharmacists or clinicians that no meaningful treatment decisions can be made in its absence. This view implies that a careful patient history is inadequate and substandard care. There is no scientific basis for this recommendation, neither for an individual woman to have medication dosages titrated so that her estrogen or progesterone levels reach a specified "target" value or that a specific ratio (often called "hormonal balancing") has been correlated with improved symptom relief or better safety as claimed. Recommended practice is to titrate estrogen or testosterone treatment based on the individual's report of symptom relief with the least side effects.

Baseline testing of hormone levels is seldom necessary and is not warranted unless the results would affect treatment decisions. Table 4 summarizes reasons for ordering laboratory tests in clinical practice.

There are few circumstances in which estrogen levels need to be measured. Estradiol and estrone levels are erratic during perimenopause. Postmenopausal women not using estrogen therapy can be assumed to have low estrogen levels. Women who do not respond to estrogen therapy may be tested to determine whether there is unusual drug absorption or metabolism. If so, using a different route of administration may be advisable.

Estrogen testing may also be considered for women who have experienced premature menopause. Although definitive data are lacking, this special population may need to achieve typical physiologic hormone levels—beyond those required to relieve symptoms alone—to maintain health over a period of years.

Commercial salivary testing for estrogen has not been proven accurate or reliable, and desired levels of hormones in postmenopausal women have not been established. Urinary estrogen levels, although useful in research, are not commonly used clinically.

Table 4. Criteria for ordering hormone testing

Estradiol	To approximate physiology when it is an appropriate goal for surgical menopause and premature ovarian failure
	When treatment failures or unusual side effects occur during treatment of peri- and postmenopausal women
Progesterone	No clinical application
Testosterone	To assess for supraphysiologic levels before adding testosterone therapy
	To ensure replacement doses do not cause excessive levels
	To evaluate treatment failures
Prolactin	To differentiate causes of amenorrhea
Inhibin B	No clinical application

Progesterone production depends on the integrity of the menstrual cycle. Early in the menopause transition, progesterone levels are usually normal. In anovulatory cycles, progesterone levels are low. During the menopause transition, progesterone is often lower than in normal-cycling women, even during ovulatory cycles. Measuring progesterone has limited value in confirming perimenopause or menopause when used as an isolated test. There are no valid reasons to test for baseline progesterone levels before initiating hormone therapy.

Testosterone levels contribute little to the diagnosis of menopause, as testosterone levels do not change during the menopause transition (from 4 y before to 2 y after). A woman who has undergone bilateral oophorectomy can be presumed to have low levels of testosterone.

As concluded by the NAMS 2005 position statement on the role of testosterone therapy, laboratory testing of testosterone levels should be used to rule out a testosterone excess state (either endogenous or secondary to testosterone treatment) rather than to diagnose testosterone insufficiency.

However, measuring women's testosterone levels in clinical practice is problematic. Serum testosterone levels reflect only a fraction of the total intracellular amount formed in situ by adrenal precursors, such as dehydroepiandrosterone (DHEA) and androstenedione. Measuring total and free or bioavailable testosterone may provide only a limited view of a woman's androgen status. Measurement of DHEA sulfate may contribute to a more complete picture of androgen activity, but this has not been proven. Measurement of the testosterone metabolites androsterone and androstenediol has also been proposed as a more complete measure of androgenic activity, but it also has not been established or correlated with androgen-related conditions or symptoms.

A further challenge for the clinician is identifying a commercial assay that can accurately measure the low serum testosterone levels found in women. Free or bioavailable testosterone values are derived from the total serum testosterone level, and they are useless if the total serum measurement is inaccurate. Recently, liquid chromatography-tandem spectrometry techniques have been developed for commercially measuring steroids and have become the gold standard for measuring testosterone. Baseline or posttreatment free or bioavailable testosterone levels should always be correlated with clinical findings. Laboratory values do not always correlate with therapeutic effect, so dosing should be based on symptom improvement as long as testosterone values remain within normal range.

A measurement of testosterone in saliva is available. However, these assays have questionable reliability and accuracy, especially to ensure the very low ranges seen in women. Furthermore, salivary concentrations of testosterone represent only a small fraction of the amount in circulation, and accurate measurement is limited by the imprecision of available assays. Their use in clinical practice is not recommended.

Thyroid function. The primary function of the thyroid gland is to produce hormones that regulate metabolism, primarily by increasing the basal metabolism rate. Thyroid hormones also affect protein synthesis, carbohydrate and lipid metabolism, and absorption of vitamins. These hormones are regulated through a complex interaction of the hypothalamus and the pituitary and thyroid glands. Much of this regulatory function is controlled by TSH, which is secreted by the anterior pituitary gland.

The thyroid gland takes iodine from the circulating blood, combines it with the amino acid tyrosine, and converts it to the thyroid hormones triiodothyronine (T_3) and thyroxine (T_4). The thyroid gland stores T_3 and T_4 until they are released into the bloodstream under the influence of TSH from the pituitary gland. Most thyroid hormones are bound to proteins. Hence, dialysis assessment of the free portion of thyroid hormone (eg, free T_3, free T_4) is desirable for accurate portrayal of thyroid function.

The USPSTF has stated that it could not determine the balance of benefits and risks of screening asymptomatic adults for thyroid disease. However, NAMS recommends that all women first presenting with irregular menses and/or vasomotor symptoms have thyroid screening, as these symptoms may have their origin in thyroid abnormality. A TSH level using a sensitive TSH assay is the initial screening test. If the TSH level is abnormal, then thyroid function should be evaluated further.

Women taking thyroxine supplements should have their serum TSH levels monitored. Measurement of free T_4 levels is not indicated for assessing the adequacy of thyroxine supplements.

See page Section E, page 158, for a comprehensive discussion about thyroid disease.

Screening for risk factors. The menopause-focused evaluation is also an opportunity to screen for risk factors of disease, including osteoporosis, CVD, DM, cancers, and STIs. Premature menopause presents its own set of long-term risks.

Osteoporosis risk. All postmenopausal women should be assessed for osteoporosis risk. This assessment requires a history, physical examination, and diagnostic tests. The goals of evaluation are the following:

- Identifying the risk of fracture
- Establishing the presence of osteoporosis
- Assessing the severity of osteoporosis
- Ruling out secondary causes of osteoporosis
- Identifying modifiable risk factors for falls and injuries

Risk factors for osteoporosis can often be identified with a simple questionnaire along with the standard physical measurements. Potentially modifiable risk factors should be noted. Risk factors may help explain contributing causes of osteoporosis or help guide therapeutic recommendations but cannot be used to diagnose osteoporosis. A detailed discussion of osteoporosis is found in Section E, page 113.

Bone mineral density (BMD) testing is the current technical standard for diagnosing osteoporosis. The current available methods of measuring BMD are found in Table 5. A complete discussion of testing recommendations is found in Section E, page 118.

Dual-energy x-ray absorptiometry (DXA) is the technical standard for measuring BMD. All the recent large, randomized, controlled clinical trials have used DXA of the hip and spine to determine therapeutic efficacy. DXA is the preferred technique because it measures BMD at the important sites of osteoporotic fractures, especially the hip. This radiation-based BMD measurement is based on the principles of x-ray densitometry or absorptiometry—the degree to which tissues absorb radiation. The greater the density, the greater the amount of energy absorbed.

Quantitative ultrasound (QUS) detects the transmission of high-frequency sound waves through or across bone, providing information on bone structure and strength. Ultrasound measurement sites include the heel (calcaneus), forearm, tibia, phalanges, and metatarsals. Of all ultrasound measurement sites, the best predictor is the heel. Studies have shown that QUS of the heel predicts hip fracture almost as well as hip DXA. The advantages of ultrasound are its low cost, portability of equipment, ease of use, and lack of ionizing radiation. Disadvantages include nonuniform reporting and the measurement of sites unresponsive to therapy.

Table 5. Tests measuring bone mineral density

Method	Body site
Dual-energy x-ray absorptiometry	Hip Spine Total body
Single-energy x-ray absorptiometry	Heel
Quantitative ultrasound	Heel Forearm Tibia Phalanges Metatarsals
Quantitative computed tomography	Spine
Peripheral dual-energy x-ray absorptiometry	Forearm Finger Heel
Peripheral quantitative computed tomography	Forearm

- *BMD scores.* To standardize values from different bone densitometry tests, results are reported as standard deviations, as either a Z-score or a T-score.

T-scores. A T-score is based on the mean peak BMD of a normal, young adult population and is expressed in terms of standard deviations from the average value of this reference population. A value above the young normal mean is expressed as a positive T-score, while a negative T-score denotes a BMD value below average (but not necessarily below normal) for young women.

Lower BMD T-scores indicate more severe osteoporosis and higher risk of fracture. Every decrease of one standard deviation from age-adjusted bone density represents approximately a 10% to 12% change in BMD and an increase in the risk of fracture by a factor of approximately 1.5. The risk of fracture, however, also depends on other factors such as age, frailty, and previous fracture. Older women are at much higher risk of fracture than are younger women with the same T-score. A woman who has had at least one vertebral fracture has four times the risk of another vertebral fracture and twice the risk of a hip fracture as a woman with the same age and BMD T-score who has not had a fracture. Diseases such as osteomalacia are also associated with low BMD and should be excluded before the diagnosis of osteoporosis is confirmed.

Interpretation and clinical application of T-scores are made after all other pertinent data are evaluated, particularly the age and fracture history of the woman. For example, at the same T-score of –2.5, a 75-year-old woman has about 8 to 10 times the hip fracture risk of a 45-year-old postmenopausal woman. Both women have the same bone mass but very different bone quality.

Z-scores. A Z-score is based on the standard deviation from the mean BMD of a reference population of the same gender, ethnicity, and age. A Z-score below –2 is generally an unexpectedly low value and suggests that factors other than age may account for the low BMD. Medical causes of bone loss (ie, not menopause-related) can be present even when Z-scores are not low.

- *Biochemical bone markers.* Biochemical markers of bone turnover cannot diagnose osteoporosis, predict bone density, or predict fracture risk. However, these tests have been studied as a means of assessment to show therapeutic response. Bone turnover changes can provide evidence of osteoporosis therapy efficacy much earlier than BMD changes (sometimes within weeks). The value of such markers in routine clinical practice, however, has not been established.

The rate of bone remodeling affects bone strength and can be examined by measuring surrogate markers of bone turnover in the blood or urine. Markers examine either bone formation or bone resorption, using serum or urine (see Table 6).

Bone formation markers are serum proteins produced by osteoblast process, and include bone alkaline phosphatase, osteocalcin, and the C- and N-terminal propeptides of type I collagen.

Bone resorption markers mostly measure breakdown products of type I collagen. These include the modified amino acids hydroxyproline and galactosyl hydroxylysine, the pyridinium cross-links pyridinoline and deoxypyridinoline, and the C-telopeptides and N-telopeptides of type I collagen associated with the cross-linking site. Collectively, pyridinoline, deoxy-pyridinoline, C-telopeptides, and N-telopeptides are referred to as "collagen cross-links."

The clinical use of bone turnover markers is not new. Total serum alkaline phosphatase has been used to indicate bone turnover; alkaline phosphatase and hydroxyproline have been used in the management of Paget's disease. Both tests have been investigated in postmenopausal women.

The biochemical estimates of both bone resorption and formation increase markedly at menopause by 30% to 100% and decrease after treatment with hormones. An increase in bone resorption precedes the increase in formation at menopause, so that information on both aspects of remodeling improves estimates of the bone loss rate.

- *Tests for secondary causes of osteoporosis.* Once osteoporosis is diagnosed, potential secondary causes of osteoporosis should be considered. Various laboratory tests can identify secondary causes of osteoporosis. (See Section E, page 117, for more about secondary causes.)

Table 6. Common biochemical bone markers of bone turnover	
Formation	**Resorption**
Serum	*Serum*
Bone alkaline phosphatase total and bone-specific (Marketed as Alkphase-B, Tandem-R Ostase)	Cross-linked N-telopeptides (marketed as Osteomark)
C-terminal propeptides of type I collagen	*Urine*
	C-telopeptides of type I collagen (marketed as CrossLaps
N-terminal propeptides of type I collagen	Deoxypyridinoline (marketed as Pyrilinks-D)
Osteocalcin	Cross-linked N-telopeptides (marketed as Osteomark)
	Pyridinoline (marketed as Pyrilinks)

Cardiovascular risk. CVD, including coronary artery disease and stroke, remains the leading cause of death and disability in US and Canadian women. More women than men die of CVD.

Recommendations for BP, lipids, and global risk targets are available. Vigilance is needed to ensure optimal achievement of these targets, even when evaluating women for conditions other than cardiac disease. In an American Heart Association survey, less than 30% of the women indicated that they had had a discussion about these topics with their physician.

Developing a standardized procedure for cardiovascular risk factor assessment and management is important for evaluating women at risk for CVD. (See Section E, page 129, for more about CVD, including guidelines.)

- *Blood pressure.* It is important to identify and manage high BP. Elevated BP is strongly related to the risk of cardiovascular, cerebrovascular, and renal diseases. Treatment and control of elevated BP in the United States has contributed substantially to the reduction in stroke and heart disease mortality during the past 30 years, especially in women.

It is important to obtain BP measurements under controlled conditions. The recommended technique from the Seventh Report of the Joint National Committee on Prevention, Detection, Evaluation, and Treatment of High Blood Pressure (JNC 7) for measuring BP is summarized below:

— Have the woman be seated quietly for at least 5 minutes with her feet on the floor and arm supported at the level of the heart.

— Be sure she did not smoke or consume caffeine 30 minutes before BP measurement.

— Use the appropriate cuff size with a bladder that encircles at least 80% of the upper arm. A properly calibrated and validated instrument should be used.

— Record systolic pressure at the first sound (phase 1) and diastolic pressure at the disappearance (phase 5) of sound.

— Obtain BP readings at two or more sittings.

• *Lipid tests.* Fasting elevated serum cholesterol levels, particularly elevated LDL-C, low HDL-C, and high triglycerides, are risk factors for CVD. The preferred optimum approach is to perform a Framingham Risk Score and treat according to Adult Treatment Panel III guidelines. (See Section E, page 133, for more about lipid testing.)

The Vertical Auto Profile (VAP) cholesterol test evaluates markers for heart disease. It measures total cholesterol, HDL-C, LDL-C, and triglycerides, as well as important lipid subclasses such as LDL-C pattern size, Lp(a), IDL, and HDL2. These allow a more accurate, direct-measured LDL-C rather than the calculated LDL-C of the routine cholesterol test.

• *Diabetes mellitus.* The presence of DM is considered to confer a risk of CVD equivalent to the risk for patients who have had a cardiac event (ie, a CVD risk equivalent). At considerably increased risk are those who have other components of the metabolic syndrome. (See Section E, page 135, for a comprehensive discussion of DM.)

• *Other tests.* Newer risk factors such as homocysteine, highly sensitive C-reactive protein, and lipoprotein(a) have been considered by an expert panel for their potential value in screening and modifying cardiovascular risk. These tests have become more commonplace in patients with intermediate risk for CVD and sway the practitioner toward recommending therapy for dyslipidemia or insulin resistance in those who meet borderline treatment criteria. In selected cases, additional risk testing may be beneficial in refining global cardiac risk.

In women whose symptoms, however atypical for angina, recur with exertion or simply involve the torso of a woman with significant CVD risk, both stress testing and referral to a cardiac specialist must be considered. Exercise stress is always preferred over pharmacologic stress if the woman is able to exercise maximally to greater than 85% maximal heart rate (measured in beats per minute as 220 minus age, in years). Submaximal stress tests can have markedly reduced sensitivity for the detection of CVD in women and should be interpreted cautiously.

Electrocardiogram (ECG) monitoring is still primarily recommended for ischemic evaluation during stress testing, but in women, it has a high false-positive rate when used without nuclear or echocardiographic imaging. ECG alone cannot be used in women with baseline ST abnormalities or conduction disease on ECG. In women who cannot achieve maximal exercise stress or have baseline ECG abnormalities, pharmacologic stress choices include inotropic agents (eg, dobutamine) or vasodilators (eg, dipyridamole, adenosine).

Additional testing for systemic atherosclerosis using the ankle-brachial index would be indicated in the patient with leg cramping on exertion that is relieved by rest. Carotid B-mode ultrasound to measure intima-medial thickness may suggest further predisposition to CVD, indicating a need for additional risk factor modification and a lower LDL-C goal for lipid therapy. Electron-beam computed tomography to assess the extent of coronary artery calcification, although nonspecific in most patients, may suggest a likelihood of CVD if levels are high.

Diabetes mellitus risk. The goal of glucose screening is to identify women who have or who are at risk for DM. For a complete discussion of DM screening, see Section E, page 136.

Cancer risk. Cancer is the second leading cause of death for women in the United States and Canada, exceeded only by heart disease.

Menopause is not associated with increased cancer risk. However, since cancer rates increase with age, women in midlife and beyond should be evaluated for their risk of cancer of the lung, breast, uterus, ovary, colon, rectum, and skin—the most common cancers that affect women.

• *Breast cancer* is the second major cause of cancer mortality in US and Canadian women. For many women, breast cancer is their primary health concern. (See Section E, page 140, for a complete discussion.)

• *Endometrial cancer* affects cells that line the inside of the uterus (the endometrium). See Section E, page 146, for a complete discussion.)

• *Cervical cancer.* In North America, the mortality rate from cervical cancer has dropped sharply over the years but remains a serious concern. (See Section E, page 149, for a complete discussion.)

• *Ovarian cancer* causes more deaths than any other cancer of the reproductive system, primarily because it usually is detected in an advanced stage. (See Section E, page 151, for a complete discussion.

• *Colorectal cancer* is the third leading cause of cancer death in US and Canadian women. (See Section E, page 152, for a complete discussion.)

- *Pancreatic cancer* is generally asymptomatic until advanced stages. Jaundice may be the first symptom if the cancer develops near the common bile duct. (See Section E, page 154, for a complete discussion.)

- *Skin cancer.* Women should be examined periodically for skin cancers and precursors to skin cancer. (See Section E, page 155, for a complete discussion.)

Sexually transmitted infections. STI testing could include screening for pathogens, including bacterial vaginosis, chlamydia, genital herpes, gonorrhea, hepatitis B virus (HBV), human papillomavirus (HPV), human immuno-deficiency virus (HIV), and syphilis. (For a complete discussion, see Section E, page 156.)

Evaluation of premature menopause. Because ovarian insufficiency has a cumulative negative effect on bone and, possibly, CVD, a timely diagnosis is warranted. (See Section D for a complete discussion.)

Suggested reading

History gathering and Physical examination

Aiello EJ, Yasui Y, Tworoger SS, et al. Effect of a yearlong, moderate-intensity exercise intervention on the occurrence and severity of menopause symptoms in postmenopausal women. *Menopause* 2004;11:382-388.

Bradley KA, Boyd-Wickizer J, Powell SH, Burman ML. Alcohol screening questionnaires in women: a critical review. *JAMA* 1998;280:166-171.

Brown WJ, Williams L, Ford JH, Ball K, Dobson AJ. Identifying the energy gap: magnitude and determinants of 5-year weight gain in midage women. *Obes Res* 2005;13:1431-1441.

Calle EE, Rodriguez C, Walker-Thurmond K, Thun MJ. Overweight, obesity, and mortality from cancer in a prospectively studied cohort of US adults. *N Engl J Med* 2003;348:1625-1638.

Calle EE, Thun MJ, Petrelli JM, Rodriguez C, Heath CW Jr. Body-mass index and mortality in a prospective cohort of US adults. *N Engl J Med* 1999;341:1097-1105.

Chobanian AV, Bakris GL, Black HR, et al, for the Joint National Committee on Prevention, Detection, Evaluation, and Treatment of High Blood Pressure. National Heart, Lung, and Blood Institute; National High Blood Pressure Education Program Coordinating Committee. Seventh report of the Joint National Committee on Prevention, Detection, Evaluation, and Treatment of High Blood Pressure. *Hypertension* 2003;42:1206-1252.

Coker AL, Smith PH, Bethea L, King MR, McKeown RE. Physical health consequences of physical and psychological intimate partner violence. *Arch Fam Med* 2000;9:451-457.

Cowie CC, Rust KF, Byrd-Holt DD, et al. Prevalence of diabetes and impaired fasting glucose in adults in the US population: National Health and Nutrition Examination Survey 1999-2002. *Diabetes Care* 2006;21:1263-1268.

Dansinger ML, Gleason JA, Griffith JL, Selker HP, Schaefer EJ. Comparison of the Atkins, Ornish, Weight Watchers, and Zone diets for weight loss and heart disease risk reduction. *JAMA* 2005;293:43-53.

Davis SR, Davison SL, Donath S, Bell RJ. Circulating androgen levels and self-reported sexual function in women. *JAMA* 2005;294:91-96.

Di Castelnuovo AD, Costanzo S, Bagnardi V, Donati MB, Iacoviello L, Gaetano G. Alcohol dosing and total mortality in men and women: an updated meta-analysis of 34 prospective studies. *Arch Intern Med* 2006;166:2437-2445.

Eckel RH, Krauss RM. American Heart Association call to action: obesity as a major risk factor for coronary heart disease. American Heart Association Nutrition Committee. *Circulation* 1998;97:2099-2100.

Family Violence Prevention Fund. *National Consensus Guidelines on Identifying and Responding to Domestic Violence Victimization in Health Care Settings.* February 2004. Available at: http://www.endabuse.org/programs/healthcare/files/Consensus.pdf. Accessed July 3, 2007.

Fiellin DA, Reid MC, O'Connor PG. Outpatient management of patients with alcohol problems. *Ann Intern Med* 2000;133:815-827.

Folsom AR, Kushi LH, Anderson KE, et al. Associations of general and abdominal obesity with multiple health outcomes in older women: the Iowa Women's Health Study. *Arch Intern Med* 2000;160:2117-2128.

Gallicchio L, Miller SR, Visvanathan V, et al. Cigarette smoking, estrogen levels, and hot flashes in midlife women. *Maturitas* 2006;53:133-143.

Gielen AC, O'Campo PJ, Campbell JC, et al. Women's opinions about domestic violence screening and mandatory reporting. *Am J Prev Med* 2000;19:279-285.

Grundy SM, Cleeman JI, Daniels SR, et al. Diagnosis and management of the metabolic syndrome: an American Heart Association/National Heart, Lung, and Blood Institute Scientific Statement. *Circulation* 2005;112:2735-2752.

Guyatt GH, Velhuyzen Van Zanten SJ, Feeny DH, Patrick DL. Measuring quality of life in clinical trials: a taxonomy and review. *CMAJ* 1989;140:1441-1448.

Health Canada. Physical Activity of Canadians: Baby Boomers Aged 40 to 54. Ottawa, ON, Canada: *National Population Health Survey Highlights*, 1999.

Howard BV, Van Horn L, Hsia J, et al, for the Women's Health Initiative Investigators. Low-fat dietary pattern and risk of cardiovascular disease: the Women's Health Initiative randomized controlled Dietary Modification Trial. *JAMA* 2006;295:655-666.

Humphreys J, Parker B, Campbell JC. Intimate partner violence against women. In: Fitzpatrick JJ, Taylor D, Woods N, eds. *Annual Review of Nursing Research.* New York: Springer Publishing, 2001:275-306.

Jakicic JM, Marcus BH, Gallagher KI, Napolitano M, Lang W. Effect of exercise duration and intensity on weight loss in overweight, sedentary women: a randomized trial. *JAMA* 2003;290:1323-1330.

Klap R, Tang L, Wells K, Starks SL, Rodriguez M. Screening for domestic violence among adult women in the United States. *J Gen Intern Med* 2007;22:579-584.

Kuller LH, Simkin-Silverman LR, Wing RR, Meilahn EN, Ives DG. Women's Healthy Lifestyle Project: a randomized clinical trial. *Circulation* 2001;103:32-37.

Kyriacou DN, Anglin D, Taliaferro E, et al. Risk factors for injury to women from domestic violence against women. *N Engl J Med* 1999;341:1892-1898.

Lindh-Astrand L, Nedstrand E, Wyon Y, Hammar M. Vasomotor symptoms and quality of life in previously sedentary postmenopausal women randomised to physical activity or estrogen therapy. *Maturitas* 2004;48:97-105.

McTigue KM, Harris R, Hemphill B, et al. Screening and interventions for obesity in adults: summary of the evidence for the US Preventive Services Task Force. *Ann Intern Med* 2003;139:933-949.

Moore T, Conlin P, Ard J, Svetky L. DASH diet is effective treatment for stage 1 isolated systolic hypertension. *Hypertension* 2001;38:155-158.

National Cholesterol Education Program/American Heart Association step I dietary pattern on cardiovascular disease. *Circulation* 2001;103:1823-1825.

National Institutes of Health Consensus Development Panel on Osteoporosis Prevention, National Women's Health Report. Women and obesity. *Natl Womens Health Rep* 2006;28:1-4.

National Institutes of Health, National Heart, Lung, and Blood Institute. Clinical guidelines on the identification, evaluation, and treatment of overweight and obesity in adults: evidence report. 1998. Available at: http://www.nhlbi.nih.gov/guidelines/obesity/ob_gdlns.pdf. Accessed July 5, 2007.

National Institutes of Health, National Heart, Lung, and Blood Institute. The Practical Guide to Identification, Evaluation, and Treatment of Overweight and Obesity in Adults: evidence report. 2000. Available at: http://www.nhlbi.nih.gov/guidelines/obesity/prctgd_c.pdf. Accessed July 2, 2007.

National Library of Medicine, National Institutes of Health. How to determine your BMI. 2006. Available at: http://www.nlm.nih.gov/medlineplus/ency/article/007196.htm. Accessed July 5, 2007.

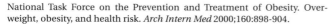

National Task Force on the Prevention and Treatment of Obesity. Overweight, obesity, and health risk. *Arch Intern Med* 2000;160:898-904.

Osteoporosis Canada. Calcium calculator. Available at: http://www.osteoporosis.ca/english/about%20osteoporosis/calcium%20calculator/default.asp?s=1). Accessed August 2, 2007.

Park HS, Lee KU. Postmenopausal women lose less visceral adipose tissue during a weight reduction program. *Menopause* 2003;10:222-227.

Ross GW, Abbott RD, Petrovitch H, et al. Association of coffee and caffeine intake with the risk of Parkinson disease *JAMA* 2000;283:2674-2679.

Schneider HJ, Glaesner H, Klotsche J, et al, for the DETECT Study Group. Accuracy of anthropometric indicators of obesity to predict cardiovascular risk. *J Clin Endocrinol Metab* 2007;92:589-594.

Snow V, Barry P, Fitterman N, Qaseem A, Weiss K, for the Clinical Efficacy Assessment Subcommittee of the American College of Physicians. Pharmacologic and surgical management of obesity in primary care: a clinical practice guideline from the American College of Physicians. *Ann Intern Med* 2005;142:525-531.

US Department of Health and Human Services, Office of Disease Prevention and Health Promotion Program. *Healthy People 2010*. Washington, DC: US Department of Health and Human Services, 2002. Available at: http://www.health.gov/healthypeople. Accessed July 2, 2007.

US Department of Health and Human Services and US Department of Agriculture. *Dietary Guidelines for Americans, 2005*, 6th ed. Washington, DC: US Government Printing Office, 2005. Available at: http://www.healthierus.gov/dietaryguidelines. Accessed August 2, 2007.

US Preventive Services Task Force. Screening for family and intimate partner violence: recommendation statement. *Ann Intern Med* 2004; 140:382-386.

US Preventive Services Task Force. Screening for obesity in adults: recommendations and rationale. *Ann Intern Med* 2003;139:930-932.

Ustun B, Compton W, Mager D, et al. WHO Study on the reliability and validity of the alcohol and drug use disorder instruments: overview of methods and results [erratum in: *Drug Alcohol Depend* 1998;50:185-186]. *Drug Alcohol Depend* 1997;47:161-169.

Utian WH, Janata JW, Kingsberg SA, Schluchter M, Hamilton JC. The Utian Quality of Life (UQOL) Scale: development and validation of an instrument to quantify quality of life through and beyond menopause. *Menopause* 2002;9:402-410.

Warren MP, Artacho CA, Hagey AR. Role of exercise and nutrition. In: Lobo RA, ed. *Treatment of the Postmenopausal Woman: Basic and Clinical Aspects*, 3rd ed. San Diego, CA: Academic Press, 2007:655-682.

Wiklund I, Dimenas E, Wahl M. Factors of importance when evaluating quality of life in clinical trials. *Control Clin Trials* 1990;11:169-179.

Winger G, Woods JH, Hofmann FG, eds. *A Handbook on Drug and Alcohol Abuse: The Biomedical Aspects*, 4th ed. New York: Oxford University Press, 2004.

Zhang SM, Lee IM, Manson JE, Cook NR, Willett WC, Buring JE. Alcohol consumption and breast cancer risk in the Women's Health Study. *Am J Epidemiol* 2007;165:667-676.

Zollner YF, Acquadro C, Schaefer M. Literature review of instruments to assess health-related quality of life during and after menopause. *Qual Life Res* 2005;14:309-327.

Diagnostic and screening tests

Alonso de Lecinana M, Egido JA, Fernandez C, et al, for the PIVE Study Investigators of the Stroke Project of the Spanish Cerebrovascular Diseases Study Group. Risk of ischemic stroke and lifetime estrogen exposure. *Neurology* 2007;68:33-38.

American Cancer Society. *Cancer Facts & Figures 2007*. Available at: http://www.cancer.org/docroot/STT/content/STT_1x_Cancer_Facts__Figures_2007.asp. Accessed July 11, 2007.

The American College of Obstetrics and Gynecologists. Primary and preventive care: periodic assessments. ACOG Committee Opinion Number 357. December 2006.

American College of Physicians. Screening for thyroid disease. Available at: http://www.acponline.org/sci-policy/thyralgo.htm. Accessed July 11, 2007.

American Diabetes Association. Screening for type 2 diabetes. *Diabetes Care* 2004;27(suppl):S11-S14.

American Heart Association. Heart disease and stroke statistics—2007 update. Available at: http://circ.ahajournals.org/cgi/content/full/circulationaha.106.179918. Accessed September 4, 2007.

Anderson GL, Judd HL, Kaunitz AM, et al, for the Women's Health Initiative investigators. Effects of estrogen plus progestin on gynecologic cancers and associated diagnostic procedures: the Women's Health Initiative randomized trial. *JAMA* 2003;290:1739-1748.

Armstrong K, Eisen A, Weber B. Assessing the risk of breast cancer. *N Engl J Med* 2000;342:564-571.

Bachmann G, Bancroft J, Braunstein G, et al. Female androgen insufficiency: the Princeton consensus statement on definition, classification, and assessment. *Fertil Steril* 2002;77:660-665.

Bachmann G, Cheng RF, Rovner E. Vulvovaginal complaints. In: Lobo RA, ed. *Treatment of the Postmenopausal Woman: Basic and Clinical Aspects*, 3rd ed. San Diego, CA: Academic Press, 2007:263-269.

Baines CJ, McFarlane DV, Miller AB. Sensitivity and specificity of first screen mammography in 15 NBSS centres. *Can Assoc Radiol J* 1988;39:273-276.

Bairey Merz CN, Johnson BD, Berga S, Braunstein G, Reis SE, Bittner V, for the WISE Study Group. Past oral contraceptive use and angiographic coronary artery disease in postmenopausal women: data from the National Heart, Lung and Blood Institute-sponsored Women's Ischemia Syndrome Evaluation. *Fertil Steril* 2006;85:1425-1431.

Berry DA, Cronin KA, Pleviritis SK, et al, for the Cancer Intervention and Surveillance Modeling Network (CISNET) Collaborators. Effect of screening and adjuvant therapy on mortality from breast cancer. *N Engl J Med* 2005;353:1784-1792.

Boyd NF, Byng JW, Jong RA, et al. Quantitative classification of mammographic densities and breast cancer risk: results from the Canadian National Breast Cancer Screening Study. *J Natl Cancer Inst* 1995;87:670-675.

Boyd NF, Dite GS, Stone J, et al. Heritability of mammographic density, a risk factor for breast cancer. *N Engl J Med* 2002;12:886-894.

Buse J, Ginsberg HN, Bakris GL, et al; American Heart Association; American Diabetes Association. Primary prevention of cardiovascular disease in people with diabetes mellitus: a scientific statement from the American Heart Association and the American Diabetes Association. *Circulation* 2007;115:114-126.

Byrne C, Schairer C, Wolfe J, et al. Mammographic features and breast cancer risk: effects with time, age, and menopause status. *J Natl Cancer Inst* 1995;87:1622-1629.

Canadian Diabetes Association. 2003 clinical practice guidelines for the prevention and management of diabetes in Canada: selected highlights. Canadian Diabetes Association. 2003. Available at: http://www.diabetes.ca/files/CPG backgrounders.pdf. Accessed July 2, 2007.

Centers for Disease Control and Prevention. *Chlamydia in the United States; April 2001*. Available at: http://www.cdc.gov/std/chlamydia/STDFact-Chlamydia.htm. Accessed August 5, 2007.

Centers for Disease Control and Prevention. Sexually transmitted diseases treatment guidelines 2002. *MMWR* 2002;51(RR-6):1-78.

Chen C-L, Weiss NS, Newcomb P, Barlow W, White E. Hormone-replacement therapy in relation to breast cancer. *JAMA* 2002;287:734-741.

Chlebowski RT, Wactawski-Wende J, Ritenbaugh C, et al, for the Women's Health Initiative Investigators. Estrogen plus progestin and colorectal cancer in postmenopausal women. *N Engl J Med* 2004;350:991-1004.

Chobanian AV, Bakris GL, Black HR, et al, for the National High Blood Pressure Education Program Coordinating Committee. The seventh report of the Joint National Committee on Prevention, Detection, Evaluation, and Treatment of High Blood Pressure: the JNC 7 report. *JAMA* 2003;289:2560-2572.

Clevenger-Hoeft M, Syrop CH, Stovall DW, et al. Sonohysterography in premenopausal women with and without abnormal bleeding. *Obstet Gynecol* 1999;94:516-520.

College of Cardiology/American Heart Association expert consensus document on electron-beam computed tomography for the diagnosis and prognosis of coronary artery disease. *J Am Coll Cardiol* 2000;36:326-340.

Creinin MD. Laboratory criteria for menopause in women using oral contraceptives. *Fertil Steril* 1996;66:101-104.

Day SJ, Deszo EL, Freund GG. Dual sampling of the endocervix and its impact on AutoCyte Prep endocervical adequacy. *Am J Clin Pathol* 2002;118:41-46.

Dijkhuizen FP, Mol BW, Brolmann HA, Heinz AP. The accuracy of endometrial sampling in the diagnosis of patients with endometrial carcinoma and hyperplasia: a meta-analysis. *Cancer* 2000;89:1765-1772.

Executive summary: Stages of Reproductive Aging Workshop (STRAW): Park City, Utah, July 2001. *Menopause* 2001;8:402-407.

Expert Panel on Detection, Evaluation, and Treatment of High Blood Cholesterol in Adults. Executive summary of the third report of the National Cholesterol Education Program (NCEP) Expert Panel on Detection, Evaluation, and Treatment of High Blood Cholesterol in Adults (Adult Treatment Panel III). *JAMA* 2001;285:2486-2497.

Fabian CJ, Kimler BF, Zalles CM, et al. Short-term breast cancer prediction by random periareolar fine-needle aspiration cytology and the Gail risk model. *J Natl Cancer Inst* 2000;92:1217-1227.

Fischbach F. *A Manual of Laboratory & Diagnostic Tests*, 7th ed. Philadelphia, PA: Lippincott Williams & Wilkins, 2003.

Fowler-Brown A, Pignone M, Pletcher M, Tice JA, Sutton SF, Lohr KN; US Preventive Services Task Force. Exercise tolerance testing to screen for coronary heart disease: a systematic review for the technical support for the US Preventive Services Task Force. *Ann Intern Med* 2004;140:W9-W24.

Fox J, Remington P, Layde P, et al. The effect of hysterectomy on the risk of an abnormal screening Papanicolaou test result. *Am J Obstet Gynecol* 1999;180:1104-1109.

Gail MH, Brinton LA, Byar DP, et al. Projecting individualized probabilities of developing breast cancer for white females examined annually. *J Natl Cancer Inst* 1989;81:1879-1886.

Garnero P, Hausherr E, Chapuy MC, et al. Markers of bone resorption predict hip fracture in elderly women: the EPIDOS Prospective Study. *J Bone Miner Res* 1996;11:1531-1538.

Gibbons RJ, Balady GJ, Bricker JT, et al. ACC/AHA 2002 guideline update for exercise testing: summary article. A report of the American College of Cardiology/American Heart Association Task Force on Practice Guidelines (Committee to Update the 1997 Exercise Testing Guidelines). *Circulation* 2002;106:1883-1892.

Girdler SS, Hinderliter AL, Wells EC, Sherwood A, Grewen KM, Light KC. Transdermal versus oral estrogen therapy in postmenopausal smokers: hemodynamic and endothelial effects. *Obstet Gynecol* 2004;103:169-180.

Godtfredsen NS, Prescott E, Osler M. Effect of smoking reduction on lung cancer risk. *JAMA* 2005;294:1505-1510.

Greendale GA, Reboussin BA, Sie A, et al, for the Postmenopausal Estrogen/Progestin Interventions (PEPI) Investigators. Effects of estrogen and estrogen-progestin on mammographic parenchymal density. *Ann Intern Med* 1999;130:262-269.

Greenland P, Smith SC, Grundy SM. Improving coronary heart disease risk assessment in asymptomatic people: role of traditional risk factors and noninvasive cardiovascular tests. *Circulation* 2001;104:1863-1867.

Grundy SM, Pasternak R, Greenland P, Smith S, Fuster V. Assessment of cardiovascular risk by use of multiple risk factor assessment equations: a statement for healthcare professionals from the American Heart Association and the American College of Cardiology. *Circulation* 1999;97:1837-1847.

Ho MH, Bhatia NN. Lower urinary tract disorders in postmenopausal women. In: Lobo RA, ed. *Treatment of the Postmenopausal Woman: Basic and Clinical Aspects*, 3rd ed. San Diego, CA: Academic Press, 2007:693-737.

Hulley S, Furberg C, Barrett-Connor E, et al, for the HERS Research Group. Noncardiovascular disease outcomes during 6.8 years of hormone therapy: Heart and Estrogen/progestin Replacement Study follow-up (HERS II). *JAMA* 2002;288:58-66.

Kannel WB, Hjortland MC, McNamara PM, Gordon T. Menopause and risk of cardiovascular disease: the Framingham study. *Ann Intern Med* 1976;85:447-452.

Kaunitz AM, Masciello A, Ostrowski M, et al. Comparison of endometrial biopsy with the endometrial Pipelle and Vabra aspirator. *J Reprod Med* 1988;33:427-431.

Kavanagh AM, Mitchell H, Giles GG. Hormone replacement therapy and accuracy of mammographic screening. *Lancet* 2000;355:270-274.

Kim YK, Wasser SK, Fujimoto VY, Klein NA, Moore DE, Soules MR. Utility of follicle stimulating hormone (FSH), luteinizing hormone (LH), oestradiol and FSH:LH ratio in predicting reproductive age in normal women. *Hum Reprod* 1997;12:1152-1155.

Knight JA, Martin LJ, Greenberg CV, et al. Macronutrient intake and change in mammographic density at menopause: results from a randomized trial. *Cancer Epidemiol Biomarkers Prev* 1999;8:123-128.

Kriege M, Brekelmans CTM, Boetes C, et al, for the Magnetic Resonance Imaging Screening Study Guide. Efficacy of MRI and mammography for breast-cancer screening in women with a familial or genetic predisposition. *N Engl J Med* 2004;351:427-437.

Labrie F, Belanger A, Cusan L, Gomez JL, Candas B. Marked decline in serum concentrations of adrenal C19 sex steroid precursors and conjugated androgen metabolites during aging. *J Clin Endocrinol Metab* 1997;82:2396-2402.

Labrie F, Luu-The V, Labrie C, Simard J. DHEA and its transformation into androgens and estrogens in peripheral target tissues: intracrinology. *Front Neuroendocrinol* 2001;22:185-212.

Ladenson PW, Singer PA, Ain KB, et al. American Thyroid Association guidelines for detection of thyroid dysfunction. *Arch Intern Med* 2000;160:1573-1575.

Langer RD, Pierce JJ, O'Hanlon KA, et al. Transvaginal ultrasonography compared with endometrial biopsy for the detection of endometrial disease. *N Engl J Med* 1997;337:1792-1798.

Laya MB, Larson EB, Taplin SH, White E. Effect of estrogen replacement therapy on the specificity and sensitivity of screening mammography. *J Natl Cancer Inst* 1996;88:643-649.

Lieberman DA, Weiss DG, Bond JH, Ahnen DJ, Garewal H, Chejfec G. Use of colonoscopy to screen asymptomatic adults for colorectal cancer. Veterans Affairs Cooperative Study Group 380. *N Engl J Med* 2000;343:162-168.

Lochner DM, Brubaker KL. Incidence of malignancy in hormone therapy users with indeterminate calcifications on mammogram. *Am J Obstet Gynecol* 2006;194:82-85.

Manson JE, Colditz GA, Stampfer MJ, et al. A prospective study of obesity and risk of coronary heart disease in women. *N Engl J Med* 1990;322:882-889.

McTiernan A, Kooperberg C, White E, et al. Recreational physical activity and the risk of breast cancer in postmenopausal women: the Women's Health Initiative Cohort Study. *JAMA* 2003;290:1331-1336.

McTiernan A, Martin CF, Peck JD, et al, for the Women's Health Initiative Mammogram Density Study Investigators. Estrogen-plus-progestin use and mammographic density in postmenopausal women: Women's Health Initiative randomized trial. *J Natl Cancer Inst* 2005;97:1366-1376.

Mosca L, Banka CL, Benjamin EJ, et al, for the Expert Panel/Writing Group. Evidence-based guidelines for cardiovascular disease prevention in women: 2007 update. *Circulation* 2007;115:1481-1501.

Mosca L, Jones WK, King KB, Ouyang P, Redberg RF, Hill MN, for the American Heart Association Women's Heart Disease and Stroke Campaign Task Force. Awareness, perception, and knowledge of heart disease risk and prevention among women in the United States. *Arch Fam Med* 2000;9:506-515.

National Cancer Institute of Canada. *Canadian Cancer Statistics* 2007. Available at: http://www.cancer.ca. Accessed July 11, 2007.

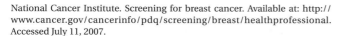

National Cancer Institute. Screening for breast cancer. Available at: http://www.cancer.gov/cancerinfo/pdq/screening/breast/healthprofessional. Accessed July 11, 2007.

The North American Menopause Society. Effects of menopause and estrogen replacement therapy or hormone replacement therapy in women with diabetes mellitus: consensus opinion of The North American Menopause Society. *Menopause* 2000;7:87-95.

The North American Menopause Society. Estrogen and progestogen use in peri- and postmenopausal women: September 2007 position statement of The North American Menopause Society. *Menopause* 2007;14:168-182.

The North American Menopause Society. Management of postmenopausal osteoporosis: 2006 position statement of The North American Menopause Society. *Menopause* 2006;13:340-367.

The North American Menopause Society. The role of calcium in peri- and postmenopausal women: 2006 position statement. *Menopause* 2006;13:862-877.

Olsen O, Gøtzsche PC. Cochrane review on screening for breast cancer with mammography. *Lancet* 2001;358:1340-1342.

Parsons AK, Londono JL. Detection and surveillance of endometrial hyperplasia and carcinoma. In: Lobo RA, ed. *Treatment of the Postmenopausal Woman: Basic and Clinical Aspects.* Philadelphia, PA: Lippincott Williams & Wilkins, 1999:513-538.

Pickhardt PJ, Choi R, Hwang I, et al. Computed tomographic virtual colonoscopy to screen for colorectal neoplasia in asymptomatic adults. *N Engl J Med* 2003;349:2191-2200.

Pisano ED, Gatsonis C, Hendrick E, et al, for the Digital Mammographic Imaging Screening Trial (DMIST) Investigators Group. Diagnostic performance of digital versus film mammography for breast-cancer screening. *N Engl J Med* 2005;353:1773-1783.

Ridker PM, Hennekens CH, Buring JE, Rifai N. C-reactive protein and other markers of inflammation in the prediction of cardiovascular disease in women. *N Engl J Med* 2000;342:836-843.

Rosenberg RD, Hunt WC, Williamson MR, et al. Effects of age, breast density, ethnicity, and estrogen replacement therapy on screening mammographic sensitivity and cancer stage at diagnosis: review of 183,134 screening mammograms in Albuquerque, New Mexico. *Radiology* 1998;209:511-518.

Roubidoux MA, Wilson TE, Orange RJ, Fitzgerald JT, Helvie MA, Packer SA. Breast cancer in women who undergo screening mammography: relationship of hormone replacement therapy to stage and detection method. *Radiology* 1998;208:725-728.

Saslow D, Boetes C, Burke W, et al, for the American Cancer Society Breast Cancer Advisory Group. American Cancer Society guidelines for breast screening with MRI as an adjunct to mammography. [Erratum in: *CA Cancer J Clin* 2007;57:185] *CA Cancer J Clin* 2007;57:75-89.

Sawaya GF, Grady D, Kerlikowske K, et al. The positive predictive value of cervical smears in previously screened postmenopausal women: the Heart and Estrogen/progestin Replacement Study (HERS). *Ann Intern Med* 2000;133:942-950.

Sawaya GF, McConnell KJ, Kulasingam SL, et al. Risk of cervical cancer associated with extending the interval between cervical-cancer screenings. *N Engl J Med* 2003;349:1501-1509.

Schaefer EJ, Lamon-Fava S, Cohn SD, et al. Effects of age, gender, and menopausal status on plasma low density lipoprotein cholesterol and apolipoprotein B levels in the Framingham Offspring Study. *J Lipid Res* 1994;35:779-792.

Schairer C, Gail M, Byrne C, et al. Estrogen replacement therapy and breast cancer survival in a large screening study. *J Natl Cancer Inst* 1999;91:264-270.

Schiffman M, Solomon D. Findings to date from the ASCUS-LSIL Triage Study (ALTS). *Arch Pathol Lab Med* 2003;127:946-949.

Schoenfeld P, Cash B, Flood A, et al, for the CONCeRN Study Investigators. Colonoscopic screening of average-risk women for colorectal neoplasia. *N Engl J Med* 2005;352:2061-2068.

Shavelle DM, Budoff MJ, LaMont DH, Shavelle RM, Kennedy JM, Brundage BH. Exercise testing and electron beam computed tomography in the evaluation of coronary artery disease. *J Am Coll Cardiol* 2000;36:32-38.

Smith RA, Cokkinides V, Eyre HJ. American Cancer Society guidelines for the early detection of cancer, 2006. *CA Cancer J Clin* 2006;56:11-25.

Smith RA, Saslow D, Sawyer KA, et al, for the Breast Cancer Advisory Group. American Cancer Society guidelines for breast cancer screening: update 2003. *CA Cancer J Clin* 2003;54:141-169.

Smith-Bindman R, Kerlikowske K, Feldstein VA, et al. Endovaginal ultrasound to exclude endometrial cancer and other endometrial abnormalities. *JAMA* 1998;280:1510-1517.

Sornay-Rendu E, Munoz F, Garnero P, Duboeuf F, Delmas PD. Identification of osteopenic women at high risk of fracture: the OFELY study. *Bone Miner Res* 2005;20:1813-1819.

Stefanick ML, Anderson GL, Margolis KL, et al, for the Women's Health Initiative Investigators. Effects of conjugated equine estrogens on breast cancer and mammography screening in postmenopausal women with hysterectomy: the Women's Health Initiative. *JAMA* 2006;295:1647-1657.

Stenson WF, Newberry R, Lorenz R, Baldus C, Civitelli R. Increased prevalence of celiac disease and need for routine screening among patients with osteoporosis. *Arch Intern Med* 2005;165:393-399.

Stovall TG, Photopulos GJ, Poston WM, Ling FW, Sandles LG. Pipelle endometrial sampling in patients with known endometrial carcinoma. *Obstet Gynecol* 1991;77:954-956.

Surks MI, Ortiz E, Daniels GH, et al. Subclinical thyroid disease: scientific review and guidelines for diagnosis and management. *JAMA* 2004;291:228-238.

Tilanus-Linthorst MM, Obdeijin IM, Bartels KC, et al. First experiences in screening women at high risk for breast cancer with MR imaging. *Breast Cancer Res Treat* 2000;63:53-60.

US Preventive Services Task Force. Screening for breast cancer: recommendations and rationale. 2002. Available at: http://www.ahrq.gov/clinic/3rduspstf/breastcancer/brcanrr.htm. Accessed July 11, 2007.

US Preventive Services Task Force. Screening for chlamydial infection. 2007. Available at: http://www.ahrq.gov/clinic/uspstf/uspschlm.htm. Accessed July 11, 2007.

US Preventive Services Task Force. Screening for coronary heart disease: Recommendation statement. 2004. Available at: http://www.ahrq.gov/clinic/3rduspstf/chd/chdrs.htm. Accessed July 11, 2007.

US Preventive Services Task Force. Screening for diabetes mellitus, adult type 2: recommendations and rationale. 2003. Available at: http://www.ahrq.gov/clinic/3rduspstf/diabscr/diabetrr.htm. Accessed July 11, 2007.

US Preventive Services Task Force. Screening for osteoporosis in postmenopausal women: recommendations and rationale. 2002. Available at: http://www.ahrq.gov/clinic/3rduspstf/osteoporosis/osteorr.htm. Accessed July 11, 2007.

US Preventive Services Task Force. Screening for thyroid disease: recommendation statement. *Ann Intern Med* 2004;140:125-127.

Warren R, Skinner J, Sala E, et al. Associations among mammographic density, circulating sex hormones, and polymorphisms in sex hormone metabolism genes in postmenopausal women. *Cancer Epidemiol Biomarkers Prev* 2006;15:1502-1508.

Weiss M, Loprinzi CL, Creagan ET, Dalton RJ, Novotny P, O'Fallon JR. Utility of follow-up tests for detecting recurrent disease in patients with malignant melanomas. *JAMA* 1995;274:1703-1705.

Wilson PW, D'Agostino RB, Levy D, et al. Prediction of coronary heart disease using risk factor categories. *Circulation* 1998;97:1837-1847.

World Health Organization. *Assessment of Fracture Risk and Its Application to Screening for Postmenopausal Osteoporosis: Report of a WHO Study Group.* Geneva, Switzerland: World Health Organization, 1994. Technical report series 843.

Prescription hormonal drugs—including contraceptives, menopause hormone therapy (HT), androgens, selective estrogen-receptor modulators (SERMs; now termed estrogen agonists/antagonists by the US Food and Drug Administration)—and over-the-counter (OTC) hormone treatments are among the treatments considered for women during perimenopause and beyond. The majority are government approved for the indication(s) for which they are most commonly prescribed (see Box), whereas some are prescribed "off label" (ie, used for an indication other than the government-approved indication). OTC hormone treatments are classified as dietary supplements ("natural health products" in Canada) and are approved differently from prescription drugs. Hormonal drugs that are custom compounded from a prescription are not government approved, although some active ingredients meet the specifications of the United States *Pharmacopeia* (USP) (see page 218 for more about custom-compounded hormones).

What Does Government Approval Mean?

In the prescription drug approval process in the United States, a manufacturer sends study information on a particular product for a particular health indication to the US Food and Drug Administration (FDA). The FDA then considers the product's effectiveness, dosage, side effects, and possible short-term and long-term risks. If FDA approval is given, the product may then be offered on the US market for the approved health indication(s), accompanied by the FDA-approved product labeling (ie, prescribing information or package insert). All advertising and education from the manufacturer must comply with the prescribing information. In Canada, a similar regulatory process exists with the Therapeutic Products Directorate of Health Canada.

Once a drug is on the market clinicians can legally prescribe it for "off-label" (unapproved) indications (eg, prescribing an oral contraceptive to treat hot flashes). This is a common medical practice that relies on additional research and clinical experience documenting safety, efficacy, and dose. Also, in certain US states with the patient's permission, a pharmacist can substitute a generic equivalent drug, if available, for the one that was prescribed

Clinicians can also legally write an individual prescription for a custom drug formulation that is mixed (compounded) by a pharmacist. Although the active ingredient(s) is government approved, the formulation is not.

OTC products are regulated differently from drugs, with the marketer not being required to prove efficacy, safety, and proper dose. These are regulated as "dietary supplements" ("natural health products" in Canada) even though they may not be used orally see Section H, page 237, for more about how dietary supplements are regulated).

Contraceptives

Despite a decline in fertility during perimenopause, pregnancy is still possible until menopause is reached. Perimenopausal women who wish to guard against an unwanted pregnancy should be counseled regarding various birth control methods (see Section C, page 29, for more about fertility and nonhormonal options for birth control). Hormonal contraceptives—both with and without estrogen—offer a viable option for more perimenopausal women. Readers are referred to standard texts for listings of available hormonal contraceptives and their respective government-approved labeling (prescribing information).

Perimenopausal women should be aware that use of oral contraceptives (OCs) or any other hormonal or intrauterine contraceptive method does not reduce the risk of acquiring sexually transmitted infections (STIs). Accordingly, women at risk should protect themselves through use of "safer sex" practices (see Section C, page 156, for more about avoiding STIs).

Combination (estrogen-progestin) contraceptives. Many oral and nonoral options are available when prescribing a combination contraceptive (ie, containing estrogen and progestin).

Labeling for all estrogen-containing contraceptives in the United States and Canada contains a black box warning that cigarette smoking increases the risk of serious cardiovascular side effects from hormonal contraceptive use, and that this risk increases with age and with heavy smoking (≥15 cigarettes/d) and is quite marked in women over age 35. Women over age 35 who smoke should not use estrogen-containing contraceptives.

Labeling also lists other contraindications. These hormonal therapies increase the risk of venous thromboembolism (VTE). Although the incidence of VTE is very low in reproductive-age women, VTE risk increases with age and body mass index. Thus, an additional contraindication for perimenopausal women is obesity (see Table 1).

Combination estrogen-progestin contraceptives are a safe, effective birth control option for healthy, lean, nonsmoking, midlife women. Of these, combination OCs have been found to provide important noncontraceptive benefits, including regulation of irregular uterine bleeding, reduction of vasomotor symptoms, decreased risk for ovarian and endometrial cancer, and maintenance of bone density (with a potential for decreased risk for postmenopausal osteoporotic fractures). Use of low-dose OCs has not been found to increase the risk of myocardial infarction or stroke in these women, nor does long-term use appear to affect the risk of breast cancer. These benefits may apply for nonoral combination contraceptives as well. (Refer to labeling for details, including side effects, for each drug.)

Table 1. Labeling contraindications for estrogen-containing contraceptives in perimenopausal women
• Cigarette smoking
• Obesity
• Thrombophlebitis or thromboembolic disorders
• Cerebrovascular or coronary artery disease (current or past history)
• Valvular heart disease with thrombogenic complications
• Thrombogenic rhythm disorders
• Hereditary or acquired thrombophilias
• Major surgery with prolonged immobilization
• Diabetes mellitus with vascular involvement
• Headaches with focal neurological symptoms such as aura
• Uncontrolled hypertension
• Known or suspected carcinoma of the breast or personal history of breast cancer
• Carcinoma of the endometrium of other known of suspected estrogen-dependent neoplasia
• Undiagnosed abnormal genital bleeding
• Cholestatic jaundice of pregnancy or jaundice with prior hormonal contraceptive use
• Hepatic adenomas or carcinomas, or active liver disease
• Known or suspected pregnancy

Oral combination contraceptives. OCs are the most commonly used combination estrogen-progestin contraceptive, and dozens are available in North America. Many consumers refer to an OC as "The Pill."

When prescribing combination OCs for perimenopausal women, some clinicians feel that prescribing ultralow-dose estrogen OCs is prudent. However, use of traditional OC formulations (21 active tablets followed by 7 hormone-free days) with 20 µg estrogen is associated with higher rates of breakthrough bleeding and spotting. Newer formulations with 25 µg estrogen and a triphasic regimen of the progestins desogestrel (Cyclessa) or norgestimate (Ortho Tricylen Lo)—both available in the United States but not Canada—appear to achieve the low rates of unscheduled bleeding and spotting characteristic of higher-estrogen OCs. Accordingly, these 25-µg estrogen formulations may be a prudent choice for perimenopausal women. Some perimenopausal women may note the occurrence of bothersome vasomotor symptoms or other symptoms during the 7-day OC pill-free interval. Use of continuous OC tablets or formulations with shorter or no pill-free intervals often reduces such symptoms.

Two 20-µg estrogen combination OCs formulated with the progestin norethindrone acetate (Lo Estrin-24 Fe) or drospirenone (Yaz) are based on a 24/4 regimen (24 active pills followed by 4 placebo days) rather than the traditional 21/7 cycle. These newer formulations, both available in the United States but not Canada, may have a better bleeding profile than other formulations containing 20 µg of estrogen, although studies are lacking in perimenopausal women.

Drospirenone differs from other synthetic progestins in that it is derived from 17α-spirolactone. The estrogen plus drospirenone OC (Yaz) has similar efficacy and safety profiles to other low-dose OCs, but seems to offer improved tolerability with regard to weight gain, acne, and mood changes. Drospirenone has antimineralocorticoid activity, including the potential for hyperkalemia in high-risk patients. Yaz, which delivers daily doses of 3 mg drospirenone plus 20 µg ethinyl estradiol, is also FDA approved for the treatment of symptoms of premenstrual dysphoric disorder (PMDD).

Use of extended-OC formulations results in withdrawal bleeding less than monthly. Two extended regimens (Seasonale, Seasonique; available in the United States but not Canada) include 84 tablets that combine 30 µg estrogen and the progestin levonorgestrel. Scheduled withdrawal bleeding occurs every 3 months.

One newer combination OC (Lybrel; available in the United States but not Canada) is designed to be taken 365 days a year, without a placebo phase or pill-free interval. Consisting of 90 µg levonorgestrel and 20 µg ethinyl estradiol, this continuous formulation OC provides a steady low dose of hormones. No scheduled withdrawal bleeding will occur with this OC. During the first few cycles, breakthrough bleeding is common, but bleeding decreases over time.

Common side effects of combination OCs include nausea and breast tenderness, which tend to resolve as OC use continues. Use of combination OCs does not cause weight gain or headaches.

Nonoral combination contraceptives. Government-approved nonoral combination contraceptives include a vaginal ring (NuvaRing; available in the United States and Canada) and a weekly patch (Ortho Evra, Evra; available in the United States but not Canada), both worn for 3 of 4 weeks. The ring releases ethinyl estradiol and etonogestrel and the patch delivers ethinyl estradiol and norelgestromin (the primary active metabolite of norgestimate). Etonogestrel and norelgestromin are the biologically active metabolites of desogestrel and norgestimate, respectively, both of which are progestins used in commonly prescribed combination OCs.

As with combination OCs, use of either the ring or patch results in cyclical monthly withdrawal bleeding. Because these methods are longer acting, patient adherence (and therefore contraceptive efficacy) may be higher than with oral combination products. Although side effects and contraindications are in general similar to those for combination OCs, breast tenderness is more common with initial use of the patch than with OCs.

Labeling indicates that the patch wearer is exposed to about 60% more estrogen versus using a typical OC containing 35 μg estrogen. As a result, labeling for the patch now contains a warning that its risk of VTE may be higher than with other combination contraceptives. One epidemiologic study found that VTE risk was similar to that of combination OCs, and another study found the risk two times higher with the patch. Because age is itself an independent risk factor for VTE, some experts believe that the ring and OCs are more appropriate contraceptive choices for perimenopausal women than the patch. (Readers are referred to the labeling for these products for more details.)

Progestin-only contraceptives. In contrast to combination contraceptives, progestin-only contraceptives can be used by some perimenopausal women for whom contraceptive doses of estrogen are contraindicated. They are, for example, an effective alternative for cigarette smokers over the age of 35, women with hypertension (controlled and uncontrolled), and those with a history of VTE. Contraindications include history of hormone-dependent cancer and unexplained abnormal uterine bleeding.

Progestin-only contraceptives are available in several routes of delivery: oral tablet, injection, subdermal implant, and intrauterine device (IUD). They also offer noncontraceptive advantages (see labeling).

Oral progestin-only contraceptives. Progestin-only OCs formulated with norethindrone or norgestrel provide effective contraception for perimenopausal women. Women using these therapies may experience irregular bleeding, spotting, or, less commonly, amenorrhea. Breakthrough bleeding is more common with these therapies than with combination contraceptives. It can be decreased by taking the pills on a strict schedule (ie, exact same time each day). Many consumers refer to this type of OC as "The Mini-Pill" or "POP" (progestin-only pill).

Injectable progestin-only contraceptives. Injectable progestin-only contraceptives are also available. The progestin medroxyprogesterone acetate (MPA) provides highly effective, long-term contraception when the hormone is administered suspended in a solution ("depot"). Depot MPA (DMPA) is available in the United States and Canada (Depo-Provera). The dose, 150 mg intramuscular (IM) injection into either the buttock or upper arm every 3 months, does not need to be adjusted for body weight. Although DMPA contraception is reversible, return of fertility after cessation of therapy can be delayed 12 to 18 months. Some DMPA users report weight gain. Less common side effects include change in libido, depression, and nervousness. Some consumers call DMPA "The Birth Control Shot."

Depo-subQ Provera 104 is the newer version, containing 31% less progestin (104 mg) than Depo-Provera IM. The dose is injected subcutaneously into the anterior thigh or abdomen every 3 months, using a smaller needle than IM administration, which may cause less pain. Depo-subQ Provera 104 is available in the United States, not Canada. It is also FDA approved for the treatment of endometriosis-related pain.

Initially, irregular bleeding or spotting is common with use of the injectable progestin-only contraceptives. After four or more injections, at least one half of users will experience amenorrhea. Use of these products suppresses ovarian estradiol production, which can reversibly lower bone mineral density (BMD). Labeling contains a black box warning of the loss of BMD. Accordingly, clinicians prescribing these injectables to perimenopausal women may wish to supplement ("add back") oral or transdermal estrogen, using doses similar to those used in conventional menopausal HT.

Implant progestin-only contraceptives. An etonogestrel subdermal contraceptive implant product (Implanon; available in the United States but not Canada), consisting of one toothpick-sized polymer capsule implanted under the skin of the inner arm by a healthcare provider, offers perimenopausal women highly effective contraception for up to 3 years. Irregular bleeding or spotting or amenorrhea may occur during implant use. The levonorgestrel subdermal implant product (Norplant), consisting of six silicone rods offering contraception for up to 5 years, is no longer available in North America.

Intrauterine device contraceptives. IUDs offer perimenopausal women highly effective, convenient, long-term contraception. The IUD is the most widely used reversible contraceptive around the world, with 85 to 100 million users. In the United States and Canada, however, the IUD is used by less than 1% of contraceptive users. The IUD may be a particularly desirable contraceptive alternative for midlife women, including those considering surgical sterilization.

One IUD available in the United States and Canada is the levonorgestrel-releasing intrauterine system (IUS; Mirena), FDA approved for 5 years of contraception (but appears to maintain high efficacy for up to 7 y). Irregular uterine bleeding and spotting are the most commonly reported side effects. These side effects become considerably less prominent as women develop either light cyclical menses; ongoing, unpredictable, light uterine bleeding or spotting; or amenorrhea.

For some perimenopausal women considering hysterectomy or endometrial ablation to treat menorrhagia, insertion of the progestin IUD may result in sufficient reduction in menstrual blood loss to allow long-term deferral or avoidance of surgery. Use of this IUD also appears as effective as GnRH agonists in treating pain associated with endometriosis. High local endometrial progestin concentrations are achieved with use of the progestin IUD. Accordingly, combining its use with systemic estrogen in menopausal HT achieves off-label treatment of vasomotor symptoms and endometrial protection.

The second IUD available in the United States is nonhormonal—the copper IUD (ParaGard T 380A), which is approved for 10 years of contraception (but appears to maintain high efficacy indefinitely). Canada has two copper IUDs (Nova-T and Flexi-T 300), each providing up to 5 years of contraception. The principal side effects associated with use of the copper IUD are increased cramping and menstrual flow. Accordingly, the copper IUD may not be an optimal choice for women who have problems with dysmenorrhea or menorrhagia at baseline.

The progesterone IUS, Progestasert, is no longer on the North American market.

Insertion of an IUD is an office-based procedure, with the procedure different for the two types. Although uterine perforation rarely occurs during insertion of modern IUDs, expulsion rates can be as high as 5% in the first months following insertion. Clinicians trained in insertion have the lowest rate of IUD expulsions and uterine perforations.

Emergency contraception. Emergency contraception (EC) refers to contraceptive measures that, if taken after coitus, may prevent pregnancy. It may be appropriate in certain cases, such as after unprotected sexual intercourse, a condom accident, an IUD partially or totally expelled, or if one or more progestin-only contraceptive pills or several combination OC pills have been missed. It is meant only for occasional use, when primary means of contraception fail, as other contraceptive methods are more reliable. The EC pill is often referred to as the "Morning-after Pill," but this phrase is figurative since these products are licensed for use up to 72 hours after sexual intercourse.

Since EC methods act before postfertilization implantation of the embryo, they are medically and legally considered forms of contraception according to the International Federation of Gynecology and Obstetrics. EC pills are not to be confused with the "Abortion Pill" (RU486, mifestone, Mifeprex).

Various oral estrogen-progestin contraceptives are government approved in the United States and Canada for safe and effective EC. Most use a dose of 120 µg ethinyl estradiol plus 0.60 mg levonorgestrel within 72 hours after unprotected intercourse, followed by another dose 12 hours later. It must be used within this time as EC has no effect once a fertilized egg has become implanted. Efficacy is approximately 75%. Nausea and vomiting are common side effects.

The progestin-only method, approved in the United States and Canada for EC, is more effective and better tolerated than the combined regimen. Marketed as Plan B, this method uses levonorgestrel in a dose of 1.5 mg, either as two 0.7-mg tablets 12 hours apart, or more recently as a single dose. The original FDA labeling indicated that Plan B reduces the risk of pregnancy by 89%. Current labeling does not include this figure, but states that if it is taken within 72 hours after coitus, 7 out of 8 women who would have become pregnant will not, and that Plan B works even better if taken within the first 24 hours after coitus. Individuals older that 18 years can purchase Plan B over the counter in the United States. Otherwise, Plan B is available by prescription. In Canada, Plan B is the only government-approved product for EC.

EC is not effective in women who are already pregnant. Inadvertent ingestion of EC during pregnancy, however, is not known to be harmful to the woman or her fetus. Concomitant administration of St. John's wort and some enzyme-inducing drugs (including certain anticonvulsants and the antibiotic rifampicin) may reduce the effectiveness of EC and larger doses of steroids may be required.

Noncontraceptive benefits of hormonal contraceptives. Perimenopausal use of combined OCs for contraception has been associated with many noncontraceptive benefits (see Table 2); these benefits may apply to other forms of estrogen-containing contraceptives.

Table 2. Noncontraceptive benefits of combined oral contraceptives for perimenopausal women
• Restoration of regular menses
• Decreased dysmenorrhea
• Reduced pain associated with endometriosis (continuous use of OCs)
• Reduced menorrhagia
• Suppression of vasomotor symptoms
• Enhanced BMD and possible prevention of osteoporotic fractures
• Decreased need for biopsies for benign breast disease
• Decreased need for surgery for benign ovarian tumors
• Prevention of endometrial and ovarian malignancies
• Possible prevention of colorectal cancer

Hormonal contraceptives (including extended-use combination OCs, injectable progestin, and the levonorgestrel-releasing IUS) are often used to reduce the frequency of menses or eliminate menstruation entirely (see Section C, page 30, for more about abnormal uterine bleeding).

Transition from hormonal contraception to HT. Some women will require HT after they have reached menopause. The clinical challenge is determining when to transition from the use of hormonal contraception to the lower hormone levels found in menopausal HT. Transitioning too soon may expose a perimenopausal woman to the risk of unintended pregnancy and result in irregular bleeding and unpleasant vasomotor symptoms. However, once it can be assured that menopause has been reached, transitioning to HT is advised so that hormone-related risks are minimized with exposure to lower levels.

Historically, monitoring the follicle-stimulating hormone (FSH) level has been used to determine when menopause is reached. However, assessing FSH is not useful in women using hormones. Some clinicians withdraw hormonal contraception, recommending use of a nonhormonal method of contraception until two FSH levels have been measured; however, some women experience unpleasant vasomotor symptoms during the hormone-free period.

Other clinicians prefer to recommend hormonal contraceptive use for a woman until she has reached an age at which she is statistically likely to be postmenopausal. In nonsmoking women, the median age of menopause is approximately 51 years—meaning that 50% of nonsmoking 51-year-old women have not reached menopause. About 90% of women will have reached menopause by age 55. Therefore, these clinicians continue contraception for women until they are age 55 or older. With this approach, women who choose to transition from hormonal contraception to HT can accomplish this without laboratory testing or any hormone-free days.

ET and EPT

The only pharmacologic therapy government approved in the United States and Canada for treating menopause-related symptoms is estrogen.

Terminology. Estrogen-containing drugs for menopausal use are divided into two categories: estrogen therapy (ET) and combined estrogen-progestogen therapy (EPT). (See Box for terminology preferred by NAMS.)

Menopausal hormone therapy terminology

Estrogen therapy (ET): unopposed estrogen prescribed for postmenopausal women who have had a hysterectomy. Close surveillance is required if ET is prescribed for women with a uterus who are intolerant of progestogens.

Estrogen plus progestogen (EPT): a combination of estrogen and progestogen (either progesterone or progestin, synthetic forms of progesterone). Although the available data suggest that the benefits of EPT are almost exclusively due to the estrogen, progestogen reduces the risk of endometrial adenocarcinoma in women with a uterus, a risk that is significantly increased in women using unopposed estrogen (see Section E, page 146, for more about endometrial cancer).

Hormone therapy (HT): encompasses both ET and EPT. The FDA, however, refers to EPT as HT.

Previously, the terms *estrogen replacement therapy* and *hormone replacement therapy* were used. However, the term *replacement* is a misnomer because postmenopausal levels of HT provide only a small fraction of the estrogen the ovaries once produced. The FDA declared that the word *replacement* can no longer be used by marketers of products available in the United States. The FDA uses ET to describe unopposed ET and HT to describe EPT. In contrast, NAMS prefers using HT to encompass all hormone therapy used for menopause, and EPT to more clearly describe combined therapy.

Marketers use various terms to describe HT that can lead to misunderstanding, particularly by the public. For example, the term *natural* is sometimes used to refer to the product source (eg, a plant) or to the chemical structure (ie, it is bioidentical to human estrogens). Some women erroneously believe that products marketed as natural, plant-based, or bioidentical are safer or better than those synthesized in a laboratory setting. Other women also erroneously believe that plant-based products, regardless of their initial derivation, are extracted from harvested crops instead of being synthesized. Healthcare providers should be aware of these beliefs and counsel women that the primary factor in determining usefulness of a hormone is not its origin or whether it is bioidentical, but its benefit-risk ratio for each individual woman.

The primary clinical question when selecting ET/EPT is to determine an individual woman's risk-benefit ratio of ET/EPT when considered for treatment of specific menopause-related symptoms and/or for disease prevention. A woman may be willing to accept certain risks of ET/EPT when therapy is used short term to treat existing symptoms as opposed to long-term use to prevent disease. Also, it is more likely to be acceptable for symptom reduction when therapy is planned to be short term in a population that is younger with presumed lower health risks. In contrast, the increased risks with ET/EPT in older women may make it less acceptable.

Estrogen therapy. The term estrogen describes a variety of chemical compounds that have an affinity for estrogen receptors α and β. (Not included in this list are selective estrogen-receptor modulators [SERMs, now called estrogen agonists/antagonists as per the FDA], which also have affinity for these receptors. See page 224 of this section for more about these compounds.)

Estrogen types. Estrogens can be divided into the following six main types.

- *Human estrogens* are those produced in the human body and include estrone (E_1), 17β-estradiol (often called estradiol or E_2), and estriol (E_3). Estradiol is the most biologically active, whereas estrone is 50% to 70% less active and estriol, an impeded estrogen, is only 10% as active as estradiol. Estradiol, the principal estrogen secreted by the ovaries, is metabolized to estrone; both estradiol and estrone can be metabolized to estriol, although exogenous estriol cannot be converted. Among the human estrogens, only 17β-estradiol is available in a government-approved, single-estrogen product.

- *Nonhuman estrogens* refer to conjugated estrogens (CE), a mixture of at least 10 estrogens obtained from natural sources (the urine of pregnant mares), occurring as the sodium salts of water-soluble estrogen sulfates. CE contains the sulfate esters of the ring B saturated estrogens—estrone (about 45%), 17β-estradiol, and 17α-estradiol—and the ring B unsaturated estrogens—equilin (about 25%), 17β-dihydroequilin, 17α-dihydroequilin, equilenin, 17β-dyhydroequilenin, 17α-dihydroequilenin, and $\Delta^{8,9}$-estrone (ie, $\Delta^{8,9}$-dehydroestrone sulfate). The pharmacologic effects of CE are a result of the sum of activities of these estrogens.

- *Synthetic estrogens* are available as two types of mixtures: esterified estrogens (which contain 75% to 85% sodium estrone sulfate) and synthetic conjugated estrogens (SCE). There are two designations of SCE: SCE-A (with a mixture of 9 of the estrogens found in CE) and SCE-B (including the estrogens found in synthetic SCE-A plus $\Delta^{8,9}$-dehydroestrone sulfate—the 10 estrogens found in CE).

- *Synthetic estrogen analogs with a steroid molecular structure* include ethinyl estradiol and estropipate (formerly called piperazine estrone sulfate).

- *Synthetic estrogen analogs without a steroid skeleton,* such as stilbesterol derivatives, are not used for menopause-related therapy.

- *Plant-based estrogens without a steroid skeleton,* also known as phytoestrogens, can have weak estrogenic as well as antiestrogenic properties, depending on the target tissue. These are not prescription products. (See Section I, page 264, for more about phytoestrogens.)

Clinical pharmacology. Endogenous estrogens exert effects on almost all cells in the body. They are largely responsible for the development and maintenance of the female reproductive system and secondary sex characteristics. By direct action, they cause growth and development of the uterus, fallopian tubes, and vagina. Along with other hormones, such as pituitary hormones and progesterone, they cause enlargement of the breasts through promotion of ductal growth, stromal development, and the accretion of fat. Estrogens are intricately involved with other hormones, especially progesterone, in the processes of the ovulatory menstrual cycle and pregnancy, and affect the release of pituitary gonadotropins. They also contribute to the shaping of the skeleton, maintenance of tone and elasticity of urogenital structures, changes in the epiphyses of the long bones that allow for the pubertal growth spurt and its termination, and pigmentation of the nipples and genitals.

Estrogens act by regulating the transcription of a number of genes. Estrogens diffuse through cell membranes, distribute themselves through the cell, and bind to and activate one or more nuclear estrogen receptors. The activated estrogen receptor(s) binds to specific DNA sequences, or hormone-response elements, which enhance the transcription of adjacent genes and, in turn, lead to the observed effects. In women, estrogen receptors have been identified in all tissues, including the reproductive tract, breast, brain, bone, and skin.

Estrogens occur naturally in several forms. The primary source of estrogen in normally cycling adult women is the ovarian follicle, which secretes 70 to 500 μg of estradiol daily, depending on the phase of the menstrual cycle. This is converted primarily to estrone, which circulates in roughly equal proportion to estradiol, and to small amounts of estriol. After menopause, most endogenous estrogen is produced by conversion of androstenedione (secreted by the adrenal cortex) to estrone by peripheral tissues. Thus, estrone and the sulfate conjugated form, estrone sulfate, are the most abundant circulating endogenous estrogens in postmenopausal women. Although circulating estrogens exist in a dynamic equilibrium of metabolic interconversions, estradiol is the principal intracellular human estrogen and is substantially more potent than estrone or estriol at the receptor.

Circulating estrogens modulate the pituitary secretion of the gonadotropins, luteinizing hormone, and FSH through a negative feedback mechanism and ET acts to reduce the elevated levels of these hormones in postmenopausal women.

Pharmacokinetics. Estrogens used in oral ET are well-absorbed from the gastrointestinal tract after release from the drug formulation. Maximum plasma concentrations are attained 4 to 10 hours after oral administration. Estrogens are also well absorbed through the skin and mucous membranes. When applied transdermally or topically in high enough doses, absorption is usually sufficient to cause systemic effects. Although systemic absorption is possible when estrogen is applied vaginally, absorption is minimal with modern low-dose treatment.

Although naturally occurring estrogens circulate in the blood largely bound to sex hormone-binding globulin (SHBG) and albumin, only unbound estrogens enter target tissue cells. The half-life of the different estrogens in CE ranges from 10 to 25 hours; the half-life of estradiol is approximately 16 hours (oral) and 4 to 8 hours (transdermal). After removal of transdermal patches, serum estradiol levels decline in about 12 to 24 hours to preapplication levels.

When orally administered, naturally occurring estrogens and their esters are rapidly metabolized in both the gut and the liver before reaching the general circulation—called the "first-pass effect." This significantly decreases the amount of estrogen (primarily estrone sulfate) available for circulation. In addition, the first pass through the liver affects other liver functions and is presumed to be one of the reasons various routes of administration impact lipid profiles differently. In contrast, synthetic estrogens are degraded very slowly in the liver and other tissues, which results in their high intrinsic potency.

Systemic estrogens administered by nonoral routes are not subject to first-pass metabolism, but they do undergo significant hepatic uptake, metabolism, and enterohepatic recycling.

Certain types of transdermal and topical preparations cause less variability in blood levels compared with oral preparations at steady state, and exhibit near zero-order pharmacokinetics. However, there may be substantial interpatient variability in blood levels.

Transdermal and topical administration produces therapeutic plasma levels of estradiol with lower circulating levels of estrone and estrone conjugates, and requires smaller total doses than oral therapy.

Marketed estrogens. Estrogens are available in many prescription preparations, both as single agents in oral preparations (see Table 3), transdermal patch or gel or topical emulsion preparations (see Table 4), vaginal preparations (see Table 5), oral and transdermal preparations in combination with a progestin (see Table 6), and

oral preparations with an androgen (see Table 7). Readers are urged to refer to product labeling prior to prescribing.

All government-approved estrogen-containing products that achieve systemic levels at recommended doses are approved in the United States and Canada for the treatment of moderate to severe vasomotor symptoms. Only some are also approved for the treatment of moderate to severe vaginal dryness and symptoms of vulvar and vaginal atrophy, although labeling states that when prescribing the product solely for vaginal symptoms, vaginal preparations should be considered. Other systemic estrogen-containing products are sometimes prescribed off label for this indication. One oral estrogen (Enjuvia) is also approved for the treatment of pain with intercourse.

Still fewer estrogen-containing systemic products have government approval for the "prevention" of post-menopausal osteoporosis because not all marketers of estrogen-containing products have funded the long-term trials to prove efficacy or they are awaiting government review of their applications (see Section E, page 120, for a chart of approved therapies). Previously, some estrogen-containing products were also approved for the "treatment" of postmenopausal osteoporosis, but this indication was withdrawn from all such products by the FDA. Off-label use of systemic estrogen-containing products for an osteoporosis indication has more risk than for vaginal symptoms.

Table 3. Oral ET products for postmenopausal use in the United States and Canada

Composition	Product Name	Available Dosages (mg)
conjugated estrogens (formerly conjugated equine estrogens)	Premarin	0.3, 0.45*, 0.625, 0.9, 1.25
synthetic conjugated estrogens, A	Cenestin*	0.3. 0.45, 0.625, 0.9, 1.25
	Congest**	0.3, 0.625, 0.9, 1.25, 2.5
	C.E.S**	0.3, 0.625, 0.9, 1.25
	PMS-Conjugated**	0.3, 0.625, 0.9, 1.25
synthetic conjugated estrogens, B	Enjuvia*	0.3, 0.45, 0.625, 0.9, 1.25
esterified estrogens	Menest*	0.3, 0.625,1.25, 2.5
	Neo-Estrone**	0.3, 0.625, 1.25
17β-estradiol	Estrace	0.5, 1.0, 2.0
	various generics	0.5, 1.0, 2.0
estradiol acetate	Femtrace*	0.45, 0.9, 1.8
estropipate (formerly piperazine estrone sulfate)	Ortho-Est*	0.625 (0.75 estropipate, calculated as sodium estrone sulfate 0.625), 1.25 (1.5), 2.5 (3.0)
	Ogen**	0.625 (0.75), 1.25 (1.5), 2.5 (3.0)
	various generics	0.625 (0.75), 1.25 (3.0)

* Available in the United States but not Canada.
** Available in Canada but not the United States.
Products not marked are available in both the United States and Canada.

All vaginal estrogen-containing therapies are government approved for treating moderate to severe vaginal dryness and symptoms of vulvovaginal atrophy. Only one vaginal product (Femring) delivers systemic doses and thus is approved for vasomotor symptoms. No vaginal product is approved for osteoporosis.

The following are the most common types of estrogen products used in prescription preparations.

• *Conjugated estrogens.* Most clinical studies have used conjugated estrogens (CE; formerly called conjugated equine estrogens [CEE]). As a result, more is known about its efficacy and safety than any other estrogen product. CE is available as Premarin in oral tablet, vaginal cream, and injectable formulations (although the latter is not used for menopausal HT) and in combination products with progestin (Premphase, Prempro in the US; Premplus in Canada). Although Premarin has been on the US market for more than 65 years, no generic equivalent has been FDA approved to date.

The standard CE oral dose is 0.625 mg daily, based on bone protection studies. Recent studies have shown that many women receive substantial benefit from lower doses (0.45 mg or 0.3 mg/d), although some women require higher doses for symptom relief and osteoporosis prevention.

• *Synthetic conjugated estrogens.* Two types of synthetic conjugated estrogen (SCE) mixtures are available, both as oral tablets—SCE-A (with 9 estrogens) and SCE-B (with 10 estrogens). The SCE-A available in the United States is Cenestin (Congest, C.E.S., and PMS-Conjugated in Canada). The SCE-B is Enjuvia, available in the United

Table 4. Transdermal and topical ET products for postmenopausal use in the United States and Canada

Composition	Product Name	Delivery Rate	Dosing (mg/day)
17β-estradiol matrix patch	Alora*	0.025, 0.05, 0.075, 0.1	twice weekly
	Climara	0.025, 0.0375*, 0.05, 0.075, 0.1	once weekly
	Esclim*	0.025, 0.0375, 0.05, 0.075, 0.1	twice weekly
	Estradot**	0.025, 0.0375, 0.05, 0.075, 0.1	twice weekly
	Menostar*	0.014	once weekly
	Oesclim**	0.05, 0.1	twice weekly
	Vivelle	0.025*, 0.0375*, 0.05, 0.075*, 0.1*	twice weekly
	Vivelle-Dot*	0.025, 0.0375, 0.05, 0.075, 0.1	twice weekly
	various generics	0.1, 0.05	once or twice weekly
17β-estradiol reservoir patch	Estraderm	0.05, 0.1	twice weekly (patch cannot be cut)
17β-estradiol transdermal gel	EstroGel 0.06%* Estrogel 0.06%**	0.035	daily application; 1 metered pump delivers 1.25 g of gel containing 0.75 mg 17β-estradiol
	Elestrin 0.06%*	0.0125	daily application; 1 metered pump delivers 0.87 g of gel containing 0.52 mg 17β-estradiol
	Divigel 0.1%*	0.003, 0.009, 0.027	daily application; 3 strengths of packets provide 0.25, 0.5, or 1.0 g of gel
17β-estradiol topical emulsion	Estrasorb*	0.05 (2 packets)	daily application of 2 packets; 1 packet = 1.74 g of emulsion
17β-estradiol transdermal spray	Evamist*	0.021 mg per 90 mcL spray (metered-dose pump)	initial: 1 spray/d of 1.7% solution, increasing to 2-3 sprays/d if needed

* Available in the United States but not Canada.
** Available in Canada but not the United States.
Products not marked are available in both the United States and Canada.

States but not Canada. The FDA does not view Cenestin or Enjuvia as generic equivalents to Premarin, even though Enjuvia contains the primary 10 estrogens included in Premarin. In Canada, C.E.S. has been approved as a generic equivalent to Premarin since 1963, although at least one study shows that it is not bioequivalent.

Both Cenestin and Enjuvia are available in the same wide range of dosages as Premarin, including ultralow-dose 0.3 mg. No synthetic CE product is government approved for osteoporosis.

- *Estradiol.* Initially, 17β-estradiol (or simply "estradiol") could be administered only by injection because it was not absorbed from the gastrointestinal tract. After micronization was developed, an oral product (Estrace) was marketed; various oral generics are also available. Subsequently, transdermal estradiol delivery systems were developed, first the reservoir patch (Estraderm), followed by the matrix patches (Alora, Climara, Esclim, Estradot, Oesclim, Vivelle, Vivelle-Dot), offering various adhesives. A few transdermal gels (Divigel, Estrogel, Elestrin), a transdermal spray (Evamist), and a topical emulsion of estradiol hemihydrate (Estrasorb) are newer options. Vaginal forms of estradiol are also available (Estrace Vaginal Cream, Estring Vaginal Ring), as well as the estradiol acetate vaginal ring (Femring) that exerts systemic effects and the estradiol hemihydrate vaginal tablet (Vagifem). Estradiol valerate is widely used in Europe, but in the United States and Canada, it is available only in an injectable formulation (Delestrogen) not used for menopausal HT. Estradiol is also used in EPT products. Estradiol is the most widely used estrogen in Europe. It is the one estrogen available commercially in government-approved formulations that can be considered bioidentical.

- *Esterified estrogens.* Esterified estrogens (Menest in the United States; Neo-Estrone in Canada) are oral products of synthetic estrogen mixtures containing 75% to 85% sodium estrone sulfate. They are not indicated for osteoporosis. Estratab, another esterified estrogens product, was withdrawn from the North American market several years ago.

- *Estropipate.* Formerly called piperazine estrone sulfate, this is an oral form of estrone sulfate that has been

Table 5. Vaginal ET Products for postmenopausal use in the United States and Canada

Composition	Product Name	Dosing
Vaginal Creams		
17β-estradiol	Estrace Vaginal Cream*	initial: 2-4 g/d for 1-2 wk maintenance: 1 g/d (0.1 mg active ingredient/g)
conjugated estrogens (formerly conjugated equine estrogens)	Premarin Vaginal Cream	0.5-2 g/d (0.625 mg active ingredient/g)
esterified estrogens	Neo-Estrone Vaginal Cream**	2-4 g/d (1 mg active ingredient/g)
Vaginal Rings		
17β-estradiol	Estring	device containing 2 mg releases 7.5 µg/d for 90 d
estradiol acetate	Femring*	device containing 12.4 mg or 24.8 mg estradiol acetate releases 0.05 mg/d or 0.10 mg/d estradiol for 90 d (systemic levels)
Vaginal Tablet		
estradiol hemihydrate	Vagifem	initial: 1 tablet/d for 2 wk maintenance: 1 tablet twice/wk (tablet containing 25.8 µg of estradiol hemihydrate equivalent to 25 µg of estradiol)

* Available in the United States but not Canada.
** Available in Canada but not the United States.
Products not marked are available in both the United States and Canada.

Table 6. Combination EPT products for postmenopausal use in the United States and Canada

Composition	Product Name	Available Dosages
Oral Continuous-Cyclic Regimen		
conjugated estrogens (E) + medroxyprogesterone acetate (P) (E alone for days 1-14, followed by E+P on days 15-28)	Premphase*	0.625 mg E + 5.0 mg P (2 tablets: E and E+P)
Oral Continuous-Combined Regimen		
conjugated estrogens (E) + medroxyprogesterone acetate (P)	Prempro*	0.3 or 0.45 mg E + 1.5 mg P (1 tablet); 0.625 mg E + 2.5 or 5.0 mg P (1 tablet)
	Premplus**	0.625 mg E + 2.5 or 5.0 mg P (2 tablets: E and P)
ethinyl estradiol (E) + norethindrone acetate (P)	femhrt*	2.5 µg E + 0.5 mg P (1 tablet); 5 µg E + 1 mg P (1 tablet)
	femHRT**	5 µg E + 1 mg P (1 tablet)
17β-estradiol (E) + norethindrone acetate (P)	Activella*	0.5 mg E + 0.1 mg P (1 tablet); 1 mg E + 0.5 mg P (1 tablet)
17β-estradiol (E) + drospirenone (P)	Angeliq*	1 mg E + 0.5 mg P (1 tablet)
Oral Intermittent-Combined Regimen		
17β-estradiol (E) + norgestimate (P) (E alone for 3 d, followed by E+P for 3 d, repeated continuously)	Prefest*	1 mg E + 0.09 mg P (2 tablets: E and E+P)
Transdermal Continuous-Combined Regimen		
17β-estradiol (E) + norethindrone acetate (P)	CombiPatch,* Estalis**	0.05 mg E + 0.14 mg P (9 cm^2 patch, twice/wk); 0.05 mg E + 0.25 mg P (16 cm^2 patch, twice/wk)
17β-estradiol (E) + levonorgestrel (P)	Climara Pro*	0.045 mg E + 0.015 mg P (22 cm^2 patch, once/wk)
Transdermal Continuous-Sequential Regimen		
17β-estradiol (E) + norethindrone acetate (P) (E alone for 2 wk, followed by E+P for 2 wk, repeated continuously)	Estalis Sequi**	0.05 mg E twice/wk (Vivelle 50 patch) for 2 wks, then 9 or 16 cm^2 Estalis patch twice/wk for 2 wk
	Estracomb**	0.05 mg E twice/wk for 2 wk, then 0.05 mg E + 0.25 mg P for 2 wk

* Available in the United States but not Canada.
** Available in Canada but not the United States.

solubilized and stabilized by piperazine. It is marketed as Ogen (in Canada, no longer in the United States) and Ortho-Est (in the United States, not Canada), as well as in generic formulations. Ogen is approved for the prevention of postmenopausal osteoporosis.

- *Ethinyl estradiol* is a synthetic steroid is widely use in combination contraceptives. It is also available in one oral EPT product (femhrt in the United States, femHRT in Canada). Estinyl, an oral ethinyl estradiol product, is no longer available in the United States and Canada.

Table 7. Oral estrogen-testosterone products for postmenopausal use in the United States and Canada

Composition	Product Name	Available Dosages
esterified estrogens (E) + methyltestosterone (T)	Estratest,* various pseudo-generics*†	1.25 mg E + 2.5 mg T
	Estratest HS,* various pseudo-generics*†	0.625 mg E + 1.25 mg T

* Available in the United States but not Canada.
† Since Estratest and Estratest HS are not FDA approved but permitted on the US market by the FDA while additional studies are being conducted, there can be no generic equivalent as defined in the regulations.

Sometimes an estrogen product is described as a "natural hormone." The word "natural" is a marketing term used in many industries, including foods, in an attempt to denote that the product is better or safer than another product. Sometimes the term is used to describe an estrogen with a plant origin. There is no evidence that so-called natural estrogen products have a different efficacy or safety profile than other hormones, although one product may be better tolerated by an individual woman.

Measuring estrogen potency presents a challenge, as estrogens vary in their dose equivalency and their effects on various target tissues. Oral micronized estradiol 1.0 mg is equivalent to CE 0.625 mg with respect to effects on liver function, whereas 0.5 mg oral micronized estradiol produces changes in bone density equivalent to CE 0.625 mg. (See Table 8 for an approximation of equivalency.) Very few head-to-head trials have compared different estrogens. Clinicians tend to view estrogen products as equivalent on a dose-for-dose basis, although data do not support this assumption; their metabolic pathways and side effects can vary in general and from woman to woman. HT must always be tailored to the individual.

Route of administration. For menopause-related therapy, estrogen can be administered orally, transdermally,

Table 8. Approximate equivalent estrogen doses for postmenopausal use

Oral	
conjugated estrogens	0.625 mg
synthetic conjugated estrogens	0.625 mg
esterified estrogens	0.625 mg
estropipate (0.75 mg)	0.625 mg
ethinyl estradiol	0.005-0.015 mg
estradiol	1.0 mg
Transdermal/topical	
estradiol patch	0.05 mg
estradiol gel	1.5 mg/2 metered doses
Vaginal	
conjugated estrogens	1.25 mg
estradiol	0.5 mg

topically, or vaginally. Intramuscular preparations are not recommended for menopause therapy because serum estrogen levels associated with injections rise to very high levels after administration.

- *Oral administration.* Oral ET remains the most widely used formulation in North America. With all oral estrogen products, estrone will be the predominant estrogen in the circulation owing to the first pass uptake and metabolism in the liver.

This hepatic effect with oral ET results in greater stimulation of certain proteins compared with transdermal therapy, including lipoproteins such as high-density lipoprotein cholesterol (HDL-C). Oral estrogen is also associated with about a 25% increase in triglycerides. Oral ET stimulates hepatic globulins, coagulation factors, and some inflammatory markers such as C-reactive protein and MMP-9, with implications for coronary disease. There also may be differences in glucose-insulin metabolism, but these data are less clearcut. Other important inflammatory markers such as E-selectin decrease with both modes of administration. The ESTHER trial suggested that oral ET but not transdermal ET is associated with an increase of VTE.

Oral estrogen and combined oral-androgen therapy affect levels of endogenous sex hormones such as testosterone, SHBG, dehypdroepiandrosterone, and androstenedione. Exogenous oral estrogen alone increases SHBG but decreases the testosterone-SHBG ratio. Combined oral estrogen-androgen treatment has the opposite effect, reducing SHBG levels but slightly increasing the testosterone-SHBG ratio. (For more about androgen therapy, see page 223.)

• *Transdermal/topical administration.* Estrogen delivered in these ways can be prescribed in lower doses than oral administration because they are not dependent on gastrointestinal absorption or subjected to first-pass hepatic metabolism. There is variation in absorption among transdermal and topical estrogens, depending on the patches are applied and the carrier vehicle.

In contrast to oral ET, transdermal/topical administration of estrogen has the advantage of not increasing triglycerides, but the disadvantage of not increasing HDL-C. Because of less liver exposure, transdermal and topical ET may have less adverse effect on gallbladder disease and coagulation factors.

Transdermal and topical ET are associated with relatively stable serum levels, unlike fluctuating serum levels found with oral estrogen. Thus, when monitoring estrogen levels is required, transdermal or topical ET is a better choice than oral ET. These methods of administration may also result in fewer headaches than oral ET.

Estraderm was the first transdermal patch approved for use in the United States and Canada, administering estradiol from a reservoir patch. Other transdermal patches are now available, each delivering estradiol from a matrix patch. Patch adhesives differ among product options. In addition, a transdermal gel, transdermal spray, and topical emulsion are available. The spray, gel, and emulsion formulations have the advantage over patches that they are less likely to cause skin irritation, but the gel and emulsion products have the disadvantage that skin-to-skin contact within 2 hours after application can lead to transfer of small amounts of estradiol. Also, sunscreen application shortly before applying transdermal and topical products may substantially increase estradiol exposure. With the spray, when sunscreen is applied before application there is no significant change in estradiol absorption or exposure. Use of sunscreen on the same area after application of transdermal estradiol has both increased and decreased estradiol absorption. The transdermal and topical ET products are listed in Table 4 on page 208.

Vaginal administration. There are several different ways to deliver estrogen vaginally—creams, rings, and tablets (see Table 5 on page 209). Vaginal creams have been available for decades; the tablet and ring products were more recently marketed. Small amounts of estrogen administered locally are effective for treating atrophic vaginitis (see Section C, page 51). Readers are advised to refer to government-approved labeling prior to prescribing. Labeling for vaginal estrogen products often includes the same warnings, contraindication, and side effects as labeling for systemic estrogen-containing products, despite the fact that low-dose vaginal ET does not typically result in systemic estrogen levels.

Except for the estradiol acetate vaginal ring (Femring), vaginal estrogens are not used for systemic effects (eg, hot flashes) although systemic absorption of vaginal estrogen cream has been documented, and women may notice breast tenderness when initiating therapy. With the vaginal ring Estring, an estrogen surge is measurable the first day the ring is in place, but then the levels remain in the menopausal range. With the vaginal tablet (Vagifem), only a small amount of estrogen is absorbed, but more than with the estradiol vaginal ring (Estring). In a head-to-head study with estrogen cream, women preferred the tablet because it was less messy.

Adding a progestogen to low-dose vaginal ET is not typically recommended. Adding a progestogen is recommended with Femring or higher doses of other vaginal ET, as enough estrogen may reach the bloodstream to potentially increase the risk of endometrial cancer.

The woman's individual needs and preference should be the primary factors in determining the estrogen delivery route. In some women, medical factors may determine the route (eg, vaginal administration to treat vaginal atrophy or transdermal administration for women with hypertriglyceridemia). Other factors include cost and insurance coverage.

Progestogen therapy and EPT. Progestogen therapy can be an option to treat hot flashes (see Section C, page 35) and other conditions of women at menopause and beyond, but the primary use in menopausal treatment is to oppose ET in women with a uterus to reduce the increased risk of endometrial hyperplasia and cancer associated with unopposed ET. (See Section E, page 146, for more about endometrial cancer.)

Terminology. The term *progestogen* refers to a wide range of hormones with the properties of the naturally occurring steroid progesterone. Progestogen includes both *progesterone* and the synthetic progestational compounds termed *progestins*.

• *Progesterone* is the steroid hormone produced by the ovary after ovulation and by the placenta during pregnancy. Exogenous progesterone is a compound identical to endogenous progesterone. It can be synthesized in the laboratory for therapeutic use, and it is available as progesterone USP (ie, it meets specifications of the USP). This is the only bioidentical progestogen. Relatively recent advances have allowed progesterone crystals to be micronized, resulting in improved oral absorption. Before micronization, the rapid inactivation and poor bioavailability of orally administered progesterone led to the development in the 1950s of progestins.

• *Progestins* are synthetic products that have progesterone-like activity but are not identical to that produced in the human body. Progestins can be classified as those more closely resembling in chemical structure either *progesterone* or *testosterone* (also called *19-nortestosterone derivatives*).

Those structurally related to progesterone are further classified into two groups: (1) *pregnane derivatives*—including those that are acetylated, such as MPA, megestrol acetate, cyproterone acetate, and chlormadinone acetate; and those that are nonacetylated, such as dydrogesterone and medrogestone—and (2) *19-norpregnane derivatives*—including those that are acetylated, such as nomegestrol and nestorone; and those that are nonacetylated, such as demegestone, trimegestone, and promegestone.

Those progestins structurally related to testosterone are further classified into two groups: (1) those that are ethinylated—including estranes, such as norethindrone (NET) (also called norethisterone), norethindrone acetate (NETA), norethylnodrel, lynestrenol, and ethynodiol diacetate; and the 18-ethylgonanes, such as levonorgestrel (LNG), norgestrel, desogestrel, gestodene, and norgestimate—and (2) those that are nonethinylated, such as dienogest and drospirenone.

Progestins obtained from a plant-derived precursor (eg, diosgenin, which is found in plants such as the wild yam or soybean) should not be referred to as *natural* progestogens because they undergo multiple chemical reactions during synthesis.

Mode of action. In the human, two progestogen receptor (PR) proteins, PR-α and PR-β, have been identified. Whether the available progestogen therapies preferentially bind to PR-α or PR-β is unclear. The primary actions of progestogen have been characterized in most detail in the uterus. In this target tissue, progestogen functions primarily as an antiestrogen, decreasing the number of nuclear estrogen receptors, most likely through down-regulation of estrogen receptors. In the endometrium, progestogen increases the activity of 17β-hydroxysteroid dehydrogenase, resulting in conversion of estradiol to estrone, a biologically weaker estrogen. These changes result in less estrogen-induced endometrial stimulation.

Marketed progestogens. A wide variety of progestogen types, modes of administration, and dosage regimens are available, each having distinct side effects as well as different actions on the endometrium and other organ systems (see Table 9). Very few clinical trials have evaluated the relative potencies of progestogens.

All government-approved progestogen formulations will provide endometrial protection if the dose and duration are adequate. Combined EPT products are available; although these are convenient and many women prefer to take one pill or use one patch, they do reduce dosing flexibility. All combined EPT products in the United States and Canada are government approved for postmenopausal use, including endometrial protection (see Table 6).

Table 9. Progestogens Used for EPT in the United States and Canada

Composition	Product Name	Available Dosages
Oral Tablet: Progestin		
medroxyprogesterone acetate	Provera, various generics	2.5, 5, 10 mg
norethindrone (formerly norethisterone)	Micronor, Nor-QD,* various generics	0.35 mg
norethindrone acetate	Aygestin,* various generics	5 mg
norgestrel	Ovrette*	0.075 mg
megestrol acetate	Megace, various generics	20*, 40 mg
Oral Capsule: Progesterone		
progesterone (in peanut oil)	Prometrium	100, 200* mg
Intrauterine System: Progestin		
levonorgestrel	Mirena	20 µg/d approx release rate (52 mg IUS has 5-y use)
Vaginal Gel: Progesterone		
progesterone	Prochieve 4%* Crinone 4%**	45 mg/ applicator

*   Available in the United States but not Canada.
** Available in Canada but not the United States.
Products not marked are available in both the United States and Canada.

Among the progestins listed in Table 9, the compound most structurally related to bioidentical progesterone is MPA. Generally speaking, progestins structurally related to testosterone are more potent than progesterone and MPA.

The FDA approval of progestogen products to oppose menopausal ET is relatively recent, although progestogens have been used for this indication for decades. The most commonly used progestogen formulation for endometrial protection among US women is the oral progestin MPA, either alone (Provera, generics) or in combination with CE (Prempro, Premphase in the United States; Premplus in Canada). It is also the most widely studied progestogen for postmenopausal use. Other progestins are combined with other estrogens in several oral and transdermal EPT products. Low doses of transdermal progestogens should have metabolic advantages over higher doses of oral therapy because they avoid the first-pass hepatic effects; however, data on this are limited.

Anecdotal data and results from the Postmenopausal Estrogen/Progestin Interventions (PEPI) trial suggest that women who experience unpleasant side effects, especially mood changes, with a synthetic progestin sometimes respond more favorably to bioidentical progesterone. Before the late 1990s, North American women seeking progesterone products had to rely on custom-compounded formulations. Prometrium, an oral capsule containing micronized progesterone, was first approved in Canada, then by the FDA for marketing in the United States. However, Prometrium should never be used by a woman allergic to peanuts, as the active ingredient is suspended in peanut oil. In addition, a small percentage of women may experience extreme dizziness and/or drowsiness during initial therapy, so women should use caution when driving or operating machinery. Bedtime dosing is advised.

Micronized progesterone formulations (eg, cream, lotion, gel, oral capsule, suppositories) are also available by prescription through custom-compounding pharmacies. (See page 218 of this section for more about custom-compounded hormones.)

It is important to note that topical cream or gel preparations with progesterone, obtained either over the counter or custom-compounded from a prescription, may not exert sufficient activity to protect the endometrium from unopposed estrogen. These products should not be used for this purpose until optimum therapeutic doses and serum levels of topical progesterone are established. (For more about topical progesterone, see page 225 of this section.)

Since vaginal administration at typical doses avoids systemic effects, vaginal progestogen is an attractive option. The vaginal bioadhesive gel containing 4% micronized progesterone provides sustained and controlled delivery of progesterone to the vaginal tissue. In a trial using cyclic administration of the gel, no hyperplasia was observed after 3 months. This product is marketed as Prochieve 4% in the United States and Crinone 4% in Canada.

The use of a progestin-releasing IUS to protect the endometrium is appealing because it delivers the progestin in the highest concentration where it is needed. Mirena, the only progestogen-containing IUS available in the United States and Canada, is not government approved for this use, although there are small studies suggesting it is effective. There is some systemic absorption of levonorgestrel with Mirena. Its relatively low dose (20 µg/d) and 5-year lifespan make it an attractive alternative for perimenopausal women. The progesterone IUD, Progestasert, is no longer on the North American market.

EPT regimens. Many types of regimens are used when prescribing EPT, and descriptive terminology is often inconsistent. The clinical goal of these EPT regimens is to provide uterine protection, maintain estrogen benefits, and minimize side effects (particularly uterine bleeding,

which is annoying to many women and often reduces compliance), although there is no consensus on how to accomplish this goal. Regimens may be classified into the following types: cyclic, cyclic-combined, continuous-cyclic, continuous long-cycle, continuous-combined, and intermittent-combined (see Table 10). With hyphenated regimen names, the first and second words denote the estrogen and progestogen components, respectively.

Table 10. Terminology defining types of EPT regimens

Regimen	Estrogen	Progestogen
Cyclic	Days 1-25	Last 10-14 days of ET cycle
Cyclic-combined	Days 1-25	Days 1-25
Continuous-cyclic (sequential)	Daily	10-14 days every mo
Continuous-cyclic (sequential) long-cycle	Daily	14 days every 2-6 mo
Continuous-combined	Daily	Daily
Intermittent-combined (pulsed-progestogen; continuous-pulsed)	Daily	Repeated cycles of 3 days on, 3 days off

Source: Adapted from NAMS Position Statement *Menopause* 2003.

- *Cyclic EPT.* In this regimen, estrogen is taken from day 1 to day 25 of the calendar month with progestogen added the last 10 to 14 days. This allows for a hormone-free interval of 3 to 6 days and is designed to mimic the normal premenopausal ovulatory cycle. Progestogen therapy should be used for 10 days or more to provide endometrial protection.

With this regimen and standard EPT dosing, about 80% of women have withdrawal uterine bleeding after the progestogen cycle. This bleeding usually starts 1 to 2 days after the last progestogen dose and continues for a few days during the therapy-free interval. Estrogen should be resumed at the beginning of the next month irrespective of whether bleeding has stopped.

Some women will experience vasomotor symptoms during the therapy-free intervals, due to the relatively short half-life of estrogens (eg, the half-life of oral estradiol has been reported to be 15-20 h).

This is the oldest of the regularly used EPT regimens and is decreasing in popularity in North America, primarily because newer regimens have lower uterine bleeding rates.

- *Cyclic-combined EPT.* For this regimen, estrogen is combined with a progestogen on days 1 to 25, followed by a hormone-free interval of approximately 5 days. This regimen provides a low rate of uterine bleeding and a high rate of tolerability in studies using oral micronized progesterone. In one trial, endometrial biopsies performed before and after 4 months of cyclic-combined EPT (2 mg/d 17β-estradiol plus 50, 100, or 200 mg/d oral micronized progesterone) showed an atrophic endometrium in all women receiving 200 mg/day oral micronized progesterone and in most women receiving 100 mg/day. Uterine bleeding occurred in the first few cycles, but decreased with time. However, the trial duration of 4 months is considered inadequate for evaluating the regimen's effect on endometrial hyperplasia.

- *Continuous-cyclic EPT.* In this regimen, sometimes referred to as *sequential EPT*, estrogen is used every day with progestogen added cyclically for 10 to 14 days during each month. The combination oral EPT product Premphase uses a sequential regimen of estrogen for 14 days followed by estrogen and progestin for 14 days, similar to oral contraceptives. In a typical continuous-cyclic regimen, progestogen is started on the 1st or 15th of the month. Starting the first day of the month makes it easier for some women to track their uterine bleeding, as the cycle day corresponds with the day of the month.

Uterine bleeding occurs in about 80% of women when the progestogen is withdrawn, although it sometimes starts 1 or 2 days earlier, depending on the dose and type of progestogen used. The main advantage of the continuous-cyclic regimen compared with the cyclic EPT is the absence of an estrogen-free period during which vasomotor symptoms may reoccur.

- *Continuous-cyclic (sequential) long-cycle EPT.* To lessen the exposure to progestogen and the incidence of uterine bleeding, a modified continuous-cyclic EPT regimen of daily estrogen with cyclic progestogen (eg, 10 mg/d MPA for 14 d during the month) added every 2 to 6 months has been evaluated. Although this regimen reduces the number of withdrawal bleeding episodes, it has resulted in heavier and longer periods.

The effect on endometrial protection is undetermined. Two studies did not find evidence of endometrial hyperplasia after 1 year in women using estrogen at standard (0.625 mg/d CE) or one half standard (0.3 mg/d CE) doses with MPA administered either quarterly or every 6 months. However, the Scandinavian Long Cycle Study, which used 2 mg/day of 17β-estradiol (twice the standard dose) with a progestin administered quarterly, was stopped after 3 of 5 scheduled years because of an increased incidence of hyperplasia compared with a monthly progestogen regimen. Until more data are available, the continuous long-cycle regimen is not recommended as standard therapy. If prescribed, endometrial monitoring is mandatory. Some clinicians utilize the high negative predictive value of a thin, distinct endometrial echo on transvaginal ultrasound in women who wish to pursue such a regimen.

- *Continuous-combined EPT.* These regimens were developed to address the withdrawal uterine bleeding, which is annoying to women and decreases continuance. In this regimen, a woman uses estrogen and progestogen every day. Within several months, the endometrium can become atrophic and amenorrhea results.

Rates of endometrial hyperplasia are low in women using currently marketed continuous-combined EPT preparations, based on short-term studies (usually no longer than 1 y). Such studies are not considered long enough to assess endometrial cancer risk. The continuous-combined regimen has been the predominant regimen used in North America.

Combined oral CE plus MPA (CE 0.625/MPA 2.5 mg/d; CE 0.45/MPA 2.5 mg/d; CE 0.45/MPA 1.5 mg/d; CE 0.3/ MPA 1.5 mg/d) produced hyperplasia rates equal to those found in the placebo arms of clinical trials (<1%). Oral continuous-combined regimens of 17β-estradiol (1 mg/d) with NETA (0.1, 0.25, or 0.5 mg/d), as well as oral ethinyl estradiol (1.0, 2.5, 5.0, or 10 µg/d) combined with NETA (0.2, 0.5, 1.0, or 1.0 mg/d, respectively), also had hyperplasia rates less than 1%. Transdermal 17β-estradiol (50 µg/d) combined with NETA (0.14 or 0.25 mg/d) did not result in any measurable hyperplasia after 1 year of treatment. A continuous-combined transdermal patch delivering 17β-estradiol (25 µg/d) and NETA (0.125 mg/d) provided endometrial protection and maintained a high rate of amenorrhea in a 2-year clinical trial.

- *Intermittent-combined EPT.* This regimen (also called *pulsed-progestogen* or *continuous-pulsed EPT*) uses estrogen daily with the progestogen dose intermittently administered in cycles of 3 days on and 3 days off, which is then repeated without interruption. This regimen (Prefest) was designed to lower the incidence of uterine bleeding while avoiding the down-regulation of progesterone receptors that continuous progestogen can produce, a mechanism that theoretically may not fully protect the endometrium. By interrupting the progestogen for 3 of every 6 or 7 days, up-regulation of progesterone receptors occurs intermittently.

In clinical trials, pulsed regimens have shown amenorrhea rates of 80% after 1 year with favorable endometrial hyperplasia safety profiles. However, almost all prospective studies of this regimen were only 1 year long. Longer-term surveillance of endometrial effects will be needed to more fully ascertain efficacy and safety.

Clinical goal of EPT. The clinical goal of progestogen in EPT is to provide endometrial protection while maintaining estrogen benefits and minimizing unwanted progestogen-induced effects, particularly uterine bleeding. EPT discontinuance correlates with uterine bleeding—women with more days of amenorrhea have higher rates of continuance.

For the postmenopausal woman using systemic ET, adding progestogen therapy to ET reduces the risk of endometrial cancer induced by ET to the level found in women not taking hormones. Data from the PEPI trial showed that women who took unopposed ET during the 3-year trial had a significantly increased risk of hyperplasia (34%) whereas those taking EPT had a risk of only 1%. A 2004 Cochrane review reports that the addition of oral progestin to ET, administered as either continuous-cyclic or continuous-combined, is associated with reduced rates of hyperplasia. Cyclic progesterone added to ET also has been shown to inhibit the development of endometrial hyperplasia. In the PEPI trial, combining CE (0.625 mg/d) with progesterone (200 mg/d for 12 d/mo) over a 3-year follow-up did not produce an increase in endometrial hyperplasia compared with placebo. Progestogen does not eliminate endometrial cancer risk because there is a risk independent of hormone use.

It has been suggested that continuous-combined EPT may not be as protective as continuous-cyclic EPT, citing the possibility that some buildup of the endometrium may not be shed, and that continuous progestogen may completely down-regulate progesterone receptors, thereby reducing endometrial protection. However, epidemiologic studies of continuous-combined EPT indicate no increased risk and may even suggest some added protection against endometrial cancer.

Studies have provided data regarding the necessary dose and duration of the progestogen course to oppose the estrogen-induced risk of endometrial hyperplasia and adenocarcinoma (see Table 11). With an oral progestin used in a cyclic regimen with a standard estrogen dose (eg, 0.625 mg CE, 1 mg oral estradiol, or 0.05 mg patch), the minimum effective dose for endometrial protection is 5 mg/day of MPA, or the equivalent, for 12 to 14 days each month. With oral micronized progesterone, the minimum effective dose is 200 mg/day for 12 to 14 days each month. Larger or smaller estrogen doses may require larger or smaller progestogen doses, respectively. A progestin-containing intrauterine device and a progesterone vaginal gel offer other possible options for endometrial protection, although long-term efficacy data are lacking regarding their endometrial cancer protection.

Use of EPT should be limited to the lowest effective dose and shortest duration consistent with treatment goals, benefits, and risks for the individual woman. Long-term surveillance is necessary, even in women receiving appropriate doses of progestogen.

Uterine bleeding with EPT. Many postmenopausal women dislike having episodes of uterine bleeding, and this hormone-related side effect decreases EPT continuance. Various regimens have been designed to lessen or eliminate bleeding.

Table 11. Minimum progestogen dosing requirements for endometrial protection with standard estrogen dosing*

	Continuous-Cyclic EPT (Daily, 12-14 days/mo)	Continuous-Combined EPT (Daily)
Oral tablets		
medroxyprogesterone acetate	5 mg	2.5 mg
norethindrone	0.35-0.7 mg	0.35 mg
norethindrone acetate	2.5 mg	0.5-1 mg
micronized progesterone	200 mg	100 mg
Intrauterine system		
levonorgestrel	—	20 µg/d
Vaginal		
progesterone gel	45 mg	45 mg

* 0.625 mg CE, 1 mg oral estradiol, 0.05 mg patch, or the equivalent. Table includes only products available in the United States and Canada.

Uterine bleeding terminology

Withdrawal uterine bleeding—predictable bleeding that often results from progestogen cessation (or withdrawal).

Breakthrough uterine bleeding—unpredictable and irregular bleeding associated with regimens using continuous progestogen.

Retrospective trials have suggested that regular uterine bleeding occurring after day 11 of a cyclic 12-day progestogen course reflects a normal secretory pattern of the endometrial tissue. However, prospective trials have not confirmed these findings, and no correlation has been established between day of bleeding onset and histologic findings. Nevertheless, most studies with cyclic administration of progestogen have shown a high percentage of regular withdrawal uterine bleeding in women with a normal secretory endometrium. Bleeding pattern is a less reliable indicator of endometrial safety when continuous-combined regimens are used.

Breakthrough uterine bleeding has been observed in 40% of women on a continuous-combined regimen during the first 3 to 6 months. The probability of achieving amenorrhea is greater if EPT is started 12 months or more after menopause; women who are recently postmenopausal exhibit more breakthrough bleeding. Most women (75%-89%) who continue therapy become amenorrheic within 12 months. However, bleeding may persist intermittently for months or years. Persistent breakthrough bleeding with continuous-combined EPT may necessitate switching to another regimen.

A study comparing two continuous-combined regimens— CE 0.625 mg/day plus MPA 2.5 mg/day and 17β-estradiol 1 mg/day plus NETA 0.5 mg/day—found that within 3 months, 71.4% of the estradiol-NETA users experienced amenorrhea compared with 40.0% of the CE-MPA users, but after 6 months, the differences were not statistically significant. This study confirmed other findings that recently postmenopausal women (within 1-2 y of last menses) experienced more bleeding than women more than 3 years postmenopausal.

Treatment with one of the 19-nortestosterone derivatives (eg, NET, NETA, LNG, norgestimate) or oral micronized progesterone tends to produce less breakthrough uterine bleeding during the first few months of use.

Among women using EPT beyond 2 years, those using a continuous-combined regimen have a lower rate of breakthrough uterine bleeding and fewer endometrial biopsies than those using the cyclic regimen. These findings confirm other studies that show decreased breakthrough uterine bleeding over time in women using the continuous-combined regimen.

The intrauterine administration of progestogen results in less bleeding than oral therapies.

Extrauterine effects of progestogens. Progestogens exhibit effects on organ systems other than the endometrium. These effects vary depending on the progestogen type, dose, route of administration, and the EPT regimen.

Although no EPT (or ET) regimen should be initiated for the primary or secondary prevention of cardiovascular disease (CVD), based on clinical trials (primarily the Women's Health Initiative [WHI] and the Heart and Estrogen/ progestin Replacement Study [HERS]) reporting significantly increased risks with EPT, some observational studies have shown that ET has beneficial effects on atheroscle -rosis, vasodilation, plasma lipids, arterial response to injury, and insulin sensitivity. Adding some progestogens may diminish these beneficial effects, but they generally do not eliminate them. All progestogens negate the beneficial effect of estrogen on blood flow. Selecting a metabolically neutral progestogen for EPT, such as micronized progesterone or norgestimate, is recommended to maintain higher plasma HDL-C. In animal studies, progestins with a higher androgenic potency reduce more of the beneficial effects of estrogens on vasodilation; progesterone and 19-norpregnane derivatives have less of an adverse effect. These beneficial endpoints do not outweigh the overall lack of CVD benefit reported in randomized controlled trials (RCTs). (For more about CVD, see Section E, page 129.)

For women with type 2 diabetes mellitus who are using EPT to treat acute menopausal symptoms, continuous-cyclic EPT regimens are recommended to minimize progestogen exposure; low-dose oral micronized progesterone is also recommended. (For more about diabetes, see Section E, page 135.)

Progestogen has limited effect on the bone-enhancing action of ET. Although adding 2.5 mg MPA or 1 mg NETA to ET slightly enhances estrogen's ability to prevent BMD loss in early postmenopausal women, estrogen alone is adequate to maintain BMD. EPT reduces spine and hip fractures, but the role of progestogen in this effect is not known. NAMS recommends that the decision to add progestogen to ET should not be based on its skeletal impact. (For more about osteoporosis, see Section E, page 113.)

Breast cancer risk is not decreased when progestogen is added to ET, and data suggest that there may be an increased risk with standard doses. Mammographic density is increased with progestogen use, although this effect will reverse with discontinuation of use. Breast discomfort and pain may increase with progestogen use. (For more about breast cancer, see Section E, page 140.)

Some progestogens may negatively affect mood, particularly in women with a history of mood disorders. Data are inadequate to recommend specific progestogens or EPT regimens for minimal adverse effects. In general, the side effects of added progestogen are mild, although they may be severe in a small percentage of women. (For more about mood disorders, see Section C, page 47.)

These findings have resulted in the consideration to prescribe less progestogen or unopposed ET for women with an intact uterus. However, there is insufficient evidence regarding endometrial safety to recommend unopposed ET or off-label use of long-cycle progestogen (ie, progestogen for 12-14 d every 3-6 mo).

Bioidentical hormones. The term "bioidentical hormones" means different things to different people. To scientists and healthcare providers, bioidentical hormones are those that are chemically identical to the hormones produced by women (primarily in the ovaries) during their reproductive years. A woman's body can make various estrogens (such as 17β-estradiol, estrone, and estriol) as well as progesterone, testosterone, and other hormones. Thus, bioidentical HT can mean a medication that provides one or more of these hormones as the active ingredient.

Some bioidentical hormones are made available in well-tested, government-approved, brand-name prescription drugs. Several government-approved drugs in the United States and Canada contain 17β-estradiol, and those that are not taken orally remain in the body as 17β-estradiol. There are two government-approved bioidentical progesterone products: oral capsules (Prometrium) and 4% vaginal gel (Prochieve 4% in the United States, Crinone 4% in Canada).

Often healthcare providers, pharmacists, and consumers use the term bioidentical hormone to describe those hormonal formulations that are custom compounded (see below).

Custom-compounded formulations. Bioidentical hormones are also offered through custom-compounded formulations sometimes referred to as BHT (bioidentical hormone therapy) or BHRT (bioidentical hormone replacement therapy). For decades, pharmacists have custom-compounded formulations, including those containing hormones, for individuals as prescribed by their clinicians. Custom compounding of hormone therapy allows individualized dosing and combinations of therapy, depending on a woman's preference or tolerance. It also allows for different modes of administration of hormones, including subdermal implants, sublingual tablets, rectal suppositories, and nasal sprays. Products can be prepared without the binders, fillers, dyes, preservatives, or adhesives that are found in patented, commercially available products. To a large extent, only those individuals with a documented need were prescribed a custom preparation.

In the wake of the WHI findings, however, compounding became much more popular as symptomatic women with concerns about patented hormone therapies have frequently become targets for unproven BHT products. Unfortunately, these products are often offered to women as safer or more effective alternatives to government-evaluated and approved medications, even though they have not been tested for effectiveness and safety. No safety information is consistently provided to these women and, as a result, many women are confused about the risks associated with treating their menopause symptoms. Standardization may be uncertain. Hormonal drugs that are custom compounded from a prescription are not government approved, although some active ingredients meet the specifications of the USP. Often, third party payors do not reimburse prescription costs for custom-compounded formulations, as they are viewed as experimental drugs.

Transdermal creams and pills of many varieties are compounded. Some of the most widely used custom estrogen products contain estriol, a weak estrogen having 5% to 10% the effect of estradiol. Limited data show that oral estriol helps to relieve hot flashes. Estriol alone or in an oral "tri-estrogen" mixture of three estrogens (usually 80% estriol, 10% estrone, and 10% estradiol, and sometimes called Tri-Est) is often promoted as providing the benefits of government-approved estrogen products without increasing the risk of breast or endometrial cancer. Although estriol is a weak estrogen, it can still have a stimulatory effect on the breast and endometrium. Claims supporting estriol or any compounded formulation as safer than the government-approved formulations have not

been substantiated by well-designed clinical trials. Until more is known, women with an intact uterus using custom-compounded estrogen should also use progestogen to counter estrogen's stimulatory effect on the endometrium.

Before the oral capsule micronized progesterone product (Prometrium) was marketed in the United States, oral micronized progesterone USP was a frequently prescribed compound. Custom products are still used and may be especially appropriate for women with peanut allergies, since Prometrium contains progesterone suspended in peanut oil. A 100-mg dose of micronized progesterone USP is equivalent to about 2.5 mg MPA.

Custom topical preparations of progesterone are also available, although the strength typically used is available in OTC products (eg, Pro-Gest cream). Topical progesterone products have not been shown to achieve adequate serum levels to counter the stimulatory effect of estrogen on the uterus (see page 225 of this section for more about topical progesterone).

Custom-compounded formulations should be used with caution and only with informed patient consent. There are individual women for whom the positives outweigh the negatives, but for the vast majority of women, government-approved hormone products will provide the appropriate therapy without assuming the risks and cost of custom preparations. More research is needed to sort out the risk-benefit ratio of using compounded hormones.

ET/EPT contraindications and warnings. ET/EPT contraindications listed in labeling for various products are often the same, regardless of whether their effects are systemic or local (see Table 12). Local ET may not actually be contraindicated in all these situations. Readers should refer to the current product labeling before prescribing any ET/EPT regimen.

Systemic and local ET/EPT products marketed in the United States have "class labeling" that includes a black box warning (indicating that the warning is significant) that ET increases the risk of endometrial cancer (for more about endometrial cancer, see Section E, page 146). Progestogen is advised when prescribing systemic ET/EPT for women with an intact uterus.

The FDA requires within the black box of all systemic ET/EPT products (and some local ET products) the notation that the WHI study found increased risks of stroke and deep vein thrombosis (DVT) in postmenopausal women (50-79 y old) during 5.6 years of treatment with oral CE (0.625 mg/d) combined with MPA (2.5 mg/d) when compared with placebo. Black box verbiage indicates that in the CE-only arm of the WHI, an increase in stroke and DVT was noted during 6.8 and 7.1 years, respectively, of treatment. (For more, see Section C, page 134.)

Table 12. Listed contraindications for ET/EPT
• Undiagnosed abnormal genital bleeding
• Known, suspected, or history of breast cancer except in appropriately selected patients being treated for metastatic disease
• Known or suspected estrogen-dependent neoplasia
• Active or history of deep vein thrombosis, pulmonary embolism
• Active or recent (within the past year) arterial thrombo-embolic disease (eg, stroke, myocardial infarction)
• Liver dysfunction or disease
• Known or suspected pregnancy
• Known hypersensitivity to ET/EPT

Table 13. Potential side effects of ET/EPT
• Uterine bleeding (starting or returning)
• Breast tenderness (sometimes enlargement)
• Nausea
• Abdominal bloating
• Fluid retention in extremities
• Changes in the shape of the cornea (sometimes leading to contact lens intolerance)
• Headache (sometimes migraine)
• Dizziness
• Mood changes with EPT, particularly with progestin

Black box labeling for all systemic ET/EPT products and some local ET products also includes the statement that ET/EPT should not be used for the prevention of cardiovascular disease or dementia. Also noted is that the Women's Health Initiative Memory Study (WHIMS), a substudy of WHI, reported an increased risk of developing probable dementia in postmenopausal women 65 or older during 5.2 years of treatment with oral CE (0.625 mg/d) alone and during 4 years of treatment with oral CE (0.625 mg/d) combined with MPA (2.5 mg/d) relative to placebo; it is unknown whether this finding applies to younger women. (For more about cognition and hormones, see Section C, page 45).

Additional black box verbiage includes the following statements: Other doses of CE and MPA, and other combinations and dosage forms of ET/EPT, were not studied in WHI, and in the absence of comparable data, these risks should be assumed to be similar. Because of these risks, ET/EPT should be prescribed at the lowest effective doses and for the shortest duration consistent with treatment goals and risks for the individual women. Close clinical surveillance of all women using ET/EPT is important, and should include endometrial sampling, when indicated. There is no evidence that the use of "natural" or "bioidentical" ET/EPT formulations will result in a different risk profile than synthetic ET/EPT products of equivalent dose.

Although not in a black box, labeling also warns of an increased risk of breast cancer with ET/EPT (for more, see Section E, page 140). Readers are referred to labeling for additional warnings for various ET/EPT products before prescribing.

ET/EPT side effects. A number of side effects are associated with ET/EPT (see Table 13), although these vary dependent on route of administration, type of progestogen, and dose (see labeling for specific products before prescribing). Side effects often lead to discontinuation of therapy sooner than desired.

Scientific evidence has absolved ET/EPT from culpability in weight gain. The Rancho Bernardo prospective cohort study found no significant differences in body weight between hormone users and nonusers after 15 years of follow-up. These results persisted even after adjustments for a number of confounding factors, including age, initial body mass index, smoking, and exercise. The results generally agree with those from the PEPI trial. A longitudinal study of perimenopausal weight gain in the Massachusetts Women's Health Study also found similar results. (See Section C, page 68, for more about weight.)

In some women, EPT causes fluid retention in the hands and feet and/or abdominal bloating with gaseous distention. A few women experience gastrointestinal irritation and nausea from oral EPT administration.

The most common side effect of transdermal patch ET/EPT is skin irritation at the patch application site. This can sometimes be alleviated by rotating the patch, putting it on the buttock, and being sure the site is very clean. Using OTC hydrocortisone cream can help as well as switching to a different ET/EPT patch which may have a different type of adhesive that will not be so irritating. Using talcum powder around the patch edge can prevent formation of dirt rings (dirt can be cleaned with mineral oil).

Women using EPT often experience uterine bleeding. Some women regard this EPT-induced bleeding as an unacceptable nuisance, although the bleeding often decreases or stops over time. Manipulating dosages and evaluating for other gynecologic disease is indicated. In studies using ultralow-dose EPT (0.3-0.45 mg CE or equivalent), bleeding is a less common side effect.

Although the vaginal estrogen ring is generally well tolerated, headache, abdominal pain, and vaginal pain, irritation, and erosion have been reported. If the ring falls out, it can be rinsed off and reinserted. The ring does not usually interfere with sexual intercourse, although it can be removed if it is uncomfortable for either partner.

Estrogen vaginal creams are considered messy by some women. There are anecdotal reports of estrogen absorption by the male partner during sexual intercourse, leading to gynecomastia.

Estrogens are partly metabolized by CYP450 3A4. Inducers of 3A4, such as St. John's wort, rifampin, or carbamazepine, may decrease estrogen concentrations and its effectiveness, while inhibitors such as itraconazole and clarithromycin may increase estrogen concentrations and its toxicity.

A number of strategies exist for dealing with other ET/EPT side effects (see Table 14). Although there is limited scientific evidence to support these tips, clinical experience has determined they are helpful in some women.

An important principle to keep in mind when prescribing HT, and especially when managing side effects, is that each woman is an individual with her own psychology and physiology. Each woman should be advised that it may take time to find the best regimen for her and that regular reevaluation with attempts to taper the dose are important. Sometimes it may take more than one or two products or regimens to find the appropriate one for an individual. A certain amount of the search is trial and error. (For more regarding counseling, see Section J.)

Women should be counseled not to expect immediate results. Clinical data suggest that relief of vasomotor symptoms with low-dose ET/EPT is not fully evident until 8 to 12 weeks of use. Setting realistic expectations about outcomes with scientific support will help prevent disappointment.

Some clinicians choose to initiate therapy always with unopposed ET to achieve the symptom benefits without any adverse effects of progestogen; after symptoms are relieved, dosage adjustments can be made and a progestogen added if the uterus is intact.

Timing of initiation. The WHI designers did not take into account that the timing of HT initiation may affect the results, and recruited mostly older, symptom-free women. Emerging data reveal that the timing of HT initiation in naturally menopausal women is important. For example, the absolute risk of coronary heart disease (CHD) is considerably lower in younger, newly postmenopausal women compared with those studied in WHI and HERS. Both ET and EPT appear to increase the risk of ischemic stroke in postmenopausal women, but RCT data are not consistent in this finding. For the women in the WHI, there were 8 additional strokes per 10,000 women per year in the EPT arm (oral CE plus MPA) and 12 additional strokes per 10,000 women per year in the ET (oral CE) arm compared to placebo. The absolute risk of stroke, however, is lower in women aged 50 to 59 years (1 additional stroke/10,000 women/y of ET) or within 5 years of menopause (3 additional strokes/10,000 women/y of EPT) than in older women more distant from menopause. (For more about stroke, see Section E, page 129.) In the WHI, heart attack risk increased during the first year of EPT use for older women, but not younger ones. Many experts now believe that HT may have beneficial effects in women whose arteries are still healthy, regardless of age.

Initiating HT during perimenopause is associated with lower risk compared to starting HT several years after menopause. The ongoing Early versus Late Intervention Trial with Estradiol (ELITE), being conducted by the National Institute of Aging, is evaluating whether the timing of ET initiation reduces subclinical atherosclerosis progression and cognitive decline in two populations of women, those less than 1 year and those more than 10 years postmenopause. As concluded in a 2007 review article by Hodis and Mack, ELITE and future studies with hypotheses guided by the results of previous RCTs of HT

Table 14. Dealing with ET/EPT side effects

Side effect	Strategy
Fluid retention	Restrict salt; maintain adequate water intake; exercise; try a mild prescription diuretic.
Bloating	Switch to low-dose nonoral estrogen; lower the progestogen dose to a level that still protects the uterus; switch to another progestin or to micronized progesterone.
Breast tenderness	Lower the estrogen dose; switch to another estrogen; restrict salt; switch to another progestin; cut down on caffeine and chocolate.
Headaches	Switch to nonoral estrogen; lower the dose of estrogen and/or progestogen; switch to a continuous-combined regimen; switch to progesterone or a 19-norpregnane derivative; ensure adequate water intake; restrict salt, caffeine, and alcohol.
Mood changes	First, investigate preexisting depression or anxiety; lower the progestogen dose; switch progestogen; switch from systemic progestin to the progestin IUS; change to a continuous-combined EPT regimen; ensure adequate water intake; restrict salt, caffeine, and alcohol.
Nausea	Take oral estrogen tablets with meals or before bed; switch to another oral estrogen; switch to nonoral estrogen; lower the estrogen or progestogen dose.

have the potential to create a new paradigm for the primary prevention of CHD in women.

Premature menopause and premature ovarian failure are conditions associated with a lower risk of breast cancer and earlier onset of osteoporosis and CHD, but there are no clear data as to whether ET or EPT will affect morbidity or mortality from these conditions. The risk-benefit ratio for younger women who initiate therapy at an early age may be more favorable but is currently unknown.

Weighing benefits and risks. After the July 2002 announcement of the first WHI results with CE plus MPA in predominantly asymptomatic postmenopausal women (mean age, 63 y), use of all systemic HT therapies for any indication declined significantly, no doubt because clinicians and their patients were concerned about the risks identified in this study. Since that time, different methods of analyzing these data and information from other trials have softened some of the concerns. In addition, lower dose products are now available that may offer similar benefits with fewer risks.

Many experts now believe that the wide-scale move away from HT during the past few years was an overreaction and that many women who could have been helped suffered needlessly. Others in the medical community disagree, saying that key questions about long-term use still are not answered. All would agree that the WHI helped to reverse a popular theory permeating women's health during the late 1990s that HT benefited every woman. Unfortunately, many women and healthcare providers still have an exaggerated view of the risks involved in using HT. This type of treatment has received inordinately greater negative exposure than other treatments with greater risk to the public health.

NAMS and other leading healthcare organizations support the use of HT in appropriate situations. Use of HT should be consistent with treatment goals, benefits, and risks for the individual woman, taking into account cause of menopause, time since menopause, symptoms, and domains (such as sexuality and sleep) that may have an impact on quality of life and the underlying risk of CVD, stroke, VTE, diabetes, and other conditions.

It may be helpful when reviewing risks with women considering HT to put its risks into perspective. As concluded in a 2007 review by Hodis and Mack, RCTs indicate that the risks of HT, including breast cancer, stroke, and VTE, are similar to other commonly used treatments. Overall, these risks are rare (<1 event/1,000 women/y) and even rarer when initiated in women less than 60 years of age or within 10 years of menopause. In addition, the literature indicates similar benefits of HT in women who initiate HT in close proximity to menopause, to other medications used for the primary prevention of CHD in women.

Importantly, the effects of eithe ET or EPT on risk of breast cancer, CHD, stroke, total CVD, and osteoporotic fracture in *perimenopausal* women with moderate to severe menopause symptoms have not been established in RCTs. The findings from trials in different populations should, therefore, be extrapolated with caution. For example, data from large studies such as the WHI and HERS should not be extrapolated to symptomatic postmenopausal women younger than 50 years of age who initiate HT at that time, as these women were not studied in those trials. The WHI and HERS involved predominantly asymptomatic postmenopausal women aged 50 years and older (mean ages, 63-67 y, respectively), the majority of whom were 10 years or more beyond menopause. HERS was conducted solely among women with known coronary artery disease. The data should not be extrapolated to women experiencing premature menopause (≤40 y) and initiating HT at that time.

Progestogen is advised for all women with an intact uterus who are using systemic ET, thereby reducing uterine cancer risk to the level of using no hormones. Lower-than-standard doses of HT should be considered (ie, daily doses of 0.3 mg oral CE or the equivalent). Different estrogens, progestogens, and routes of administration offer potential advantages for some women. In the absence of clinical trial data for each estrogen and progestogen, however, the clinical trial results for one agent may be generalized to all agents within the same family. Caution is advised when considering custom-compounded HT products.

Systemic HT is the most effective treatment for moderate to severe vasomotor symptoms. Since these symptoms are generally short-term, recommending HT for this indication has low risk.

No HT regimen should be used for the primary or secondary prevention of CVD or stroke, and HT should be avoided for women who have an elevated baseline for stroke.

There is strong evidence of the efficacy of both ET and EPT in reducing the risk of postmenopausal osteoporotic fracture through long-term treatment. (In the WHI, the trial that first demonstrated fracture protection, daily 0.625 mg oral CE with or without 5 mg MPA was used; fracture protection with other therapies and lower doses still remains to be determined.) For women who require drug therapy for osteoporosis risk reduction (including women at high risk of fracture during the next 5-10 y), HT can be considered an option, weighing its risks and benefits as well as those of other government-approved therapies. (See Section E, page 119, for more.)

Extended use of the lowest effective dose for treatment goals of systemic HT is acceptable under the following circumstances, provided that the woman is well aware of the potential risks and benefits and that there is clinical supervision:

- For the woman for whom, in her own opinion, the benefits of menopause symptom relief outweigh risks, notably after failing an attempt to stop HT.

- For women who are at high risk of osteoporotic fracture and also have moderate to severe menopause symptoms.

- For further prevention of bone loss in the woman with established reduction in bone mass when alternate therapies are not appropriate for that woman or cause side effects or when the outcomes of the extended use of alternate therapies are unknown.

When considering HT, various modes of administration are associated with different potential pros and cons (see Table 15).

When a decision is made to discontinue systemic HT, there are no definitive data to support abrupt cessation versus tapering the dose. There seems to be little difference in terms of return of menopause symptoms. Symptoms have an approximate 50% chance of recurring when therapy is discontinued, independent of age and duration of HT use. The decision to continue HT should be individualized on the basis of severity of symptoms and current risk-benefit ratio considerations, provided the woman in consultation with her healthcare provider believes that continuation of therapy is warranted.

Low-dose vaginal ET is generally recommended for postmenopausal women whose only menopause-related symptom is vaginal atrophy. For symptomatic vaginal atrophy that does not respond to nonhormonal vaginal lubricants and moisturizers, low-dose vaginal ET is effective and well tolerated while limiting vaginal absorption. Progestogen is generally not indicated. Low-dose, local ET should be continued so long as distressful vaginal symptoms remain. For women treated for non-hormone-dependent cancer, management of vaginal atrophy is similar to that for women without a cancer history. For women with a history of hormone-dependent cancer, management recommendations are dependent upon each woman's preference in consultation with her oncologist.

Monitoring therapy. Clinical monitoring of women using HT includes ongoing evaluation for potential adverse effects. At least yearly return visits are recommended, during which time the woman and her clinician should review the decision to use HT, including a discussion of any new research findings. More often visits may be required, especially for women just starting HT or for those having bothersome side effects. Annual mammography is indicated. Endometrial surveillance is not required for women using systemic ET and adequate progestogen. Data are insufficient to recommend annual endometrial surveillance in asymptomatic women using low-dose vaginal ET for the treatment of vaginal atrophy. If a woman is at high risk for endometrial cancer, is using a greater dose of vaginal ET, or is having symptoms (spotting, break-through bleeding), closer surveillance may be required. The clinical goal is to use the lowest effective HT dose for the shortest time consistent with treatment goals.

Table 15. Potential pros and cons of HT routes of administration

Oral estrogen

Pros:
- Familar, easy
- Beneficial effect on HDL-C, LDL-C, and total cholesterol
- Large amount of data
- Usually relatively low cost

Cons:
- Risk of thrombosis, stroke
- Increase in triglycerides, C-reactive protein, other hepatic proteins
- Risk of reducing libido through SHBG impact

Transdermal/topical estrogen

Pros:
- Avoids hepatic first pass effect
- Less increase on triglycerides than oral ET
- Less effect on C-reactive protein than oral ET
- Perhaps less risk of thrombosis than oral ET
- Less risk of reducing libido than oral ET
- Fewer GI side effects than oral ET
- Topical emulsion is moisturizing

Cons:
- Patch adhesive sensitivity/residue
- Patch is less private
- Usually relatively higher cost

Vaginal (local) estrogen

Pros:
- Vaginal benefit at lower dose
- Low-dose therapy typically avoids adverse systemic effects

Cons:
- Increase in vaginal discharge
- Some may consider less convenient to use
- Lack of long-term uterine safety data for low-dose products

Progestogens

Pros:
- Reduces adverse effect of estrogen on endometrium
- Some progestogens reduce adverse effect of oral estrogen on triglycerides
- Progesterone dosed at night can improve insomnia

Cons:
- Some progestogens increase risk of breast cancer
- Some progestogens reduce beneficial effect of oral estrogen on HDL-C
- Adverse side effects, such as bloating
- Dysphoric effect for some women

Androgen

Although androgens are defined as hormones that promote the development and maintenance of male secondary sex characteristics and structures, they are important for women as well. Androgens are the immediate precursors for estrogen biosynthesis. In addition, androgens affect sexual desire, muscle mass and strength, BMD, distribution of adipose tissue, energy, and psychological well-being.

The major androgens in women, as in men, are testosterone, androstenedione, dehydroepiandrosterone (DHEA), and the peripheral metabolite, dihydrotestosterone. Androgens are synthesized primarily in the ovary and adrenal glands, although significant peripheral conversion occurs. Most circulating testosterone is tightly bound to SHBG. Only the free, or unbound, fraction is bioactive (approximately 1%-2% of the circulating testosterone). Serum testosterone concentrations in women are approximately 10% of those in men.

While production of both ovarian and adrenal androgens decreases with age, there is no abrupt decline in these hormones with menopause, as occurs with ovarian estradiol production. Surgical menopause is an exception, because testosterone levels decrease by approximately 50% following bilateral oophorectomy. In addition to oophorectomy, a number of factors cause reduced androgen concentrations in women, including hypopituitarism, adrenal insufficiency, corticosteroid use, and the use of drugs that increase SHBG concentrations (eg, oral ET), resulting in decreased bioavailable testosterone.

Oral ET and combined oral-androgen therapy affect levels of endogenous sex hormones such as testosterone, SHBG, DHEA, and androstenedione. Exogenous oral ET alone increases SHBG but decreases the testosterone-SHBG ratio. Combined oral estrogen-androgen treatment has the opposite effect, reducing SHBG levels but slightly increasing the testosterone-SHBG ratio.

Potential benefits. Androgen therapy is receiving increasing attention for treating postmenopausal women suffering from sexual dysfunction. In women with surgically induced menopause, high doses of intramuscular testosterone have significantly improved sexual desire, fantasy, and arousal compared with either estrogen alone or placebo. In several studies, postmenopausal women randomized to treatment with oral esterified estrogens (EE) plus methyltestosterone reported significantly improved sexual sensation and desire compared with estrogen alone. Oral administration of the adrenal androgen DHEA also has been shown to improve sexual interest and satisfaction in women with adrenal insufficiency, but not in those experiencing natural menopause.

In several large, randomized, double-blind, placebo-controlled clinical trials, testosterone administered via a transdermal patch significantly increased the frequency of satisfying sexual activity and desire in estrogen-treated, surgically induced and naturally menopausal women with sexual dysfunction. For more about clinical evaluation of sexual function, see Section C, page 57. See Section F, page 191, for more about measuring testosterone levels.

Androgen therapy may play a role in the maintenance of BMD and body composition in women. In a 9-week randomized study of estrogen alone versus combined estrogen-methyltestosterone therapy, both treatments reduced urinary markers of bone resorption, but only combined estrogen-androgen therapy resulted in an increase in serum markers of bone formation. In a study of testosterone and estradiol therapy administered by implants, women randomized to combined estradiol and testosterone had significantly greater BMD increases than those who received estradiol alone. In addition, women who received both estradiol and testosterone implants experienced an increase in fat-free mass and a reduced ratio of fat mass to fat-free mass.

Androgen products. Currently, there are no FDA-approved androgen-containing prescription products for treating sexual dysfunction in women. The only androgen-containing product available in the United States is a combination of esterified estrogens (EE) and methyltestosterone, marketed as Estratest (1.25 mg EE and 2.5 mg methyltestosterone) and Estratest HS (0.625 mg EE and 1.25 mg methyltestosterone)(see Table 7 on page 211 of this section). These oral tablets are indicated for the treatment of moderate to severe vasomotor symptoms unresponsive to estrogen. Estratest, available for 40 years, is one of hundreds of older drugs that are not officially FDA approved. In recent years, the FDA indicated that the product could continue on the market while additional FDA-required studies are being conducted. The marketer submits ongoing safety and efficacy data annually to the FDA, similar to FDA-approved drugs. Several "pseudo-generic" EE plus methyltestosterone products (eg, Covaryx) are available using Estratest data; since there is no FDA-approved brand product, these products are not truly generic equivalents according to federal regulations.

In Canada, one oral testosterone prescription drug is used off label in women, although it is not government approved for women: testosterone undecanoate (Andriol). It is typically used at 40 mg/day; however, the optimal dosing for women is yet to be determined.

Testosterone administered by IM injection often results in supraphysiologic levels, with the highest levels occurring near the time of administration.

Custom-compounded preparations of micronized testosterone USP are available, although no definitive studies have determined absorption and utilization rates and these preparations are not government approved. As with IM testosterone, compounded implants often yield supraphysiologic levels, particularly just after implantation. (See page 218 of this section for more about custom compounding.)

If the goal is improving libido, custom-compounded topical 2% testosterone USP (cream, ointment) may be applied directly to the vagina and clitoral area, or any skin surface, several times weekly. Testosterone is well absorbed through the skin; supraphysiologic levels will be obtained if large amounts are applied. Extensive anecdotal evidence supports use of this therapy for improving libido; however, no controlled studies have confirmed the safety or efficacy of topical testosterone for sexual dysfunction in women.

Prescription androgen-containing products formulated for men, including skin patches (Androderm, Testoderm) and gels (Androgel), are inappropriately dosed for women and should not be used.

In the United States, DHEA is available as an oral dietary supplement and may be purchased without a prescription. It is not available in Canada. Although the typical dose for women with low androgen levels is 50 mg per day, there is limited regulation of available products and great variability in the actual amount of hormone present in each tablet. (See page 226 of this section for more information about DHEA.)

Several prescription androgen products, including testosterone patches and gels appropriately dosed for women, are under investigation for use in postmenopausal women with sexual dysfunction.

Monitoring therapy. Clinical monitoring of women using androgens includes a subjective assessment of sexual response and satisfaction. Women also should be evaluated for potential adverse effects, including hirsutism and acne. Intermittent monitoring of lipids and liver function tests may be prudent. Annual mammography is indicated. Measuring the free testosterone level or free androgen index (total testosterone/SHBG) in women using topical testosterone therapies will not help with the assessment of efficacy, but it may be used as a safety measure, with the goal of keeping the value within the normal range for women of reproductive age. However, commercial laboratory measurements of testosterone levels in women are quite variable.

The cause of sexual dysfunction is often multifactorial and may include psychological problems (eg, depression or anxiety disorders), conflict within the relationship, fatigue, stress, lack of privacy, issues relating to prior physical or sexual abuse, medications, or physical problems that make sexual activity uncomfortable (eg, endometriosis or atrophic vaginitis). It is very important to assess and treat other potential causes of sexual dysfunction before considering a trial of androgen therapy.

Potential risks. The potential risks of androgen therapy for women are not well defined. When recommending such therapy, clinicians should fully inform women of potential risks and monitor for adverse reactions. These include acne, weight gain, excess facial and body hair, permanent lowering of the voice, clitoral enlargement, changes in emotion (eg, increased anger), and adverse changes in lipids and liver function tests. Such effects are unlikely if androgen levels are maintained within normal physiologic ranges. Estrogenic risks and side effects are also possible because androgens are converted to estrogens. Whether androgen use in postmenopausal women will increase the risk of CVD or breast cancer is unknown. A report from the Nurses' Health Study suggested an increased risk of breast cancer in current users of testosterone therapies. If risk exists, it is likely to be minimal.

Limited research is available on the use of androgens in women not using concurrent ET. Because androgen does not protect the endometrium against estrogen-induced hyperplasia, a progestogen should be added to the estrogen-androgen regimen in women with a uterus. (For more about endometrial cancer and progestogen therapy to reduce risk, see Section E, page 148.)

Selective estrogen-receptor modulators

Selective estrogen-receptor modulators, commonly referred to as SERMs, are estrogen-like compounds that act as weak estrogen agonists in some organ systems and as estrogen antagonists, depending on the SERM and the target tissue. In this way, they differ from endogenous human estrogen, which affects most receptors in a similar stimulatory manner.

SERMs now called estrogen agonists/antagonists by FDA

In mid-2007, the FDA disallowed the term "selective estrogen-receptor modulator" (SERM), preferring "estrogen agonist/antagonist." No acronym has yet been suggested. In this guidebook, "SERM" is used to avoid confusion until the new terminology is more widely recognized and accepted.

Because they can distinguish among different estrogren receptors, SERMs can be used to selectively target, prevent, and treat a number of diseases, including cancer, osteoporosis, and CVD. Consumers are often confused regarding SERMs, erroneously believing that they provide all the benefits of ET without any of the risks.

SERMs currently available in the United States and Canada include raloxifene and tamoxifen. Tibolone, a SERM widely used around the world for several menopause-related indications, is not available in the United States or Canada. More SERMs and SERM combinations are forthcoming, with lasofoxifene and bazedoxifene anticipated in the near future.

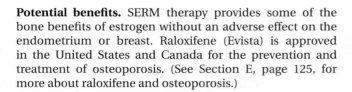

Potential benefits. SERM therapy provides some of the bone benefits of estrogen without an adverse effect on the endometrium or breast. Raloxifene (Evista) is approved in the United States and Canada for the prevention and treatment of osteoporosis. (See Section E, page 125, for more about raloxifene and osteoporosis.)

SERMs have moved into the clinical realm for the primary prevention of breast cancer. Tamoxifen (Nolvadex), the first clinically significant SERM, has been approved for some years to decrease the incidence of contralateral breast cancer in postmenopausal women with ER-positive breast cancers.

In older women with osteopenia or osteoporosis, raloxifene therapy is associated with a significant reduction in the incidence of ER-positive breast cancer. The Study of Tamoxifen and Raloxifene (STAR) revealed that raloxifene is equivalent to tamoxifen in reducing the incidence of invasive breast cancer in postmenopausal women at high risk for the disease. Raloxifene also significantly reduced the incidence of ER-positive breast cancer in the RUTH trial. Unlike the SERM tamoxifen, indicated for breast cancer, raloxifene does not adversely affect the endometrium. In mid-2007, the FDA approved raloxifene for preventing invasive breast cancer. (See Section E, page 145, for more about breast cancer and SERMs.)

Contraindications and risks. Raloxifene labeling includes the statement that the drug should not be used for the primary or secondary prevention of CVD or in premenopausal women. A black box warning emphasizes that the drug is contraindicated in women with an active or past history of VTE and that women at risk for stroke should use raloxifene only after evaluating the risk-benefit ratio.

Raloxifene was associated with fewer VTE events and pulmonary emboli than tamoxifen in a direct comparison trial. Use of each of these agents should be discontinued prior to and during prolonged immobilization. Raloxifene should be used with caution in women with hepatic impairment. Concomitant use with systemic ET is not recommended.

The optimal duration of use of raloxifene has not been established. The most commonly reported side effects of raloxifene are hot flashes (increased frequency or severity), leg cramps, peripheral edema, athralgia, flu syndrome, and sweating.

Tamoxifen is associated with an increased risk for endometrial cancer. In a direct comparison trial with tamoxifen, raloxifene was associated with a 36% reduction in endometrial cancer. Readers should refer to the product labeling before prescribing these therapies.

Over-the-counter (OTC) hormones

Three OTC hormone preparations require special mention: topical progesterone, DHEA, and melatonin. These steroid-containing products are not government regulated as drugs, but as dietary supplements (see Section H, page 237, for more about dietary supplements).

Topical progesterone. Many brands of topical progesterone can be purchased without a prescription in lotion, gel, and cream preparations. Progesterone is the progestogen secreted by the human ovary and hence is called *bioidentical* or *natural* to distinguish it from synthetic progestogens (ie, progestins). Although bioidentical to endogenous progesterone, the "natural" progesterone used for therapy is synthesized commercially by a chemical process using plants such as soybeans and wild yam (*Dioscorea villosa*).

Topical progesterone preparations vary widely in dosages, formulations, additional ingredients, and recommended application sites. In addition, the concentration of the OTC brands vary as well (eg, creams range from no active ingredient to ≥450 mg progesterone/oz, compared with prescription custom-compounded progesterone cream that usually contains 400-450 mg progesterone/oz).

American and Canadian women purchase millions of dollars of various OTC topical progesterone creams each year, and use appears to be growing. Marketers claim progesterone cream balances the hyperestrogenic surges of perimenopause (so-called "estrogen dominance") and thus relieves hot flashes and other menopause-related symptoms. Some marketers tout other benefits, including protection against osteoporosis and breast cancer, and even breast enlargement.

Although clinical experience is extensive, scientific evidence of efficacy for menopause-related symptoms is limited. In three RCTs evaluating use of topical progesterone cream for hot flashes, results were insufficient to support a claim of efficacy. Nonetheless, some practitioners recommend using creams that contain more than 400 mg progesterone per ounce (either OTC or custom compounded) for perimenopausal women to achieve physiologic (not pharmacologic) levels of progesterone during the time of estrogen dominance. Progesterone cream can be applied to the palms, inner arms, chest, or inner thighs, although applying to palms seems inadvisable as transference to others, including infants and children, is theoretically possible.

Both anecdotal and limited clinical trial evidence suggest that absorption of topical progesterone cream is minimal and varies from woman to woman. These studies have shown that progesterone in cream formulations can be absorbed through the skin. However, serum levels of progesterone were low. Also, no improvement was seen for endpoints of BMD, cardiovascular markers, or endometrial protection.

Topical progesterone cream should not be recommended to lower the risk for osteoporosis or any other serious disease. Neither should it be used to prevent estrogen-induced endometrial hyperplasia.

No adverse effects associated with use of OTC progesterone creams have been reported in the medical literature. It is unclear if they are safe for women with a history of a hormone-dependent neoplasm.

OTC topical creams made from the wild yam plant are marketed as containing a progesterone precursor (diosgenin) that has the ability to provide the health benefits attributed to progesterone cream. However, diosgenin cannot be converted into progesterone within the body.

Some wild yam creams contain progesterone that has been produced in the laboratory from the diosgenin extracted from wild yam and then added to the cream. But many wild yam creams contain only progesterone precursors and thus do not provide any absorbable progesterone.

Data do not support any menopause-related health claims for wild yam creams. Diosgenin has been found to have an estrogenic effect on mouse mammary epithelium, although no studies have been conducted in humans. Health risks and side effects are unknown.

DHEA. DHEA and its sulfoconjugate, dehydroepiandrosterone sulfate (DHEAS), are androgen prohormones. In women, endogenous DHEA is produced by the adrenal glands (90%) and the ovaries (10%). Almost all DHEA is converted to DHEAS, which degrades more slowly than does DHEA. DHEA levels peak in women at age 25, with levels declining steadily after age 30 until it becomes almost undetectable by age 70. A temporary increase in the rate of decline appears to be related to menopause. The fall in secretion of DHEA and DHEAS by the adrenal gland parallels the decline in formation of androgen and estrogen by steroidogenic enzymes in specific-target peripheral tissues.

Having no known receptors, DHEA and DHEAS serve as precursors to androgens such as testosterone and dihydrotestosterone, both of which have steroid receptors and are biologically active.

Because DHEA production declines with advancing years, supplements containing DHEA are promoted by marketers for their ability to ward off a variety of age-related symptoms. However, no relationship between decreasing DHEA levels and accelerated aging has been proven.

Most often, DHEA is sold as a single-ingredient oral supplement, although it is sometimes packaged with herbs or other ingredients. Although DHEA is a hormone, it is government regulated as a dietary supplement, not a drug. Products vary widely in amount of DHEA. An analysis of 16 DHEA-containing dietary supplements found that only 7 of the 16 products contained DHEA within 90% to 110% of the product specifications stated on the product label.

Long-term oral DHEA treatment is innately suboptimal because oral DHEA must first undergo significant hepatic first-pass metabolism, the rate of which unpredictably accelerates over time. The dose of DHEA must thus be increased, resulting in an increase in adverse side effects. Transdermal or vaginal DHEA offers more promise for future research.

Few clinical trials of DHEA have been conducted. Most trials have evaluated its use to treat adrenal insufficiency, and it appears to be effective for this use. Other results indicate that DHEA increases physical and psychological well-being and energy, although not all studies have demonstrated a clear relationship between DHEA and psychological variables. In general, women with physiologic, age-related declines in DHEA secretion have shown little benefit from exogenous DHEA.

Oral DHEA (50 mg/d) given to 60 symptomatic perimenopausal women for 6 months resulted in little improvement of perimenopausal symptoms or well-being when compared with placebo. Improvement of behavioral symptoms in postmenopausal women is believed to be mediated by neuroendocrine effects of DHEAS or its active metabolites on pituitary beta-endorphin secretion. DHEA supplementation in early and late postmenopausal women is also associated with an increase in growth hormone and insulin-like growth factor levels.

Topical application of DHEA for 2 weeks to postmenopausal women significantly increased serum testosterone levels with little change in estradiol and estrone levels. Oral administration was associated with an increase in estradiol and estrone levels in addition to an increase in testosterone levels, likely due to the hepatic first-pass effect.

A 2007 update of a Cochrane review of four studies measuring cognition (three in normal older women and men, and one in perimenopausal women with decreased well-being) found no evidence of an improvement in memory or other aspects of cognitive function after DHEA treatment (typically 25 mg/d for women, 50 mg/d for men).

Administration of oral DHEA to women results in a slight decrease in HDL-C, but its effect on CVD risk is unknown. Long-term studies are needed to elucidate the role of DHEA in altering the risk of CVD in postmenopausal women. Observational studies of DHEA levels in individuals with CVD are inconsistent. In studies to date involving transdermal DHEA administration, there are no reports of significant adverse effects.

Increased hip BMD was noted in a small group (N = 14) of women aged 60 to 70 years who used topical 10% DHEA cream, but the results could not be replicated in a 6-month trial of 100 mg oral DHEA.

DHEA appears to have no benefit as an antiobesity drug, although some clinical data support the contention that DHEA supplementation improves lean body mass and glucose tolerance.

The effects of DHEA on sexual function are being explored. In an RCT among women with naturally occurring adrenal insufficiency, oral DHEA (50 mg/d for 4 mo) demonstrated significant increases in sexual function (frequency of thoughts and fantasies, interest, level of mental/physical satisfaction). In another RCT of postmenopausal women (N = 16), oral DHEA (single dose of 300 mg) demonstrated significant increases in mental and physical sexual arousal ratings.

Some complementary and alternative medicine clinicians recommend a daily oral intake of 50 mg or less of DHEA to postmenopausal women with a loss of vitality and/or low libido. It is believed that, at this level, DHEA is converted to more potent androgens, including testosterone. At pharmacologic levels of 1,600 mg daily, DHEA will be converted to estrone and estradiol.

At doses of 25 to 50 mg/day, DHEA appears to be well tolerated in older women. Few adverse effects have been reported at these doses, although in some women, androgenic side effects (eg, facial hair growth, acne) may occur. Nausea, vomiting, dermatitis, and jaundice have been noted with chronic use of low-dose DHEA. With higher doses of DHEA, side effects reported by women include jaundice, elevated liver function tests, virilization, adverse effect on lipids and the breast, depressed mood, and, possibly, hepatocarcinogenicity. Clinical trials are needed to support these safety observations.

DHEA is contraindicated in women of reproductive age, especially if they are at any risk of pregnancy, because of possible masculinization of a female fetus. DHEA is also contraindicated in women who have hormone-responsive tumors. The National Institute on Aging recommends against taking DHEA supplements to reverse the effects of aging.

See page 223 of this section for more about androgen.

Melatonin. Melatonin (N-acetyl-5-methoxytryptamine), an endogenous pineal gland hormone, is widely used by women as a self-medication, but its effects on sleep and behavioral sedation are inconsistent in studies. There are, however, no data that melatonin provides relief from menopause-related sleep disturbances nor that melatonin retards aging. Melatonin may have uses other than for sleep, ie, to prevent or treat jet lag symptoms, particularly in those who have crossed several time zones. (See Section C, page 40, for more about sleep disturbances.)

Although melatonin is a hormone, it is government regulated as a dietary supplement, not a drug. Melatonin is available OTC in most pharmacies and health food stores. However, the lack of regulation and its availability in small doses with increased vehicle-to-drug ratio increases the likelihood of misformulation and poor release of melatonin.

Melatonin regulates the "central clock" and the rest-activity cycles. It is produced from its precursor, tryptophan, with the process regulated by the suprachiasmatic nucleus of the hypothalamus. Endogenous melatonin levels are highest in childhood, drop significantly during puberty, and decline steadily thereafter throughout life.

From a circadian perspective, light suppresses melatonin secretion during the day to a level that is virtually not measurable. Melatonin blood levels begin to increase in the evening and peak between midnight and 3:00 AM, resulting in a direct sedative effect and drop in body temperature, thus promoting sleep. In postmenopausal versus premenopausal women under constant routine conditions, melatonin was shown to peak earlier in the night without differences in time of melatonin onset or amplitude.

The active urinary metabolite of melatonin, 6-sulfatoxy-melatonin, is significantly lower in individuals with insomnia than in those without insomnia, suggestive that melatonin suppression or deficit might be responsible for sleep difficulties, particularly in older adults. Melatonin augments benzodiazepine-induced sleep and may be useful in weaning patients from long-term benzodiazepine use. In one study, discontinuation of benzodiazepine therapy in patients with insomnia was achieved using a 2-mg controlled-release melatonin formulation for 6 weeks, with good sleep quality preserved at 6 months.

The optimal dose of melatonin or safety of long-term melatonin therapy is not known as data are sparse. It has been used in doses varying from 0.3 to 10 mg daily, although continuous daily use is not recommended. Melatonin is available in two formulations: quick-release and sustained-release. Since melatonin has a short half-life of approximately 30 to 60 minutes, a sustained-release formulation is likely beneficial when taken at night to replicate physiology and sustain sleep.

Certain pharmacologic agents such as nonsteroidal anti-inflammatory drugs, benzodiazepines, and beta-adrenergic receptor blockers can inhibit endogenous melatonin synthesis. Acute and chronic alcohol use, tryptophan deficiency, and caffeine are also associated with decreased melatonin function. Monoamine oxidase inhibitors, noradrenergic uptake inhibitors, selective serotonin-reuptake inhibitors, neuroleptics, and psoralens enhance melatonin function.

Adverse effects, such as abdominal cramps, hangover effects, dizziness, fatigue, irritability, and impaired balance are associated with high doses (>3 mg/d) of melatonin. High doses also exacerbate depression; its use is best avoided in women with a history of mental illness. Melatonin should be used with caution in the elderly since it can affect the activity of various neurotransmitters that are altered with advancing age, such as dopamine, serotonin, GABA, and opioid peptides.

Melatonin does not appear to regulate cerebral blood flow. However, in animal studies, melatonin has caused coronary and cerebral artery vasoconstriction. Data regarding its use in postmenopausal women with diabetes are conflicting.

Suggested reading

Contraceptives

Abrams LS, Skee D, Natarajan J, Wong FA. Pharmacokinetic overview of Ortho Evra/Evra. *Fertil Steril* 2002;77(2 Suppl 2):S3-S12.

Ahrendt HJ, Nisand I, Bastianelli C, et al. Efficacy, acceptability and tolerability of the combined contraceptive ring, NuvaRing, compared with an oral contraceptive containing 30 microg of ethinyl estradiol and 3 mg of drospirenone. *Contraception* 2006;74:451-457.

Anderson FD. Safety and efficacy of an extended-regimen oral contraceptive utilizing continuous low-dose ethinyl estradiol. *Contraception* 2006; 73:229-234.

Andersson K, Mattson LA, Rybo G, Stadberg E. Intrauterine release of levonorgestrel—a new way of adding progestogen in hormone replacement therapy. *Obstet Gynecol* 1992;79:963-967.

Archer DF, Jensen JT, Johnson JV, Borisute H, Grubb GS, Constantine GD. Evaluation of a continuous regimen of levonorgestrel/ethinyl estradiol: phase 3 study results. *Contraception* 2006;74:429-445.

Audet MC, Moreau M, Koltun WD, et al. Evaluation of contraceptive efficacy and cycle control of a transdermal contraceptive patch vs an oral contraceptive: a randomized clinical trial. *JAMA* 2001;285:2347-2354.

Bachmann G, Sulak PJ, Sampson-Landers C, Benda N, Marr J. Efficacy and safety of a low-dose 24-day combined oral contraceptive containing 20 micrograms ethinylestradiol and 3 mg drospirenone. *Contraception* 2004;70:191-198.

Bagger YZ, Tanko LB, Alexandersen P, et al. Two to three years of hormone replacement treatment in healthy women have long-term preventive effects on bone mass and osteoporotic fractures: the PERF study. *Bone* 2004;34:728-735.

Bairey Merz CN, Johnson BD, Berga S, Braunstein G, Reis SE, Bittner V, for the WISE Study Group. Past oral contraceptive use and angiographic coronary artery disease in postmenopausal women: data from the National Heart, Lung and Blood Institute-sponsored Women's Ischemia Syndrome Evaluation. *Fertil Steril* 2006;85:1425-1431.

Barad D, Kooperberg C, Wactawski-Wende J, Liu J, Hendrix SL, Watts NB. Prior oral contraception and postmenopausal fracture: a Women's Health Initiative observational cohort study. *Fertil Steril* 2005;84:374-383.

Burger HG, Dudley EC, Hopper JL, et al. Prospectively measured levels of serum follicle-stimulating hormone, estradiol, and the dimeric inhibins during the menopausal transition in a population-based cohort of women. *J Clin Endocrinol Metab* 1999;84:4025-4030.

Chu MC, Cosper P, Nakhuda GS, Lobo RA. A comparison of oral and transdermal short-term estrogen therapy in postmenopausal women with metabolic syndrome. *Fertil Steril* 2006;86:1669-1675.

Clarke SC, Kelleher J, Lloyd-Jones H, Slack M, Schofiel PM. A study of hormone replacement therapy in postmenopausal women with ischaemic heart disease: the Papworth HRT atherosclerosis study. *BJOG* 2002;109:1056-1062.

Cole JA, Norman H, Doherty M, Walker AM. Venous thromboembolism, myocardial infarction, and stroke among transdermal contraceptive system users. *Obstet Gynecol* 2007;109:339-346.

Creinin MD. Laboratory criteria for menopause in women using oral contraceptives. *Fertil Steril* 1996;66:101-104.

Crosignani PG, Vercellini P, Mosconi P, et al. Levonorgestrel-releasing intrauterine device versus hysteroscopic endometrial resection in the treatment of dysfunctional uterine bleeding. *Obstet Gynecol* 1997; 90:257-263.

Foldart JM, Sulak PJ, Schellschmidt I, Zimmermann D, for the Yasmin Extended Regimen Study Group. The use of an oral contraceptive containing ethinylestradiol and drospirenone in an extended regimen over 126 days. *Contraception* 2006;73:34-40.

Hubacher D, Grimes DA. Noncontraceptive health benefits of intrauterine devices: a systematic review. *Obstet Gynecol Surv* 2002;57:120-128.

Hubacher D, Lara-Ricalde R, Taylor DJ, Guerra-Infante F, Guzman-Rodriguez R. Use of copper intrauterine devices and the risk of tubal infertility among nulligravid women. *N Engl J Med* 2001;345:561-567.

Hurskainen R, Teperi J, Rissanen P, et al. Clinical outcomes and costs with the levonorgestrel-releasing intrauterine system or hysterectomy for treatment of menorrhagia: randomized trial 5-year follow-up. *JAMA* 2004;291:1456-1463.

Kaunitz AM. Combination oral contraceptives. *Contemp Clin Obstet Gynecol* 2001;1:149-166.

Kaunitz AM. Depo-Provera's black box: time to reconsider? *Contraception* 2005;72:165-167.

Kaunitz AM. Menstruation: choosing whether…and when. *Contraception* 2000;62:277-284.

Kaunitz AM. Noncontraceptive health benefits of oral contraceptives. *Rev Endocr Metab Disord* 2002;3:277-283.

Kaunitz AM. Oral contraceptive use in perimenopause. *Am J Obstet Gynecol* 2001;185:32-37.

Kaunitz AM. Use of hormonal contraception in women with coexisting medical conditions. *Obstet Gynecol* 2006;6:1453-1472.

Lewandowski KC, Komorowski J, Mikhalidis DP, et al. Effects of hormone replacement therapy type and route of administration on plasma matrix metalloproteinases and their tissue inhibitors in postmenopausal women. *J Clin Endocrinol Metab* 2006;91:3123-3130.

Lobo RA, Cassidenti DL. Pharmacokinetics of oral 17 beta-estradiol. *J Reprod Med* 1992;37:77-84.

Mueck AO, Genazzani AR, Samsioe G, Vukovic-Wysocki I, Seeger H. Low-dose continuous combinations of hormone therapy and biochemical surrogate markers for vascular tone and inflammation: transdermal versus oral application. *Menopause* 2007;14:1-7.

Nakajima ST, Archer DF, Ellman H. Efficacy and safety of a new 24-day oral contraceptive regimen of norethindrone acetate 1 mg/ethinyl estradiol 20 micro g (Loestrin 24 Fe). *Contraception* 2007;75:16-22.

Pearlstein TB, Bachmann GA, Zacur HA, Yonkers KA. Treatment of premenstrual dysphoric disorder with a new drospirenone-containing oral contraceptive formulation. *Contraception* 2005;72:414-421.

Petta CA, Ferriani RQ, Abrao MS, et al. Randomized clinical trial of a levonorgestrel-releasing intrauterine system and a depot GnRH analogue for the treatment of chronic pelvic pain in women with endometriosis. *Hum Reprod* 2005;20:1993-1998.

Potts RO, Lobo RA. Transdermal drug delivery: clinical considerations for the obstetrician-gynecologist. *Obstet Gynecol* 2005;105(5 Pt 1):953-961.

Power J, French R, Cowan F. Subdermal implantable contraceptives versus other forms of reversible contraceptives or other implants as effective methods of preventing pregnancy. *Cochrane Database Syst Rev* 2007;3:CD001326.

Rapkin AJ, Winer SA. Drospirenone: a novel progestin. *Expert Opin Pharmacother* 2007;8:989-999.

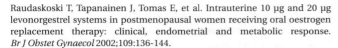

Raudaskoski T, Tapanainen J, Tomas E, et al. Intrauterine 10 μg and 20 μg levonorgestrel systems in postmenopausal women receiving oral oestrogen replacement therapy: clinical, endometrial and metabolic response. *Br J Obstet Gynaecol* 2002;109:136-144.

Raudaskoski TH, Lahti EI, Kauppila AJ, et al. Transdermal estrogen with a levonorgestrel-releasing intrauterine device for climacteric complaints: clinical and endometrial responses. *Am J Obstet Gynecol* 1995;172:114-119.

Raymond EG, Trussell J, Polis CB. Population effect of increased access to emergency contraceptive pills: a systematic review. *Obstet Gynecol* 2007;109:181-186.

Roumen FJ, Apter D, Mulders TM, Dieben TO. Efficacy, tolerability and acceptability of a novel contraceptive vaginal ring releasing etonogestrel and ethinyl estradiol. *Hum Reprod* 2001;16:469-475.

Salpeter SR, Walsh JME, Ormiston TM, Greyber E, Buckley NS, Salpeter EE. Meta-analysis: effect of hormone-replacement therapy of components of the metabolic syndrome in postmenopausal women. *Diabetes Obes Metab* 2006;8:538-554.

Scott RT Jr, Ross B, Anderson C, Archer DF. Pharmacokinetics of percutaneous estradiol: a crossover study using a gel and a transdermal system in comparison with oral micronized estradiol. *Obstet Gynecol* 1991;77:758-764.

Shulman LP. Safety and efficacy of a new oral contraceptive containing drospirenone. *J Reprod Med* 2002;47(11 Suppl):981-984.

Slater CC, Hodis HN, Mack WJ, Shoupe D, Paulson RJ, Stanczyk FZ. Markedly elevated levels of estrone sulfate after long-term oral, but not transdermal, administration of estradiol in postmenopausal women. *Menopause* 2001;8:200-203.

Sulak PJ, Kuehl TJ, Coffee A, Willis S. Prospective analysis of occurrence and management of breakthrough bleeding during an extended oral contraceptive regimen. *Am J Obstet Gynecol* 2006;195:935-941.

Sumino H, Ichikawa S, Kasama S, et al. Different effects of oral conjugated estrogen and transdermal estradiol on arterial stiffness and vascular inflammatory markers in postmenopausal women. *Atherosclerosis* 2006;189:436-442.

US Food and Drug Administration. FDA approves over-the-counter access for Plan B for women 18 and older; prescription remains required for those 17 and under. 2006. Available at: http://www.fda.gov/bbs/topics/NEWS/2006/NEW01436.html. Accessed September 21, 2007.

Van den Heuvel MW, van Bragt AJ, Alnabawy A, Kaptein MC. Comparison of ethinylestradiol pharmacokinetics in three hormonal contraceptive formulations: the vaginal ring, the transdermal patch, and an oral contraceptive. *Contraception* 2005;72:168-174.

Westhoff C. Clinical practice. Emergency contraception. *N Engl J Med* 2003;349:1830-1835.

Westhoff C. Depot-medroxyprogesterone acetate injection (Depo-Provera): a highly effective contraceptive option with proven long-term safety. *Contraception* 2003;68:75-87.

White T, Ozel B, Jain JK, Stanczyk FZ. Effects of transdermal and oral steroidal contraceptives on estrogen-sensitive hepatic proteins, levonorgestrel, serum-binding globulins, and C-reactive protein. *Contraception* 2006;74:293-296.

Wildemeersch D, Schacht E, Wildemeersch P, Calleweart K, Pylyser K, De Wever N. Endometrial safety with a low-dose intrauterine levonorgestrel-releasing system after 3 years of estrogen substitution therapy. *Maturitas* 2004;48:65-70.

Yonkers KA, Brown C, Pearlstein TB, Foegh M, Sampson-Landers C, Rapkin A. Efficacy of a new low-dose oral contraceptive with drospirenone in premenstrual dysphoric disorder. *Obstet Gynecol* 2005;106:492-501.

Zanger D, Yang BK, Ardans J, et al. Divergent effects of hormone therapy on serum markers of inflammation in postmenopausal women with coronary artery disease on appropriate medical management. *J Am Coll Cardiol* 2000;36:1797-1802.

ET and EPT

Akhrass F, Evans AT, Wang Y, et al. Hormone replacement therapy is associated with less coronary atherosclerosis in postmenopausal women. *J Clin Endocrinol Metab* 2003;88:5611-5614.

Al-Azzawi F, Buckler HM, for the United Kingdom Vaginal Ring Investigator Group. Comparison of a novel vaginal ring delivering estradiol acetate versus oral estradiol for relief of vasomotor symptoms. *Climacteric* 2003;6:118-127.

Anderson GL, Judd HL, Kaunitz AM, et al, for the Women's Health Initiative Investigators. Effects of estrogen plus progestin on gynecologic cancers and associated diagnostic procedures: the Women's Health Initiative Randomized Trial. *JAMA* 2003;290:1739-1748.

Arana A, Varas C, González-Pérez A, Gutiérrez L, Bjerrum L, García Rodgríguez LA. Hormone therapy and cerebrovascular events: a population-based nested case-control study. *Menopause* 2006;13:730-735.

Archer DF, Dorin M, Lewis V, Schneider DL, Pickar JH. Effects of lower doses of conjugated equine estrogens and medroxyprogesterone acetate on endometrial bleeding. *Fertil Steril* 2001;75:1080-1087.

Archer DF, Furst K, Tipping D, Dain MP, Vandepol C. A randomized comparison of continuous combined transdermal delivery of estradiol-norethindrone acetate and estradiol alone for menopause. CombiPatch Study Group. *Obstet Gynecol* 1999;94:498-503.

Archer DF, Pickar JH, Bottiglioni F, for the Menopause Study Group. Bleeding patterns in postmenopausal women taking continuous combined or sequential regimens of conjugated estrogens with medroxyprogesterone acetate. *Obstet Gynecol* 1994;83:686-692.

Badimon L, Bayes-Genis A. Effects of progestogens on thrombosis and atherosclerosis. *Hum Reprod Update* 1999;5:191-199.

Baracat E, Haidar M, Lopez FJ, Pickar J, Dey M, Negro-Villar A. Estrogen activity and novel tissue selectivity of delta8,9-dehydroestrone sulfate in postmenopausal women. *J Clin Endrocinol Metab* 1999;84:2020-2027.

Barnabei VM, Cochrane BB, Aragaki AK, et al, for the Women's Health Initiative Investigators. Menopausal symptoms and treatment-related effects of estrogen and progestin in the Women's Health Initiative. *Obstet Gynecol* 2005;105(5 pt 1):1063-1073.

Barnes BB, Levrant SG. Pharmacology of estrogens. In: Lobo, RA, ed. *Treatment of the Postmenopausal Woman: Basic and Clinical Aspects*, 3rd ed. San Diego, CA: Academic Press, 2007:767-777.

Barrett-Connor E, Slone S, Greendale G, et al. The Postmenopausal Estrogen/Progestin Interventions Study: primary outcomes in adherent women. *Maturitas* 1997;27:261-274.

Barrett-Connor E, Wehren LE, Siris ES, et al. Recency and duration of postmenopausal hormone therapy: effects on bone mineral density and fracture risk in the National Osteoporosis Risk Assessment (NORA) study. *Menopause* 2003;10:412-419.

Belisle S, Derzko C. Hormone replacement therapy and cancer: Canadian consensus on menopause and osteoporosis. *J SOGC* 2001;23:1198-1203.

Beral V, for the Million Women Study Collaborators. Ovarian cancer and hormone replacement therapy in the Million Women Study. *Lancet* 2007;369:1703-1710.

Beral V, Bull D, Reeves G, for the Million Women Study Collaborators. Endometrial cancer and hormone-replacement therapy in the Million Women Study. *Lancet* 2005;365:1543-1551.

Bhavnani BR. Pharmacokinetics and pharmacodynamics of conjugated equine estrogens: chemistry and metabolism. *Proc Soc Exp Biol Med* 1998;217:6-16.

Bhavnani BR, Nisker JA, Martin J, Aletebi F, Watson L, Milne JK. Comparison of pharmacokinetics of a conjugated equine estrogen preparation (Premarin) and a synthetic mixture of estrogens (C.E.S.) in postmenopausal women. *J Soc Gynecol Investig* 2000;7:175-1783.

Bjarnason K, Cerin A, Lindgren R, Weber T. Adverse endometrial effects during long cycle hormone replacement therapy. Scandinavian Long Cycle Study Group. *Maturitas* 1999;32:161-170.

Bolaji II, Mortimer G, Grimes H, Tallon DF, O'Dwyer E, Fottrell PF. Clinical evaluation of near-continuous oral micronized progesterone therapy in estrogenized postmenopausal women. *Gynecol Endocrinol* 1996;10:41-47.

Brunner RL, Gass M, Aragaki A, et al, for the Women's Health Initiative Investigators. Effects of conjugated equine estrogen on health-related quality of life in postmenopausal women with hysterectomy. *Arch Intern Med* 2005;165:1976-1986.

Brynhildsen J, Hammar M. Low dose transdermal estradiol/norethisterone acetate treatment over 2 years does not cause endometrial proliferation in postmenopausal women. *Menopause* 2002;9:137-144.

Buck A, Shen L, Kelly S, et al. Steady-state bioavailability of estradiol from two matrix transdermal delivery systems, Alora and Climara. *Menopause* 1998;5:107-112.

Buckler H, Al-Azzawi F, for the UK VR Multicentre Trial Group. The effect of a novel vaginal ring delivering oestradiol acetate on climacteric symptoms in postmenopausal women. *Br J Obstet Gynaecol* 2003;110:753-759.

Buist DSM, Newton KM, Miglioretti DL, et al. Hormone therapy prescribing patterns in the United States. *Obstet Gynecol* 2004;104:1042-1050.

Burry KA, Patton PE, Hermsmeyer K. Percutaneous absorption of progesterone in postmenopausal women treated with transdermal estrogen. *Obstet Gynecol* 1999;180:1504-1511.

Buyon JP, Petri MA, Kim MY, et al. The effect of combined estrogen and progesterone hormone replacement therapy on disease activity in systemic lupus erythematosus: a randomized trial. *Ann Intern Med* 2005;142:953-962.

Canonico M, Oger E, Plu-Bureau G, et al, for the Estrogen and Thromboembolism Risk (ESTHER) Study Group. Hormone therapy and venous thromboembolism among postmenopausal women: impact of the route of estrogen administration and progestogens—the ESTHER Study. *Circulation* 2007;115:840-845.

Casper RF, Chapdelaine A. Estrogen and interrupted progestin: a new concept for menopausal hormone replacement therapy. *Am J Obstet Gynecol* 1993;168:1188-1196.

Chan JA, Meyerhardt JA, Chan AT, Giovannucci EL, Colditz GA, Fuchs CS. Hormone replacement therapy and survival after colorectal cancer diagnosis. *J Clin Oncol* 2006;24:5680-5686.

Chen CL, Weiss NS, Newcomb P, Barlow W, White E. Hormone replacement therapy in relation to breast cancer. *JAMA* 2002;287:734-741.

Chen WY, Manson JE, Hankinson SE, et al. Unopposed estrogen therapy and the risk of invasive breast cancer. *Arch Intern Med* 2006;166:1027-1032.

Chen Z, Bassford T, Green SB, et al. Postmenopausal hormone therapy and body composition—a substudy of the estrogen plus progestin trial of the Women's Health Initiative. *Am J Clin Nutr* 2005;82:651-656.

Chetkowski RJ, Meldrum DR, Steingold KA, et al. Biologic effects of transdermal estradiol. *N Engl J Med* 1986;314:1615-1620.

Chlebowski RT, Hendrix SL, Langer RD, et al, for the WHI investigators. Influence of estrogen plus progestin on breast cancer and mammography in healthy postmenopausal women: the Women's Health Initiative randomized trial. *JAMA* 2003;289:3243-3253.

Cicinelli E, Di Naro E, De Ziegler D, et al. Placement of the vaginal 17β-estradiol tablets in the inner or outer one third of the vagina affects the preferential delivery of 17β-estradiol toward the uterus or periurethral areas, thereby modifying efficacy and endometrial safety. *Am J Obstet Gynecol* 2003;189:55-58.

Cirigliano M. Bioidentical hormone therapy: a review of the evidence. *J Womens Health* 2007;16:600-631.

Conner P, Svane G, Azavedo E, et al. Mammographic breast density, hormones, and growth factors during continuous combined hormone therapy. *Fertil Steril* 2004;81:1617-1623.

Cooper A, Spencer C, Whitehead MI, Ross D, Barnard GJ, Collins WP. Systemic absorption of progesterone from Progest cream in postmenopausal women [letter]. *Lancet* 1998;351:1255-1256.

Corson SL, Richart RM, Caubel P, et al. Effect of a unique constant-estrogen, pulsed-progestin hormone replacement therapy containing 17β-estradiol and norgestimate on endometrial histology. *Int J Fertil* 1999;44:279-285.

Curb JD, Prentice RL, Bray PF, et al, for the Women's Health Initiative Investigators. Venous thrombosis and conjugated equine estrogen in women without a uterus: data from the Women's Health Initiative. *Arch Int Med* 2006;166:772-780.

Cushman M, Kuller LH, Prentice R, et al, for the Women's Health Initiative Investigators. Estrogen plus progestin and risk of venous thrombosis. *JAMA* 2004;292:1573-1580.

CYP3A and drug interactions. *Med Lett Drugs Ther* 2005;47:54-55.

Daly E, Vessey MP, Hawkins MM, Carson JL, Gough P, Marsh S. Risk of venous thromboembolism in users of hormone replacement therapy. *Lancet* 1996;348:977-980.

Darj E, Nilsson S, Axelsson O, Hellberg D. Clinical and endometrial effects of oestradiol and progesterone in post-menopausal women. *Maturitas* 1991;13:109-115.

de Lignieres B. Endometrial hyperplasia: risks, recognition and the search for a safe hormone replacement regimen. *J Reprod Med* 1999;44:191-196.

de Ziegler D, Ferriani R, Moraes LA, Bulletti C. Vaginal progesterone in menopause: Crinone 4% in cyclical and constant combined regimens. *Hum Reprod* 2000;15(Suppl):S149-S158.

Dessole S, Rubattu G, Ambrosini G, et al. Efficacy of low-dose intravaginal estriol on urogenital aging in postmenopausal women. *Menopause* 2004;11:49-56.

Diem S, Grady D, Quan J, et al. Effects of ultralow-dose transdermal estradiol on postmenopausal symptoms in women aged 60 to 80 years. *Menopause* 2006;13:130-138.

Doherty JA, Cushing-Haugen KL, Saltzman BS, et al. Long-term use of postmenopausal estrogen and progestin hormone therapies and the risk of endometrial cancer. *Am J Obstet Gynecol* 2007;197:139.e1-e7.

Dupont A, Dupont P, Cusan L, et al. Comparative endocrinological and clinical effects of percutaneous estradiol and oral conjugated estrogen as replacement therapy in menopausal women. *Maturitas* 1991;13:297-311.

Eriksen BC. A randomized, open, parallel-group study on the preventive effect of an estradiol-releasing vaginal ring (Estring) on recurrent urinary tract infections in postmenopausal women. *Am J Obstet Gynecol* 1999;180:1072-1079.

Espeland MA, Rapp SR, Shumaker SA, et al, for the Women's Health Initiative Memory Study Investigators. Conjugated equine estrogens and global cognitive function in postmenopausal women: Women's Health Initiative Memory Study. *JAMA* 2004;291:2959-2968.

Ettinger B, Ensrud KE, Wallace R, et al. Effects of ultralow-dose transdermal estradiol on bone mineral density: a randomized clinical trial. *Obstet Gynecol* 2004;104:443-451.

Ettinger B, Grady D, Tosteson ANA, Pressman A, Macer JL. Effect of the Women's Health Initiative on women's decisions to discontinue postmenopausal hormone therapy. *Obstet Gynecol* 2003;102:1225-1232.

Ettinger B, Li DK, Klein R. Continuation of postmenopausal hormone replacement therapy: comparison of cyclic versus continuous combined schedule. *Menopause* 1996;3:185-189.

Ettinger B, Li DK, Klein R. Unexpected vaginal bleeding and associated gynecologic care in postmenopausal women using hormone therapy: comparison of cyclic versus continuous combined schedules. *Fertil Steril* 1998;69:865-869.

Ettinger B, Pressman A, Van Gessel A. Low-dosage esterified estrogen opposed by progestin at 6-month intervals. *Obstet Gynecol* 2001;98:205-211.

Ettinger B, Selby J, Citron JT, et al. Cyclic hormone replacement therapy using quarterly progestin. *Obstet Gynecol* 1994;83:693-700.

Fanchin R, de Ziegler D, Bergeron C, Righini C, Torrisi C, Frydman R. Transvaginal administration of progesterone. *Obstet Gynecol* 1997;90:396-401.

Ferreira E, Brown TER. Pharmacotherapy: Canadian consensus on menopause and osteoporosis. *J Obstet Gynaecol Can* 2001;23:1105-1114.

Fitzpatrick LA, Good A. Micronized progesterone: clinical indications and comparison with current treatments. *Fertil Steril* 1999;72:389-397.

Fletcher AS, Erbas B, Kavanagh AM, Hart S, Rodger A, Gertig DM. Use of hormone replacement therapy (HRT) and survival following breast cancer diagnosis. *Breast* 2005;14:192-200.

Fournier A, Berrino F, Riboli E, Avenel V, Clavel-Chapelon F. Breast cancer risk in relation to different types of hormone replacement therapy in the E3N-EPIC cohort. *Intl J Cancer* 2005;114:448-454.

Freeman EW, Sammel MD, Lin H, Nelson DB. Associations of hormones and menopausal status with depressed mood in women with no history of depression. *Arch Gen Psychiatry* 2006;63:375-382.

Gambrell RD. Progesterone skin cream and measurements of absorption [editorial]. *Menopause* 2003;10:1-3.

Gambrell RD Jr. Strategies to reduce the incidence of endometrial cancer in postmenopausal women. *Am J Obstet Gynecol* 1997;177:1196-1204.

Gillet JY, Andre G, Faguer B. Induction of amenorrhea during hormone replacement therapy: optimal micronized progesterone dose: a multicenter study. *Maturitas* 1994;19:103-115.

Girdler SS, Hinderliter AL, Wells EC, Sherwood A, Grewen KM, Light KC. Transdermal versus oral estrogen therapy in postmenopausal smokers: hemodynamic and endothelial effects. *Obstet Gynecol* 2004;103:169-180.

Gordon S, Walsh BW, Ciaccia AV, Siddhanti S, Rosen AS, Plouffe L. Transition from estrogen-progestin to raloxifene in postmenopausal women: effect on vasomotor symptoms. *Obstet Gynecol* 2004;103:267-273.

Graff-Iversen S, Hammar N, Thelle DS, Tonstad S. Hormone therapy and mortality during a 14-year follow-up of 14,324 Norwegian women. *J Intern Med* 2004;256:437-445.

Greenspan SL, Resnick NM, Parker RA. The effect of hormone replacement on physical performance in community-dwelling elderly women. *Am J Med* 2005;118:1232-1239.

Greiser C, Greiser EM, Dören M. Menopausal hormone therapy and risk of breast cancer: a meta-analysis of epidemiological studies and randomized controlled trials. *Hum Reprod Update* 2005;11:561-573.

Grodstein F, Lifford K, Resnick NM, Curhan GC. Postmenopausal hormone therapy and risk of developing urinary incontinence. *Obstet Gynecol* 2004;103:254-260.

Grodstein F, Manson JE, Stampfer MJ. Hormone therapy and coronary heart disease: the role of time since menopause and age at hormone initiation. *J Womens Health* 2006;15:35-44.

Grodstein F, Stampfer MJ. The epidemiology of coronary heart disease and estrogen replacement in postmenopausal women. *Prog Cardiovasc Dis* 1995;38:199-210.

Grodstein F, Stampfer MJ, Colditz GA, et al. Postmenopausal hormone therapy and mortality. *N Engl J Med* 1997;336:1769-1775.

Grodstein F, Stampfer MJ, Goldhaber SZ, et al. Prospective study of exogenous hormones and risk of pulmonary embolism in women. *Lancet* 1996;348:983-987.

Grodstein F, Stampfer MJ, Manson JE, et al. Postmenopausal estrogen and progestin use and the risk of cardiovascular disease. *N Engl J Med* 1996;335:453-461.

Guetta V, Cannon RO III. Cardiovascular effects of estrogen and lipid-lowering therapies in postmenopausal women. *Circulation* 1996;93:1928-1937.

Gutthann SP, Rodriguez LAG, Castellsague J, et al. Hormone replacement therapy and risk of venous thromboembolism: population based case-control study. *BMJ* 1997;314:796-800.

Haas S, Walsh B, Evans S, Krache M, Ravnikar V, Schiff I. The effect of transdermal estradiol on hormone and metabolic dynamics over a six-week period. *Obstet Gynecol* 1988;71:671-676.

Haimov-Kochman R, Barak-Glantz E, Arbel R, et al. Gradual discontinuation of hormone therapy does not prevent the reappearance of climacteric symptoms: a randomized prospective study. *Menopause* 2006;13:370-376.

Hall G, Blomback M, Landgren BM, Bremme K. Effects of vaginally administered high estradiol doses on hormonal pharmacokinetics and hemostasis in postmenopausal women. *Fertil Steril* 2002;78:1172-1177.

Harvey J, Scheeurer C, Kawakami FT, Quebe-Fehling E, de Palacios PI, Ragavan VV. Hormone replacement therapy and breast density changes. *Climacteric* 2005;8:185-192.

Hendrix SL, Cochrane BB, Nygaard IE, et al. Effects of estrogen with and without progestin on urinary incontinence. *JAMA* 2005;293:935-948.

Hendrix SL, Wassertheil-Smoller S, Johnson KC, et al, for the WHI Investigators. Effects of conjugated equine estrogen on stroke in the WHI. *Circulation* 2006;113:2425-2434.

Hersh AL, Stefanick ML, Stafford RS. National use of postmenopausal hormone therapy: annual trends and response to recent evidence. *JAMA* 2004;291:47-53.

Hill DA, Weiss NA, Beresford SA, et al. Continuous combined hormone replacement therapy and risk of endometrial cancer. *Am J Obstet Gynecol* 2000;183:1456-1461.

Hodis HN, Mack WJ. Postmenopausal hormone therapy in clinical perspective. *Menopause* 2007;14:944-957.

Holmberg L, Anderson H, for the HABITS steering and data monitoring committees. HABITS (hormonal replacement therapy after breast cancer—is it safe?), a randomised comparison: trial stopped. *Lancet* 2004;363:453-455.

Holmgren PA, Lindskog M, von Schoultz B. Vaginal rings for continuous low-dose release of oestradiol in the treatment of urogenital atrophy. *Maturitas* 1989;11:55-63.

Holzer G, Riegler E, Honigsmann H, Farokhnia S, Schmidt JB. Effects and side-effects of 2% progesterone cream on the skin of peri- and postmenopausal women: results from a double-blind, vehicle-controlled, randomized study. *Br J Dermatol* 2005;153:626-634.

Hsia J, Langer RD, Manson JE, et al, for the Women's Health Initiative Investigators. Conjugated equine estrogens and coronary heart disease: the Women's Health Initiative. *Arch Intern Med* 2006;166:357-365.

Hulley S, Grady D, Bush T, et al. Randomized trial of estrogen plus progestin for secondary prevention of coronary heart disease in postmenopausal women: Heart and Estrogen/progestin Replacement Study (HERS) Group. *JAMA* 1998;280:605-613.

Jick H, Darvy LE, Myers MW, et al. Risk of hospital admission for idiopathic venous thromboembolism among users of postmenopausal estrogens. *Lancet* 1996;348:981-983.

Johnson JV, Davidson M, Archer D, Bachmann G. Postmenopausal uterine bleeding profiles with two forms of combined continuous hormone replacement therapy. *Menopause* 2002;9:16-22.

Jondet M, Maroni M, Yaneva H, Brin S, Peltier-Pujol F, Pelissier C. Comparative endometrial histology in postmenopausal women with sequential hormone replacement therapy of estradiol and either chlormadinone acetate or micronized progesterone. *Maturitas* 2002;41:115-121.

Kendall A, Dowsett M, Folkherd E, Smith I. Caution: Vaginal estradiol appears to be contraindicated in postmenopausal women on adjuvant aromatase inhibitors. *Ann Oncol* 2006;17:584-587.

Kotsopoulos J, Lubinski J, Neuhausen SL, et al. Hormone replacement therapy and the risk of ovarian cancer in *BRCA1* and *BRCA2* mutation carriers. *Gynecol Oncol* 2006;100:83-88.

Kritz-Silverstein D, Barrett-Connor E. Long-term postmenopausal hormone use, obesity, and fat distribution in older women. *JAMA* 1996;275:987-988.

Kurman RJ, Felix JC, Archer DF, Nanavati N, Arce J, Moyer DL. Norethindrone acetate and estradiol-induced endometrial hyperplasia. *Obstet Gynecol* 2000;96:373-379.

Lacy JV Jr, Brinton LA, Lubin JH, Sherman ME, Schatzkin A, Schairer C. Endometrial carcinoma risks among menopausal estrogen plus progestin and unopposed estrogen users in a cohort of postmenopausal women. *Cancer Epidemiol Biomarkers Prev* 2005;14:1724-1731.

Lemaitre RN, Weiss NS, Smith NL, et al. Esterified estrogen and conjugated equine estrogen and the risk of incident of myocardial infarction and stroke. *Arch Intern Med* 2006;166:399-404.

Lethaby A, Farquhar C, Sarkis A, Roberts H, Jepson R, Barlow D. Hormone replacement therapy in postmenopausal women: endometrial hyperplasia and irregular bleeding. *Cochrane Database Syst Rev* 2004;3:CD000402.

Levine H, Watson N. Comparison of the pharmacokinetics of Crinone 8% administered vaginally versus Prometrium administered orally in postmenopausal women. *Fertil Steril* 2000;73:516-521.

Lobo RA. Clinical aspects of hormone replacement. In Lobo RA, ed. *Treatment of the Postmenopausal Woman: Basic and Clinical Aspects*, 2nd ed. Philadelphia, PA: Lippincott Williams & Wilkins, 1999:125-139.

Lobo RA, Zacur HZ, Caubel P, et al. A novel intermittent regimen of norgestimate to preserve the beneficial effects of 17β-estradiol on lipid and lipoprotein profiles. *Am J Obstet Gynecol* 2000;182:41-49.

Lochner DM, Brubaker KL. Incidence of malignancy in hormone therapy users with indeterminate calcifications on mammogram. *Am J Obstet Gynecol* 2006;194:82-85.

Lord C, Buss C, Lupien SJ, Pruessner JC. Hippocampal volumes are larger in postmenopausal women using estrogen therapy compared to past users, never users and men: a possible window of opportunity effect. *Neurobiol Aging* 2006 Oct 6; [Epub ahead of print].

Lyytinen H, Pukkala E, Ylikorkala O. Breast cancer risk in postmenopausal women using estrogen-only therapy. *Obstet Gynecol* 2006;108:1354-1360.

Margolis KL, Bonds DE, Rodabough RJ, et al, for the Women's Health Initiative Investigators. Effect of oestrogen plus progestin on the incidence of diabetes in postmenopausal women: results from the Women's Health Initiative Hormone Trial. *Diabetologia* 2004;47:1175-1187.

McTiernan A, Martin CF, Peck JD, et al, for the Women's Health Initiative Mammogram Density Study Investigators. Estrogen-plus-progestin use and mammographic density in postmenopausal women: Women's Health Initiative randomized trial. *J Natl Cancer Inst* 2005;97:1366-1376.

Melamed M, Castano E, Notides A, Sasson S. Molecular and kinetic basis for the mixed agonist/antagonist activity of estriol. *Mol Endocrinol* 1997; 11:1868-1878.

Miles RA, Press MF, Paulson RJ, Dahmoush L, Lobo RA, Sauer MV. Pharmacokinetics and endometrial tissue levels of progesterone after administration by intramuscular and vaginal routes: a comparative study. *Fertil Steril* 1994;62:485-490.

Million Women Study Collaborators. Breast cancer and hormone-replacement therapy in the Million Women Study. *Lancet* 2003;362:419-427.

Nachtigall LE. Clinical trial of the estradiol vaginal ring in the US. *Maturitas* 1995;22(Suppl):S43-S47.

Naessen T, Rodriguez-Macias K. Menopausal estrogen therapy counteracts normal aging effects on intima thickness, media thickness and intima/media ratio in carotid and femoral arteries. *Atherosclerosis* 2006;189:387-392.

Naessen T, Rodriguez-Macias K. Endometrial thickness and uterine diameter not affected by ultralow doses of 17beta-estradiol in elderly women. *Am J Obstet Gynecol* 2002;186:944-947.

Neven P, Quail D, Levrier M, et al. Uterine effects of estrogen plus progestin therapy and raloxifene: adjudicated results from the EURALOX study. *Obstet Gynecol* 2004;103:881-891.

Nielsen TF, Ravn P, Pitkin J, Christiansen C. Pulsed estrogen therapy improves postmenopausal quality of life: a 2-year placebo-controlled study. *Maturitas* 2006;53:184-190.

The North American Menopause Society. Clinical challenges of perimenopause: consensus opinion of The North American Menopause Society. *Menopause* 2000;7:5-13.

The North American Menopause Society. Estrogen and progestogen use in peri- and postmenopausal women: March 2007 position statement of The North American Menopause Society. *Menopause* 2007;14:168-182.

The North American Menopause Society. *Understanding the Controversy: Hormone Testing and Bioidentical Hormones*. Proceedings from the Postgraduate Course at the 17th Annual Meeting. Cleveland, OH: The North American Menopause Society, 2006.

The North American Menopause Society. Role of progestogens in hormone replacement therapy for postmenopausal women: position statement of The North American Menopause Society. *Menopause* 2003;10:113-132.

Ockene JK, Barad DH, Cochrane BB, et al. Symptom experience after discontinuing use of estrogen plus progestin. *JAMA* 2005;294:183-193.

Odmark I-S, Bixo M, Englund D, Risberg B, Jonsson B, Olsson S-E. Endometrial safety and bleeding pattern during a five-year treatment with long-cycle hormone therapy. *Menopause* 2005;12:699-707.

Paganini-Hill A, Corrada MM, Kawas CH. Increased longevity in older users of postmenopausal estrogen therapy: the Leisure World Cohort Study. *Menopause* 2006;13:12-18.

Pelissier C, Maroni M, Yaneva H, Brin S, Peltier-Pujol F, Jondet M. Chlormadinone acetate versus micronized progesterone in the sequential combined hormone replacement therapy of the menopause. *Maturitas* 2001;40:85-94.

Phillips A, Demarest K, Hahn DW, et al. Progestational and androgenic receptor binding affinities and in vivo activities of norgestimate and other progestins. *Contraception* 1990;41:399-410.

Pickar JH, Yeh I-T, Wheeler JE, Cunnane MF, Speroff L. Endometrial effects of lower doses of conjugated equine estrogens and medroxyprogesterone acetate: two-year substudy results. *Fertil Steril* 2003;80:1234-1240.

Prior JC. Progesterone as a bone-tropic hormone. *Endocr Rev* 1990; 11:386-398.

Ravdin PM, Cronin KA, Howlader N, et al. The decrease in breast-cancer incidence in 2003 in the United States. *N Engl J Med* 2007;356:1670-1674.

Raz R, Stamm W. A controlled trial of intravaginal estriol in postmenopausal women with recurrent urinary tract infections. *N Engl J Med* 1993; 329:753-756.

Rebbeck TR, Friebel T, Wagner T, et al. Effect of short-term hormone replacement therapy on breast cancer risk reduction after bilateral prophylactic oophorectomy in BRCA1 and BRCA2 mutation carriers: the PROSE Study Group. *J Clin Oncol* 2005;23:7804-7810.

Rejnmark L, Vestergaard P, Tofteng CL, et al. Response rates to oestrogen treatment in perimenopausal women: 5-year data from the Danish Osteoporosis Prevention Study (DOPS). *Maturitas* 2004;48:307-320.

Reubinoff BE, Wurtman J, Rojansky N, et al. Effects of hormone replacement therapy on weight, body composition, fat distribution, and food intake in early postmenopausal women: a prospective study. *Fertil Steril* 1995; 64:963-968.

Rosenberg L, Palmer JR, Wise LA, Adams-Campbell LL. A prospective study of female hormone use and breast cancer among black women. *Arch Intern Med* 2006;166:760-765.

Ross AH, Boyd ME, Colgan TJ, Ferenczy A, Fugere P, Lorrain J. Comparison of transdermal and oral sequential progestogen in combination with transdermal estradiol: effects on bleeding patterns and endometrial histology. *Obstet Gynecol* 1993;82:773-779.

Ross D, Cooper AJ, Pryse-Davies J, Bergeron C, Collins WP, Whitehead MI. Randomized, double-blind, dose-ranging study of the endometrial effects of a vaginal progesterone gel in estrogen-treated postmenopausal women. *Am J Obstet Gynecol* 1997;177:937-941.

Rossouw JE, Prentice RL, Manson JE, et al. Post-menopausal hormone therapy and risk of cardiovascular disease by age and years since menopause. *JAMA* 2007;297:1465-1477.

Salpeter SR, Walsh JME, Greyber E, Salpeter EE. Coronary heart disease events associated with hormone therapy in younger and older women: a meta-analysis. *J Gen Intern Med* 2006;21:363-366.

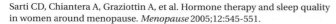

Sarti CD, Chiantera A, Graziottin A, et al. Hormone therapy and sleep quality in women around menopause. *Menopause* 2005;12:545-551.

Scarabin P-Y, Oger E, Plu-Bureau G, for the EStrogen and THromboEmbolism Risk (ESTHER) Study Group. Differential association of oral and transdermal oestrogen-replacement therapy with venous thromboembolism risk. *Lancet* 2003;362:428-432.

Schairer C, Byrne GM, Rosenberg PS, et al. Estrogen replacement therapy and breast cancer survival in a large screening study. *J Nat Cancer Inst* 1999; 91:264-270.

Schiff I, Tulchinsky D, Cramer D, Ryan KJ. Oral medroxyprogesterone in the treatment of postmenopausal symptoms. *JAMA* 1980;244:1443-1445.

Schoonen WG, Joosten JW, Kloosterboer HJ. Effects of two classes of progestagens, pregnane and 19-nortestosterone derivatives, on cell growth of human breast tumor cells: I. MCF-7 cell lines. *J Steroid Biochem Mol Biol* 1995;55:423-437.

Sellers TA, Mink PJ, Cerhan JR, et al. The role of hormone replacement therapy in the risk for breast cancer and total mortality in women with a family history of breast cancer. *Ann Intern Med* 1997;127:973-980.

Shantakumar S, Terry MB, Paykin A, et al. Age and menopausal effects of hormonal birth control and hormone replacement therapy in relation to breast cancer risks. *Am J Epidemiol* 2007;165:1187-1198.

Shau WY, Hsieh CC, Hsieh TT, Hung TH, Huang KE. Factors associated with endometrial bleeding in continuous hormone replacement therapy. *Menopause* 2002;9:188-194.

Shoupe D, Meme D, Mezrow G, Lobo RA. Prevention of endometrial hyperplasia in postmenopausal women with intrauterine progesterone. *N Engl J Med* 1991;325:1811-1812.

Shumaker SA, Legault C, Kuller L, et al, for the Women's Health Initiative Memory Study Investigators. Conjugated equine estrogens and incidence of probable dementia and mild cognitive impairment in postmenopausal women: Women's Health Initiative Memory Study. *JAMA* 2004; 291:2947-2985.

Shumaker SA, Legault C, Rapp SR, et al, for the WHIMS Investigators. Estrogen plus progestin and the incidence of dementia and mild cognitive impairment in postmenopausal women: the Women's Health Initiative Memory Study: a randomized controlled trial. *JAMA* 2003;289:2651-2662.

Sidelmann JJ, Jespersen J, Andersen LF, Skouby SO. Hormone replacement therapy and hypercoagulability: results from the prospective Danish Climacteric Study. *Br J Obstet Gynecol* 2003;110:541-547.

Simon JA, Bouchard C, Waldbaum A, Utian W, Zborowski J, Snabes MC. Low dose of transdermal gel for treatment of symptomatic postmenopausal women: a randomized controlled trial. *Obstet Gynecol* 2007;109:588-596.

Smith NL, Heckbert SR, Lemaitre RN, et al. Esterified estrogen and conjugated equine estrogens and the risk of venous thrombosis. *JAMA* 2004;292:1581-1587.

Speroff L, Rowan J, Symons J, Genant H, Wilborn W, for the CHART Study Group. The comparative effect on bone density, endometrium, and lipids of continuous hormones as replacement therapy (CHART Study): a randomized controlled trial. *JAMA* 1996;276:1397-1403.

Speroff L, Whitcomb RW, Kempfert NJ, Boyd RA, Paulissen JB, Rowan JP. Efficacy and local tolerance of a low-dose, 7-day matrix estradiol transdermal system in the treatment of menopausal vasomotor symptoms. *Obstet Gynecol* 1996;88:587-592.

Stanczyk FZ. Structure-function relationships, pharmacokinetics, and potency of orally and parenterally administered progestogens. In: Lobo, RA, ed. *Treatment of the Postmenopausal Woman: Basic and Clinical Aspects*, 3rd ed. San Diego, CA: Academic Press, 2007:779-798.

Stefanick ML, Anderson GL, Margolis KL et al, for the Women's Health Initiative Investigators. Effects of conjugated equine estrogens on breast cancer and mammography screening in postmenopausal women with hysterectomy: the Women's Health Initiative. *JAMA* 2006;295:1647-1657.

Steiner AZ, Hodis HN, Lobo RA, Shoupe D, Xiang M, Mack WJ. Postmenopausal oral estrogen therapy and blood pressure in normotensive and hypertensive subjects: the Estrogen in the Prevention of Atherosclerosis Trial. *Menopause* 2005;12:728-733.

Sturdee DW, Ulrich LG, Barlow DH, et al. The endometrial response to sequential and continuous combined oestrogen-progestogen replacement therapy. *Br J Obstet Gynecol* 2000;107:1392-1400.

Suhonen SP, Allonen HO, Lahteenmaki P. Sustained-release estradiol implants and a levonorgestrel-releasing intrauterine device in hormone replacement therapy. *Am J Obstet Gynecol* 1995;172:562-567.

Suhonen SP, Holmstrom T, Allonen HO, Lahteenmaki P. Intrauterine and subdermal progestin administration in postmenopausal hormone replacement therapy. *Fertil Steril* 1995;63:336-342.

Tamimi RM, Hankinson SE, Chen WY, Rosner B, Colditz GA. Combined estrogen and testosterone use and risk of breast cancer in postmenopausal women. *Arch Intern Med* 2006;166:1483-1489.

Tempfer CB, Riener EK, Hefler LA, Huber JC, Muendlein A. DNA microarray-based analysis of single nucleotide polymorphisms may be useful for assessing the risks and benefits of hormone therapy. *Fertil Steril* 2004;82:132-137.

Utian WH. Hormone therapy and risk of gynecologic cancers [letter]. *JAMA* 2004;291:42-43.

Utian WH, Burry KA, Archer DF, et al. Efficacy and safety of low, standard, and high dosages of an estradiol transdermal system (Esclim) compared with placebo on vasomotor symptoms in highly symptomatic menopausal patients: the Esclim Study Group. *Am J Obstet Gynecol* 1999;181:71-79.

Utian WH, Gass MLS, Pickar JH. Body mass index does not influence response to treatment, nor does body weight change with lower doses of conjugated estrogens and medroxyprogesterone acetate in younger, postmenopausal women. *Menopause* 2004;11:306-314.

Utian WH, Shoupe D, Bachmann G, Pinkerton JV, Pickar JH. Relief of vasomotor symptoms and vaginal atrophy with lower doses of conjugated equine estrogens and medroxyprogesterone acetate. *Fertil Steril* 2001; 75:1065-1079.

van Haaften M, Donker G, Sie-Go D, et al. Biochemical and histological effects of vaginal estriol and estradiol applications on the endometrium, myometrium and vagina of postmenopausal women. *Gynecol Endocrinol* 1997;11:175-185.

Varila E, Wahlström T, Rauramo I. A 5-year follow-up study on the use of levonorgestrel intrauterine system in women receiving hormone replacement therapy. *Fertil Steril* 2001;76:969-973.

Vasilakis C, Jick H, del Mar Melero-Montes M. Risk of idiopathic venous thromboembolism in users of progestagens alone. *Lancet* 1999; 354:1610-1611.

Vickers MR, MacLennan AH, Lawton B, et al. Main morbidities recorded in women's international study of long duration oestrogen after menopause (WISDOM): a randomised controlled trial of hormone replacement therapy in postmenopausal women. *BMJ* 2007;335:239.

von Schoultz E, Rutqvist LE, for the Stockholm Breast Cancer Study Group. Menopausal hormone therapy after breast cancer: the Stockholm Randomized Trial. *J Natl Cancer Inst* 2005;97:533-535.

Vooijs G, Geurts T. Review of the endometrial safety during intravaginal treatment with estriol. *Eur J Obstet Gynecol Reprod Biol* 1995;62:101-106.

Wagner TM, Moslinger RA, Muhr D, et al. BRCA1-related breast cancer in Austrian breast and ovarian cancer families: specific BRCA1 mutations and pathological characteristics. *Int J Cancer* 1998;77:354-360.

Walsh BW, Paul S, Wild RA, et al. The effects of hormone replacement therapy and raloxifene on C-reactive protein and homocysteine in healthy postmenopausal women: a randomized, controlled trial. *J Clin Endocrinol Metab* 2000;85:214-218.

Warren MP. A comparative review of the risks and benefits of hormone replacement therapy regimens. *Am J Obstet Gynecol* 2004;190:1141-1157.

Weiderpass E, Adami H-O, Baron JA, et al. Risk of endometrial cancer following estrogen replacement with and without progestins. *J Natl Cancer Inst* 1999;91:1131-1137.

Weisberg E, Ayton R, Darling G, et al. Endometrial and vaginal effects of low-dose estradiol delivered by vaginal ring or vaginal tablet. *Climacteric* 2005;8:83-92.

White VE, Bennett L, Raffin S, Emmett K, Coleman MJ. Use of unopposed estrogen in women with uteri: prevalence, clinical implications, and economic consequences. *Menopause* 2000;7:123-128.

The Women's Health Initiative Steering Committee. Effects of conjugated equine estrogen in postmenopausal women with hysterectomy: the Women's Health Initiative randomized controlled trial. *JAMA* 2004;291:1701-1712.

The Writing Group for the PEPI Trial. Effects of estrogen or estrogen/progestin regimens on heart disease risk factors in postmenopausal women. *JAMA* 1995;273:199-208.

The Writing Group for the PEPI Trial. Effects of hormone replacement therapy on endometrial biopsy in postmenopausal women. *JAMA* 1996;275:370-375.

The Writing Group for the PEPI. Effects of hormone therapy on bone mineral density: results from the postmenopausal estrogen/progestin interventions (PEPI) trial. *JAMA* 1996;276:1389-1396.

Androgen

Arlt W, Justl HG, Callies F, et al. Oral dehydroepiandrosterone for adrenal androgen replacement: pharmacokinetics and peripheral conversion to androgens and estrogens in young healthy females after dexamethasone suppression. *J Clin Endocrinol Metab* 1998;83:1928-1934.

Barrett-Connor E, Young R, Notelovitz M, et al. A two-year, double-blind comparison of estrogen-androgen and conjugated estrogens in surgically menopausal women: effects on bone mineral density, symptoms and lipid profiles. *J Reprod Med* 1999;44:1012-1020.

Barry NN, McGuire JL, van Vollenhoven RF. Dehydroepiandrosterone in systemic lupus erythematosus: relationship between dosage, serum levels, and clinical response. *J Rheumatol* 1998;25:2352-2356.

Basson R, ed. Update on sexuality at menopause and beyond: normative, adaptive, problematic, dysfunctional. *Menopause* 2004;11(pt 2 of 2):707-788.

Bell RJ, Davison SL, Paplia MA, et al. Endogenous androgen levels and cardiovascular risk profile in women across the adult life span. *Menopause* 2006;14:630-638.

Braunstein GD. Safety of testosterone treatment in postmenopausal women. *Fertil Steril* 2007;88:1-17.

Buster JE, Kingsberg S, Aguirre O, et al. Testosterone patch for low sexual desire in surgically menopausal women: a randomized trial. *Obset Gynecol* 2005;105:944-952.

Davis SR. Intervention: androgens. In: Lobo, RA, ed. *Treatment of the Postmenopausal Woman: Basic and Clinical Aspects*, 3rd ed. San Diego, CA: Academic Press, 2007:799-812.

Davis SR, Davison S, Donath S, Bell R. Circulating androgen levels and self-reported sexual function in women. *JAMA* 2005;294:91-96.

Davis SR, McCloud P, Strauss BJ, Burger H. Testosterone enhances estradiol's effects on postmenopausal bone density and sexuality. *Maturitas* 1995;21:227-236.

Davison S, Bell R, Donath S, Montalto J, Davis S. Androgen levels in adult females: changes with age, menopause, and oophorectomy. *J Clin Endocrinol Metab* 2005;90:3847-3853.

Dimitrakakis C, Jones RA, Liu A, Bondy CA. Breast cancer incidence in postmenopausal women using testosterone in addition to usual hormone therapy. *Menopause* 2004;11:531-535.

Graves G, Lea R, Bourgeois-Law G. Menopause and sexual function: Canadian consensus on menopause and osteoporosis. *J SOGC* 2001;23:849-852.

Judd HL, Lucas WE, Yen SS. Effect of oophorectomy on circulating testosterone and androstenedione levels in patients with endometrial cancer. *Am J Obstet Gynecol* 1974;118:793-798.

Laumann EO, Paik A, Rosen RC. Sexual dysfunction in the United States: prevalence and predictors. *JAMA* 1999;281:537-544.

Lobo RA. Androgens in postmenopausal women: production, possible role, and replacement options. *Obstet Gynecol Survey* 2001;56:361-376.

Morales AJ, Nolan JJ, Nelson JC, Yen SS. Effects of replacement dose of dehydroepiandrosterone in men and women of advancing age. *J Clin Endocrinol Metab* 1994;78:1360-1367.

Nathorst-Boos J, von Schoultz B. Psychological reactions and sexual life after hysterectomy with and without oophorectomy. *Gynecol Obstet Invest* 1992;4:97-101.

The North American Menopause Society. The role of testosterone therapy in postmenopausal women: position statement of the North American Menopause Society. *Menopause* 2005;12:497-511.

Raisz LG, Wiita B, Artis A, et al. Comparison of the effects of estrogen alone and estrogen plus androgen on biochemical markers of bone formation and resorption in postmenopausal women. *J Clin Endocrinol Metab* 1996;81:37-43.

Rannevik G, Jeppsson S, Johnell O, Bjerre B, Laurell-Borulf Y, Svanberg L. A longitudinal study of the perimenopausal transition: altered profiles of steroid and pituitary hormones, SHBG and bone mineral density. *Maturitas* 1995;21:103-113.

Sarrel P, Dobay B, Wiita B. Estrogen and estrogen-androgen replacement in postmenopausal women dissatisfied with estrogen-only therapy. *J Reprod Med* 1998;43:847-856.

Sherwin BB, Gelfand MM, Brender W. Androgen enhances sexual motivation in females: a prospective, crossover study of sex steroid administration in the surgical menopause. *Psychosom Med* 1985;47:339-351.

Shifren JL, Braunstein GD, Simon JA, et al. Transdermal testosterone treatment in women with impaired sexual function after oophorectomy. *N Engl J Med* 2000;343:682-688.

Shifren JL, Davis SR, Moreau M, Waldbaum A, Bouchard C, DeRogatis L, Derzko C, Bearnson P, Kakos N, O'Neill S, Levine S, Wekselman K, Buch A, Rodenberg C, Kroll R. Testosterone patch for the treatment of hypoactive sexual desire disorder in naturally menopausal women: results from the Intimate NM1 study. *Menopause* 2006;13:770-779.

Simon J, Braunstein G, Nachtigall L, et al. Testosterone patch increases sexual activity and desire in surgically menopausal women with hypoactive sexual desire disorder. *J Clin Endocrinol Metab* 2005;90:5226-5233.

Sutton-Tyrrell K, Wildman RP, Matthews KA, et al. Sex hormone-binding globulin and the free androgen index are related to cardiovascular risk factors in multiethnic premenopausal and perimenopausal women enrolled in the Study of Women Across the Nation (SWAN). *Circulation* 2006;111:1242-1249.

Tamimi RM, Hankinson SE, Chen WY, Rosner B, Colditz GA. Combined estrogen and testosterone use and risk of breast cancer in postmenopausal women. *Arch Intern Med* 2006;166:1483-1489.

Wierman ME, Basson R, Davis SR, et al. Androgen therapy in women: an Endocrine Society clinical practice guideline. *J Clin Endocrinol Metab* 2006;91:3697-3710.

Selective estrogen-receptor modulators

Barrett-Connor E, Mosca L, Collins P, et al, for the Raloxifene Use for the Heart (RUTH) Trial Investigators. Effects of raloxifene on cardiovascular events and breast cancer in postmenopausal women. *N Engl J Med* 2006;355:125-137.

Cuzick J, Forbes JF, Sestak I, et al. Long-term results of tamoxifen prophylaxis for breast cancer–96 month follow-up of the IBIS-1 trial. *J Natl Cancer Inst* 2007;99:272-282.

Gordon S, Walsh BW, Ciaccia AV, Siddhanti S, Rosen AS, Plouffe L. Transition from estrogen-progestin to raloxifene in postmenopausal women: effect on vasomotor symptoms. *Obstet Gynecol* 2004;103:267-273.

Grady D, Ettinger B, Moscarelli E, et al, for the Multiple Outcomes of Raloxifene Evaluation Investigators. Safety and adverse effects associated with raloxifene: multiple outcomes of raloxifene evaluation. *Obstet Gynecol* 2004;104:837-844.

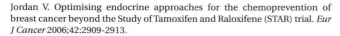

Jordan V. Optimising endocrine approaches for the chemoprevention of breast cancer beyond the Study of Tamoxifen and Raloxifene (STAR) trial. *Eur J Cancer* 2006;42:2909-2913.

Martino S, Cauley JA, Barrett-Connor B, et al, for the CORE Investigators. Continuing outcomes relevant to Evista: breast cancer incidence in postmenopausal osteoporotic women in a randomized trial of raloxifene. *J Natl Cancer Inst* 2004;96:1751-1761.

Powles TJ, Ashley S, Tidy A, Smith IE, Dowsett M. Twenty-year follow-up of the Royal Marsden randomized, double-blinded tamoxifen breast cancer prevention trial. *J Natl Cancer Inst* 2007;99:283-290.

Vogel VG, Constantino JP, Wickerham DL, et al, for the National Surgical Adjuvant Breast and Bowel Project (NSABP). Effects of tamoxifen vs raloxifene on the risk of developing invasive breast cancers and other disease outcomes: the NSABP Study of Tamoxifen and Raloxifene (STAR) P-2 Trials. *JAMA* 2006;295:2727-2741.

Over-the-counter hormones

Arendt J, Skene DJ, Middleton B, Lockley SW, Deacon S. Efficacy of melatonin treatment in jet lag, shift work, and blindness. *J Biol Rhythms* 1997;12:604-617.

Arlt W, Callies F, Allolio B. DHEA replacement in women with adrenal insufficiency; pharmacokinetics, bioconversion and clinical effects on well-being, sexuality and cognition. *Endocr Res* 2000;26:505-511.

Barnhart KT, Freeman E, Grisso JA, et al. The effect of DHEA supplementation to symptomatic perimenopausal women on serum endocrine profiles, lipid parameters, and health-related quality of life. *J Clin Endocrinol Metab* 1999;84:3896-3902.

Bellipanni G, Di Marzo F, Blasi F, Di Marzo A. Effects of melatonin in perimenopausal and menopausal women: our personal experience. *Ann N Y Acad Sci.* 2005;1057:393-402.

Blask DE, Sauer LA, Dauchy RT, et al. Melatonin inhibition of cancer growth in vivo involves suppression of tumor fatty acid metabolism via melatonin receptor-mediated signal transduction events. *Cancer Res* 1999;59:4693-4701.

Buscemi N, Vandermeer B, Hooton N, et al. Efficacy and safety of exogenous melatonin for secondary sleep disorders and sleep disorders accompanying sleep restriction: meta-analysis. *BMJ* 2006;332:385-393.

Cagnacci A, Arangino S, Renzi A, et al. Influence of melatonin administration on glucose tolerance and insulin sensitivity of postmenopausal women. *Clin Endocrinol* 2001;54:339-346.

Callies F, Fassnacht M, van Vlijmen JC, et al. Dehydroepiandrosterone replacement in women with adrenal insufficiency: effects on body composition, serum leptin, bone turnover, and exercise capacity. *J Clin Endocrinol Metab* 2001;86:1968-1972.

Casson PR, Anderson RN, Herrod HG, et al. Oral dehydroepiandrosterone in physiologic doses modulates immune function in postmenopausal women. *Am J Obstet Gynecol* 1993;169:1536-1539.

Clore NJ. Dehydroepiandrosterone and body fat. *Obes Res* 1995;3(Suppl): 613S-616S.

Diamond P, Cusan L, Gomez JL, et al. Metabolic effects of 12-month percutaneous dehydroepiandrosterone replacement therapy in postmeno-pausal women. *J Endocrinol* 1996;150:S43-S50.

Dudley SD, Buster JE. Alternative therapy: dehydroepiandrosterone for menopausal hormone replacement. In: Lobo, RA, ed. *Treatment of the Postmenopausal Woman: Basic and Clinical Aspects*, 3rd ed. San Diego, CA: Academic Press, 2007:821-828.

Garfinkel D, Loudon M, Nof D, Zisapel N. Improvement of sleep quality in elderly people by controlled-release melatonin. *Lancet* 1995;346:541-544.

Garfinkel D, Zisapel N, Wainstein J, Laudon M. Facilitation of benzodiazepine discontinuation by melatonin: a new clinical approach. *Arch Intern Med* 1999;159:2456-2460.

Hackbert L, Heiman JR. Acute dehydroepiandrosterone (DHEA) effects on sexual arousal in postmenopausal women. *J Womens Health Gend Based Med* 2002;11:155-162.

Hahm H, Kujawa J, Augsburger L. Comparison of melatonin products against USP's nutritional supplements standards and other criteria. *J Am Pharm Assoc* 1999;39:27-31.

Haimov I, Laudon M, Zisapel N, et al. Sleep disorders and melatonin rhythms in elderly people. *BMJ* 1994;309:167.

Harrod CG, Bendok BR, Hunt Batjer H. Interactions between melatonin and estrogen may regulate cerebrovascular function in women: clinical implications for the effective use of HRT during menopause and aging. *Med Hypotheses* 2005;64:725-735.

Hermann AC, Nafziger AN, Victory J, Kulawy R, Rocci ML, Jr, Bertino JS Jr. Over-the-counter progesterone cream produces significant drug exposure compared to a food and drug administration-approved oral progesterone product. *J Clin Pharmacol* 2005;4:614-619

Huppert FA, Van Niekerk JK. Dehydroepiandrosterone (DHEA) supplemen-tation for cognitive function. *Cochrane Database Syst Rev* 2007;3:CD000304.

Katz D, McHorney CA. Clinical correlates of insomnia in patients with chronic illness. *Arch Intern Med* 1998;158:1099-1107.

Khaw KT. Dehydroepiandrosterone, dehydroepiandrosterone sulfate and cardiovascular disease. *J Endocrinol* 1996;150(Suppl):S149-S153.

Labrie F, Belanger A, Cusan L, Candas B. Physiological changes in dehydro-epiandrosterone are not reflected by serum levels of active androgens and estrogens but of their metabolites: intracrinology. *J Clin Endocrinol Metab* 1997;82:2403-2409.

Labrie F, Diamond P, Cusan L, Gomez JL, Bélanger A, Candas B. Effect of 12-month dehydroepiandrosterone replacement therapy on bone, vagina, and endometrium in postmenopausal women. *J Clin Endocrinol Metab* 1997;82:3498-3505.

Labrie F, Luu-The V, Lin SX, et al. Intracrinology: role of the family of 17 beta-hydroxysteroid dehydrogenases in human physiology and disease. *J Mol Endocrinol* 2000;25:1-16.

Lamberg L. Melatonin potentially useful but safety, efficacy remain uncertain. *JAMA* 1996;276:1011-1014.

Leonetti HB, Longo S, Anasti JN. Transdermal progesterone cream for vasomotor symptoms and postmenopausal bone loss. *Obstet Gynecol* 1999;94:225-228.

Lobo RA. The future of therapy and the role of hormone therapy. In: Lobo, RA, ed. *Treatment of the Postmenopausal Woman: Basic and Clinical Aspects*, 3rd ed. San Diego, CA: Academic Press, 2007:875-880.

Lovas K, Gebre-Medhin G, Trovik TS, et al. Replacement of dehydroepi-androsterone in adrenal failure: no benefit for subjective health status and sexuality in a 9-month, randomized, parallel group clinical trial. *J Clin Endocrinol Metab* 2003;88:1112-1118.

Morales AJ, Haubrich RH, Hwang JY, et al. The effect of six months treatment with a 100 mg daily dose of dehydroepiandrosterone (DHEA) on circulating sex steroids, body composition, and muscle strength in age-advanced men and women. *Clin Endocrinol* 1998;49:421-432.

Morales AJ, Nolan JJ, Nelson JC, Yen SS. Effects of replacement dose of dehydroepiandrosterone in men and women of advancing age. *J Clin Endocrinol Metab* 1994;78:1360-1367.

Mortola JF, Yen SS. The effects of oral dehydroepiandrosterone on endocrine-metabolic parameters in postmenopausal women. *J Clin Endocrinol Metab* 1990;71:696-704.

Naguib M, Samarkandi AH. Premedication with melatonin: a double-blind, placebo-controlled comparison with midazolam. *Br J Anaesth* 1999;82:875-880.

Nair KS, Rizza RA, O'Brien P, et al. DHEA in elderly women and DHEA or testosterone in elderly men. *New Engl J Med* 2006;355:1647-1659.

The North American Menopause Society. Estrogen and progestogen use in peri- and postmenopausal women: March 2007 position statement of The North American Menopause Society *Menopause* 2007;14:168-182.

The North American Menopause Society. The role of testosterone therapy in postmenopausal women: position statement of the North American Menopause Society. *Menopause* 2005;12:497-511.

The North American Menopause Society. The role of local vaginal estrogen for treatment of vaginal atrophy in postmenopausal women: 2007 position statement of The North American Menopause Society. *Menopause* 2007; 14:357-369.

Orentreich N, Brind J, Rizer R, Vogelmen JH. Age changes and sex differences in serum dehydroepiandrosterone sulfate concentration throughout adulthood. *J Clin Endocrinol Metab* 1984;59:551-555.

Parasrampuria J, Schwartz K, Petesch R. Quality control of DHEA dietary supplement products [letter]. *JAMA* 1998;280:1565.

Parsons TD, Kratz KM, Thompson E, et al. DHEA supplementation and cognition in postmenopausal women. *Int J Neurosci* 2006;116:141-155.

Penev PD, Zee PC. Melatonin: a clinical perspective. *Ann Neurol* 1997; 42:545-553.

Reiter RJ. Melatonin and human reproduction. *Ann Intern Med* 1998; 39:103-108.

Resta O, Caratozzolo G, Pannacciulli N, et al. Gender, age and menopause effects on the prevalence and the characteristics of obstructive sleep apnea in obesity. *Eur J Clin Invest* 2003;33:1084-1089.

Rohr UD, Herold J. Melatonin deficiencies in women. *Maturitas* 2002; 41(Suppl 1):S85-S104.

Secreto G, Chiechi LM, Amadori A, et al. Soy isoflavones and melatonin for the relief of climacteric symptoms: a multicenter, double-blind, randomized study. *Maturitas* 2004;47:11-20.

Spitzer RL, Terman M, Williams JB, et al. Jet lag: clinical features, validation of a new syndrome-specific scale, and lack of response to melatonin in a randomized, double-blind trial. *Am J Psychiatry* 1999;156:1392-1396.

Stomati M, Rubino S, Spinetti A, et al. Endocrine, neuroendocrine and behavioral effects of oral dehydroepiandrosterone sulfate supplementation in postmenopausal women. *Gynecol Endocrinol* 1999;13:15-25.

Travis RC, Allen DS, Fentiman IS, Key TJ. Melatonin and breast cancer: a prospective study. *J Natl Cancer Inst* 2004;96:475-482.

Vallareal DT, Holloszy JO. Effect of DHEA on abdominal fat and insulin action in elderly women and men. *JAMA* 2004;292:2243-2248.

van der Helm-van Mil AH, van Someren EJ, van den Boom R, et al. No influence of melatonin on cerebral blood flow in humans. *J Clin Endocrinol Metab* 2003;88:5989-5994.

van Diest R. Subjective sleep characteristics as coronary risk factors: their association with type A behavior and vital exhaustion. *J Psychosom Res* 1990;34:415-426.

van Vollenhoven RF, Park JL, Genovese MC, West JP, McGuire JL. A double-blind, placebo-controlled, clinical trial of dehydroepiandrosterone in severe systemic lupus erythematosus. *Lupus* 1999;8:181-187.

Vashisht A, Wadsworth F, Carey A, Carey B, Studd J. A study to look at hormonal absorption of progesterone cream used in conjunction with transdermal estrogen. *Gynecol Endocrinol* 2005;21:101-105.

Walters JF, Hampton SM, Ferns GA, Skene DJ. Effect of menopause on melatonin and alertness rhythms investigated in constant routine conditions. *Chronobiol Int* 2005;22:859-872.

Wolf OT, Neumann O, Hellhammer DH, et al. Effects of a two-week physiological dehydroepiandrosterone substitution on cognitive performance and well-being in healthy elderly men and women. *J Clin Endocrinol Metab* 1997;82:2363-2367.

Wren BG, Champion SM, Willetts K, Manga RZ, Eden JA. Transdermal progesterone and its effect on vasomotor symptoms, blood lipid levels, bone metabolism markers, moods, and quality of life for postmenopausal women. *Menopause* 2003;10:13-18.

Wren BG, McFauland K, Edwards L, et al. Effect of sequential transdermal progesterone cream on endometrium, bleeding pattern, and plasma progesterone levels in postmenopausal women. *Climacteric* 2000;3:155-166.

Yen S, Morales A, Khorram O. Replacement of DHEA in aging men and women: potential remedial effects. *Ann NY Acad Sci* 1995;774:128-142.

Zhdanova IV, Wurtman RJ, Regan MM, Taylor JA, Shi JP, Leclair OU. Melatonin treatment for age-related insomnia. *J Clin Endocrinol Metab* 2001;86:4727-4730.

Zimmerman RC, Olcese JM. Melatonin. In: Lobo, RA, ed. *Treatment of the Postmenopausal Woman: Basic and Clinical Aspects*, 3rd ed. San Diego, CA: Academic Press, 2007:829-836.

This section of the textbook discusses the major nonprescription therapies considered by women at menopause and beyond, including vitamins and minerals, other nonbotanical dietary supplements available over the counter (OTC), vaginal lubricants and moisturizers, and topical agents used for sexual pleasure. Botanical supplements are discussed in Section I.

NAMS recommends use of some of these nonprescription therapies, when indicated, with appropriate oversight from a healthcare provider. However, the public frequently self-medicates with little guidance or knowledge of the efficacy and safety of the products they use. Few OTC therapies have patient package inserts (user information sheets that explain the evidence for the claimed efficacy and safety of the product). This document, required by the US Food and Drug Administration (FDA) for all marketed prescription medications, provides vital information on how to take a drug safely, identify its negative side effects, and avoid potentially dangerous interactions with other drugs.

Safety may not be mentioned at all in a nonprescription product's advertising or label, although the word "natural" is often seen, and is often misinterpreted by the public as being without risk of adverse effects. In addition, dietary supplements—a common type of OTC therapy—are government regulated in the United States and Canada differently from prescription drugs with regard to allowed health claims, causing confusion among the public and sometimes healthcare providers as well. Thus, OTC therapies present challenges to the menopausal woman and her healthcare providers.

> NAMS understands that nonprescription therapies have not been proven to be as effective as prescription therapies when treating certain health conditions. Yet, since the basic tenet of the Hippocratic Oath is to do no harm and nonpharmacologic treatments typically do little harm, NAMS often suggests nonpharmacologic treatments as "first-line" treatments as they have the least risk.

Government regulations for dietary supplements

This section of the textbook presents the current government regulations for dietary supplements in the United States and Canada—essential information for both the healthcare provider and the public.

Terminology. In the United States, the term *dietary supplement* includes OTC vitamins, minerals, amino acids, enzymes, herbs, plants in various forms (such as extracts), and combinations intended for ingestion as an addition to the diet. In the United States, according to the 1994 Dietary Supplement Health and Education Act (DSHEA), a dietary supplement is defined as a pill, capsule, tablet, or liquid that contains a "dietary ingredient." However, other products that are not ingested also fall within the dietary supplement guidelines (eg, topical progesterone cream).

In Canada, the term *natural health product* (NHP) is used in place of dietary supplement as defined by the Natural Health Products Regulations, which came into effect in 2004. NHPs include vitamins and minerals, probiotics, and other products such as amino acids and essential fatty acids. Also classified as NHPs are herbal products, homeopathic medicines, and traditional medicines such as Traditional Chinese Medicine (see Section I for more about complementary and alternative medicine [CAM] therapies).

United States. In the United States, government regulations regarding whether a dietary supplement is effective and safe are less strict than those for prescription drugs. Under the DSHEA, the manufacturer (not the FDA) is responsible for determining that any representations or claims made about its products are substantiated by adequate evidence to show that they are not false or misleading. Dietary supplement marketers can make health claims for so-called "natural conditions" (eg, hot flashes, age-related memory loss) without providing documentation for efficacy and safety to the government. However, they cannot claim that a product prevents, treats, or cures a disease (eg, prevents heart attacks or osteoporosis, cures depression) unless the FDA approves the claim.

DSHEA further states that the manufacturer (not the FDA) is responsible for ensuring that labels on packages of dietary supplements are truthful and not misleading, that they contain enough information for consumers to make an informed choice, that the serving size ("dose") is appropriate, and that all the dietary ingredients in the product are accurately listed.

Demonstrating safety is not required before a dietary supplement is approved for sale. Under DSHEA, dietary supplement manufacturers are responsible for substantiating the safety of the ingredients used in a product. The FDA is responsible for taking action against any unsafe dietary supplement product after it reaches the market. This regulatory agency accomplishes its responsibilities through monitoring safety literature, dietary supplement adverse-event reports, and product information.

Although many manufacturers have rigorous quality control measures in place, many products are not monitored for purity or level of active ingredient. As a result, strength and quality can be unpredictable. If a product is suspected of causing harm, the FDA can halt sales and have it analyzed.

Botanicals (eg, soy, isoflavones, black cohosh) are classified by the FDA as a food, drug, or dietary supplement (see Section I for more about CAM therapies). There are numerous quality control concerns with some botanicals, including misidentification, "underlabeling" (ie, including prescription drugs in OTC products), adulteration, substitution, and contamination. In addition, analytic-method standards are lacking for many products, leading to difficulty when attempting to assess product quality.

Marketers use different methods to determine the levels of "active ingredient" in their products.

To address these concerns, the FDA established a rule, effective August 24, 2007, for good manufacturing practices for dietary supplements. This rule will help ensure that these products are produced in a quality manner, do not contain contaminants or impurities, and are accurately labeled. Manufacturers are required to evaluate the identity, purity, strength, and composition of their dietary supplements. The rule has a 3-year phase-in, with the largest companies having until June 2008 to comply with the regulations; the smallest companies have until June 2010. In addition, by the end of 2007, manufacturers will be required to report all serious adverse events to the FDA.

In the United States, products designated "USP" (*United States Pharmacopeia*) or "NSF" (National Sanitation Foundation) are generally reliable indicators of good quality control. It is also preferable to choose specific brands that have been used in clinical trials.

Canada. In Canada, it is the role of the Natural Health Products Directorate to ensure access to safe, effective, high-quality NHPs. The experience has been similar to that in the United States, with most of the responsibility placed on the government to prove that products were unsafe or ineffective. The Canadian regulations, released in 2004 and being implemented in stages until 2010, require that all NHPs have a product license before they can be sold in Canada.

All licensed NHPs in Canada display a product identification number preceded by the prefix "NPN" (or "DIN-HM" for homeopathic medicine) assigned once the product is authorized for sale. All manufacturers, packagers, labelers, and importers are required to obtain site licensing and practice product safety and quality. Standard labeling requirements ensure that customers can make informed choices. An adverse-reaction reporting system is assisting in issuing advisories to the public.

Until the transition is complete, Canadian consumers are advised to purchase products displaying a "DIN" (drug identification number) or "NPN" on their labels, which indicates that the product has undergone and passed a review of its formulation, labeling, and instructions for use. A list of licensed natural health products in Canada is available at http://www.hc-sc.gc.ca.

Vitamins and minerals

The human body requires more than 45 vitamins and minerals to maintain health. Often, the daily diet does not contain all the nutrients required for optimal health. Every woman may benefit from a good-quality, daily multivitamin and mineral supplement. This textbook will provide a brief overview of the nutrients of most interest to women in midlife and beyond.

As stated in the *2005 Dietary Guidelines for Americans*, nutrient needs should be met primarily through consuming foods or nutrient-fortified foods. Dietary supplements, while recommended in some cases, cannot replace a healthful diet.

Daily recommended dietary intakes. Since 1994, the National Academy of Sciences in the United States and Health Canada have collaborated in the revision of the dietary reference standards known as *Dietary Reference Intakes (DRIs)*. This provides a set of four nutrient-based reference values designed to replace the Recommended Dietary Allowances in the United States and the Recommended Nutrient Intakes in Canada. The DRIs include recommended intakes for individuals, estimated average requirements, adequate intakes, and tolerable upper intake levels (ULs). Table 1 lists selected recommended intakes and ULs for women aged 51 to 70 years and 19 to 70 years, respectively.

Table 1. Selected dietary reference intake recommendations for women

Nutrient	Recommended dietary reference intakes (for women 51-70 y)	Tolerable upper intake levels (for women 19-70 y)
- Vitamins		
Vitamin A	700 µg (2,330 IU)	3,000 µg (10,000 IU)
Vitamin C	—	2,000 mg
— nonsmokers	75 mg	—
— smokers	110 mg	—
Vitamin D	—	50 µg (2,000 IU)
— age 51-69	10 µg (400 IU)	—
— age 70+	15 µg (600 IU)	—
Vitamin E (α-tocopherol)	15 mg (22 IU)	1,000 mg (1,500 IU)
Folate	400 µg	1,000 mg
Vitamin B_6 (pyridoxine)	1.5 mg	100 mg
Vitamin B_{12}	2.4 µg	No UL established
Minerals		
Calcium	1,200 mg	2,500 mg
Magnesium	320 mg	350 mg
Phosphorus	700 mg	4,000 mg

Source: National Academy of Sciences 2004.

Vitamins. A balanced diet low in saturated fat and high in whole grains, fruits, and vegetables, with adequate water, vitamins, and minerals, contributes to good health. Vitamins are any of various organic substances essential in small quantities to the nutrition of most animals and some plants. They act especially as coenzymes and precursors of coenzymes in the regulation of metabolic processes but do not provide energy or serve as building units. They are present in natural foodstuffs or sometimes are produced within the body. The DRIs provided in this section are for women aged 51 to 70 years.

Vitamin A. Vitamin A is necessary for the health of skin, mucous membranes, retinal function, and immune function. Vitamin A deficiency is associated with significant eye problems, including night blindness and conjunctival dryness.

The DRI for vitamin A is 700 µg (2,330 IU). Recommended intake may be increased in malabsorption syndromes associated with pancreatic insufficiency or in any condition in which fat malabsorption occurs, including diets that drastically restrict fat-containing foods. Absorption requires the presence of bile salts, pancreatic lipase, protein, and dietary fat. Requirements for vitamin A may also be increased in those receiving cholestyramine, colestipol, mineral oil, and neomycin.

Food sources include organ meats, sweet potato, pumpkin, carrots, spinach, collards, kale, turnip greens, egg yolk, milk, cheese, and butter.

As a fat-soluble vitamin, oversupplementation can cause buildup, with potential for toxic effects. Prolonged high doses may cause bleeding from the gums, dry or sore mouth, or drying, cracking, or peeling of the lips. Excessive intake (>10,000 IU/d) may stimulate bone loss and counteract the effects of calcium supplements and can cause hypercalcemia, hair loss, and hepatotoxicity.

B vitamins. B_1 (thiamin), B_2 (riboflavin), B_3 (niacin), B_5 (pantothenic acid), B_6 (pyridoxine), B_9 (folic acid), and B_{12} (cyanocobalamine) are water-soluble vitamins. B vitamin supplements are available either in combination or individually.

Simple nutritional deficiency of any one of the B vitamins is rare, since inadequate nutritional intake usually results in multiple deficiencies. Supplementation may be necessary in malnutrition because of inadequate dietary intake or in those undergoing rapid weight loss. B vitamins may be supplemented after bariatric surgery.

- *Vitamin B_1 (thiamin)* is a coenzyme in the metabolism of carbohydrates and branched-chain amino acids.

  Food sources include whole grain products, fortified cereals, legumes, pork, beef, yeast, and fresh vegetables. The DRI for thiamin is 1.1 mg. Increased doses may be needed with hemodialysis and in persons with malabsorption syndromes. There is no known toxicity.

- *Vitamin B_2 (riboflavin)* is a coenzyme in numerous reactions that are necessary for normal tissue respiration. It is also needed for activation of pyridoxine and for conversion of tryptophan to niacin. Absorption may be decreased when probenecid is used.

  Food sources are organ meats, milk, whole grain breads, and fortified cereals. The DRI for riboflavin is 1.1 mg for women. Excess riboflavin can cause the urine to turn bright yellow. There is no known toxicity.

- *Vitamin B_3 (niacin, niacinamide).* Niacin, after conversion to niacinamide, is a component of coenzymes necessary for tissue respiration, glycogenolysis, and lipid, amino acid, protein, and purine metabolism.

  Niacin (but not niacinamide) is used in the treatment of hyperlipidemia. It improves all major lipid parameters, reducing low-density lipoprotein (LDL) cholesterol and triglycerides and increasing high-density lipoprotein (HDL) cholesterol. In a meta-analysis of five trials involving 432 patients, the difference in LDL and triglyceride reduction in women was greater than in men at all doses.

  Food sources of vitamin B_3 include meat, fish, poultry, enriched and whole-grain breads, and fortified cereals. The DRI for niacin for women is 14 mg.

  Adverse effects include flushing, itching, and gastrointestinal (GI) discomfort. These are more commonly experienced when therapeutic rather than nutritional doses are taken, especially when beginning therapy. Niacin should be taken with the evening meal. Flushing may be minimized by taking aspirin 1 hour earlier, by increasing the niacin dose gradually, or by using the extended-release form.

- *Vitamin B_6 (pyridoxine)* acts as a coenzyme for various metabolic functions affecting protein, carbohydrate, and lipid utilization. It is involved in the conversion of tryptophan to niacin or serotonin and of glycogen to glucose, in the synthesis of γ-aminobutyric acid within the central nervous system, and in red blood cell synthesis.

  Food sources of pyridoxine are whole grains, fortified cereals, and organ meats. Pyridoxine supplements have been used to treat a variety of conditions (eg, premenstrual syndrome, depression, carpal tunnel syndrome, and diabetic neuropathy) with varied results.

  The DRI for pyridoxine is 1.5 mg. Recommended intakes may be increased if a woman is taking any of the following medications: cycloserine, hydralazine, immunosuppressants, isoniazid, or estrogen-containing contraceptives. Increased intake is typically not required with standard doses of menopausal hormone therapy. Although it is generally nontoxic, high doses of pyridoxine (2-6 g/d) taken for several months have caused severe sensory neuropathy with residual weakness.

- *Vitamin B_9 (folate, folic acid)* is converted in the liver and plasma into its metabolically active form, tetrafolic acid, in the presence of ascorbic acid. This vitamin is necessary for normal erythropoiesis, synthesis, and metabolism of various amino acids, and for other metabolic processes.

Deficiency may produce megaloblastic and macrocytic anemias.

Folate occurs naturally in food; dietary sources include dark green leafy vegetables, whole-grain breads, and fortified cereals. Folic acid is the synthetic form of folate that is found in supplements and added to fortified foods. Folic acid is almost completely absorbed, primarily in the upper duodenum, but absorption is impaired in malabsorption syndromes.

Folic acid supplements are routinely recommended preconception and during pregnancy, as this nutrient reduces the incidence of neural tube defects in the newborn.

The DRI for this vitamin is 400 µg. Requirements may be increased in those receiving estrogen-containing contraceptives. No side effects other than allergic reactions have been reported with folic acid administration, even at doses up to ten times the DRI for a month. Higher doses than the DRI are generally not recommended until the diagnosis of pernicious anemia has been ruled out, because they correct the hematologic manifestations of pernicious anemia while allowing neurologic damage to progress irreversibly.

- *Vitamin B_{12} (cyanocobalamin)* acts as a coenzyme for various metabolic functions. It is necessary for growth, hematopoiesis, and myelin synthesis. Dietary B_{12} is released from the proteins to which it is bound by gastric acid and pancreatic proteases, then bound to intrinsic factor and absorbed from the lower half of the ileum.

Deficiency may lead to macrocytic, megaloblastic anemia and possible irreversible neurologic damage (with pernicious anemia caused by either lack of or inhibition of intrinsic factor).

Food sources are fish, seafood, egg yolk, milk, and fermented cheeses. Bacteria found on vegetables may be a source of B_{12} for strict vegetarians (vegans). Ordinary cooking temperatures will not cause loss of B_{12} from foods, but severe heating should be avoided to maintain B_{12} levels.

Deficiency may be the result of inadequate nutrition or intestinal malabsorption. It can occur in vegans, since vitamin B_{12} is found in animal protein and not in vegetables. Additional causes of deficiency are alcoholism, gastritis with achlorhydria, lack of intrinsic factor, and gastrectomy.

The oral route is useful for treating nutritional B_{12} deficiency when absorption is normal, but it is not useful in small-bowel disease, in malabsorption syndromes, or after total gastrectomy or ileal resection. For treating deficiency resulting from lack of absorption, vitamin B_{12} is given by injection (either intramuscularly or deep subcutaneously). It is also available in a sublingual dosage form. B_{12} plasma concentration determination is recommended before treatment of deficiency and between the 5th and 7th day of therapy.

The DRI for B_{12} is 2.4 µg. Recommended intakes may be increased by medications, including colchicine, erythropoietin, and metformin. Toxicity is not a problem, although hypokalemia is possible during the first 48 hours of treatment for megaloblastic anemia. B_{12} administration may mask folic acid deficiency.

Vitamin C (ascorbic acid). Ascorbic acid, a water-soluble vitamin, is needed for collagen formation and tissue repair as well as metabolism of folic acid, iron, phenylalanine, tyrosine, norepinephrine, and histamine; utilization of carbohydrates; synthesis of lipids and proteins; immune function; hydroxylation of serotonin; and preservation of blood vessel integrity. Ascorbic acid enhances absorption of nonheme iron. It is absorbed from the jejunum.

Dietary sources include citrus fruits, green vegetables (peppers, broccoli, cabbage), tomatoes, and potatoes. Vitamin C supplements gradually lose potency with storage and in foods the nutrient is rapidly destroyed by exposure to air, by drying or salting, and up to 50% in ordinary cooking.

The DRI is 75 mg. Requirements may be increased in acquired immunodeficiency syndrome, gastrectomy, ileal resection, surgery, and tuberculosis, and in individuals who are heavy smokers.

Toxicity can occur in individuals with a history of oxalate-containing renal stones. High-dose ascorbic acid (but not sodium ascorbate) may decrease urine pH, causing renal tubular reabsorption of oxalate with the possibility of precipitation of oxalate stones in the urinary tract. High doses may cause diarrhea. Withdrawal scurvy may occur after prolonged administration of 2 to 3 g/day.

Vitamin D. Vitamin D is a sterol-like compound synthesized in nature by interaction between 7-dehydrocholesterol and ultraviolet (UAB) light which, by a photochemical reaction, opens up the B ring of the steroid nucleus. Typically, this synthesis takes place in the skin of many animals, including humans. This compound—also called *vitamin D_3* or *cholecalciferol*—is biologically inactive.

After cutaneous synthesis, cholecalciferol is absorbed into the bloodstream where it is transported to the liver and rapidly hydroxylated at the 25 position to produce 25-hydroxycholecalciferol [25(OH)D], commonly considered to be inactive as well, although this issue is not completely resolved. The 25(OH)D is measurable in serum, and as such it serves as the functional indicator for vitamin D status and probably also as the principal storage form of the vitamin in the body.

The final step in the activation of the molecule is further hydroxylation at the 1 position of the A-ring to produce

1,25-dihydroxycholecalciferol or calcitriol. Calcitriol is one of the most potent biological molecules known, working at submicrogram levels. It has been recognized for some years that the calcitriol circulating in the blood is synthesized in the kidney in response to fibroblast growth factor 23, parathyroid hormone (PTH), and hypophosphatemia. Secreted calcitriol goes to the intestinal mucosa, where it induces the synthesis of a calcium transport protein in the mucosal cell which mediates the active absorption of calcium from food into the bloodstream.

Also included as vitamin D is a similar compound, ergocalciferol or vitamin D_2, which, in experimental animals, has an ability to prevent rickets roughly similar to that of cholecalciferol. Ergocalciferol is produced synthetically by irradiation of a product of ergot mold.

Both forms of vitamin D (D_2 and D_3) are measured in International Units (IUs), with 1 µg of cholecalciferol being equivalent to 40 IU. Until recently, these forms had been considered to be equipotent, but it is now clear that vitamin D_3 is substantially more potent than vitamin D_2 by a factor of at least 4.

Vitamin D is essential for the efficient intestinal absorption of calcium and thus for bone health. In women with a severe vitamin D deficiency, gross absorption of dietary calcium is no more than 10%. Calcium absorption efficiency varies inversely with serum 25(OH)D up to levels of about 80 nmol/L (32 ng/mL), above which further increases in vitamin D status produce no further improvement in absorption efficiency. Similarly, in a population-based study of the National Health and Nutrition Examination Survey III data, both bone mineral density (BMD) and lower-extremity neuromuscular function improved as vitamin D status improved up to levels above 80 nmol/L (32 ng/mL). However, such a small fraction of the population has values above 80 nmol/mL that it is not clear from the available data whether a plateau is reached; it is possible that even higher values for serum 25(OH)D may be needed to optimize bone and neuromuscular health.

Studies have found that vitamin D (≥700 IU/d) with supplemental calcium can reduce the rate of postmeno-pausal bone loss, especially in older women. More recent results from the Women's Health Initiative randomized controlled trial (RCT) found that participants taking calcium (1,000 mg/d) plus vitamin D (400 IU/d) had a small but significant 1% improvement in hip BMD. Vitamin D supplementation also has been found to improve muscle strength and balance, and to reduce the risk of falling. A meta-analysis of RCTs in postmenopausal women (mean ages, 71-85 y) found that a vitamin D dosage of 700 to 800 IU/day was associated with significant reductions in the risk of both hip and nonverteberal fractures. No significant changes were found in outcomes for either of those fracture sites in trials that used only 400 IU/day. (See Section E, page 113, for more about osteoporosis.)

It has recently become clear that the 1-α-hydroxylation step occurs, not solely in the kidney but in many other tissues as well, and that the calcitriol synthesized in those tissues serves an autocrine function, ie, it acts (and is degraded) locally in the cells and tissues concerned. It links extra-cellular stimuli to transcription of the genetic code for the synthesis for a variety of cell-specific products. In the intestinal mucosa, as previously noted, the product concerned is a calcium transport protein, but in many other tissues where calcitriol binding occurs, the proteins concerned are related primarily to cell differentiation, cell proliferation, cell apoptosis, and various aspects of the immune response.

Most clinicians do not measure vitamin D nutritional status, but it can be evaluated by measuring serum 25(OH)D. Some uncertainty remains with respect to the level of serum 25(OH)D that signifies the bottom end of the healthy range, but it is clear that the published laboratory reference ranges are not coextensive with the healthy range. There is a near-consensus that the bottom end of that healthy range is at least as high as 75 to 80 nmol/L (30-32 ng/mL), and some of the cancer and autoimmune studies suggest that the bottom end of the healthy range may be as high as 100 to 125 nmol/L (40-50 ng/mL). Measurement of calcitriol levels is not usually helpful for diagnostic purposes, as calcitriol has a very short half-life in the blood and it reflects effective calcium intake status rather than vitamin D status. Calcitriol will normally be high on a low calcium intake, and normally low on a high calcium intake.

Total metabolic consumption of vitamin D at a serum 25(OH)D level of 80 nmol/L (32 ng/mL) is approximately 4,000 IU (100 µg)/day. It is difficult to establish a true intake requirement, since most of the vitamin D that individuals use every day probably comes by way of cutaneous synthesis within their own bodies. This source varies by degree of skin exposure to the sun, the time of day at which such exposure occurs, the latitude at which one lives, the age of the person concerned, and the skin pigmentation. Thus, urban blacks at midlatitudes and above are at a substantial disadvantage. In all studies published to date, they have values for serum 25(OH)D substantially lower than those of light-skinned individuals, and as a group they must be considered to be vitamin D deficient.

For the typical US Caucasian individual living in the Northeast, sunlight exposure of 5 to 15 minutes on the arms and legs between the hours of 10 am and 3 pm two to three times a week may be adequate. Women with dark-colored skin may require as much as 5 to 10 times longer skin exposure because their darker skin pigment markedly reduces vitamin D production from sunlight. Wearing a sunscreen with a sun protection factor of 8 or more blocks the skin's ability to produce vitamin D by 95%.

The recommended adequate dietary intake for vitamin D is 400 IU/day for women aged 51 to 70 years and 600

IU/day for women older than age 70. New (2007) guidelines from the National Osteoporosis Foundation recommend 800 to 1,000 IU/day of vitamin D_3 for adults age 50 and over. Doses as high as 2,000 IU/day are safe. In Canada, the recommended vitamin D intake for women under 50 years is 400 IU/day and 800 IU/day for women over age 50. In the absence of sunlight, most experts agree that at least 800 IU and preferably 1,000 IU/day of vitamin D is needed to maintain a healthy serum level of 25(OH)D of at least 30 ng/mL. In Canada, vitamin D synthesis in the skin is absent during the winter months of October to March, and thus for part of the year, Canadians must rely on dietary sources of vitamin D.

The actual requirement for additional oral intake, therefore, will vary from person to person, although it will be similar within the various different ages and ethnic groups. The goal must be to provide enough of a regular input of vitamin D to ensure maintenance of a serum 25(OH)D level of 80 nmol (32 ng/mL) or higher. As a rough guide, the serum 25(OH)D level, under steady-state dosing, will rise by about 1 nmol/L per µg cholecalciferol/day. Thus, an individual with a serum 25(OH)D value of 50 nmol/L (20 ng/mL) will typically need at least 30 µg of additional vitamin D_3/day (1,200 IU) to reach a level of 80 nmol/L (32 ng/mL)—or, to use the units commonly reported in the United States, serum 25(OH)D will rise by about 1 ng/mL for every 100 IU/day of additional cholecalciferol.

Various studies have shown that 60% to nearly 100% of individuals—whether institutionalized or free-living, or whether using vitamin D supplements or not—have serum 25(OH)D values below 80 nmol/L (32 ng/mL). Vitamin D insufficiency is nearly universal among individuals over age 90.

The current UL is 2,000 IU/day, according to a report of the Food and Nutrition Board in 1997. Experts consider this level very conservative, as a 1999 analysis of the toxicity data by Vieth et al and a subsequent 2007 study by Hatchcock et al found no concerns at regular intakes below 40,000 IU/day, concluding that 10,000 IU/day is safe for essentially all the adult population. Although there are no reasons to use as much as 10,000 IU/day on a regular basis, it is useful to know that such a dose is safe.

The principal source of vitamin D is cutaneous synthesis. Curiously, although low latitudes are associated with a greater UVB irradiance, the prevalence of vitamin D insufficiency is no different in the southern tier of US states than in the northern, possibly because there is more sun avoidance in Southern states.

A few food sources are available—primarily oily fish (eg, salmon). But only wild-caught fish (deriving their vitamin D from ingested phytoplankton) are good sources; farm-raised fish have far less vitamin D. Fish liver oil has long been the classical source of vitamin D, and years ago cod and halibut liver oils were used as mainstays in the prevention of rickets in children. For decades, milk has been fortified with a small amount of vitamin D (100 IU per 8-oz serving), and more recently some orange juices have been fortified to the same level. Small amounts of vitamin D have been added to certain ready-to-eat cereals.

Current daily requirements can usually be met with an oral multivitamin supplement (typically containing 400 IU vitamin D) plus moderate sun exposure. However, older women (>65 y) who have little or no sun exposure and rely on diet alone for vitamin D intake will have suboptimal 25(OH)D levels. Because vitamin D must be metabolized before it is biologically active, taking vitamin D at the same time as a calcium supplement is not necessary. However, some calcium supplements contain vitamin D, providing the convenience of obtaining adequate levels of both nutrients.

The principal high-potency form of the vitamin available to clinicians was once 50,000 IU of vitamin D_2, as an oral prescription product. Now there are several OTC products containing 1,000 to 10,000 IU vitamin D_3 per dose, allowing consumers to obtain the vitamin D they need.

With both fortified foods and supplements, reading the labels is important. Until recently, vitamins D_2 and D_3 were thought to be equally potent, and manufacturers were free to choose either form of the vitamin. D_3 is much more effective for treating vitamin D deficiency.

Vitamin E (α-tocopherol). This fat-soluble vitamin acts in conjunction with selenium as an antioxidant, protecting polyunsaturated fatty acids in various cell structures and protecting red blood cells from hemolysis. Deficiency of this vitamin is rare.

Food sources include nuts, seeds, whole grains, vegetable oil, and wheat germ. The DRI for vitamin E is 15 mg. High dietary intake of polyunsaturated fatty acids may increase this requirement.

The National Institutes of Health recommends basing the DRI on the α-tocopherol form of vitamin E because it is the most active, usable form. The expression of vitamin E activity has been changed from IUs to α-tocopherol equivalents, with 1.5 IU equal to 1 mg α-tocopherol-equivalent.

According to the 2004 NAMS position statement on the management of vasomotor symptoms, clinical trial results are insufficient to either support or refute efficacy for vitamin E in treating hot flashes; however, no serious side effects have been associated with short-term use and the paper thus concluded that oral vitamin E (400-800 IU/d) is an option to recommend. (See Section C, page 35, for more about vasomotor symptoms.)

Vitamin E oil, used topically, may be helpful for relieving vulvovaginal itching and irritation as well as for providing vaginal lubrication to ease penetration during intercourse.

(See Section C, page 51, for more about vulvovaginal symptoms.)

High antioxidant intake from food and supplement sources of vitamin E, vitamin C, and carotene has been associated with delaying cognitive decline in the elderly. However, the association of low serum vitamin E with cognition merits further exploration. (See Section C, page 45, for more about cognition.)

Among healthy adults, no acute adverse effects have been noted with vitamin E use at doses of up to 1,200 IU/day. However, a meta-analysis of 19 trials among patients with chronic diseases found a statistically significant relationship between high-dosage (defined as ≥400 IU/d) vitamin E and all-cause mortality, although the trials were often small. The authors commented that whether these findings should be generalized to healthy adults is uncertain.

General guidelines caution that vitamin E doses over 400 IU/day are to be avoided in people taking warfarin and related anticoagulants because of its interference with platelet function, which can have an additive effect, decreasing blood clotting (see Box below). However, this was questioned in the NAMS 2004 vasomotor symptoms position statement, which pointed out that the perception that vitamin E increases bleeding risk may result from the fact that individuals with vitamin K deficiency may experience increased bleeding with high doses of vitamin E. A generalized increase in bleeding risk has not been observed in studies designed to assess bleeding risk, even with vitamin E dosages up to 1,200 IU/day for 1 month in individuals on chronic warfarin doses.

Precautions when using OTC anticoagulant therapies

- Use is contraindicated in individuals with active bleeding (eg, abnormal uterine bleeding, peptic ulcer, intracranial bleeding) or a history of bleeding (hemostatic disorders), drug-related hemostatic problems, and in those taking prescription anticoagulant medications (eg, warfarin [Coumadin], or antiplatelet agents, such as ticlopidine, clopidogrel, dipyridamole).

- Caution is advised when using more than one OTC anticoagulant therapy, including aspirin (including low-dose aspirin for cardiovascular benefits), aspirin-containing products, nonsteroidal anti-inflammatory drugs (NSAIDs), vitamin E, fish oil, dong quai, evening primrose oil, feverfew, garlic, ginger, and *Ginkgo biloba*).

- Use should be discontinued 7 to 10 days before dental or surgical procedures; use can usually be resumed after discharge.

Vitamin K. Supplementation with vitamin K (1 mg/d) seems to be associated with beneficial effects on bone turnover and BMD. Taking vitamin K as part of a daily multivitamin supplement may contribute to reducing postmenopausal bone loss, especially in the hip, but further validation is needed to define its contribution. Vitamin K supplements are contraindicated in women taking warfarin. The DRI for vitamin K is 90 μg.

Antioxidant vitamins and prevention of cardiovascular disease or cancer. The antioxidants vitamin E, vitamin C, and beta-carotene (a form of vitamin A) have been examined in regard to their effects on markers of cardiovascular disease (CVD) as well as for primary prevention and effects on existing CVD and cancer. The following trials found no role for either of these effects.

- *Homocysteine Studies Collaboration.* There has been a continuing debate regarding the relation between homocysteine concentrations and CVD and whether treatments that decrease homocysteine concentration affect disease outcomes. This meta-analysis of prospective and retrospective studies examined homocysteine and vascular disease risk in ischemic heart disease and stroke. Homocysteine blood concentrations were more strongly associated with outcome variables in retrospective studies of patients with CVD than in prospective studies of patients with no history of disease. The authors suggested that elevated homocysteine may be a modest independent predictor of ischemic heart disease and stroke risk. However, the patient population at risk needs to be determined. Of note, those with the most relevant, highly elevated homocysteine concentration seem to be a very small portion of the population.

- *Vitamin Intervention for Stroke Prevention.* This RCT conducted over 2 years examined the effect of higher compared with lower doses of folic acid, pyridoxine, and cobalamine to reduce the risk of events in 3,680 patients with nondisabling cerebral infarction. No significant difference between the two groups was found for either primary or secondary outcome measurements.

- *Heart Outcomes Prevention Evaluation (HOPE).* The HOPE study examined vitamin E supplementation and cardiovascular events in high-risk patients. This was based on the belief that oxidation of the LDL molecule is important in the development and progression of atherosclerosis; thus, antioxidants might be useful in the treatment of CVD. It was a double-blind study of secondary prevention, with more than 4,000 patients in each of the vitamin E and placebo groups over 4.5 years. Patients were age 55 years or older and were at high risk for cardiovascular events, from either CVD or diabetes mellitus (DM). The study compared vitamin E, 400 IU/day, or placebo and either an angiotensin-converting enzyme inhibitor or placebo. The study demonstrated that vitamin E had no apparent benefit in patients at high risk for cardiac events.

- *Heart Protection Study Collaborative Group.* In a second study in a large group of patients that mirrored the HOPE trial, 20,536 patients at risk for cardiovascular events were randomized to receive antioxidant vitamin supplementation with vitamin E, vitamin C, and beta-carotene or placebo. Outcomes examined were major coronary events. Antioxidant levels were monitored. The daily antioxidant regimen had no benefit, on the basis of the outcome parameters measured over 5 years. This study addressed whether combined antioxidant therapy would be beneficial compared with single-antioxidant therapy.

- *Massachusetts Women's Health Study.* This study evaluated vitamin E taken long term in the primary prevention of CVD and cancer. A total of 39,876 women were randomized to receive either 600 IU vitamin E or placebo, and 100 mg aspirin or placebo every other day. The average follow-up was 10.1 years. Results demonstrated a nonsignificant 7% risk reduction for nonfatal myocardial infarction (MI), nonfatal stroke, or cardiovascular death. No difference was seen in total mortality. No significant difference between groups was noted regarding frequency of cancer.

- *HOPE-TOO.* In this extension of the HOPE trial, effects of long-term vitamin E supplementation on cardiovascular events and cancer were examined. Study patients were age 55 and older and had a history of coronary or peripheral arterial disease, stroke, or DM, plus one other cardiovascular risk factor. Patients were randomized to receive either 400 IU/day vitamin E or placebo, and median follow-up was 7 years. Results demonstrated no significant difference in the primary outcomes of MI, stroke, or cardiovascular death. However, the patients receiving vitamin E had a higher risk of heart failure. Vitamin E had no effect on occurrence of cancer.

Minerals. Trace elements and metals in biologic fluids are essential nutrients for humans. They act as "biochemical triggers," some forming complexes with enzymes and helping in the binding of biologic ligands. Some of the major minerals are discussed here.

Calcium. This divalent, cationic element is the fifth most abundant element on earth, present in pearls and marble, ivory and antlers, corals and bone. Calcium is also the most abundant mineral in the human body. An adult human body contains 1,000 to 1,200 g calcium, 99% of which is in bones and teeth. As an element, calcium can neither be synthesized nor degraded as it moves through the processes of cellular and organ-level metabolism.

Calcium requirements for skeletal maintenance fluctuate throughout a woman's life. During the teen years, calcium requirements are high because of the demands of a rapidly growing skeleton. During a woman's reproductive years, less calcium is required for bone health as bone turnover stabilizes (ie, bone formation and resorption rates become balanced) and peak adult bone mass is achieved and maintained.

Calcium requirements remain stable until menopause when the bone resorption rate increases because of the decrease in ovarian estrogen production. Calcium needs rise at that time because of decreased efficiency in the utilization of dietary calcium, which is owing, in large part, to estrogen-related shifts in intestinal calcium absorption and renal conservation.

The amount of calcium needed is also affected by the decrease in intestinal absorption that occurs with age. Gross calcium absorption averages 20% to 30%, with transient increases during adolescent growth spurts and pregnancy. By age 65, calcium absorption efficiency is typically 50% below adolescent peak absorption.

One factor that may limit calcium absorption is a lack of vitamin D resulting from age-related declines in several functions, including ingestion, cutaneous synthesis of the parent vitamin, renal synthesis of the active form of the vitamin (1,25-dihydroxyvitamin D [25(OH)D]), and intestinal responsiveness. Dietary factors limiting calcium absorption include consumption of oxalic acid (found in spinach, rhubarb, and some other green vegetables), large amounts of grains that contain phytates (eg, wheat bran, soy protein isolates), and, possibly, tannins (found in tea). Evidence indicates that other dietary components, such as fat, phosphorus, magnesium, and caffeine, have negligible effects on calcium absorption at generally applicable intake levels.

In RCTs, calcium plus vitamin D has been shown to reduce or halt bone loss in healthy postmenopausal women and in postmenopausal women with substantial bone loss or previous fracture, especially in those 5 or more years past menopause. A review of more than 20 studies found that postmenopausal women receiving calcium supplementation had bone losses of 0.014% per year compared with 1.0% per year in untreated women. In longer-term trials, the beneficial effects of calcium supplementation were sustained for up to 4 years.

Older studies found that, in the presence of adequate vitamin D, calcium also reduced the incidence of spine, hip, and other fractures. Some more recent, large, RCTs did not show significant efficacy of daily oral calcium supplements in preventing fracture. Three studies of calcium and vitamin D and one study on calcium alone found no efficacy in reducing fracture risk using prespecified intent-to-treat analysis. However, in two of the studies, baseline calcium intake was already at or close to the response threshold, and calcium intake for the other two was not reported. Additionally, treatment adherence was poor (35%-55%) in two of the studies, but when analysis was confined to treatment-adherent participants, significant reductions in fracture risk were found. The 2006 NAMS osteoporosis position statement, which reached the conclusion that primary analysis (intent-to-treat) of the effect of calcium intake on fractures did not show efficacy, did conclude that secondary evidence (patient compliance) revealed benefit.

Calcium seems to potentiate the effect of exercise on BMD in postmenopausal women, primarily in those with daily calcium intake above 1,000 mg.

Calcium, either alone or with vitamin D, is not as effective as pharmacotherapy with either menopausal estrogen alone (ET) or estrogen combined with a progestogen (EPT), a selective estrogen-receptor modulator (SERM), or a bisphosphonate. However, supplemental calcium substantially improves the efficacy of these agents in reducing menopause-related bone loss. Because of the well-established need for adequate calcium intake, all key clinical trials with either a SERM or a bisphosphonate have provided supplemental calcium to both treatment and placebo arms. Although it is likely that calcium potentiates the positive BMD effects of SERMs and bisphosphonates as it does for ET/EPT, this conclusion can only be surmised. (Note that the FDA now disallows the term "selective estrogen-receptor modulator" [SERM], preferring "estrogen agonist/antagonist.")

As discussed in the 2006 NAMS position statement on calcium, the importance of an adequate calcium intake for skeletal health is well established. NAMS notes that calcium has also been associated with beneficial effects in several nonskeletal disorders, primarily colorectal cancer, hypertension, nephrolithiasis, and obesity, although the extent of those effects and the mechanisms involved have not been fully elucidated.

Calcium nutritional status is very difficult to assess using usual laboratory tests. Serum calcium is maintained in the normal range in most cases, even with the presence of severe deficiency. Some combination of a history of low calcium intake, coupled with decreased bone mass for age, increased bone remodeling indices, and high serum PTH will usually be characteristic of calcium deficiency; however, each of these associated changes can be produced by other causes. Because inadequate calcium intake is prevalent, it is safe to assume that most patients need more calcium.

Women with low 25(OH)D levels are unlikely to absorb calcium optimally. Given the fact that low serum vitamin D levels are linked to calcium deficiency, laboratory tests for vitamin D are being used more often in lieu of specific tests for calcium deficiency. (See page 240 for more about vitamin D.)

Recommended intakes for nutrients have been established in the United States by the Institute of Medicine (IOM). In 1997, the IOM published revised calcium requirements for North American residents. The National Institutes of Health and Osteoporosis Canada (previously the Osteoporosis Society of Canada) have also published calcium intake guidelines. Recommendations related to peri- and postmenopausal women are presented in Table 2. A woman's calcium requirement rises at menopause (or whenever estrogen is lost). This is because calcium

Table 2. Recommended intakes for daily calcium for peri- and postmenopausal women	
Institute of Medicine	
Aged 31-50 years	1,000 mg
Aged 51 and older	1,200 mg
National Institutes of Health	
Premenopausal women aged 25-50	1,000 mg
Postmenopausal women younger than age 65 and using estrogen therapy	1,000 mg
Postmenopausal women not using estrogen therapy	1,500 mg
All women aged 65 and older	1,500 mg
Osteoporosis Canada	
Premenopausal women	1,000 mg
"Menopausal" women	1,500 mg

Source: Adapted from the Institute of Medicine, the National Institutes of Health, and Osteoporosis Canada.

absorption efficiency and renal conservation are both estrogen dependent, and both deteriorate in the estrogen-deprived state.

Such intakes are probably sufficient for most individuals to maintain skeletal mass during the peak adult years and to minimize age-related bone loss during involution. These recommendations are based mainly on several RCTs in which intakes of 1,500 to 2,500 mg/day, coupled with adequate vitamin D status and protein intake, reduced PTH secretion to premenopausal normal values, stopped (or slowed) age-related bone loss, and reduced osteoporotic fractures by up to 55%. Intakes that would be optimal for other health/disease endpoints are less well studied, but such data as are available indicate an intake requirement at least as high as that for the protection of bone mass. The 2006 NAMS position statement on calcium concluded that the target calcium intake for most postmenopausal women is 1,200 mg/day.

It is currently difficult to pin down the calcium intake status of the population because of the rapidly changing environment with respect to food fortification and supplement use. From food sources alone, median calcium intakes for women aged 40 to 60 years are under 600 mg/day and have been approximately stable at that level for many years, despite education and other campaigns to improve calcium intake. This leaves a substantial gap that ranges from 400 to 900 mg/day to be filled by fortified foods, supplements, or both. Specific populations of postmenopausal women at extra risk for inadequate calcium intake include women who are lactose intolerant, follow a pure vegetarian diet (vegan; typically getting only 250 mg/d of calcium), or have poor eating habits. This low probability of adequacy led the 2005 Dietary Guidelines Advisory Committee to classify calcium as a "shortfall" nutrient.

It has been shown, moreover, that clinician attention to recommending an adequate calcium intake has dropped by nearly 50% since the introduction of the bisphosphonate drugs for osteoporosis in 1995. Because patients tend to find nutritional advice from their clinicians more credible than the comparable advice they get from all other sources, it is critically important that clinicians continue to emphasize the importance of getting an adequate calcium intake.

Dietary sources are the preferred means of obtaining adequate calcium intake because there are other essential nutrients in high-calcium foods.

For most US residents, dairy products (eg, milk, cheese, yogurt, ice cream) are the major contributors of dietary calcium, providing approximately 70% of the total calcium intake of postmenopausal women aged 60 years and older. An 8-oz serving of milk or yogurt, or a 1- to 1.5-oz cube of hard cheese, contains about 300 mg calcium. All other (nondairy) foods combined contribute a total of only 150 to 250 mg calcium to a typical adult diet. Hence, meeting current intake recommendations from typical foods requires consumption of approximately three servings of dairy food per day. Reduced-fat or low-fat products contain at least as much calcium per serving as high-fat dairy products, and they offer an alternative for women concerned about body weight and lipid profiles.

Because many people will not choose to achieve the recommended three dairy servings a day, food manufacturers have introduced a variety of calcium-fortified products, including fruit juices, breakfast cereals, and breads. These foods are not equally well engineered, as the added calcium may exhibit reduced bioavailability or such poor physical properties as to cause the fortificant to settle into the bottom of the carton (as with soy beverages). Thus, while calcium fortification of foods is a welcomed improvement in the nutritional value of available foods, it still functions in a climate of "buyer beware," and the consumer would be well advised to attempt to choose brands that have demonstrated fortificant bioavailability.

Since labeling of calcium can be misleading, the best way to understand the calcium content of a tablet or food item is to look at the label. A total of 100% of the daily value equates with 1,000 mg, so that if the label shows that the item contains 40% of the daily value, the amount of calcium is 400 mg.

An estimated 25% of the US population and 70% of the world's population exhibit some degree of "lactase non-persistence" (ie, inability to metabolize lactose in dairy products), which in some individuals may produce diarrhea, bloating, and gas when dairy products are consumed (ie, "lactose intolerance"). Lactase nonpersistence is more common among people of East Asian, African, and South American descent. Other GI problems (eg, celiac disease, irritable bowel syndrome, Crohn's disease, GI infection), or their treatment with intestinal antibiotics, can cause lactose intolerance, either temporary or permanent. Many women with lactase nonpersistence can tolerate milk normally if they have never stopped drinking it since youth or if they increase intake gradually, thereby conditioning their intestinal flora to produce lactase. The National Medical Association has issued a consensus report recommending three servings of dairy per day for all African Americans. Those few who remain intolerant may substitute yogurt and lactase-treated milk. True milk intolerance or allergy is rare. Calcium supplements or calcium-fortified foods should be considered if dietary preferences or lactase nonpersistence restricts consumption of dairy foods.

Calcium supplements offer a convenient alternative to women unable to consume enough calcium from diet alone. Their use should be confined to what their name denotes, *supplementing* an already nearly adequate diet. Dependence upon supplements for basal intake is not wise and probably not effective, since a low calcium intake is commonly a marker for a globally poor diet, and fixing only the calcium component is an inadequate response to a patient's need. Nevertheless, calcium supplements do play an important role, particularly as adjuvants in the treatment of existing disease, such as osteoporosis. As with food fortification, not all supplements are engineered equally. In the past, some calcium tablets did not disintegrate in the body to release the nutrient. Since calcium supplements, like calcium-fortified foods, are not regulated as drugs, "buyer beware" is advised. Brands that have demonstrated calcium bioavailability are the best choices.

Calcium supplements vary in type of calcium salt (and hence calcium content), formulation, price, and, to some extent, absorbability.

- The two most often used calcium supplement types contain either calcium carbonate or calcium citrate, but a wide variety of calcium salts is found in calcium supplements, including calcium acetate, calcium citrate malate, calcium gluconate, calcium lactate, calcium lactogluconate, and calcium phosphate (a collective term that describes supplements consisting of either the monobasic, dibasic, or tribasic phosphate salt of calcium). Calcium is also available in bone meal (basically calcium phosphate), as well as dolomite or oyster shell (both basically calcium carbonate) supplements. In the past, some of these have contained toxic contaminants, especially lead; however, a more recent analysis of the most commonly used brands did not reveal toxic levels of contaminants.

- Different calcium salts may contain different percentages of calcium. Calcium carbonate provides the highest percentage (40%); thus, 1,250 mg of calcium carbonate provides 500 mg of calcium. Calcium citrate (tetra-hydrated form) contains 21% calcium; 2,385 mg of calcium citrate therefore provides 500 mg of calcium. All marketed calcium supplements list the actual calcium content.

- Various formulations of calcium supplements are available, including oral tablets, chewable tablets, dissolvable oral tablets, and liquids. Another formulation for individuals with difficulty swallowing is an effervescent calcium supplement, typically calcium carbonate combined with materials such as citric acid that facilitate dissolving in water or orange juice.

- Calcium supplements also vary by price. Calcium carbonate products are typically less expensive than most other types of calcium supplements.

- Absorbability is also a concern. Contrary to popular belief, calcium carbonate and calcium citrate are equally well absorbed if taken with meals, the normal way of assimilating any nutrient. Calcium citrate malate is highly bioavailable, as are supplements containing calcium that is chelated to an amino acid (eg, bisglycinocalcium), but both these lesser-used supplements are typically more expensive than calcium carbonate. Studies comparing various commonly used calcium compounds found little differences in their bioavailability when supplements were taken with food. Calcium absorption is optimized if taken with meals and intake is spread out over the day, but contrary to previous advice, there is no practical limit to the amount that can be taken at one time. Consumption of calcium supplements with meals can also minimize the potential for rare GI side effects (ie, gaseousness, constipation). Pharmaceutical formulation of the supplement (ie, the other ingredients in the tablet and how they are packed together) actually makes more of a difference in absorbability than does the chemical nature of the calcium salt.

The side effect profile from recommended levels of calcium intake is insignificant. Calcium intervention trials have not reported any serious adverse events. Nevertheless, some women have difficulty swallowing a large tablet or have GI adverse effects. Tolerability can be addressed by getting most or all the requirement from food, or by switching the type of calcium or reducing the dose. GI adverse effects are often related to a woman's taking more calcium than required, not dividing doses, or perhaps confusing supplemental intake with recommended total daily intake.

There are no reported cases of calcium toxicity from food calcium sources, even in pastoral populations whose calcium intake may be in excess of 6,000 mg/day (almost entirely from dairy sources). All reported cases of calcium intoxication have come from the prolonged use of calcium supplement sources, principally calcium carbonate. Even from this source, intakes associated with toxicity have usually been above 4,500 mg/day, taken over prolonged periods. Intake of more than 2,500 mg/day (the UL for healthy adults set by the IOM) can increase the risk of hypercalcemia, which, in extreme cases, can lead to kidney damage. It is not necessary to measure urine calcium excretion before increasing calcium intake to recommended

levels in women who have not had a renal calculus. But a woman diagnosed with renal calculi should not consume calcium supplements above the level recommended for her age until the specific cause has been determined.

Chromium. Chromium helps to maintain normal blood glucose levels. No DRI has been established; the adequate intake established by the National Academy of Sciences for women age 50 and older is 20 μg/day.

Food sources include cereals, meats, poultry, fish, and beer. Promotion of high doses of chromium supplements for weight loss has become popular, but valid trials of both safety and efficacy are lacking. The role of chromium supplements in individuals with chromium deficiency or glucose intolerance has not been defined.

Iron. Iron serves numerous important functions in the body relating to the metabolism of oxygen, not the least of which is its role in hemoglobin transport of oxygen to tissues. Almost two thirds of iron in the body is found in hemoglobin.

Excess iron results in cellular dysfunction, leading to toxicity and even death. Although earlier research linked high iron stores with increased rates of MI in men, more recent studies have not supported such an association.

A reduction in iron negatively affects the function of oxygen transport in red blood cells. The World Health Organization considers iron deficiency the number-one nutritional disorder in the world. As many as 80% of the world's population may be iron deficient, while 30% may have iron deficiency anemia. Iron deficiency severity ranges from iron depletion, which yields little physiologic damage, to iron deficiency anemia, which can affect the function of numerous organ systems.

The most common causes of iron deficiency anemia are GI bleeding or excess menstrual flow. During perimenopause, women experiencing prolonged or repeated heavy uterine bleeding may need additional iron if they develop iron deficiency anemia. After menopause, most women should not choose a multivitamin/mineral supplement containing iron because iron is no longer lost through menstrual bleeding. The DRI of elemental iron for menstruating women is 18 mg/day; after menopause, the amount is 8 mg/day. Women who use multivitamins should be advised to use the appropriate formulation.

In addition to GI bleeding and excess menstrual flow, other conditions associated with a high risk of developing iron deficiency anemia include kidney failure (especially those on dialysis); chronic infectious, inflammatory, or malignant disorders (eg, arthritis and cancer); and GI malabsorption diseases (eg, Celiac and Crohn's disease). Not all these conditions will respond to iron supplementation.

Many individuals (particularly menstruating women and vegetarians) who engage in regular, intense exercise have marginal or inadequate iron status, requiring iron supplementation.

Signs of iron deficiency anemia include fatigue and weakness, decreased work performance, difficulty maintaining body temperature, decreased immune function, and glossitis (inflamed tongue).

Iron is readily available in food (eg, organ meats, beef, turkey, clams, oysters, oatmeal, beans) and fortified foods (eg, breakfast cereals). When iron deficiency anemia is diagnosed, OTC or prescription oral iron supplements are often recommended. Prescription intravenous iron therapy may be called for in some cases.

There are two forms of dietary iron: heme and nonheme. Heme iron, derived from hemoglobin, is found in animal foods that originally contained hemoglobin, such as red meats, poultry, and fish. Plant foods such as rice, maize, black beans, lentils, soybeans, and wheat contain nonheme iron, the form added to iron-fortified foods. Although heme iron is absorbed better than nonheme iron, most dietary iron is nonheme iron. Absorption of heme iron ranges from 15% to 35% and is not significantly affected by diet. In contrast, only 2% to 20% of nonheme iron in plant foods is absorbed. Concomitant intake of calcium, tannins (found in tea), or phytates (found in legumes and whole grains) can decrease absorption.

Total dietary iron intake in vegetarian diets may meet recommended levels; however, that iron is less available for absorption than in diets that include meat.

Supplemental iron is available in two forms: ferrous and ferric. Ferrous iron salts (ferrous fumarate, ferrous sulfate, and ferrous gluconate) are the best absorbed forms of iron supplements. "Elemental iron" is the amount of iron in a supplement that is available for absorption.

Magnesium. This nutrient is a divalent, cationic element and, like calcium, it is relatively abundant on earth. An adult human body contains between 25 and 35 g magnesium, approximately one half of which is in the skeleton. Also like calcium, magnesium is a chemical element that can neither be synthesized nor degraded in the process of its utilization by living organisms.

Magnesium is a necessary cofactor for numerous cellular enzymes involved in intermediary and energy metabolism. In magnesium deficiency, global cellular functions are impaired, although there is no discrete disease syndrome that is characteristic of magnesium deficiency. Magnesium is said to function as a physiologic calcium channel blocker, modulating the entry of calcium into the cytosol of various functioning tissues. When magnesium is deficient, cell calcium rises, with resultant hypertonia, muscle cramps, and elevated vascular tone.

Magnesium absorption from the diet is much more efficient than that of calcium, with net absorption usually in the range of 40% to 60% of ingested intake. Urinary magnesium can be reduced sharply with inadequate intake, but may rise substantially in uncontrolled DM and with certain diuretics.

With severe magnesium deficiency, calcium homeostasis is seriously disrupted. The parathyroid glands are not able to respond to hypocalcemia by secretion of PTH, and the bone resorptive apparatus is not able to respond to PTH. Hence, hypocalcemia, refractory to any intervention other than magnesium repletion, ensues. Clinically recognizable magnesium deficiency occurs when there is excessive loss of body electrolytes through the intestine (eg, intestinal fistulas and various hypersecretory malabsorption syndromes), as well as during recovery from alcoholism. Milder degrees of deficiency, to the extent they occur, are presumably due either to inadequate dietary intake or to hypermagnesiuria induced, for example, by DM or certain diuretics. The full extent of the clinical expression of magnesium deficiency is uncertain but seems to include a higher risk of hypertensive CVD, excessive platelet aggregation and platelet-induced thrombosis, and, at least in some individuals, osteoporosis.

Magnesium is sometimes mentioned as a necessary supplement for the protection of bone health, for absorption of calcium, or both. However, in most trials focused on BMD or osteoporotic fracture, benefits of calcium were observed without magnesium supplements. Moreover, a study with calcium absorption as the endpoint found that adding 789 to 826 mg/day of magnesium, more than double the daily average magnesium intake (280 mg) for postmenopausal women, had no effect on calcium absorption. There are, however, two lines of evidence suggesting that subclinical magnesium deficiency may complicate the osteoporotic disease process in certain individuals.

Celiac disease is not simply a syndrome of malabsorption, but of excess electrolyte loss through the intestine, and a nonnegligible fraction of patients with osteoporosis have silent celiac disease as a cause of, or contributor to, their osteoporosis. These individuals clearly need calcium supplementation, but available evidence suggests that they benefit from magnesium supplementation as well. Patients with osteoporosis, even though they lack overt intestinal symptoms and nevertheless have positive endomysial antibodies, would not be harmed by magnesium supplementation, and might be helped.

A second line of evidence comes from the demonstration that many patients with vitamin D deficiency fail to show the expected PTH response to their inefficient calcium absorption. These individuals have presumptive magnesium deficiency by virtue of a positive magnesium tolerance test and response of PTH to supplementation with magnesium citrate. The cause of the magnesium deficiency in these individuals is unknown, and the ultimate significance of their silent magnesium deficiency remains unclear.

Taken daily, magnesium and some other nonprescription preventive medications (eg, riboflavin, coenzyme Q10) may be effective and safe for migraine sufferers.

The DRI for magnesium is 320 mg/day for women. The evidence supporting this recommendation is weak, as there are no generally agreed-upon indicators of optimal magnesium status. For the most part, this estimate is based on the amount of ingested magnesium needed to maintain zero magnesium balance.

Median magnesium intake in adult US women is approximately 230 mg/day, and roughly 60% to 70% of the US population regularly has an intake below the DRI. This ostensible shortfall is about as large as the intake gap for calcium and vitamin D, but its clinical significance is much less clear. Until firmer evidence becomes available, it would seem both prudent and safe to attempt to improve magnesium intake status for most adults.

Magnesium is fairly widely distributed in a variety of foods, the richest sources being nuts, certain seeds, legumes, and various marine fish. Dairy foods are also good sources of magnesium and in typical diets will often be the major source of magnesium. If a woman reaches the target figure noted elsewhere for calcium (3 dairy servings/d), she would automatically receive, from that source alone, roughly 40% of her recommended daily intake of magnesium.

Several popular calcium supplements combine calcium and magnesium. There is popular lore to the effect that magnesium must be present for calcium to be absorbed, which is the ostensible rationale for a combination supplement product. That statement is correct, however, only for severe magnesium deficiency (as in malabsorption syndromes) and has been shown to be incorrect for typical adults. In controlled trials using isotopically labeled calcium sources, even a doubling of magnesium intake had no influence on calcium absorption efficiency. Moreover, all the trials establishing the efficacy of calcium in slowing age-related bone loss and reducing osteoporotic fracture risk were performed without supplementing magnesium intake.

In women with excessive magnesium loss, usually due to GI disease (eg, diarrhea, vomiting), magnesium supplementation would be appropriate.

There are no known cases of magnesium toxicity from food sources. Magnesium taken by mouth as various salts tends to have a cathartic effect, and one such preparation (magnesium citrate) has routinely been used as a means of cleaning out the GI tract before endoscopy or surgery. Anything more-than-modest supplementation with magnesium salts is likely to elicit some degree of catharsis. The UL published by the Food and Nutrition Board for magnesium applies only to supplemental sources and not to food sources. That value has been set at 350 mg of supplemental magnesium per day.

Zinc. Found in almost every cell, zinc is an essential mineral that stimulates the activity of approximately 100 enzymes. Zinc is involved in nucleic acid and protein synthesis and degradation, is needed for DNA synthesis and wound healing, supports the immune system, and helps maintain the senses of taste and smell. The DRI for zinc is 8 mg.

Zinc is found in a wide variety of foods. Zinc absorption is greater from a diet high in animal protein than a diet rich in plant proteins. Vegetarians may need as much as 50% more zinc than nonvegetarians because of the lower absorption of zinc from plant foods.

Oysters contain more zinc per serving than any other food, but red meat and poultry provide the majority of zinc in the North American diet. Other good food sources of zinc include beans, nuts, certain seafood, whole grains, dairy products, and fortified breakfast cereals.

Zinc toxicity has been seen in both acute and chronic forms. Intakes of 150 to 450 mg/day have been associated with low copper status, altered iron function, reduced immune function, and reduced levels of HDL cholesterol.

There is no single laboratory test that adequately measures zinc nutritional status. If zinc deficiency is suspected in a woman, causes to consider are inadequate caloric intake, alcoholism, and digestive diseases. Low zinc status has been observed in 30% to 50% of alcoholics due to loss of zinc in urine and an unacceptable variety or amount of food.

Women who experience chronic diarrhea should be careful to add sources of zinc to their daily diet and may benefit from zinc supplementation. As well, anyone who has had GI surgery or digestive disorders that result in malabsorption, Crohn's disease, or short bowel syndrome, are at greater risk of zinc deficiency and should be evaluated for a zinc supplement if diet alone fails to maintain normal zinc levels.

The effect of zinc treatments on the severity or duration of cold symptoms is controversial. A study of over 100 employees of the Cleveland Clinic indicated that OTC zinc lozenges decreased the duration of colds by one half, although no differences were seen in duration of fevers or level of muscle aches.

Iron fortification programs for iron deficiency anemia may affect the absorption of zinc and other nutrients. Fortification of foods with iron does not significantly affect zinc absorption, but large amounts of iron supplements (>25 mg) may decrease zinc absorption. Taking iron supplements between meals will help decrease its effect on zinc.

Other minerals. For most individuals, additional vitamins or minerals such as the ones listed below will be present in a wholesome diet that includes five or more servings of fruits and vegetables per day. However, supplementation may be required.

- *Boron* acts as a cofactor in magnesium metabolism and thus helps in bone regulation. There is no DRI for boron. Food sources are potatoes, legumes, milk, avocado, and peanuts. A daily multivitamin and mineral supplement containing between 3 and 9 mg is adequate. Overdose can cause nausea, vomiting, and diarrhea.

- *Copper* is a component of enzymes involved in iron metabolism. The DRI is 900 µg daily. Food sources include organ meats, seafood, nuts, seeds, wheat bran, whole grain products, and cocoa.

- *Manganese* is involved in bone formation as well as in enzymes in amino acid, cholesterol, and carbohydrate metabolism. Adequate intake is 1.8 mg daily.

- *Phosphorus* is an important mineral for bones, with too much or too little resulting in bone loss. One symptom of phosphorus deficiency is bone pain. Low phosphorus levels can result from poor eating habits, intestinal malabsorption, and excessive use of antacids that bind to phosphorus. Food sources include milk, yogurt, ice cream, cheese, peas, meat, eggs, some cereals, and breads. Soft drinks are an additional source. The DRI for women age 50 and older is 700 mg, with ULs set at 4,000 mg/day for those aged 50 to 70 years and 3,000 mg/day for women older than age 70.

- *Selenium* acts to defend against oxidative stress and the reduction and oxidation of vitamin C and other substances, and in regulation of thyroid hormone action. Food sources include organ meats, seafood, and plants (depending on soil content). The DRI is 55 µg. Overdose results in hair and nail brittleness and loss.

Other supplements

A few of the currently popular nonbotanical dietary supplements and NHPs are discussed here.

Coenzyme Q10. This fat-soluble, vitamin-like compound—often called CoQ10 or ubiquinone—is found in humans and other mammals. First identified in 1957, CoQ10 is involved in energy production reactions in human physiology and functions as an antioxidant, protecting against free radical damage within mitochondria.

CoQ10, as oral tablets and capsules, is marketed OTC in the United States and Canada as a dietary supplement and an NHP, respectively. As such, evidence for safety and efficacy is limited. Most information available is from anecdotal reports, case reports, and uncontrolled clinical studies.

Widely used throughout Europe and Asia, CoQ10 is claimed to be of benefit in CVD, including angina, congestive heart failure, and hypertension, as well as musculoskeletal disorders, DM, and obesity. Because of its cellular energy-related functions, it has been investigated in Parkinson's disease for symptom reduction, but showed no significant changes in primary or secondary outcomes when compared with placebo.

CoQ10 supplementation is commonly used by individuals with congestive heart failure in an attempt to replace levels lost in myocardial cells. The extent of CoQ10 deficiency correlates with degree of severity. Many small studies of this use have been published, but most were uncontrolled and unblinded. One well-designed, RCT examining its effects on peak oxygen consumption, exercise duration, and ejection fraction concluded that CoQ10 was no better than placebo in patients receiving standard medical therapy. More randomized controlled trials, evaluating not only objective measures of cardiac performance but also clinical outcomes, are needed before supplementation can be justified.

One provocative study investigated the relation between hypercholesterolemic patients treated with statin drugs who developed statin-associated myopathies and decreased CoQ10 levels. Muscle biopsies and blood tests showed underlying genetically related metabolic muscle diseases in many of the patients. More research is needed before CoQ10 therapy is recommended for all patients using statins.

In a 2005 RCT, CoQ10 was compared with placebo in 42 migraine patients. CoQ10 was found superior to placebo for attack frequency, headache days, and days with nausea and was well tolerated.

Interest in the potential effect of CoQ10 in cancer began after lesser amounts were noted in the blood of patients with breast cancer. Animal studies suggestive of protective action against cardiotoxicity from doxorubicin have led to limited investigation in humans. Animal studies also suggest that it produces immune-stimulating effects. No RCT of CoQ10 as a treatment for cancer has been published in a peer-reviewed, scientific journal. Caution has been suggested because of its potential for interfering with the effectiveness of chemotherapy.

Adverse effects of CoQ10 have been reported, including nausea, epigastric pain, dizziness, photophobia, insomnia, irritability, headache, heartburn, and fatigue. One study reported liver enzyme elevation after extended periods of use, but no liver toxicity.

Significant drug interactions with CoQ10 include increased insulin response in DM patients and decreased response to the anticoagulant warfarin. In increasing cardiac contractility, CoQ10 may increase already elevated blood pressure. Lipid-lowering agents including simvastatin, atorvastatin, and gemfibrozil can decrease serum CoQ10 levels, as can the oral hypoglycemic agents glyburide and tolazamide.

Fish oil/omega-3 and omega-6 fatty acids. Essential nutrients for humans include the parent fatty acids of the omega-3 and omega-6 families of polyunsaturated fatty acids, α-*linolenic acid* and *linoleic acid*, respectively.

The body converts α-linolenic acid into eicosapentaenoic acid (EPA) and docosahexaenoic acid (DHA), all often referred to as omega-3 fatty acids. They are components of fish oil. These compounds are associated with cardiovascular and other health benefits. Because the conversion process may be inefficient, nutritional sources must be relied upon for an optimal level.

The most abundant sources of α-linolenic acid (omega-3 fatty acids) are fatty fish, such as salmon, sardines, herring, mackerel, black cod, and bluefish. It is also available in leafy green vegetables, nuts, and vegetable oils such as canola, soy, and especially flaxseed. Sources of linoleic acid (omega-6 fatty acids) include plant-based oils. Most American diets provide at least 10 times more omega-6 than omega-3 fatty acids. It is not known whether a desirable ratio of omega-6 to omega-3 fatty acids exists or to what extent high intakes of omega-6 fatty acids interfere with any benefit of omega-3 fatty acids consumption.

Dietary supplementation of omega-3 fatty acids has been suggested as useful in a variety of conditions. These include CVD, asthma, dementia and cognitive performance with aging, multiple sclerosis, Parkinson's disease, pre-menstrual syndrome, rheumatoid arthritis, systemic lupus erythematosus, irritable bowel disease, renal disease, and various skin conditions. As with many supplements, the quality of studies is variable. With the exception of effects on CVD and its risk factors, study results have been either insignificant or inconclusive.

Three prospective randomized trials assessing omega-3 fatty acids for the secondary prevention of cardiac events showed positive results. In the largest trial, more than 11,000 postinfarction patients who received 850 mg/day of omega-3 fatty acids experienced a 45% reduction in the rate of sudden cardiac death and a 20% reduction in the total mortality rate. These benefits occurred in patients already receiving "standard" postinfarction therapy (eg, angiotensin-converting enzyme inhibitors, beta-blockers, or antiplatelet agents). It is theorized that these effects are the result of the membrane-stabilizing effect of these oils. Though these results are impressive in women with established CVD, no large trials have yet addressed the use of omega-3 fatty acids as a means of primary prevention in postmenopausal women who are at risk.

Fish oil capsules containing varying amounts of omega-3 and omega-6 fatty acids are available as an OTC dietary supplement and NHP in the United States and Canada, respectively. In the United States, the FDA has approved a prescription form of omega-3 fatty acids (marketed as Omacor) as an adjunct to diet for treatment of persons having very high triglycerides. The American Heart Association advises that treating very high triglycerides be done under a clinician's care.

When considering fish oil for treatment of dyslipidemia, it is important to note that it does not affect HDL cholesterol and produces either no change or an increase in LDL cholesterol. The most effect on lowering triglycerides is in persons having very high baseline levels. As with any supplement used medically, the advantage of a prescription product insures consistent quality and purity.

Supplements of fish oil have the potential to slow blood clotting and potentially increase bleeding by decreasing platelet aggregation (see Box on page 243 for precautions when using OTC anticoagulant therapies).

Glucosamine and chondroitin. Glucosamine is an amino-monosaccharide that is present in almost all human tissues, especially cartilaginous tissues. Chondroitin is a complex carbohydrate that helps cartilage retain water.

OTC supplements of these agents have been promoted for pain relief, primarily in osteoarthritis (OA). These agents are sometimes taken individually but primarily in combination, and they are used as alternatives or along with analgesics and NSAIDs. In the United States and Canada, glucosamine and chondroitin are sold as dietary supplements and as NHPs, respectively; thus, they are not regulated as drugs.

Glucosamine is converted to one of two salts for supplement use. Glucosamine sulfate is the most tested form, although the hydrochloride salt may be just as effective. Individuals may respond differently to the two salts. Chondroitin is converted to the sulfate salt.

Glucosamine sulfate (alone and with chondroitin sulfate) has been shown to be symptomatically effective in a number of studies and may have a structure-modifying effect on knee OA. In animal studies, most of the oral dose is absorbed and incorporated into biologic structures, including the liver, kidneys, and articular cartilage. It is assumed that glucosamine sulfate supplementation facilitates the production and regeneration of cartilage.

Clinical studies have been conducted on glucosamine sulfate for OA for more than 20 years, primarily in Europe, where it is available by prescription for the treatment of OA. Two meta-analyses, one a Cochrane review, have found clinical trial evidence supporting the safety and efficacy of glucosamine sulfate for relieving pain and improving function in patients with OA. The Cochrane review found 16 RCTs evaluating glucosamine in OA. In 13 placebo-controlled trials, glucosamine sulfate was found to be superior to placebo in all but one. In four trials comparing glucosamine sulfate and NSAIDs, glucosamine was superior in two and equivalent in two. Nearly all trials used glucosamine at a dose of 500 mg three times daily.

The reported side effect profile for glucosamine was similar to that for placebo, although some studies noted GI complaints and sleepiness. No serious adverse events were reported. Although the preponderance of results were positive for glucosamine, the Cochrane review cautioned that more research is needed to confirm long-term effectiveness and toxicity.

Glucosamine used in supplements is obtained from chitin, extracted from marine exoskeletons. Thus, for women with seafood allergies, this supplement should be used with caution, depending on the severity of the allergy.

Chondroitin is used in an attempt to influence cartilage loss, with the assumption that because it is partially absorbed in the intestine, some of it may reach joints. Few studies have been done examining the effect on joint space; more have looked at pain relief. There has been some speculation that chondroitin has anti-inflammatory effects, but evidence is lacking. In vitro studies suggest that chondroitin may inhibit some of the cartilage-degrading enzymes. No large RCTs have addressed the efficacy of chondroitin alone in the treatment of OA.

The Glucosamine/chondroitin Arthritis Intervention Trial (GAIT), the first large-scale, multicenter clinical trial in the United States, examined the combination of glucosamine hydrochloride and chondroitin sulfate for relief of mild pain in knee OA. In this 6-month study, these substances were compared separately or in combination with each other, to celecoxib and with placebo. Glucosamine hydrochloride and chondroitin sulfate together or alone did not provide statistically significant pain relief.

In recent years, several randomized controlled studies have assessed the structure-modifying effect of glucosamine sulfate and chondroitin sulfate using plain radiography to measure joint space narrowing over several years. A meta-analysis by Bruyere et al found that there is some evidence to suggest that these agents, in combination, do have a structure-modifying effect, thereby interfering with progression of OA. The authors also concluded that combined glucosamine sulfate (but not glucosamine hydro-chloride) and chondroitin sulfate have small to moderate symptomatic efficacy in OA, although this is debated.

Concerns have been raised that these agents may interfere with glycemic control in women with DM since animal models have demonstrated such effects. An RCT of 35 individuals with type 2 DM showed no changes in glycemic control from daily therapy with 1,500 mg glucosamine sulfate and 1,200 mg chondroitin sulfate.

Inferior oral supplements of glucosamine (alone and with chondroitin) may also contain a large quantity of sodium chloride and/or potassium chloride, unneeded but less expensive "salts." These products should be avoided. Liquid glucosamine and chondroitin administration is preferred by some clinicians instead of the oral tablet form due to low absorption issues with tablets.

Supplements of glucosamine (alone and with chondroitin) are well tolerated.

S-adenosyl methionine (SAM-e). S-adenosyl methionine can be found in every living cell. Via enzymatic trans-methylation, it plays a role in the formation, activation, or metabolism of neurotransmitters, hormones, proteins, and phospholipids. This chemical is available as an oral supplement, marketed as an OTC dietary supplement in the United States and as an NHP in Canada. In some European countries, SAM-e is a prescription drug.

SAM-e is used as a mood enhancer and for joint and liver health. In August 2002, the US Agency for Healthcare Research and Quality published a comprehensive meta-analysis of 102 published studies on SAM-e. The following is a synopsis of their findings.

- To date, there are at least 48 clinical trials using SAM-e in the treatment of depression. Compared with placebo, SAM-e significantly improved scores on the Hamilton Rating Scale for Depression after 3 weeks, although risk ratios could not be calculated for either a 25% or a 50% improvement on the scale. When compared with conventional antidepressant therapy, SAM-e had statistically similar outcomes on the rating scale. Dosage for depression is usually 400 mg/day.

- SAM-e was significantly more effective than placebo in decreasing the pain of OA. Comparisons with NSAIDs showed similar outcomes. Dosage for OA is usually 1,200 mg/day.

- Intrahepatic cholestasis patients treated with SAM-e were twice as likely as placebo-treated patients to have a reduction in pruritis. Studies were inadequate to make a comparison with prescription therapies. Dosage for liver disorders is usually 200 to 400 mg/day.

Supplementation with SAM-e is well tolerated, with a side effect profile that includes occasional nausea and GI upset. Anecdotal reports have associated the product with reduced estrogen levels. More RCTs are needed to conclusively document efficacy and safety.

Vaginal lubricants and moisturizers

First-line management for women with estrogen-related vaginal dryness and mild vaginal atrophy includes nonhormonal vaginal lubricants and moisturizers, as well as regular sexual activity. Nonhormonal vaginal lubricants and moisturizers for the treatment of vaginal dryness are often available OTC.

Water-based *vaginal lubricants* (eg, Astroglide, Intimate Options, K-Y Personal Lubricant, Lubrin, Moist Again, and Silk E) coat the vagina. Their use is limited to easing penetration during intercourse. *Vaginal moisturizers* (eg, K-Y Long-Lasting Vaginal Moisturizer, Replens) offer the benefit of longer duration of effect by replenishing and maintaining water content in the vaginal vault. Vaginal moisturizers may be preferred by women who have symptoms of irritation, itching, and burning that are not limited to episodes of sexual exchange.

Women seeking therapy for vaginal dryness should be advised to use only products designed solely for vaginal use. Ingredients such as alcohol and perfume, which are contained in hand creams, can exacerbate some atrophic symptoms, such as burning and itching. Oil-based products, such as petroleum jelly and baby oil, can cause irritation, damage condoms and diaphragms, and, because they tend to cling to vaginal tissue, can also provide a habitat for abnormal vaginal and bladder bacteria. One exception to this rule is vitamin E oil. It provides vaginal lubrication to ease penetration during sexual intercourse and may relieve itching and irritation without untoward effects.

For women who want to lower vaginal pH, OTC repHresh vaginal gel may help reduce minor vaginal irritations and odors and can be use after intercourse and/or after any uterine bleeding (as both semen and menstrual blood are more alkaline).

Although all postmenopausal women should be counseled on the vaginal changes that occur with both menopause and aging, it is equally important to counsel perimenopausal women about adverse urogenital symptoms that may result from these changes. Recommendations to alleviate vaginal discomfort are especially important since vaginal atrophy left untreated may predispose women to dyspareunia. Sexual activity and/or stimulation should be encouraged for those women who want to maintain the capacity for intercourse because fewer atrophic vaginal changes are noted in sexually active women than in abstinent women.

For severe vaginal atrophy unresponsive to nonhormonal interventions, low-dose vaginal ET may be required to restore vaginal epithelium. Local vaginal estrogen is an appropriate option when vaginal atrophy is the sole symptom of diminished estrogen. In some cases, a nonhormonal method of maintaining vaginal lubrication can be used once vaginal atrophy is ameliorated or reversed. Unlike age-related changes in the urogenital tissues, most vaginal effects of diminished estrogen levels can be reversed. (See Section C, page 51, for more information on vulvovaginal symptoms.)

Topical agents for sexual pleasure

A variety of OTC agents are promoted to increase sexual pleasure when topically applied to the female genitalia. These agents are regulated in the United States as dietary supplements and in Canada as NHPs.

One such product (marketed in the United States as Zestra Feminine Arousal Fluid) is a blend of several botanical oils and extracts, including borage seed and evening primrose

oils, that when metabolized in the skin is generally recognized to cause increased blood flow and nerve conduction. A small (N = 20), double-blind, placebo-controlled, crossover study among women (aged 31-57 y), including 10 with sexual arousal disorder, found that all participants reported the 1-ml doses improved level of desire, satisfaction with level of sexual arousal, genital sensation, sexual pleasure, and ability to have orgasms. Treatment was well tolerated.

Suggested reading

Government regulations for dietary supplements

Health Canada. Natural health products. Available at: http://www.hc-sc.gc.ca/dhp-mps/prodnatur/index_e.html. Accessed September 4, 2007.

MacLean D. Nova Scotia Heart Health Program, Health and Welfare Canada, Nova Scotia Department of Health. *The Report of the Nova Scotia Nutrition Survey*. Halifax, NS, Canada, 1993.

National Academy of Sciences. Dietary reference intakes (DRIs): Recommendations for individuals, vitamins. Food and Nutrition Board, Institute of Medicine, National Academies. 2004. Available at: http://www.iom.edu/Object.File/Master/21/372/DRI%20Tables%20after%20electrolytes%20plus%20micro-macroEAR_2.pdf. Accessed August 5, 2007.

Office of Dietary Supplements. National Institutes of Health. Dietary supplements: background. Available at: http://ods.od.nih.gov/factsheets/dietarysupplements.asp. Accessed September 5, 2007.

US Department of Agriculture. Nutrition.gov. Dietary supplements. Available at: http://www.nutrition.gov/index.php?mode=subject&subject=ng_supplements&d_subject=Dietary%20Supplements. Accessed August 5, 2007.

Vitamins and minerals

Alaimo K, McDowell MA, Briefel RR, et al. Dietary intake of vitamins, minerals, and fiber of persons ages 2 months and over in the United States: Third National Health and Nutrition Examination Survey, Phase 1, 1988-91. *Adv Data* 1994;259:1-28.

Aloia JF, Vaswani A, Yeh JK, Ross PL, Flaster E, Dilmanian FA. Calcium supplementation with and without hormone replacement therapy to prevent postmenopausal bone loss. *Ann Intern Med* 1994;120:97-103.

Balk EM, Raman G, Tatsioni A, Chung M, Lau J, Rosenberg IH. Vitamin B_6, B_{12}, and folic acid supplementation and cognitive function: a systematic review of randomized trials. *Arch Intern Med* 2007;167:21-30.

Baron JA, Beach M, Mandel JS, et al. Calcium supplements for the prevention of colorectal adenomas. *N Engl J Med* 1999;340:101-107.

Bischoff HA, Dawson-Hughes B, Willett WC, et al. Effect of vitamin D on falls: a meta-analysis. *JAMA* 2004;291:1999-2006.

Bischoff HA, Stähelin HB, Dick W, et al. Effects of vitamin D and calcium supplementation on falls: a randomized controlled trial. *J Bone Miner Res* 2003;18:343-351.

Bischoff-Ferrari HA, Dietrich T, Orav EJ, et al. Higher 25-hydroxyvitamin D concentrations are associated with better lower-extremity function in both active and inactive persons aged ≥60 y. *Am J Clin Nutr* 2004;80:752-758.

Bischoff-Ferrari HA, Dietrich T, Orav EJ, Dawson-Hughes B. Positive association between 25-hydroxy vitamin D levels and bone mineral density: a population-based study of younger and older adults. *Am J Med* 2004; 116:634-639.

Bischoff-Ferrari HA, Giovannucci E, Willett WC, Dietrich T, Dawson-Hughes B. Estimation of optimal serum concentrations of 25-hydroxyvitamin D for multiple health outcomes. *Am J Clin Nutr* 2006;84:18-28.

Bischoff-Ferrari HA, Willett WC, Wong JB, Giovannucci E, Dietrich T, Dawson-Hughes B, Fracture prevention with vitamin D supplementation: a meta-analysis of randomized controlled trials. *JAMA* 2005;293:2257-2264.

Bodnar LM, Simhan HN, Powers RW, Frank MP, Cooperstein E, Roberts JM. High prevalence of vitamin D insufficiency in black and white pregnant women residing in the northern United States and their neonates. *J Nutr* 2007;137:305-306.

Borghi L, Schianchi T, Meschi T, et al. Comparison of two diets for the prevention of recurrent stones in idiopathic hypercalciuria. *N Engl J Med* 2002;346:77-84.

Bourgoin BP, Evans DR, Cornett JR, Lingard SM, Quattrone AJ. Lead content in 70 brands of dietary calcium supplements. *Am J Public Health* 1993;83:1155-1160.

Braam LA, Knapen MH, Geusens P, et al. Vitamin K1 supplementation retards bone loss in postmenopausal women between 50 and 60 years of age. *Calcif Tissue Int* 2003;73:21-26.

Brown JP, Josse RG, for the Scientific Advisory Board of the Osteoporosis Society of Canada. 2002 clinical practice guidelines for the diagnosis and management of osteoporosis. *CMAJ* 2002;167(10 Suppl):S1-S34.

Chapuy MC, Arlot ME, Duboeuf F, et al. Vitamin D3 and calcium to prevent hip fractures in elderly women. *N Engl J Med* 1992;327:1637-1642.

Chapuy MC, Preziosi P, Maamer M, et al. Prevalence of vitamin D insufficiency in an adult normal population. *Osteoporos Int* 1997;7:439-443.

Chevalley T, Rizzoli R, Nydeggar V, et al. Effects of calcium supplements on femoral bone mineral density and vertebral fracture rate in vitamin-D-replete elderly patients. *Osteoporos Int* 1994;4:245-252.

Cummings SR, Black DM, Thompson DE, et al. Effect of alendronate on risk of fracture in women with low bone density but without vertebral fractures: results from the Fracture Intervention Trial. *JAMA* 1998;280:2077-2082.

Daniele ND, Carbonelli MC, Candeloro N, Iacopino L, De Lorenzo A, Andreoli A. Effect of supplementation on calcium and vitamin D on bone mineral density and bone mineral content in peri- and post-menopausal women: a double-blind, randomized, controlled trial. *Pharmacol Res* 2004; 50:637-641.

Dawson-Hughes B, Dallal GE, Krall EA, Sadowski L, Sahyoun N, Tannenbaum S. A controlled trial of the effect of calcium supplementation on bone density in postmenopausal women. *N Engl J Med* 1990;323:878-883.

Dawson-Hughes B, Harris SS, Krall EA, Dallal GE. Effect of calcium and vitamin D supplementation on bone density in men and women 65 years of age and older. *N Engl J Med* 1997;337:670-676.

Dawson-Hughes B, Seligson FH, Hughes VA. Effects of calcium carbonate and hydroxyapatite on zinc and iron retention in postmenopausal women. *Am J Clin Nutr* 1986;44:83-88.

Deehr MS, Dallal GE, Smith KT, Taulbee JD, Dawson-Hughes B. Effects of different calcium sources on iron absorption in postmenopausal women. *Am J Clin Nutr* 1990;51:95-99.

Delmas PD, Bjarnason NH, Mitlak BH, et al. Effects of raloxifene on bone mineral density, serum cholesterol concentrations, and uterine endometrium in postmenopausal women. *N Engl J Med* 1997;337:1641-1647.

Devine A, Dick IM, Heal SJ, Criddle RA, Prince RL. A 4-year follow-up study of the effects of calcium supplementation on bone density in elderly postmenopausal women. *Osteoporos Int* 1997;7:23-28.

Durlach J, Bac P, Durlach V, Rayssiguier Y, Bara M, Guiet-Bara A. Magnesium status and ageing: an update. *Magnes Res* 1998;11:25-42.

Elders PJ, Lips P, Netelenbos JC, et al. Long-term effect of calcium supplementation on bone loss in perimenopausal women. *J Bone Miner Res* 1994;9:963-970.

Elders PJ, Netelenbos JC, Lips P, et al. Calcium supplementation reduces vertebral bone loss in perimenopausal women: a controlled trial in 248 women between 46 and 55 years of age. *J Clin Endocrinol Metab* 1991;73:533-540.

Evans RA, Somers NM, Dunstan CR, Royle H, Kos S. The effect of low-dose cyclical etidronate and calcium on bone mass in early postmenopausal women. *Osteoporos Int* 1993;3:71-75.

Falchuk KH. Disturbances in trace elements. In: Fauci A, Braunwald E, Isselbacher KJ, et al, eds. *Harrison's Principles of Internal Medicine*, 14th ed. New York: McGraw-Hill, 1998:490-491.

Fleming KH, Heimbach JT. Consumption of calcium in the US: food sources and intake levels. *J Nutr* 1994;124(Suppl 8):1426S-1430S.

Fogelman I, Ribot C, Smith R, Ethgen D, Sod E, Reginster JY, for the BMD-MN Study Group. Risedronate reverses bone loss in postmenopausal women with low bone mass: results from a multinational, double-blind, placebo-controlled trial. *J Clin Endocrinol Metab* 2000;85:1895-1900.

Ford ES, Mokdad AH. Dietary magnesium intake in a national sample of US adults. *J Nutr* 2003;133:2879-2882.

Gallagher JC, Kinyamu HK, Fowler SE, et al. Calciotropic hormones and bone markers in the elderly. *J Bone Miner Res* 1998;13:475-482.

Gallagher JC, Riggs BL, Eisman J, Hamstra A, Arnaud SB, DeLuca HF. Intestinal calcium absorption and serum vitamin D metabolites in normal subjects and osteoporotic patients: effect of age and dietary calcium. *J Clin Invest* 1979;64:729-736.

Garland CF, Garland FC, Gorham ED, et al. The role of vitamin D in cancer prevention. *Am J Public Health* 2006;96:252-261.

Garnero P, Munoz F, Sornay-Rendu E, Delmas PD. Associations of vitamin D status with bone mineral density, bone turnover, bone loss and fracture risk in healthy postmenopausal women. The OFELY study. *Bone* 2006;40:716-722.

Goldberg AC. A meta-analysis of randomized controlled studies on the effects of extended-release niacin in women. *Am J Cardiol* 2004;94:121-124.

Gorham ED, Garland CF, Garland FC, et al. Optimal vitamin D status for colorectal cancer prevention: a quantitative meta analysis. *Am J Prev Med* 2007;32:210-216.

Grant AM, Anderson FH, Avenell A, et al, for the RECORD Trial group. Oral vitamin D3 and calcium for secondary prevention of low-trauma fractures in elderly people (Randomised Evaluation of Calcium Or Vitamin D, RECORD): a randomised placebo-controlled trial. *Lancet* 2005;365:1621-1628.

Grey AB, Stapleton JP, Evans MC, Tatnell MA, Ames RW, Reid IR. The effect of the antiestrogen tamoxifen on bone mineral density in normal late postmenopausal women. *Am J Med* 1995;99:636-641.

Hathcock JN, Shao A, Vieth R, Heaney RP. Risk assessment for vitamin D. *Am J Clin Nutr* 2007;85:6-18.

Health Canada. List of licensed natural health products. Available at: http://www.hc-sc.gc.ca/dhp-mps/prodnatur/applications/licen-prod/lists/listapprnhp-listeapprpsn_e.html. Acessed September 4, 2007.

Health Canada. Vitamin D and health: information update. Available at: http://hc-sc.gc.ca/ahc-asc/media/advisories-avis/2007/2007_72_e.html. Accessed July 11, 2007.

Health Canada. Vitamin D for people over 50: background. Available at: http://www.hc-sc.gc.ca/fn-an/food-guide-aliment/context/evid-fond/vita_d_e.html. Accessed July 11, 2007.

Heaney RP. Is the paradigm shifting? *Bone* 2003;33:457-465.

Heaney RP. Bone mass, nutrition, and other lifestyle factors. *Nutr Rev* 1996;54:3-10.

Heaney RP. Vitamin D: role in the calcium economy. In: Feldman D, Glorieux FH, Pike JW, eds. *Vitamin D*, 2nd ed. San Diego, CA: Academic Press, 2005: 773-787.

Heaney RP. The vitamin D requirement in health and disease. *J Steroid Biochem Mol Biol* 2005;97:13-19.

Heaney RP. Vitamin D, nutritional deficiency, and the medical paradigm. *J Clin Endocrinol Metab* 2003;88:5107-5108.

Heaney RP, Dowell MS, Barger-Lux MJ. Absorption of calcium as the carbonate and citrate salts, with some observations on method. *Osteoporos Int* 1999;9:19-23.

Heaney RP, Dowell MS, Hale CA, Bendich A. Calcium absorption varies within the reference range for serum 25-hydroxyvitamin D. *J Am Coll Nutr* 2003;22:142-146.

Heaney RP, Recker RR, Stegman MR, Moy AJ. Calcium absorption in women: relationships to calcium intake, estrogen status, and age. *J Bone Miner Res* 1989;4:469-475.

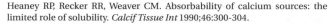

Heaney RP, Recker RR, Weaver CM. Absorbability of calcium sources: the limited role of solubility. *Calcif Tissue Int* 1990;46:300-304.

Heart Protection Study Collaborative Group. MRC/BHF Heart Protection Study of antioxidant vitamin supplementation in 20,536 high-risk individuals: a randomised placebo-controlled trial. *Lancet* 2002;360:23-33.

Holick MF. High prevalence of vitamin D inadequacy and implications for health. *Mayo Clin Proc* 2006;81:353-373.

Holick MF. Sunlight and vitamin D for bone health and prevention of autoimmune diseases, cancers, and cardiovascular disease. *Am J Clin Nutr* 2004;80(Suppl 6):1678S-1688S.

Holick MF. Vitamin D deficiency. *N Engl J Med* 2007;357:266-281.

Holick MF, Matsuoka LY, Wortsman J. Age, vitamin D, and solar ultraviolet [letter]. *Lancet* 1989;2:1104-1105.

Holick MF, Siris ES, Binkley N, et al. Prevalence of vitamin D inadequacy among postmenopausal North American women receiving osteoporosis therapy. *J Clin Endocrinol Metab* 2005;90:3215-3224.

Homocysteine Studies Collaboration. Homocysteine and the risk of ischemic heart disease and stroke: a meta-analysis. *JAMA* 2002; 288:2015-2022.

Ilich-Ernst JZ, McKenna AA, Badenhop NE, et al. Iron status, menarche, and calcium supplementation in adolescent girls. *Am J Clin Nutr* 1998;68:880-887.

Institute of Medicine, Standing Committee on the Scientific Evaluation of Dietary Reference Intakes, Food and Nutrition Board. *Dietary Reference Intakes for Calcium, Magnesium, Phosphorus, Vitamin D, and Fluoride.* Washington, DC: National Academy Press, 1997.

Ito MK, Cheung RJ, Gupta EK, et al. Key articles, guidelines, and consensus papers relative to the treatment of dyslipidemias—2005. *Pharmacotherapy* 2006;26:939-1010.

Jackson RD, LaCroix AZ, Gass M, et al, for the Women's Health Initiative Investigators. Calcium plus vitamin D supplementation and the risk of fractures. *N Engl J Med* 2006;354:669-683.

Kang JH, Cook N, Manson J, Buring JE, Grodstein F. A randomized trial of vitamin E supplementation and cognitive function in women. *Arch Intern Med* 2006;166:2462-2468.

Kim JM, White RH. Effect of vitamin E on the anticoagulant response to warfarin. *Am J Cardiol* 1996;77:545-546.

Lappe JM, Davies KM, Travers-Gustafson D, Heaney RP. Vitamin D status in a rural postmenopausal female population. *J Am Coll Nutr* 2006;25:395-402.

Lappe JM, Travers-Gustafson D, Davies KM, Recker RR, Heaney RP. Vitamin D and calcium supplementation reduces cancer risk. *Am J Clin Nutr* 2007;85:1586-1591.

Lee IM, Cook NR, Gaziano JM, et al. Vitamin E in the primary prevention of cardiovascular disease and cancer: the Women's Health Study: a randomized controlled trial. *JAMA* 2005;294:56-65.

Liu PT, Stenger S, Li H, et al. Toll-like receptor triggering of a vitamin D-mediated human antimicrobial response. *Science* 2006;311:1770-1773.

Lonn E, Bosch J, Yusef S, et al, for the HOPE and HOPE-TOO Trial Investigators. Effects of long-term vitamin E supplementation on cardiovascular events and cancer: a randomized controlled trial. *JAMA* 2005;293:1338-1347.

Lonn E, Yusef S, Arnold MJ, et al, for the Heart Outcomes Prevention Evaluation (HOPE) 2 Investigators. Homocysteine lowering with folic acid and B vitamins in vascular disease. *N Engl J Med* 2006;354:1567-1577.

Looker AC, Dawson-Hughes B, Calvo MS, Gunter EW, Sahyoun NR. Serum 25-hydroxyvitamin D status of adolescents and adults in two seasonal subpopulations from NHANES III. *Bone* 2002;30:771-777.

Lufkin EG, Whitaker MD, Nickelsen T, et al. Treatment of established postmenopausal osteoporosis with raloxifene: a randomized trial. *J Bone Miner Res* 1998;13:1747-1754.

Lukacs JL, Booth S, Kleerekoper M, Ansbacher R, Rock CL, Reame NE. Differential associations for menopause and age in measures of vitamin K, osteocalcin, and bone density: a cross-sectional exploratory study in healthy volunteers. *Menopause* 2006;13:799-808.

MacLean D. Nova Scotia Heart Health Program, Health and Welfare Canada, Nova Scotia Department of Health. *Report of the Nova Scotia Nutrition Survey.* Halifax, NS, Canada, 1993.

Matsumoto T, Miki T, Hagino H, et al. A new active vitamin D, ED-71, increases bone mass in osteoporotic patients under vitamin D supplementation: a randomized, double-blind, placebo-controlled trial. *J Clin Endcrinol Metab* 2005;90:5031-5036.

Matsuoka LY, Ide L, Wortsman J, MacLaughlin JA, Holick MF. Sunscreens suppress cutaneous vitamin D₃ synthesis. *J Clin Endocrinol Metab* 1987;64:1165-1168.

Melhus H, Michaëlsson K, Kindmark A, et al. Excessive dietary intake of vitamin A is associated with reduced bone mineral density and increased risk for hip fracture. *Ann Intern Med* 1998;129:770-778.

Meunier PJ, Vigno E, Garnero P, et al, for the Raloxifene Study Group. Treatment of postmenopausal women with osteoporosis or low bone density with raloxifene. *Osteoporos Int* 1999;10:330-336.

Meydani SN, Meydani M, Blumberg JB, et al. Assessment of the safety of supplementation with different amounts of vitamin E in healthy older adults. *Am J Clin Nutr* 1998;68:311-318.

Miller ER 3rd, Pastor-Barriuso R, Dalal D, Riemersma RA, Appel LJ, Guallar E. Meta-analysis: high-dosage vitamin E supplementation may increase all-cause mortality. *Ann Intern Med* 2005;4:142:37-46.

Napoli N, Thompson J, Civitelli R, Armamento-Villareal RC. Effects of dietary calcium compared with calcium supplements on estrogen metabolism and bone mineral density. *Am J Clin Nutr* 2007;85:1428-1433.

National Center for Complementary and Alternative Medicine. Health information. Available at: http://www.nccam.nih.gov/health/. Accessed August 5, 2007.

National Institutes of Health. NIH Consensus Development Panel on Optimal Calcium Intake. Optimal calcium intake. *JAMA* 1994;272:1942-1948.

National Osteoporosis Foundation. National Osteoporosis Foundation's Updated recommendations for calcium and vitamin D₃ intake. 2007. Available at: http://www.nof.org/prevention/calcium_and_VitaminD.htm. Accessed July 16, 2007.

National Osteoporosis Foundation. *Physician's Guide to Prevention and Treatment of Osteoporosis.* Washington, DC: National Osteoporosis Foundation, 2003.

Nesby-O'Dell S, Scanlon KS, Cogswell ME, et al. Hypovitaminosis D prevalence and determinants among African American and white women of reproductive age: third National Health and Nutrition Examination Survey, 1988-1994. *Am J Clin Nutr* 2002;76:3-4.

Nieves JW, Komar L, Cosman F, Lindsay R. Calcium potentiates the effect of estrogen and calcitonin on bone mass: review and analysis. *Am J Clin Nutr* 1998;67:18-24.

Nordin BE. Calcium and osteoporosis. *Nutrition* 1997;13:664-686.

The North American Menopause Society. Management of osteoporosis in postmenopausal women: 2006 position statement of The North American Menopause Society. *Menopause.* 2006;13:340-367.

The North American Menopause Society. The role of calcium in peri- and postmenopausal women: 2006 position statement of The North American Menopause Society. *Menopause* 2006;13:862-877.

The North American Menopause Society. Treatment of menopause-associated vasomotor symptoms: position statement of the North American Menopause Society. *Menopause* 2004;11:11-33.

O'Brien KO, Abrams SA, Liang LK, Ellis KJ, Gagel RF. Increased efficiency of calcium absorption during short periods of inadequate calcium intake in girls. *Am J Clin Nutr* 1996;63:579-583.

Office of Dietary Supplements. National Institutes of Health. Available at: http://ods.od.nih.gov. Accessed September 5, 2007.

Passeri G, Pini G, Troiano L, et al. Low vitamin D status, high bone turnover, and bone fractures in centenarians. *J Clin Endocrinol Metab* 2003;88: 5109-5115.

Peacock M, Liu G, Carey M, et al. Effect of calcium or 25OH vitamin D3 dietary supplementation on bone loss at the hip in men and women over the age of 60. *J Clin Endocrinol Metab* 2000;85:3011-3019.

Pfeifer M, Begerow B, Minne HW, Abrams C, Nachtigall D, Hansen C. Effects of a short-term vitamin D and calcium supplementation on body sway and secondary hyperthyroidism in elderly women. *J Bone Miner Res* 2000;15:1113-1118.

Porterhouse J, Cockayne S, King C, et al. Randomised controlled trial of calcium and supplementation with cholecalciferol (vitamin D$_3$) for prevention of fractures in primary care. *BMJ* 2005;330:1003-1009.

Prince RL, Devine A, Dhaliwal SS, Dick IM. Effects of calcium supplementation on clinical fracture and bone structure: results of a 5-year, double-blind, placebo-controlled trial in elderly women. *Arch Intern Med* 2006;166:869-875.

Recker RR, Hinders S, Davies KM, et al. Correcting calcium nutritional deficiency prevents spine fractures in elderly women. *J Bone Miner Res* 1996;11:1961-1966.

Reid IR, Ames RW, Evans MC, Gamble GD, Sharpe SJ. Effect of calcium supplementation on bone loss in postmenopausal women. *N Engl J Med* 1993;328:460-464.

Reid IR, Ames RW, Evans MC, Gamble GD, Sharpe SJ. Long-term effects of calcium supplementation on bone loss and fractures in postmenopausal women: a randomized controlled trial. *Am J Med* 1995;98:331-335.

Riggs BL, O'Fallon WM, Muhs J, O'Connor MK, Kumar R, Melton LJ III. Long-term effects of calcium supplementation on serum parathyroid hormone level, bone turnover, and bone loss in elderly women. *J Bone Miner Res* 1998;13:168-174.

Ross EA, Szabo NJ, Tebbett IR. Lead content of calcium supplements. *JAMA* 2000;284:1425-1429.

Rude RK, Olerich M. Magnesium deficiency: possible role in osteoporosis associated with gluten-sensitivity enteropathy. *Osteoporos Int* 1996;6:453-461.

Ryan PJ, Blake GM, Davie M, Haddaway M, Gibson T, Fogelman I. Intermittent oral disodium pamidronate in established osteoporosis: a 2-year double-masked placebo-controlled study of efficacy and safety. *Osteoporos Int* 2000;11:171-176.

Sahota O, Mundey MK, San P, Godber IM, Hosking DJ. Vitamin D insufficiency and the blunted PTH response in established osteoporosis: the role of magnesium deficiency. *Osteoporos Int* 2006;17:1013-1021.

Sebaldt RJ, Ioannidis G, Adachi JD, et al. 36 month intermittent cyclical etidronate treatment in patients with established corticosteroid induced osteoporosis. *J Rheumatol* 1999;26:1545-1549.

Shechter M, Merz CN, Paul-Labrador M, et al. Oral magnesium supplementation inhibits platelet-dependent thrombosis in patients with coronary artery disease. *Am J Cardiol* 1999;84:152-156.

Shechter M, Paul-Labrador MJ, Rude RK, Bairey Merz CN. Intracellular magnesium predicts functional capacity in patients with coronary artery disease. *Cardiology* 1998;90:168-172.

Skinner HG, Michaud DS, Giovannucci E, Willett WC, Colditz GA, Fuchs CS. Vitamin D intake and the risk for pancreatic cancer in two cohort studies. *Cancer Epidemiol Biomarkers Prev* 2006;15:1688-1695.

Slovik DM, Rosenthal DI, Doppelt SH, et al. Restoration of spinal bone in osteoporotic men by treatment with human parathyroid hormone (1-34) and 1,25-dihydroxyvitamin D. *J Bone Miner Res* 1986;1:377-381.

Song Y, Sesso HD, Manson JE, Cook NR, Buring JE, Liu S. Dietary magnesium intake and risk of incident hypertension among middle-aged and older US women in a 10-year follow-up study. *Am J Cardiol* 2006;98:1616-1621.

Specker BL. Evidence for an interaction between calcium intake and physical activity on changes in bone mineral density. *J Bone Miner Res* 1996;11:1539-1544.

Stafford RS, Drieling RL, Hersh AL. National trends in osteoporosis visits and osteoporosis treatment, 1988-2003. *Arch Intern Med* 2004;164:1525-1530.

Standing Committee on the Scientific Evaluation of Dietary Reference Intakes. *Dietary Reference Intakes for Calcium, Phosphorus, Magnesium,*

Vitamin D, and Fluoride. National Academy of Sciences, Institute of Medicine. Washington, DC: National Academy Press, 2000. Available at: http://books. nap.edu/books/0309063507/html/index.html. Accessed August 5, 2007.

Standing Committee on the Scientific Evaluation of Dietary Reference Intakes. *Dietary Reference Intakes for Thiamin, Riboflavin, Niacin, Vitamin B6, Folate, Vitamin B12, Pantothenic Acid, Biotin, and Choline.* National Academy of Sciences, Institute of Medicine. Washington, DC: National Academy Press, 1998. Available at: http://books.nap.edu/books/ 0309065542/html/index.html. Accessed August 5, 2007.

Standing Committee on the Scientific Evaluation of Dietary Reference Intakes. *Dietary Reference Intakes for Vitamin A, Vitamin K, Arsenic, Boron, Chromium, Copper, Iodine, Iron, Manganese, Molybdenum, Nickel, Silicon, Vanadium, and Zinc.* National Academy of Sciences, Institute of Medicine. Washington, DC: National Academy Press, 2000. Available at: http://books. nap.edu/catalog/10026.html. Accessed August 5, 2007.

Standing Committee on the Scientific Evaluation of Dietary Reference Intakes. *Dietary Reference Intakes for Vitamin C, Vitamin E, Selenium, and Carotenoids.* National Academy of Sciences, Institute of Medicine. Washington, DC: National Academy Press, 2000. Available at: http://books. nap.edu/books/0309069351/html/index.html. Accessed August 5, 2007.

Steingrimsdottir L, Gunnarsson O, Indridason OS, Franzson L, Sigurdsson G. Relationship between serum parathyroid hormone levels, vitamin D sufficiency, and calcium intake. *JAMA* 2005;294:2336-2341.

Stolzenberg-Solomon RZ, Vieth R, Azad A, et al. A prospective nested case-control study of vitamin D status and pancreatic cancer risk in male smokers. *Cancer Res* 2006;66:10213-10219.

Suarez FL, Savaiano DA, Levitt MD. A comparison of symptoms after the consumption of milk or lactose-hydrolyzed milk by people with self-reported severe lactose intolerance. *N Engl J Med* 1995;333:1-4.

Suarez FL, Savaiano DA, Levitt MD. The treatment of lactose intolerance. *Aliment Pharmacol Ther* 1995;9:589-597.

Thomas MK, Lloyd-Jones DM, Thadhani RI, et al. Hypovitaminosis D in medical inpatients. *N Engl J Med* 1998;338:777-783.

Toole JF, Malinow MR, Chambless LE, et al. Lowering homocysteine in patients with ischemic stroke to prevent recurrent stroke, myocardial infarction, and death: the Vitamin Intervention for Stroke Prevention (VISP) randomized controlled trial. *JAMA* 2004;291:565-575.

US Department of Health and Human Services and US Department of Agriculture. *Dietary Guidelines for Americans*, 2005, 6th ed. Washington, DC: US Government Printing Office, 2005. Available at: http://www.health.gov/ dietaryguidelines/dga2005/document/. Accessed August 5, 2007.

US Department of Health and Human Services. *Bone Health and Osteoporosis: A Report of the Surgeon General*. Rockville, MD: US Department of Health and Human Services, Office of the Surgeon General, 2004.

US Food and Drug Administration Center for Food Safety and Applied Nutrition. Dietary Supplement Current Good Manufacturing Practices (CGMPs) and Interim Final Rule (IFR) Facts. Available at: http://www.cfsan. fda.gov/~dms/dscgmps6.html. Accessed July 10, 2007.

US Food and Drug Administration Center for Food Safety and Applied Nutrition. Dietary Supplement Health and Education Act of 1994. Available at: http://vm.cfsan.fda.gov/~dms/dietsupp.html. Accessed August 5, 2007.

US Pharmacopeial Convention. *US Pharmacopeia Dispensing Information*, 20th ed. Drug Information for the Health Professional, vol 1. Englewood, CO: Micromedex, 2000.

Vieth R. Vitamin D supplementation, 25-hydroxyvitamin D concentrations, and safety. *Am J Clin Nutr* 1999;69:842-856.

Volpe SL, Taper LJ, Meacham S. The relationship between boron and magnesium status and bone mineral density in the human: a review. *Magnes Res* 1993;6:291-296.

Wactawski-Wende J, Morley Kotchen J, Anderson GL, et al, for the Women's Health Initiative Investigators. Calcium plus vitamin D supplementation and the risk of colorectal cancer. *N Engl J Med* 2006;354:684-696.

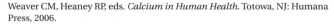

Weaver CM, Heaney RP, eds. *Calcium in Human Health*. Totowa, NJ: Humana Press, 2006.

Wooten WJ, Price W. Consensus report of the National Medical Association: the role of dairy and dairy nutrients in the diet of African Americans. *J Natl Med Assoc* 2004;96(Suppl 12):5S-31S.

Yusuf S, Dagenais G, Pogue J, Bosch J, Sleight P, for the Heart Outcomes Prevention Evaluation Study Investigators. Vitamin E supplementation and cardiovascular events in high-risk patients. *N Engl J Med* 2000;342:154-160.

Other supplements

Agency for Healthcare Research and Quality. *S-Adenosyl-L-Methionine for Treatment of Depression, Osteoarthritis, and Liver Disease. Summary, Evidence Report/Technology Assessment: Number 64*. AHRQ Publication No. 02-E033. Agency for Healthcare Research and Quality, Rockville, MD: 2002. Available at: http://www.ahrq.gov/clinic/epcsums/samesum.htm. Accessed August 5, 2007.

Bhattacharya A, Rahman M, Sun D, Fernandes G. Effect of fish oil on bone mineral density in aging C57BL/6 female mice. *J Nutr Biochem* 2007;18: 372-379.

Bruyere O, Reginster JY. Glucosamine and chondroitin sulfate as therapeutic agents for knee and hip osteoarthritis. *Drugs Aging* 2007;24:573-580.

Burr ML, Fehily AM, Gilber JF, et al. Effects of changes in fat, fish, and fibre intakes on death and myocardial reinfarction: diet and reinfarction trial. *Lancet* 1989;2:757-761.

Caruso I, Pietrogrande V. Italian double-blind multicenter study comparing S-adenosylmethionine, naproxen, and placebo in the treatment of degenerative joint disease. *Am J Med* 1987;83:66-71.

Clegg DO, Reda DJ, Harris CL, et al. Glucosamine, chondroitin sulfate, and the two in combination for painful knee osteoarthritis. *N Engl J Med* 2006;354:795-808.

Danesh J, Appleby P. Coronary heart disease and iron status: meta-analysis of prospective studies. *Circulation* 1999;99:852-854.

Dhanasekaran M, Ren J. The emerging role of coenzyme Q-10 in aging, neurodegeneration, cardiovascular disease, cancer and diabetes mellitus. *Curr Neurovasc Res* 2005;2:447-459.

DiPiro J, Talbert R, Yee GC, et al, eds. *Pharmacotherapy: A Pathophysiologic Approach*, 6th ed. New York: McGraw-Hill Medical Publishing Division, 2005.

Engeset D, Alsaker E, Lund E, et al. Fish consumption and breast cancer risk. The European Prospective Investigation into Cancer and Nutrition (EPIC). *Int J Cancer* 2006;119:175-182.

Garland ML, Hagmeyer KO. The role of zinc lozenges in treatment of the common cold. *Ann Pharmacother* 1998;32:63-69.

Hodgson JM, Watts GF, Playford DA, Burke V, Croft KD. Coenzyme Q10 improves blood pressure and glycaemic control: a controlled trial in subjects with type 2 diabetes. *Eur J Clin Nutr* 2002;56:1137-1142.

Kagan BL, Sultzer DL, Rosenlicht N, Gerner RH. Oral S-adenosylmethionine in depression: a randomized, double-blind, placebo-controlled trial. *Am J Psychiatry* 1990;147:591-595.

Karapanagiotidis IT, Bell MV, Little DC, Yakupitiyage A. Replacement of dietary fish oils by alpha-linolenic acid-rich oils lowers omega 3 content in tilapia flesh. *Lipids* 2007;42:547-559.

Khatta M, Alexander B, Krichten C, et al. The effect of coenzyme Q10 in patients with congestive heart failure. *Ann Intern Med* 2000;132:636-640.

Lim A, Manley K, Roberts M, Fraenkel M. Fish oil for kidney transplant recipients. *Cochrane Database Syst Rev* 2007:CD005282.

Ma J, Stampfer MJ. Body iron stores and coronary heart disease. *Clin Chem* 2002;48:601-603.

Marcoff L, Thompson PD. The role of coenzyme Q10 in statin-associated myopathy: a systematic review. *J Am Coll Cardiol* 2007;49:2231-2237.

Marshall PD, Poddar S, Tweed EM, Brandes L. Clinical inquiries: do glucosamine and chondroitin worsen blood sugar control in diabetes? *J Fam Pract* 2006;55:1091-1093.

McKenney JM, Sica D. Role of prescription omega-3 fatty acids in the treatment of hypertriglyceridemia. *Pharmacotherapy* 2007;27:715-728.

Metcalf RG, James MJ, Gibson RA, et al. Effects of fish-oil supplementation on myocardial fatty acids in humans. *Am J Clin Nutr* 2007;85:1222-1228.

Mourente G, Good JE, Thompson KD, Bell JG. Effects of partial substitution of dietary fish oil with blends of vegetable oils, on blood leucocyte fatty acid compositions, immune function and histology in European sea bass (*Dicentrarchus labrax L.*). *Br J Nutr* 2007;30:1-10.

Najm WI, Reinsch S, Hoehler F, Tobis JS, Harvey PW. S-Adenosyl methionine (SAMe) versus celecoxib for the treatment of osteoarthritis symptoms: a double-blind cross-over trial. [ISRCTN36233495] *BMC Musculoskelet Disord* 2004;5:6.

Office of Dietary Supplements. National Institutes of Health. Dietary supplements: background information. Available at: http://ods.od.nih.gov/factsheets/DietarySupplements_pf.asp. Accessed September 5, 2007.

Office of Dietary Supplements. National Institutes of Health. Dietary supplement fact sheet: iron. Available at: http://ods.od.nih.gov/factsheets/iron.asp. Accessed September 7, 2007.

Office of Dietary Supplements. National Institutes of Health. Facts about dietary supplements: zinc. Available at: http://ods.od.nih.gov/factsheets/cc/zinc.html. Accessed September 7, 2007.

O'Keefe JH, Harris WS. From Inuit to implementation: omega-3 fatty acids come of age. *Mayo Clin Proc* 2000;75:607-614.

Reichenbach S, Sterchi R, Scherer M, et al. Meta-analysis: chondroitin for osteoarthritis of the knee and hip. *Ann Intern Med* 2007;146:580-590.

Rosenfeld FL, Pepe S, Linnane A, et al. Coenzyme Q10 protects the aging heart against stress: studies in rats, human tissues, and patients. *Ann N Y Acad Sci* 2002;959:355-359.

Rundek T, Naini A, Sacco R, Coates K, DiMauro S. Atorvastatin decreases the coenzyme Q10 level in the blood of patients at risk for cardiovascular disease and stroke. *Arch Neurol* 2004;61:889-892.

Sandor PS, Di Clemente L, Coppola G, et al. Efficacy of coenzyme Q10 in migraine prophylaxis: a randomized controlled trial. *Neurology* 2005;64: 713-715.

Sempos CT, Looker AC, Gillum RF, Makuc DM. Body iron stores and the risk of coronary heart disease. *N Engl J Med* 1994;330:1119-1124.

Singh RB, Niaz MA, Sharma JP, Kumar R, Rastogi V, Moshiri M. Randomized, double-blind, placebo-controlled trial of fish oil and mustard oil in patients with suspected acute myocardial infarction: the Indian experiment of infarct survival—4. *Cardiovasc Drugs Ther* 1997;11:485-491.

Storch A, Jost WH, Vieregge P, et al. Randomized, double-blind, placebo-controlled trial on symptomatic effects of coenzyme Q10 in Parkinson disease. *Arch Neurol* 2007;64:938-944.

Towheed TE, Maxwell L, Anastassiades TP, et al. Glucosamine therapy for treating osteoarthritis. *Cochrane Database Syst Rev* 2005;2:CD002946.

Turner D, Zlotkin SH, Shah P, Griffiths A. Omega 3 fatty acids (fish oil) for maintenance of remission in Crohn's disease. *Cochrane Database Syst Rev* 2007:CD006320.

Yokoyama M, Origasa H, Matsuzaki M, et al, for the Japan EPA Lipid Intervention Study (JELIS) Investigators. Effects of eicosapentaenoic acid on major coronary events in hypercholesterolaemic patients (JELIS): a randomised open-label, blinded endpoint analysis. *Lancet* 2007;369: 1090-1098.

Vaginal lubricants and moisturizers

Bachmann G, Cheng RF, Rovner E. Vulvovaginal complaints. In: Lobo RA, ed. *Treatment of the Postmenopausal Woman: Basic and Clinical Aspects*, 3rd ed. San Diego, CA: Academic Press, 2007:263-269.

Gorodeski GI. Vaginal-cervical epithelial permeability decreases after menopause. *Fertil Steril* 2001;76:753-761.

Nachtigall LE. Comparative study: Replens versus local estrogen in menopausal women. *Fertil Steril* 1994;61:178-180.

The North American Menopause Society. The role of local vaginal estrogen for treatment of vaginal atrophy in postmenopausal women: 2007 position statement of The North American Menopause Society. *Menopause* 2007;14:355-369.

Society of Obstetricians and Gynaecologists of Canada. SOCG clinical practice guidelines. The detection and management of vaginal atrophy. *Int J Gynaecol Obstet* 2005;88:222-228.

Suckling J, Lethaby A, Kennedy R. Local oestrogen for vaginal atrophy in postmenopausal women. *Cochrane Database Syst Rev* 2003;6:CD001500.

Willhite LA, O'Connell MB. Urogenital atrophy: prevention and treatment. *Pharmacotherapy* 2001;21:464-480.

Topical agents for sexual pleasure

Ferguson DM, Steidle CP, Singh GS, Alexander JS, Crosby MG. Randomized, placebo-controlled, double blind, crossover design trial of the efficacy and safety of Zestra for Women in women with and without female sexual arousal disorder. *J Sex Marital Ther* 2003;29(Suppl 1):33-44.

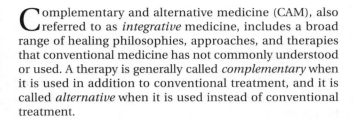

Complementary and alternative medicine (CAM), also referred to as *integrative* medicine, includes a broad range of healing philosophies, approaches, and therapies that conventional medicine has not commonly understood or used. A therapy is generally called *complementary* when it is used in addition to conventional treatment, and it is called *alternative* when it is used instead of conventional treatment.

Conventional therapies are those that are widely accepted and practiced by the mainstream medical community, including holders of MD (doctor of medicine) or DO (doctor of osteopathy) degrees, some of whom may also practice CAM. Other terms for conventional medicine are allopathic, Western, modern, and mainstream medicine, and biomedicine.

Traditional medicine refers to historical and indigenous systems of medicine that have been used for centuries. Therapies used in traditional medicine are sometimes called *natural*. Many CAM therapies are termed *holistic*, which generally means they consider the whole person, including the physical, mental, emotional, and spiritual aspects.

As reported in 2004 by the National Institutes of Health (NIH), a national survey conducted in 2002 found that 36% of Americans use some form of CAM. (When megavitamin use and prayer for health reasons are included in the definition of CAM, the percentage rises to 62%.) In a study conducted in 2003, 20% of Canadians age 12 and older reported consulting an alternative care provider in the past year. 70% of Canadians reported use of "natural health products," including herbal products, vitamin and mineral supplements, and homeopathic medicines as well as traditional medicine.

Many women who choose CAM therapies do so because these healthcare approaches mirror their own values, beliefs, and philosophic orientations toward health and life. Some turn to CAM therapies because of their dissatisfaction with conventional medicine, but most CAM users also use conventional methods. Consumers often believe that "natural" therapies are safe. However, it is unrealistic to believe that a treatment can provide benefit without the potential for negative effects.

Despite the broad use of CAM therapies, more substantial scientific information is needed to demonstrate convincingly that CAM practices are effective and safe. In 1998, the US Congress established the National Center for Complementary and Alternative Medicine (NCCAM) at the NIH to stimulate, develop, and support research on CAM for the benefit of the public. The mission of NCCAM is to provide the American public with reliable information about the safety and effectiveness of CAM practices and train CAM medicine researchers; NCCAM is not a referral agency for alternative medical treatments or individual practitioners. NCCAM can be reached through its consumer clearinghouse (toll-free at 1-888-644-6226) and through its Web site (http://nccam.nih.gov).

NCCAM groups CAM therapies into five major domains: (1) alternative medical systems, (2) mind-body medicine, (3) manipulative and body-based methods, (4) energy medicine, and (5) biologically based treatment. Brief descriptions of these systems follow.

In Canada, CAM products are regulated by the Natural Health Products Directorate (NHPD). The mission of the NHPD is to ensure access to natural health products that are safe, effective, and of high quality while respecting freedom of choice and philosophic and cultural diversity. Drugs and natural health products that are authorized for sale in Canada carry an eight-digit Drug Identification Number (DIN), a Natural Product Number (NPN), or a Drug Identification Number for Homeopathic Medicine (DIN-HM) on the label, indicating that the products have been assessed by Health Canada.

CAMline is an evidence-based Web site (www.camline.ca) for both healthcare professionals and the public that provides a specific Canadian focus.

The practice of CAM modalities is regulated individually by each Canadian province, which creates diversity regarding who is regulated and how. Naturopathy is regulated in only 4 out of 13 provinces and territories (British Columbia, Saskatchewan, Manitoba, and Ontario); traditional Chinese medicine is regulated in British Columbia only; and homeopathy is not regulated anywhere in Canada.

Alternative medical systems

Alternative medical systems include complete systems of theory and practice that have evolved independent of and often prior to the conventional biomedical approach. Many are traditional systems of medicine practiced by individual cultures throughout the world, including a number of venerable Asian approaches.

Traditional Chinese Medicine (TCM). This system of healing dates back to 200 BC in written form. TCM emphasizes the proper balance of two opposing and inseparable forces: yin and yang. Yin represents the cold, slow, or passive principle, and yang represents the hot, excited, or active principle. Any imbalance of these two forces is thought to lead to blockage in the flow of qi (pronounced "chee" and meaning vital energy) and of blood along pathways known as meridians. TCM consists of a group of techniques and methods, including acupuncture, herbal medicine, oriental massage, and qi gong, to bring the body back into harmony.

The *Chinese Materia Medica* is a standard reference book of information on medicinal substances that are used in Chinese herbal medicine. Herbal compositions are usually adjusted according to individualized diagnoses in TCM, making research on TCM herbs difficult. Many factors (eg, geographic location, harvest season, processing, storage) could impact the concentration of bioactive compounds in herbs or botanicals. In TCM, multiple herbs are usually used in combinations called "formulas," which also make standardization of herbal preparations difficult.

TCM includes menopause as part of a phenomenon that involves an imbalance of body energy. The TCM practitioner may use herbs, meditative or breathing exercises, massage, or diet to help a woman balance the energy and, therefore, reduce menopause symptoms. Acupuncture is also used by TCM practitioners in treating menopause.

Acupuncture involves stimulating specific anatomic points in the body for therapeutic purposes, usually by puncturing the skin with a needle. Acupuncture is widely practiced in North America. The US Food and Drug Administration (FDA) approved the use of acupuncture needles by licensed practitioners in 1996.

The most common acupuncture procedures use sterile, thin, solid, metallic needles that the practitioner inserts into the skin to stimulate acupuncture points. The pins are manipulated either manually or by electrical stimulation to relieve pain or prevent a broad spectrum of other health conditions. Few complications have been reported. Those that do occur are usually the result of inadequate sterilization of needles or improper needle insertion. The FDA requires manufacturers to label acupuncture needles for single use only.

Most studies evaluating the efficacy of acupuncture do not provide comparable results due to problems with design, sample size, and other factors. The results are further complicated by inherent difficulties in the use of appropriate controls, such as sham acupuncture groups.

Some specific uses for acupuncture include: pain relief; treatment of organic, mental, and emotional dysfunctions; treatment of energy disturbances; prevention of illness (eg, immune system support); induction of analgesia; treatment of addictions; and performance enhancement.

Preclinical studies have not been able to fully explain how acupuncture works within the framework of Western medicine. It is proposed that acupuncture works by conducting electromagnetic signals at a greater-than-normal rate, aiding the activity of pain-killing biochemicals. A study by Lee et al suggests that acupuncture may also alter brain chemistry by changing the release of neurotransmitters and neurohormones and affecting the parts of the central nervous system related to sensation and involuntary body functions, such as immune reactions and body regulation of temperature and of blood pressure and flow.

Acupuncture has shown efficacy in relieving the nausea and vomiting associated with surgery or chemotherapy, and it is FDA-approved for this purpose.

Studies also have shown acupuncture to be effective for postoperative dental pain. Some evidence exists for its efficacy in relieving pain associated with menstrual cramps, epicondylitis (tennis elbow), and fibromyalgia. In comparison with the side effects and iatrogenic risks of pharmaceutical therapy, which is usually prescribed for these conditions, acupuncture provides a relatively benign option.

In 1997, the NIH Consensus Development Panel on Acupuncture stated that acupuncture may be a useful adjunct or alternative therapy and it may be included in a comprehensive management program for a number of conditions, including addiction, stroke rehabilitation, headache, menstrual cramps, epicondylitis, fibromyalgia, myofascial pain, osteoarthritis, low back pain, carpal tunnel syndrome, and asthma.

Anecdotal evidence and some clinical trials support the effectiveness of acupuncture in relieving hot flashes in some women. A 2006 prospective, randomized, placebo-controlled trial (RCT) by Huang et al found that acupuncture significantly reduced severity of nocturnal hot flashes, compared with placebo. A 2007 randomized, placebo-controlled, pilot study of 29 postmenopausal women found that acupuncture significantly decreased the severity but not the frequency of hot flashes compared to placebo.

A 2007 prospective, randomized, single-blind, sham-controlled clinical trial by Vincent et al found that medical acupuncture was no better at reducing hot flashes than sham acupuncture. Acupuncture has not been shown to ameliorate general psychological distress associated with vasomotor symptoms. Future studies are merited.

Other cultural systems. Ayurveda is India's traditional system of medicine. Ayurvedic medicine (meaning "science of life") is a comprehensive system of medicine that places equal emphasis on body, mind, and spirit, and strives to restore the innate harmony of the individual. Some of the primary Ayurvedic treatments include diet, exercise, meditation, herbs, massage, exposure to sunlight, and controlled breathing.

Ayurvedic treatments have been developed in India for diseases such as diabetes, cardiovascular conditions, and neurological disorders. However, Indian medical literature suggests that the quality of clinical trials of such treatment does not meet contemporary methodological standards regarding randomization, sample size, and controls.

Other traditional medical systems have been developed by Native American, Aboriginal, African, Middle Eastern, Tibetan, and Central and South American cultures.

This textbook does not address the approach to menopause treatment using these systems.

Homeopathic medicine. Homeopathy is an unconventional Western system that is based on the principle that "like cures like" (ie, large doses of a particular substance may produce symptoms of an illness, very small doses will cure it). Minute doses of specially prepared plant extracts and minerals are used to stimulate the body's defense mechanisms and healing processes to treat illness. The approach focuses on the links among an individual's physical, emotional, and mental symptoms.

For peri- and postmenopausal women, homeopathic remedies include substances that address a group of symptoms and also enhance feelings of well-being. The three most commonly prescribed homeopathic remedies for menopausal symptoms are lachesis (derived from venom of the South American bushmaster snake), pulsatilla (derived from the wildflower *Anemone pulsatilla*), and sepia (derived from cuttlefish ink). Clinical trial results are contradictory, and systematic reviews and meta-analyses have not found homeopathy to be a definitively proven treatment for any medical condition, although homeopathic remedies generally appear safe.

Naturopathic medicine. In naturopathic medicine, disease is viewed as a manifestation of alterations in the processes by which the body naturally heals itself, and emphasizes health restoration rather than disease treatment. Naturopathic physicians employ an array of healing practices, including diet and clinical nutrition; homeopathy; acupuncture; herbal medicine; hydrotherapy; spinal and soft-tissue manipulation; physical therapies involving electric currents, ultrasound, and light therapy; therapeutic counseling; and pharmacology.

Naturopathic physicians provide primary care diagnosis and therapy. Formal training for the doctor of naturopathy (ND) degree mirrors the course work of allopathic physicians (MDs and DOs), including such areas as minor surgery, clinical pharmacology, and obstetrics, as well as classroom and clinical instruction in most of the CAM modalities. Naturopathic medicine is practiced throughout North America, Europe, Australia, and New Zealand. NDs are not licensed to practice in any of the 50 US states and are licensed in only a few of the 13 Canadian provinces and territories.

Naturopathic physicians offer a unique service, ranging from integrative medicine to lifestyle education. Individuals may choose NDs as their primary care providers, with allopathic physicians serving as specialist referrals. Most often, naturopathic physicians function as collaborators with internists, family care practitioners, and gynecologists, providing for a responsible medical care continuum. As with other CAM services, ND services are not covered by all health insurance policies.

Practice guidelines established by the American Association of Naturopathic Physicians (AANP) reflect the posture of other national medical organizations and obligate the ND to make referrals as requested by the individual or when such action is clearly in the person's best interest. Safety and efficacy of physician practice and treatment are assessed by the AANP and by peer-reviewed journals dedicated to the specific modalities themselves.

Mind-body medicine

Mind-body medicine focuses on the interactions among the brain, mind, body, and behavior, and the powerful ways in which emotional, mental, social, spiritual, and behavioral factors can directly affect health. It is an approach that respects and enhances each person's capacity for self-knowledge and self-care, and emphasizes techniques that are grounded in this approach.

Mind-body medicine includes techniques such as hypnosis; dance, music, and art therapy; prayer and mental healing; relaxation and visual imagery; meditation; and yoga. Clinical research now supports the effectiveness of mind-body interventions used in addition to conventional medicine to improve quality of life and reduce anxiety and pain.

Biofeedback can also be included in this category. Biofeedback techniques have been used with some success to control hot flashes. In addition, studies have shown that women with stress incontinence can reduce the frequency of incontinence episodes by 80% to 90% after bladder-sphincter biofeedback. Complete cures have been noted in nearly one fourth of the patients. A 2005 study by Dannecker et al found that biofeedback-assisted pelvic-floor-muscle training was effective in treating stress urinary or mixed incontinence. After the study, 71% of participants reported a persistent improvement in their incontinence symptoms. Biofeedback can also be helpful with some types of headaches.

Frequently, mind-body medicine is used in response to musculoskeletal complaints, particularly arthritis and fibromyalgia, anxiety and depression, and stress or emotional health. Major advantages to mind-body interventions are the lack of side effects and minimal health risks.

Manipulative and body-based methods

This category includes methods that are based on manipulation and/or movement of structures and systems of the body, including bones and joints, the soft tissues, and the circulatory and lymphatic systems. For example, chiropractors focus on the relation between structure (primarily the spine) and function, and the way that relation affects the preservation and restoration of health, using manipulative therapy as an integral treatment tool.

Some manipulative and body-based practices were derived from traditional systems of medicine from China, India, or Egypt, whereas others (chiropractic practices and osteopathic manipulation) were developed in the last 150 years.

There is much variation in the training and approaches of manipulative and body-based providers, but they share certain principles, such as the belief that the human body is self-regulating and has the ability to heal itself.

Osteopathic physicians (DOs) who place particular emphasis on the musculoskeletal system (believing that all the body's systems work together and that disturbances in one system may affect function elsewhere in the body) practice osteopathic manipulation. Massage therapists manipulate the soft tissues of the body to "normalize" those tissues.

Reflexology is a method of foot (and sometimes hand) massage in which pressure is applied to "reflex" zones mapped out on the feet (or hands) and can play a valuable role in inducing relaxation. Other practices include the Feldenkrais method, Trager Approach bodywork, the Alexander technique, the Bowen technique, craniosacral therapy, Rolfing, and tui na.

Energy medicine

Energy therapies focus on either energy fields originating within the body (putative energy fields, which cannot be measured, also called biofields) or those from other sources (veritable energy fields that involve the use of measurable wavelengths and frequencies, also called electromagnetic fields).

Putative energy medicine. These therapies are intended to affect the energy fields that are believed to surround and penetrate the human body. Some forms of energy therapy manipulate putative energy fields by applying pressure and/or manipulating the body by placing the practitioner's hands in, or through, these fields. Examples include qi gong, reiki, intercessory prayer, and healing touch. Qi gong is a component of TCM that combines movement, meditation, and regulation of breathing to enhance the flow of vital energy (qi) in the body, improve blood circulation, and enhance immune function. Reiki, the Japanese word representing universal life energy, is based on the belief that by channeling spiritual energy through the practitioner, the spirit is healed and it, in turn, heals the physical body. In intercessory prayer, a person intercedes through prayer on behalf of another. Healing touch is derived from the ancient technique of "laying-on of hands" and is based on the premise that it is the healing force of the therapist that affects the individual's recovery and that healing is promoted when the body's energies are in balance. By passing their hands over the individual, healers identify energy imbalances.

These approaches are some of the most controversial CAM therapies because neither the energy fields nor their therapeutic effects have been convincingly proven to exist. However, a National Center for Health Statistics survey showed that about 1% of participants had used Reiki, 0.5%

had used qi gong, and 4.6% had used some kind of healing ritual.

Veritable energy medicine. These types of therapies involve the unconventional use of electromagnetic fields to treat disease (eg, asthma, cancer) or manage pain or migraine headaches. A standard use for pulsating electromagnetic therapy is to enhance the healing of nonunion fractures; it has been claimed that this therapy is effective in treating osteoarthritis, migraine headaches, and sleep disorders. Other studies have suggested that sound-energy therapy (eg, music, wind chime, and tuning fork therapy) can help reduce pain and anxiety.

This textbook does not address the approach to menopause treatment by using these therapies.

Biologically based treatment

This category of CAM includes biologically based practices, interventions, and products, many of which overlap with conventional medicine's use of dietary supplements. Included are special dietary, orthomolecular, and individual biologic therapies, as well as herbal therapies.

Special diet therapies (eg, those proposed by Drs. Atkins, Ornish, Pritikin, and Weil) are believed to prevent and/or control illness as well as promote health. A 2007 study found that premenopausal overweight and obese women following the Atkins diet lost more weight and had more favorable metabolic effects after 12 months than women following the Zone, Ornish, or LEARN (Lifestyle, Exercise, Attitudes, Relationships and Nutrition) diets. However, questions about long-term safety and efficacy remain.

Orthomolecular therapies aim to treat disease with varying concentrations of chemicals, such as magnesium, melatonin, and megadoses of vitamins. Biologic therapies include, for example, the use of laetrile and shark cartilage to treat cancer, and bee pollen to treat autoimmune and inflammatory disease. Herbal therapies employ individual or mixtures of herbs for therapeutic value. This textbook covers botanical products used to treat menopause-related conditions.

Unlike modern plant-derived drugs, botanical therapies are complex mixtures of preparations made from the whole plant or plant part, such as root, leaves, gum, resin, or essential oil. Most botanical therapies are medicinal herbs. A medicinal herb is a plant or plant part that produces and contains chemical substances that act upon the body.

Since the early termination of the estrogen plus progestin arm of the Women's Health Initiative because of adverse events, there has been a marked increase in the use of botanical therapies by peri- and postmenopausal women to treat menopause-related symptoms. The increased use has resulted in a proliferation of new products and the need for better understanding of these botanical therapies by healthcare providers.

Herbal therapies are administered in a variety of ways, and include the following preparations that are intended for ingestion:

- Tea infusions (soft, aromatic parts of the plant are steeped, not boiled, in water)
- Tea decoctions (barks and roots, boiled in water)
- Essential oils (highly concentrated)
- Tinctures and fluid extracts (herbs macerated into water-alcohol mixtures)
- Dried standardized extracts (these typically contain part of a plant but can contain the whole plant; extracts are standardized to one ingredient only)
- Homeopathic preparations (extremely diluted)

Because of the different ways that herbal therapies are available, "recommended doses" are not provided for many of the herbs mentioned in this textbook.

Many herbal drugs were included in the *United States Pharmacopeia* (USP) from the first edition published in 1820 until the 1930s, when most of the herbal ingredients were deleted due to a "lack of general use." Yet herb products have been available, mostly as teas, and since the 1970s, as over-the-counter (OTC) capsules, tablets, and extracts. In OTC supplements, herbal therapies are standardized to one ingredient or, in the case of mixtures, to more than one ingredient. However, the content and biologic activity of the herbal therapies offered in supplement form may vary according to the production process.

Thus, clinicians and consumers must not assume that all herbal treatments labeled as containing a certain herb (eg, black cohosh) are the same. It is advisable to choose only those treatments using the same extraction process, standardized to the same ingredient(s), used in clinical trials.

In 1972, the OTC Review at the FDA evaluated all ingredients used in OTC products, requiring a higher standard of evidence (ie, controlled clinical trials) for determining safety and efficacy. Most herbs had not been subjected to clinical investigation in the United States, and the FDA's OTC expert panels did not seek data from foreign studies. Thus, most of these herbal ingredients were deemed to be in a Category III level of evidence (ie, not enough information to determine safety or efficacy) and were eventually moved to Category II (ie, banned because the ingredient was either unsafe or ineffective) because the government could not allow an ingredient of undetermined safety or efficacy to be continued on the market in OTC drug products.

Nevertheless, there was increased demand for herbal medicines in the United States. In 1994, the Dietary Supplement Health and Education Act was passed, creating a dietary supplement category that includes herbs, plants in various forms (such as extracts), enzymes, amino acids, and organ tissues as well as vitamins and minerals (see Government regulations for dietary supplements in Section H, page 237).

There are a few herbs that are still FDA approved as safe and effective ingredients in OTC drugs (eg, aloe, capsicum, cascara, ipecac, psyllium, witch hazel). Scant US governmental recognition has been given to other herbs, some of which are clinically tested and are approved as OTC medicines in other industrialized Western nations. However, the Office of Dietary Supplements (ODS), in collaboration with NCCAM—two components of the NIH—has established several Centers for Dietary Supplement Research with an emphasis on botanicals. The ODS also created an International Bibliographic Information on Dietary Supplements database, available at its Web site. More information on herbal therapies will be forthcoming.

A number of adverse events have been associated with herbal therapies. They can interact with prescription drugs, resulting in enhanced or diminished effects of the herb, the drug, or both. It is possible that a new effect may be observed that is not seen with either substance taken alone. However, the validity of many reported adverse herb-drug interactions is questionable, as some of the products used were not tested for purity.

Pharmacokinetic interactions may also occur. Mucilage-rich herbs may interfere with drug absorption. St. John's wort, an inducer of the hepatic enzyme CYP3A4, has been shown to decrease the rate of metabolism of a number of drugs. Diuretic herbs that alter sodium resorption in the renal tubule can increase plasma levels of many drugs, including lithium; women who use lithium should be asked if they are using any "slimming therapies" purchased OTC. Pharmacodynamic interactions between agonists and antagonists at receptor sites are also possible, resulting in an inhibitory or additive effect.

Dramatic quantitative and qualitative differences in drug effects may result from genetic variability in metabolizing drugs and/or herbs.

Although many drug-herb interactions are not likely to be clinically significant, caution should be exercised, particularly when prescribing drugs that have a narrow therapeutic index and serious toxicity (eg, warfarin [Coumadin]) or when the medication is necessary for life (eg, cyclosporine). Women with a disease that can be fatal if undertreated (eg, epilepsy) also require close observation.

The American College of Obstetricians and Gynecologists has issued a warning that a number of herbs, in addition to nonsteroidal anti-inflammatory drugs (NSAIDs), can cause excessive bleeding if they are taken by patients who are also taking anticoagulants. Other herbs can reduce the effectiveness of anticoagulants.

A number of herbs have been found to inhibit platelet aggregation, including dong quai, evening primrose oil, ginkgo, ginger, garlic, and feverfew (among others). Ginseng has been found to decrease platelet aggregation. (See Table 1 for a popular way of remembering four herbs that may interact with warfarin.) Combining any of these with an anticoagulant, such as warfarin, aspirin (including low-dose aspirin for cardiovascular benefits), or vitamin E, is not recommended. Women using warfarin should be told about these effects. If a woman insists on continuing herbal therapy, extra blood tests are advised, with adjustment of drug dose, when indicated. These botanicals should be avoided in women experiencing abnormal uterine bleeding. To be safe, healthcare providers should advise all women to discontinue all herbal therapy (in fact, all OTC therapies) 7 to 10 days before surgery; botanicals can usually be resumed after discharge. For more precautions when using anticoagulants, see Section H, page 243.

Table 1. Some herbs that may interact with warfarin ("the four Gs")

- Garlic
- Ginger
- *Ginkgo biloba* (may increase the anticoagulation effect)
- Ginseng (may decrease the effect)

Many herbs have hypoglycemic activity. Women who are taking insulin or oral hypoglycemics should closely monitor their blood glucose levels when adding new herbal therapies.

Biologically based CAM therapies used most often by peri- and postmenopausal women include phytoestrogens (eg, soy) and herbs (eg, black cohosh).

Phytoestrogens. The most studied of the botanicals for menopause-related conditions are compounds often termed *phytoestrogens*. They are plant-derived compounds with estrogen-like biologic activity and a chemical structure similar to that of estradiol. There are three principal groups of phytoestrogens: isoflavones, coumestans, and lignans.

Isoflavones comprise the most widely used phytoestrogens for menopause. Isoflavones are a class of phytochemicals, a broad group of nonsteroidal compounds of diverse structure that bind to estrogen receptors (ERs) in animals and human beings. Isoflavones have greater affinity for ER-β than for ER-α and possess both estrogen-agonist and estrogen-antagonist properties. The isoflavones include the biochemicals genistein, daidzein, glycitein, biochanin A, and formononetin. Genistein and daidzein are found in high amounts in soybeans and soy products as well as in red clover (see page 266 for more about red clover).

Peri- and postmenopausal women are confronted with numerous foods and supplements referred to by a variety of terms such as *phytoestrogens* or *plant estrogens, soy, soy protein*, and *isoflavones*. Unfortunately, the terms are often incorrectly used interchangeably.

Soy is the most widely used isoflavone-containing food. The term *soy* usually refers to a product derived from the whole soy (or soya) bean. *Soy protein* refers to a product derived by extracting the protein out of the whole bean.

The common soy foods and their isoflavone content are listed in Table 2. The isoflavone content of each soy food can vary considerably depending on growing conditions and processing. In Southeast Asia, many soy foods are manufactured from fermentation of soy beans (eg, miso and tempeh). This process tends to concentrate the isoflavones. Other processing to remove fats, taste, and color tends to remove isoflavones.

Table 2. Isoflavone content of foods

Food	Mean mg isoflavone per 100 g food
Soybeans, green, raw	151.17
Soy flour	148.61
Soy protein isolate	97.43
Miso soup	60.39
Tempeh	43.52
Soybeans, spouted, raw	40.71
Tofu, silken	27.91
Tofu yogurt	16.30
Soy hot dog	15.00
Soy milk	9.65
Soy sauce, shoyu	1.64

Source: Adapted from USDA-Iowa State University Database on the Isoflavone Content of Foods 1999.

Soy and other isoflavone supplements are regulated in the United States as dietary supplements; their effectiveness has not been well established, and they are not monitored for purity, amount of active ingredient, or health claims (see Government regulations for dietary supplements in Section H, page 237).

Functionally, isoflavones can exert both estrogenic and antiestrogenic effects, depending on their concentration, the concentration of endogenous sex hormones, and the specific end organ involved. Some effects of these molecules may result from interactions with pathways of cellular activity that do not involve the ERs. In addition, it is not clear whether the putative health effects in human beings are attributable to isoflavones alone or to isoflavones plus other components in whole foods.

Coronary heart disease. CHD remains the major cause of morbidity and mortality in adult women. Over the past decade there has been intense research on the potential benefit of soy protein and soy isoflavones on plasma lipids and lipoproteins as a means of reducing CHD.

Based on animal research and human epidemiologic evidence, many experts believed that consumption of soy protein and soy isoflavones could potentially reduce plasma cholesterol concentrations and reduce the risk of CHD. In 1999, the FDA approved the health claim that 25 g/day of soy protein, as part of a diet low in saturated fat and cholesterol, may reduce the risk of heart disease. Later, in 2001, the American Heart Association (AHA) recommended dietary soy protein and isoflavones for decreasing the risk of CHD. In 2006, however, the AHA reversed its recommendation and concluded that soy/soy isoflavones had such small effects on plasma lipid profiles that they probably did not reduce CHD risk.

Much of the early interest in the potential cardiovascular benefits of soy resulted from a meta-analysis of 38 studies published in 1995, which concluded that consumption of 31 to 47 g/day of soy protein could reduce plasma concentrations of both total cholesterol and low-density lipoprotein cholesterol (LDL-C). That meta-analysis was followed by a number of reports on the effect of soy protein on the plasma lipid profiles of postmenopausal women, some claiming benefits although others found no effects. There have been two well-controlled studies that seem to have placed the subject in proper perspective. A 2002 study from Tufts University concluded that the regular intake of high levels of soy protein (>50 g/d) had just a modest effect on blood cholesterol levels and only in subjects with elevated LDL-C levels (>4.14 mmol/L), although soy protein was potentially helpful when used to replace animal products in the diet. The second study, conducted in 2004 in the Netherlands, administered 25.6 g of soy protein containing 99 mg of isoflavones to postmenopausal women daily for 12 months. They found no significant effect of the soy supplementation on plasma concentrations of total cholesterol, LDL-C, high-density lipoprotein cholesterol (HDL-C), triglycerides, nor lipoprotein(a).

Those conclusions were consistent with a 2006 report by Dewell et al on the effect of soy protein and soy isoflavones on plasma lipid profiles, largely in postmenopausal women. They considered 17 studies involving soy protein and 9 studies focusing on soy isoflavone extracts. The authors concluded that both soy protein and soy isoflavone extracts caused only very small reductions in total plasma cholesterol concentrations—primarily LDL-C values—and no changes in HDL-C levels, and that these decreases were likely too small to be clinically beneficial.

Their finding was consistent with the 2006 AHA advisory on soy and cardiovascular health, which reviewed 22 randomized trials to compare isolated soy-protein isoflavones with milk and other proteins. It reported

that soy reduced plasma concentrations of LDL-C about 3% on average, with no significant effects on HDL-C, triglycerides, lipoprotein(a), or blood pressure. The panel also considered 19 studies involving purified soy isoflavone extract, and found no consistent effects on LDL-C or other plasma lipid risk factors. The overall conclusion was that any cardiovascular benefit from soy protein or isoflavone supplements would be "minimal at best."

Despite the review by Dewell and coworkers and the AHA advisory, healthcare professionals should not rush to judgment about whether soy has cardiovascular benefits, as the clinical picture is still evolving. Plasma lipid concentrations are but one surrogate marker for atherosclerosis progression and the development of CHD. In a 2007 report from Johns Hopkins, soy supplementation changed lipoprotein subclasses of postmenopausal women. There was a significant decrease in LDL-C particle number, a stronger indicator of CHD progression than LDL-C plasma concentration. Additionally, although isoflavone treatment of postmenopausal women tends not to improve plasma lipid concentrations, the isoflavones do result in significant improvement in arterial compliance and arterial stiffness, measurements closely associated with degree of atherosclerosis. Furthermore, the presence of oxidized LDL-C in artery walls enhances the accumulation of macrophage-derived foam cells in the atherosclerotic plaque, resulting in more complex and possibly less stable plaques. Interestingly, studies have found reductions in markers of LDL-C oxidation in humans consuming soy protein with isoflavones or isoflavone pills.

Whether isoflavone-containing soy protein treatment reduces the progression of atherosclerosis in postmenopausal women to an extent greater than its minimal effect on plasma lipids will soon be determined by the results of a prospective, RCT. The NIH is supporting the Women's Isoflavone Soy Health (WISH) Trial, which will end in 2009, with a primary endpoint focusing on change in carotid artery intima media thickness.

Vasomotor symptoms. There has been a major effort to determine if and to what extent soy/soy isoflavones provide benefits in the control of menopause-related vasomotor symptoms. The original basis for that effort was the observation that only 10% to 20% of Asian women have hot flashes whereas 70% to 80% of North American women experience them. It seemed reasonable to speculate that the isoflavones present in the high soy diets of Asian women were providing some protection by their binding to ERs and thus might be comparable with the well-known benefits of prescription estrogen. Up until 2006, there had been 16 RCTs conducted and reported to evaluate the effect of soy or soy isoflavones on vasomotor symptoms. Small benefits were found in half the trials and no benefits in the other half. There is no clear explanation for the conflicting outcomes; however, most of the trials lasted for 12 weeks or fewer and it has been claimed that longer trials are necessary to obtain reliable outcome data. Consequently, the following recent trials are described, one lasting 12 weeks and another lasting 12 months.

In 2007, Cheng et al reported a double-blind, prospective study in which 60 healthy postmenopausal women (40-69 y) were randomized to a placebo group and a group that was given a soy drink containing 60 mg/day of soy isoflavones. The treatment period was 12 weeks. Both hot flashes and night sweats were significantly decreased in the soy isoflavone–treated groups.

In 2006, Newton et al described a 12-month RCT of 351 women aged 45 to 55 years, of whom 52% were perimeno-pausal and 48% were postmenopausal. First, the authors evaluated a multibotanical intervention, then the effect of the addition of a soy diet to that intervention; then both were compared with traditional menopausal hormone therapy (HT). The soy diet provided 12 to 20 g/day of soy protein. The results of the interventions on hot flashes and night sweats, respectively, showed that the addition of the soy diet had no effect while HT was highly effective.

Another source of isoflavones, red clover, has been studied mainly for hot flashes. Six trials of two types of red clover isoflavones provided data for a meta-analysis by Nelson et al. This included Promensil (40 mg/d, 80-82 mg/d, 160 mg/d) and Rimostil (57 mg/d). The combined weighted mean difference in the number of daily hot flashes for red clover isoflavones compared with placebo was –0.44 (95% confidence interval [CI], –1.47-0.58) and was not statistically significant. Quality of trials and type of red clover isoflavone did not influence results.

Vaginal dryness. Two recent studies have explored the potential benefits of isoflavones for the treatment of postmenopausal vaginal dryness. An experienced group of investigators at the Helsinki University Central Hospital conducted a double-blind, randomized, placebo-controlled crossover trial. The isoflavone treatment consisted of 114 mg/day of isoflavones for 3 months. The investigators concluded that the isoflavones had no effect on subjective perception of vaginal dryness or on objective findings in the vagina.

A year later, the results of a study of peri- and postmenopausal women was reported by a group from Bangkok. This study was also a randomized crossover trial, and women were given either placebo or 25 g/day of soy. The authors concluded that a soy-rich diet did not relieve the urogenital symptoms, restore the vaginal epithelium, nor improve vaginal health of peri- and postmenopausal Thai women.

Breast and uterine effects. The trial by Cheng et al is the only study of soy and vasomotor symptoms to have reported on important safety issues. The investigators performed breast biopsies before and after 12 weeks of soy isoflavone treatment. The expression levels of ER-α, -β, and -βcx and progesterone receptors (PRs) A and B and proliferation rates,

as measured by the proliferation marker Ki67, did not change as a result of the soy treatment, suggesting no estrogen-agonist effect of the soy isoflavones on breast tissue. That observation is consistent with extensive studies done in monkeys and reported by Wood et al. Endometrial thickness was also measured by ultrasound, with histology at sampling, before and after 12 weeks of soy isoflavone treatment. As for the breast, ERs and PRs were evaluated before and after treatment as was proliferation using the Ki67 marker. There were no changes in any of these measures before or after the soy isoflavone treatment. Again, their observations on the endometrium are consistent with extensive studies of monkeys and should allay any concerns for the endometrial safety of soy isoflavones.

Bone metabolism. Over the past decade, there has been encouraging evidence that soy and soy isoflavones might have beneficial effects in retarding postmenopausal bone loss. Numerous studies with ovariectomized rats found that soy and soy isoflavones increased bone mineral density (BMD). The expectation of bone benefits for soy was heightened by the elucidation of a possible molecular mechanism; genistein and equol bind to ER-β and thus offer a rationale for a bone effect. Initially, there were about equal numbers of short-term clinical trials finding that soy isoflavones increased bone mineral content and BMD versus those that found no benefit. Recently, however, strong evidence has been reported indicating no benefits of soy or soy isoflavones on postmenopausal bone loss. Gallagher et al reported in 2004 that for postmenopausal women (mean age, 55 y) neither soy containing 52 mg/day nor 96 mg/day of isoflavones for 15 months had any benefits for BMD compared with soy protein having only traces of isoflavones. In that same year, Kreijkamp-Kaspers et al found no effect on BMD in postmenopausal women given a soy protein supplement that provided 99 mg/day of isoflavones.

Perhaps the most definitive evidence for a lack of effect of soy and soy isoflavones comes from a 2007 report by Cheong et al. A novel approach capable of detecting even trivial effect on bone was used: that of labeling the bones of postmenopausal women with 41Ca, a long-lived radiotracer, and then measuring the urinary excretion of the labeled Ca compared with the unlabeled Ca. In a crossover design, they compared 0, 97.5, and 135.5 mg/day of soy isoflavones. Additionally, they compared those effects with one woman who took HT. Neither dose of soy isoflavones had any effect, whereas the woman given HT had a major change in the urinary ratio of labeled to unlabeled calcium.

Cognitive function. Favorable effects of soy and soy isoflavones on cognitive function of postmenopausal women may emerge as their best documented health benefit. In 2003, Kritz-Silverstein et al reported the results of an RCT in which postmenopausal women aged 55 to 74 years were treated for 6 months with 110 mg/day of soy isoflavones. The study found a significant improvement in category fluency and a trend toward improvement in verbal memory among the soy isoflavone–treated women compared with those given placebo. In 2005, File et al reported the results of a double-blind, placebo-matched trial in which postmenopausal women aged 51 to 66 years were treated with 60 mg/day of soy isoflavones. The soy isoflavone treatment resulted in significant improvement in mental flexibility and planning ability. In 2006, Casini et al found similar improvements in cognitive function of postmenopausal women treated with 60 mg/day of soy isoflavones.

Summary. Whether and to what extent soy and soy isoflavones may have beneficial effects on cardiovascular health remain uncertain. There is now good evidence that they have no clinically significant effect on plasma concentrations of lipids and lipoproteins; however, they may inhibit the progression of atherosclerosis by other mechanisms, such as by prevention of oxidation of LDL-C particles, changes in LDL-C particle size, or direct artery effects on compliance or stiffness. An ongoing clinical trial should provide an answer.

Soy and soy isoflavones may have small benefits in the treatment of vasomotor symptoms in the short term (12 wk) but not for longer periods (6-12 mo). There is now good evidence that use of soy for treatment of vasomotor symptoms is "safe" for breast and endometrium. There is also strong evidence that neither soy nor soy isoflavones provide any benefit in the prevention of postmenopausal bone loss.

The most promising use of soy and soy isoflavones by postmenopausal women appears to be on maintaining cognitive function. Additional studies are needed to better understand soy's effect on cognitive function.

Herbs. A number of herbs have been used to treat acute menopause-related symptoms, including black cohosh and dong quai, plus a wide variety of multiherbal products. Herbs are generally not considered for the prevention or treatment of diseases, such as osteoporosis.

Many OTC products contain mixtures of various herbs that are advertised for relief of menopause-related symptoms. Although anecdotal evidence may support efficacy, there are scant clinical trial data to document safety or efficacy for most.

Many women and some healthcare providers believe that herbal therapies are safer than prescription drugs because they are "natural," but herbs can have pharmacologic effects and adverse side effects. RCTs are needed to document the safety and efficacy of these products. In addition, there are no studies regarding concomitant use with traditional postmenopausal HT or bone-specific agents. Because of the lack of clinical trial data, it is prudent to exercise caution with these therapies.

Marketed herb products are regulated in the United States as dietary supplements. Although some manufacturers have rigorous quality control measures in place, many products are not monitored for purity, levels of active/marker compounds, or health claims. Proprietary brand information is provided in this section to distinguish the tested herbal formulas from untested brands; however, this does not imply that these brands are better than other brands (see Government regulations for dietary supplements in Section H, page 237).

The following sections present information on some of the more commonly used herbs for treating peri- and postmenopausal women. Herbs are listed alphabetically.

Black cohosh. Preparations made from the rhizomes (underground stems) of black cohosh (botanical name *Cimicifuga racemosa* or *Actaea racemosa*) have been used by North American Indians for medicinal purposes for hundreds of years. Europeans have been using this native North American plant to treat menopause-related symptoms for more than 50 years. In 1989, the respected German Federal Institute for Drugs and Medical Devices approved black cohosh for menopause-related complaints, as well as for premenstrual syndrome and dysmenorrhea.

Although a number of the plant's constituents have been identified, its precise mechanism of action is unknown.

Black cohosh is the most widely studied herb for the treatment of menopause-related symptoms. As with most herbal supplements, not all brands are identical. Most older clinical trials have used the preparation marketed as Remifemin. The formulation and strength have changed during the past 40 years; thus, studies performed with earlier versions of Remifemin may not be applicable to the currently marketed preparation. The currently marketed tablet contains 20 mg of black cohosh isopropanolic extract, which has 1 mg triterpenes (standardized to triterpene glycoside 27-deoxyactein).

In three randomized, placebo-controlled clinical trials comparing black cohosh with estrogen for treating hot flashes, results were inconclusive. A 12-month federally funded 2006 study by Newton et al failed to find any benefit for one type of black cohosh (160 mg/d ethanolic extract) over placebo in relieving hot flashes. A 2006 RCT by Uebelhack et al found that a fixed combination of black cohosh and St. John's wort was better than placebo in treating menopausal symptoms, including those with a strong psychological component. Two trials of shorter duration showed no advantage over placebo using either Remifemin (40 mg/d) or BNO 1055 (Klimadynon, Menofem), a standardized black cohosh preparation (dose equivalent to 40 mg/d). The third trial found that an earlier formulation of Remifemin was more effective than either estrogen or placebo in relieving hot flashes.

A 24-week clinical trial by Liske et al that evaluated the effects of Remifemin black cohosh (39 mg/d or 127.3 mg/d) on vaginal cytology and reproductive hormone levels found that its benefit in relieving hot flashes was not associated with systemic estrogen-agonistic effects. While Remifemin appears to have little or no estrogenic activity, the overall effect on breast cancer is unknown.

A 3-month RCT in 2007 examining the effect of black cohosh (160 mg/d) on lipids, fibrinogen, glucose, and insulin in women aged 45 to 55 years concluded that there were no statistical differences between herbal groups and placebo.

No vaginal bleeding has been reported in study periods of up to 6 months. In a study by Raus et al, no increases in endometrial thickness as measured by ultrasound were observed after 52 weeks of treatment. A yearlong study failed to note any significant adverse events with 160 mg/day of an ethanolic extract. Some experts believe that longer trials are required to ensure endometrial safety.

The incidence of adverse events with black cohosh is relatively low, particularly with single-agent supplements. Side effects include occasional gastrointestinal (GI) discomfort, nausea, vomiting, dizziness, frontal headache, and bradycardia. The gastrointestinal disturbances are primarily with first use.

There have been more than 50 case reports that suggest a possible link between liver failure and black cohosh use. This prompted the Australian Therapeutic Goods Authority and Health Canada to require cautionary statements on all retail black cohosh product labels. The USP Dietary Supplements Panel has recommended a cautionary warning on black cohosh products that states, "In rare cases black cohosh may affect the liver. Consult a healthcare practitioner prior to use if you have a liver disorder or if you develop symptoms of liver trouble, such as abdominal pain, dark urine, extreme fatigue, or jaundice." While a cause and effect cannot be stated with certainty, practitioners should be alert to the possibility and counsel patients appropriately.

With the supplement Remifemin, a daily dose of 40 mg is the recommended dose. Results should be evident within 8 to 12 weeks.

In the United States, Remifemin and other supplements containing black cohosh are marketed and regulated as dietary supplements. In Canada, these supplements are Natural Health Products.

Cranberry. The juice of cranberries, also known as *Vaccinium macrocarpon*, has been used as a home remedy for urinary tract infections. Although it was formerly thought to work via acidification of the urine, current research demonstrates that it works primarily by preventing bacterial adherence to the urinary epithelia. In a 1994 study of elderly women

(mean age, 78.5 y) by Avorn et al, cranberry juice recipients had significantly lower odds of having bacteria with pyuria than they did when they received the placebo (27% vs 42%). A 2007 study by Bailey et al found that a concentrated cranberry preparation could reduce the recurrence of urinary tract infections in women with a history of recurring infections.

Dong quai. This aromatic herb, also known as *Angelica sinensis*, Chinese angelica, tang kuei, or dang gui, has been used as a medicinal herb in China for at least 1,200 years. Among Chinese therapies, it is the most extensively used herb for treating gynecologic conditions. It is also used to stimulate the circulation.

Different effects are observed when the root is extracted with different solvents. Water extracts first stimulate the myometrium, then relax it, whereas alcohol extracts (tinctures) exert only a relaxant effect. Some practitioners caution against using dong quai in women who have heavy menstrual flow, as it will tend to increase bleeding.

Efficacy for the relief of hot flashes has not been confirmed in controlled clinical trials. In the only double-blind, randomized, placebo-controlled trial to date (71 women), Hirata et al found that 4.5 g/day of dong quai used for 6 months was no more helpful than placebo in relieving hot flashes. It did not affect estrogenization of vaginal epithelial cells or endometrial thickness, as measured by transvaginal ultrasound. Practitioners trained in TCM counter that dong quai is not meant to be used alone, but rather in an individually tailored mixture of herbs. More research is needed to determine its efficacy and safety.

Side effects include photosensitivity and anticoagulation. Dong quai can trigger heavy uterine bleeding and should never be used in women who have fibroids, hemophilia, or other blood-clotting problems. It is contraindicated for use with anticoagulants.

Evening primrose oil. This plant, also called *Oenothera biennis*, produces seeds that are rich in oils containing γ-linolenic acid. Preparations made from the oils are reported to improve atopic eczema, reduce hypercholesterolemia, and relieve mastalgia.

Evening primrose oil is also promoted as relieving hot flashes; however, the only RCT (Chenoy et al) found no benefit over placebo for treating menopause-related hot flashes in 56 women.

The usual dose of evening primrose oil in oral supplement form is 1,500 to 3,000 mg daily. Reported side effects include inflammation, thrombosis, immunosuppression, nausea, and diarrhea. It may increase the risk of seizures in patients diagnosed with schizophrenia who are taking antipsychotics. It should not be used with phenothiazines. Evening primrose is also available in a topical preparation.

Ginkgo. This herb, also known as *Ginkgo biloba*, has been used as a medicinal agent for at least three millenia. Standardized extracts of the leaf have been used to treat many conditions, including vertigo, tinnitus, intermittent claudication, short-term memory loss, macular degeneration, and asthma. Ginkgo is thought to act by dilating blood vessels, reducing blood viscosity, modifying neurotransmitters, and acting as a potent antioxidant.

The primary use of ginkgo is to treat cerebral function disorders, including age-related cognitive decline, and slowing the progress of neurodegenerative disorders such as Alzheimer's disease. A 2007 updated Cochrane review reported trials showing improvement in cognition, activities of daily living, and mood. The review concludes that although there is promising evidence of efficacy, overall there are no compelling trial data showing that ginkgo improves cognition or cerebral function. There were also no significant differences in adverse events between ginkgo and placebo.

The most serious adverse event purportedly associated with ginkgo use is bleeding. However, whether ginkgo actually increases the risk of bleeding is not known. An RCT by Bal Dit Sollier et al evaluated 32 young, healthy, male volunteers for the effect of three doses (120, 240, and 480 mg/d) of *Ginkgo biloba* extract (Egb761) on hemostasis, coagulation, and fibrinolysis. After 14 days of repeated administration, ginkgo did not induce any significant modification of bleeding time, platelet function, or coagulation when compared with placebo. Subdural hematoma and other bleeding complications have been reported when ginkgo is used by patients receiving anticoagulant therapies; however, a recent study in healthy adults demonstrated that, when taken at recommended doses, ginkgo did not alter the international numeralized ratio (INR) or the pharmacokinetics or pharmacodynamics of warfarin when the patients were given a single, large dose of warfarin (25 mg) after 1 week of pretreatment with ginkgo.

The most common adverse effects reported with ginkgo use are GI distress and headache. Large doses may cause restlessness, anxiety, allergic skin reactions, sleep disturbances, and GI upset, including diarrhea, nausea, and vomiting.

The extracts used in most clinical trials are standardized to contain 24% flavonoids and 6% terpenes. The usual dose is 40 to 80 mg standardized-extract capsules three times daily. Treatment should be continued for at least 6 weeks to evaluate therapeutic effect. Among ginkgo supplements, the specific brands reported to have been used in most clinical trials are Tebonin (marketed in the United States as Ginkgold and Ginkoba) and Kaveri (marketed in the United States as Ginkai).

Ginseng. The most common types of ginseng are Chinese (or Korean or Asian) ginseng (*Panax ginseng*) and American ginseng (*Panax quinquefolius*). Eleuthero, also known as "Siberian ginseng" (*Eleutherococcus senticosus*) is not a true ginseng as it is not in the *Panax* genus. The various types of ginseng exhibit different effects. It is the multibranched root of these perennial, shade-loving plants that is used in botanical medicine.

Preparations of Asian ginseng root have been held in high esteem in TCM for thousands of years. More recently, marketers of ginseng supplements have promoted the products for women and men to build stamina and resistance to disease, although there is no strong documentation for these claims.

Ginseng contains more than a dozen terpenoids, especially a group of compounds called ginsenosides. Ginseng may exert estrogenic effects, although the plant does not actually contain phytoestrogens. Most clinical trials have used the ginseng supplement with the trade name Ginsana.

Ginseng has been studied for menopause-related complaints. The only RCT (Wiklund et al) found that a ginseng extract had no overall effect on vasomotor symptoms, serum levels of estrogen or follicle-stimulating hormone, or endometrial thickness in 384 postmenopausal women. Also, overall quality of life was not improved, although there was improvement in subsets involving depression, general health, and well-being.

Although ginseng is generally well tolerated, reported side effects have included nervousness, insomnia, dizziness, and hypertension. Mastalgia with diffuse breast nodularity also has been reported.

Although case reports suggest that ginseng can raise blood pressure, studies in animals and humans have found either no effect on blood pressure or a mild blood-pressure–lowering effect. In addition, several clinical trials have shown that ginseng can lower blood glucose levels. Ginseng should be used with caution by those with cardiovascular disease, diabetes, or bipolar disorder.

Case reports have associated ginseng with uterine bleeding. These reports, however, did not examine the ginseng products for adulterants. Adulteration and substitution of ginseng products has been a significant problem for many years, given the high price of the root in the international market.

In an RCT by Yuan et al, 2 weeks of American ginseng administration to subjects receiving warfarin significantly reduced the INR when compared with placebo. However, a pharmacokinetics study performed in rats did not reveal alterations in warfarin levels or impact on prothrombin time after administration of Asian ginseng. Though these herbs are related, they contain different constituents that may, in part, account for the differences in the data. Practitioners should counsel patients to exercise caution if taking anticoagulant therapy. Some experts contraindicate the use of ginseng with antihypertensives or stimulants, including dietary supplement remedies containing ma huang, ephedrine, or guarana.

Doses of standardized extracts used in clinical trials range from 100 to 600 mg/day (standardized to 4% ginsenoside).

Kava. Kava rhizome, also known as *Piper methysticum*, is used for treating anxiety, hot flashes, and sleep disruption. Active constituents in kava include the kavalactones (also called kavapyrones). Kava is ingested as a tea or as a dietary supplement. In two small studies of kava in postmeno-pausal women, significant improvements were seen in symptoms on several scales, including the Depression Status Inventory.

Laitain (sometimes called Laitan) is the brand of kava supplement that has been tested in most clinical studies. This product is not imported into the United States.

Kava has been linked with cases of severe hepatotoxicity, including active liver failure, cholestatic hepatitis, and cirrhosis of the liver. As a result, some countries (eg, Canada, United Kingdom, Germany, Australia) have banned kava supplements. In March 2002, the FDA issued a warning recommending that kava products not be used before consulting a physician. The FDA has not concluded whether kava has a causal relationship to liver disease. Although kava is still sold in the United States, many manufacturers stopped selling it due to concerns of possible litigation and inability to obtain product liability insurance.

Kava should not be used with alcohol, psychotropic medication, antihistamines, or any substance that may cause sleepiness or confusion. Reported side effects include minor GI upset, headache, sedation, or restlessness in a small percentage of users. Heavy, chronic use of kava may cause yellowing of the skin and an ichthyosiform (fish scale–like) eruption known as kava dermopathy, often accompanied by eye irritation.

Given the hepatotoxicity concerns, it may be advisable to avoid use altogether until more is known.

Licorice. The root of the licorice plant, also known as *Glycyrrhiza glabra*, contains coumarins, flavonoids, and terpenoids. The most well-known ingredients of licorice are glycyrrhizinic acid and its derivatives.

Although it is mostly used for its anti-inflammatory, antibacterial, antiviral, and expectorant properties, small amounts of licorice are often included in TCM formulations for postmenopausal women. Any therapeutic benefit may be due to the mild estrogenic activity of the compound beta-sitosterol.

Licorice root tinctures, extracts, capsules, and lozenges are available. Most licorice candies manufactured in the United States do not contain licorice but are flavored with anise, whereas imported candies usually contain real licorice. Licorice is also found in many teas and OTC cough remedies that are sold in the United States.

In TCM, licorice is always used as part of a mixture. The synergistic effects of mixtures, and perhaps dose limitations, may prevent side effects. The vast majority of reported cases of licorice-induced adverse events have been from licorice-containing candies, gums, laxatives, or chewing tobacco, not from the use of licorice as herbal medicine.

Large, chronic doses of licorice may result in pseudoprimary aldosteronism with symptoms that may include edema, hypertension, and hypokalemia. Cardiac arrhythmias and cardiac arrest, including two known deaths, have occurred in chronic consumers of licorice candy products. Cardiomyopathy, hypokalemic myopathy, and pulmonary edema have also been reported. Hypokalemia due to licorice may be potentiated by the use of diuretics, so the combination should be avoided.

A proposed warning from the USP states the following: "Excessive amounts or long-term chronic use of licorice may cause high blood pressure or low potassium. Licorice can exacerbate kidney failure, cirrhosis and congestive heart failure. Diuretic use may increase risk. If you are pregnant or nursing a baby, seek the advice of a health professional before using this product."

Sage. Some women use sage, or *Salvia officinalis*, to help with hot flashes and night sweats. While the teas are likely safe, the ethanolic extracts are not generally recommended owing to the toxicity of at least one of its components, a volatile oil called thujone. Prolonged or excessive doses of herbs that contain thujone can cause vomiting, vertigo, kidney damage, and convulsions.

St. John's wort. In Germany, St. John's wort, also known as *Hypericum perforatum*, is the most popular treatment for mild to moderate depression, and a growing number of women are taking it alone in supplement form or in combination with black cohosh to ease hot flashes.

One RCT (Uebelhack et al) found the combination of black cohosh and St. John's wort to be more effective than placebo for relieving hot flashes. In March 2006, the NIH began conducting a clinical trial evaluating the effectiveness of St. John's wort for alleviating hot flashes in women with nonmetastatic breast cancer.

Many European RCTs have been conducted on this herb. Its mechanism of action is unknown, although some studies suggest that it may be similar to that of prescription antidepressant medications. Hyperforin is the most frequently cited active constituent, as it is known to exhibit sedative effects.

In a 2005 updated database review, the Cochrane group identified 37 trials involving 2,291 patients using St. John's wort to treat mild to moderately severe depressive disorders. Most trials were 4 to 6 weeks long. The data indicate that St. John's wort was superior to placebo and was as effective as standard antidepressants. Side effects were reported by 26.3% of those on St. John's wort compared with 44.7% on antidepressants.

Of the 37 trials examined, some were placebo comparisons and some were synthetic standard antidepressant comparisons. In large trials of patients with major depression, the combined response rate ratio for hypericum extracts compared with placebo was 1.15 (95% CI, 1.02-1.29). In large trials not restricted to patients with major depression, the response rate ratio was 1.71 (95% CI, 1.40-2.09).

A 2006 review of common botanicals used for treatment of mood and anxiety disorders in peri- and postmenopausal women (Geller et al) found that five of seven trials of St. John's wort for mild to moderate depression showed significant improvement.

The results of several trials comparing St. John's wort with the selective serotonin reuptake inhibitors (SSRIs), which are government approved for the treatment of depression, were mixed. In 2002, an RCT by the Hypericum Depression Trial Study Group found that neither St. John's wort nor the SSRI sertraline performed significantly better than placebo in treating patients with major depressive disorder.

In 2005, two studies comparing St. John's wort with SSRIs found it at least as effective as paroxetine (Szegedi et al) and significantly more effective than fluoxetine (Fava et al) for moderate to severe and major depression. Studies in 2006 found it to be as efficacious as citalopram (Gastpar et al) for moderate depression and paroxetine (Anghelescu et al) for preventing relapse after recovery from moderate to severe depression. In several of the studies, St. John's wort was reported to be better tolerated than SSRIs in patients.

The brands of St. John's wort supplements used in most clinical trials include Jarsin (manufactured by Lichtwer and marketed in the United States by Abkit as Kira), Neuroplant (manufactured by Schwabe and marketed in the United States by Nature's Way as Perika and by Pharmaton as Movana), and Remotiv (manufactured by Bayer and marketed in the United States as St. John's wort by GNC). (Exact information is provided to distinguish the tested herbal formulas from untested brands; however, this does not imply that these brands are better than other brands.)

The usual dose of St. John's wort in supplement form is 300 to 600 mg (standardized to contain 3%-5% hyperforin, 0.3% hypericin, or both) three times daily. Onset of action occurs in 2 to 4 weeks. Many CAM practitioners avoid using this herb for longer than 2 years.

Gastrointestinal side effects have been reported with St. John's wort, although dosing with food minimizes upset. Fatigue is also associated with use of this herb and, in rare cases, it can increase sensitivity to sunlight. Combined with sunlight, it may also contribute to cataract formation. Those using St. John's wort should avoid sunbathing and wear sunblock, a hat, and sunglasses.

St. John's wort should not be used concomitantly with psychotropic medications. Taken with SSRIs, it may result in too much serotonin (called "serotonin syndrome"), causing dizziness, restlessness, and muscle twitching. St. John's wort may decrease serum levels of warfarin, digoxin, theophylline, indinavir, cyclosporine, and phenprocoumon. Breakthrough vaginal bleeding has occurred when St. John's wort was used with an oral contraceptive containing ethinyl estradiol and desogestrel.

Valerian. Preparations are made from the roots and underground plant parts of valerian, or *Valeriana officinalis*. This herb is used primarily to treat nervousness and insomnia and is recognized by the German health authorities and the World Health Organization for these purposes. A systematic review of RCTs of valerian for improving sleep quality (Bent et al) showed a statistically significant benefit and suggested that valerian may improve sleep quality without producing side effects.

The brand of valerian supplement tested in clinical studies is Sedonium (marketed in the United States under the same name by Abkit).

No substantial side effects of valerian have been noted with recommended dosages, although long-term administration may be associated with headache, restlessness, sleeplessness, and cardiac disorders. Unlike other sedatives, it does not appear to interact with alcohol to intensify drowsiness.

Valerian improves subjective experiences of sleep when taken nightly for 1 to 2 weeks and it appears to be a safe hypnotic sedative choice in patients with mild to moderate insomnia. The evidence for single-dose efficacy is contradictory. A number of studies indicate that a single dose is no better than placebo for sedation and that it must be taken for at least 5 to 7 days for effect. However, if a woman suffers from stress or chronic insomnia, the underlying factors should be assessed.

The usual daily dose of valerian extract is 100 to 1,800 mg.

Vitex. This herb, also known as *Vitex agnus-castus*, is commonly used for premenstrual syndrome, irregular menstruation, and cyclical mastalgia and is approved by the German health authorities for all three conditions. Vitex is generally standardized to its iridoid glycoside content, calculated as agnoside. Side effects are mild and include nausea, headache, gastrointestinal disturbances, menstrual disorders, acne, pruritus, and erythematous rash (Daniele et al).

A two-part study conducted in 2000 and 2002 (Lucks et al) found that participants taking vitex experienced strong symptomatic relief of some common menopausal symptoms. RCTs have shown it improves symptoms of premenstrual syndrome, normalizes luteal-phase length, and increases luteal-phase progesterone levels. Some herbalists recommend the herb to reduce the heavy, irregular uterine bleeding experienced by some peri-menopausal women.

Vitex is reputed to have a libido-reducing effect in both women and men, and this effect is responsible for its other names: chaste-tree berry (or chasteberry) and monk's pepper. Although clinicians who recommend vitex indicate that this effect is rare, they advise that women with low libido should not be given this herb.

The usual daily dose of vitex is approximately 250 mg of crude herb. The dose of standardized extracts (12:1 ratio) is 20 mg/day.

Suggested reading

Alternative medical systems

Andrews GJ, Boon H. CAM in Canada: places, practices, research. *Complement Therap Clin Practice* 2005;11:21-27.

Berman BM, Swyers JP, Hartnoll SM, Singh BB, Bausell B. The public debate over alternative medicine: the importance of finding a middle ground. *Altern Ther Health Med* 2000;6:98-101.

Buckman R, Lewith G. What does homeopathy do—and how? *BMJ* 1994;309:103-106.

Cohen SM, Rousseau ME, Carey BL. Can acupuncture ease the symptoms of menopause? *Holist Nurs Pract* 2003;17:295-299.

Dower C, O'Neil EH, Hough HJ. *Profiling the Professions: A Model for Evaluating Emerging Health Professions*. San Francisco, CA: Center for the Health Professions, University of California, San Francisco, 2001.

Ernst E. Is homeopathy a placebo? *Br J Clin Pharmacol* 1990;30:173-174.

Fugh-Berman A. Herbs, phytoestrogens, and other CAM therapies. In: Lobo RA, ed. *Treatment of the Postmenopausal Woman: Basic and Clinical Aspects*, 3rd ed. San Diego, CA: Academic Press, 2007:684-690.

Health Canada Office of Natural Health Products. Available at: http://www.hc-sc.gc.ca/hpfb-dgpsa/nhpd-dpsn/index_e.html. Accessed August 28, 2007.

Huang MI, Nir Y, Chen B, Schnyer R, Manber R. A randomized controlled pilot study of acupuncture for postmenopausal hot flashes: effect on nocturnal hot flashes and sleep quality. *Fertil Steril* 2006;86:700-710.

Ikenze I, Akenze A. *Menopause & Homeopathy: A Guide for Women in Midlife*. Berkeley, CA: North Atlantic Books, 1999.

Irvin JH, Friedman R, Zuttermeister PC, et al. The effect of relaxation response training on menopausal symptoms. *J Psychosom Obstet Gynecol* 1996;17:201-207.

Lee BY, LaRiccia PJ, Newberg AB. Acupuncture in theory and practice. *Hosp Physician* 2004;40:11-18.

Linde K, Clausius N, Ramirez G, et al. Are the clinical effects of homeopathy placebo effects? A meta-analysis of placebo-controlled trials. *Lancet* 1997;350:834-843.

Linde K, Jonas WB, Melchart D, Willich S. The methodological quality of randomized controlled trials of homeopathy, herbal medicines and acupuncture. *Int J Epidemiol* 2001;30:526-531.

Lockie A, Geddes L. *The Woman's Guide to Homeopathy*. London, UK: Penguin Group, 1992.

MacEoin B. *Homeopathy for Menopause*. Rochester, VT: Healing Arts Press, 1997.

Murray MT, Pizzorno JE, eds. *Encyclopedia of Natural Medicine*, 2nd ed. Rocklin, CA: Prima Publishing, 1998.

National Center for Complementary and Alternative Medicine. Get the facts: what is complementary and alternative medicine (CAM)? Available at: http://nccam.nci.nih.gov/health/whatiscam/. Accessed August 28, 2007.

National Center for Complementary and Alternative Medicine. Research report: acupuncture. Available at: http://nccam.nih.gov/health/acupuncture/. Accessed August 28, 2007.

National Institutes of Health Office of Alternative Medicine, Practice and Policy Guidelines Panel. Clinical practice guidelines in complementary and alternative medicine. An analysis of opportunities and obstacles. *Arch Fam Med* 1997;6:149-154.

NIH Consensus Conference. Acupuncture. *JAMA* 1998;280:1518-1524.

Park J. Use of alternative health care. *Health Reports* 2005;16:39-41.

Reilly DT, Taylor MA, Beattie NG, et al. Is evidence for homeopathy reproducible? *Lancet* 1994;344:1601-1606.

Sandberg M, Wijma K, Wyon Y, Nedstrand E, Hammar M. Effects of electro-acupuncture on psychological distress in postmenopausal women. *Complement Ther Med* 2002;10:161-169.

Vincent A, Barton D, Mandrekar J, et al. Acupuncture for hot flashes: a randomized, sham-controlled clinical study. *Menopause* 2007;14:45-52.

Wyon Y, Lindgren R, Lundeberg T, Hammar M. Effects of acupuncture on climacteric vasomotor symptoms, quality of life, and urinary excretion of neuropeptides among postmenopausal women. *Menopause* 1995;2:3-12.

Zell B, Hirata J, Marcus A, et al. Diagnosis of symptomatic postmenopausal women by traditional Chinese medicine practitioners. *Menopause* 2000;7:129-134.

Mind-body medicine

Burgio KL, Locher JL, Goode PS, et al. Behavioral vs drug treatment for urge urinary incontinence in older women: a randomized controlled trial. *JAMA* 1998;280:1995-2000.

Burns PA, Pranikoff K, Nochajski T, et al. A comparison of effectiveness of biofeedback and pelvic muscle exercise treatment of stress incontinence in older community-dwelling women. *J Gerontol* 1993;48:167-174.

Cardozo LD. Biofeedback in overactive bladder. *Urology* 2000;55(suppl): S24-S28.

Dannecker C, Wolf V, Raab R, Hepp H, Anthuber C. EMG-biofeedback assisted pelvic floor muscle training is an effective therapy of stress urinary or mixed incontinence: a 7-year experience with 390 patients. *Arch Gynecol Obstet* 2005;273:93-97.

Godfrey, JR. Toward Optimal Health: Eva Selhub, MD, discusses mind-body medicine for women. *J Womens Health* 2006:15:111-115.

Manipulative and body-based methods

National Center for Complementary and Alternative Medicine Health Information. Available at: http://www.nccam.nih.gov/health/. Accessed August 28, 2007.

O'Mathuna DP. Reflexology for relaxation. *Alternative Ther in Women's Health*. 2007;3:17-21.

Energy medicine

Barnes P, Powell-Griner E, McFann K, Nahin R. Complementary and alternative medicine use among adults: United States, 2002. CDC *Advance Data Report* #343. 2004.

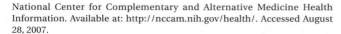

National Center for Complementary and Alternative Medicine Health Information. Available at: http://nccam.nih.gov/health/. Accessed August 28, 2007.

Vallbona C, Richards T. Evolution of magnetic therapy from alternative to traditional medicine. *Phys Med Rehabil Clin North Am* 1999;10:729-754.

Biologically based treatment

The American College of Obstetricians and Gynecologysts. ACOG Practice Bulletin No. 84: Prevention of deep vein thrombosis and pulmonary embolism. *Obstet Gynecol* 2007;110(2 Pt 1):429-440.

Gardner CD, Kiazand A, Alhassan S, et al. Comparison of Atkins, Zone, Ornish, and LEARN diets for change in weight and related risk factors among overweight premenopausal women: the A to Z Weight Loss Study: a randomized trial. *JAMA* 2007;297:969-977.

Office of Dietary Supplements. International Bibliographic Information on Dietary Supplements (IBIDS) database. Available at: http://www.ods.od.nih.gov/Health_Information/IBIDS.aspx. Accessed August 29, 2007.

Phytoestrogens

Adlercreutz H. Epidemiology of phytoestrogens. *Baillieres Clin Endocrinol Metab* 1998;12:605-623.

Albertazzi P, Pansini F, Bonaccorsi G, Zanotti L, Forini E, de Aloysio D. The effect of dietary soy supplementation on hot flushes. *Obstet Gynecol* 1998;91:6-11.

Allen JK, Becker DM, Kwiterovich PO, Lindenstruth KA, Curtis C. Effect of soy protein-containing isoflavones on lipoproteins in postmenopausal women. *Menopause* 2007;14:106-114.

Anderson JW, Johnstone BM, Cook-Newell ML. Meta-analysis of the effects of soy protein intake on serum lipids. *N Engl J Med* 1995;333:276-282.

Baird DD, Umbach DM, Lansdell L, et al. Dietary intervention study to assess estrogenicity of dietary soy among postmenopausal women. *J Clin Endocrinol Metab* 1995;80:1685-1690.

Casini ML, Marelli G, Papaleo E, Ferrari A, D'Ambrosio F, Unfer V. Psychological assessment of the effects of treatment with phytoestrogens on postmenopausal women: a randomized, double-blind, crossover, placebo-controlled study. *Fertil Steril* 2006;85:972-978.

Cheng G, Wilczek B, Warner M, Gustafsson J, Landgren B. Isoflavone treatment for acute menopausal symptoms. *Menopause* 2007;14:1-6.

Cheong JMK, Martin BR, Jackson GS, et al. Soy isoflavones do not affect bone resorption in postmenopausal women: a dose-response study using a novel approach with 41Ca. *J Clin Endocrinol Metab* 2007;92:577-582.

Dewell A, Hollenbeck PL, Hollenbeck CB. Clinical review: a critical evaluation of the role of soy protein and isoflavone supplementation in the control of plasma cholesterol concentrations. *J Clin Endocrinol Metab* 2006;91:772-780.

Erdman JW. AHA science advisory: soy protein and cardiovascular disease: a statement for healthcare professionals from the Nutrition Committee of the AHA. *Circulation* 2000;102:2555-2559.

File SE, Hartley DE, Elsabagh S, Duffy R, Wiseman H. Cognitive improvement after 6 weeks of soy supplements in postmenopausal women is limited to frontal lobe function. *Menopause* 2005;12:193-201.

Gallagher JC, Satpathy R, Rafferty K, Haynatzka V. The effect of soy protein isolate on bone metabolism. *Menopause* 2004;11:290-298.

Howes JB, Sullivan D, Lai N, et al. The effects of dietary supplementation with isoflavones from red clover on the lipoprotein profiles of post menopausal women with mild to moderate hypercholesterolaemia. *Atherosclerosis* 2000;152:143-147.

Hudson T. *Women's Encyclopedia of Natural Medicine*. Los Angeles, CA: Keats Publishing, 1999.

Ingram D, Sanders K, Kolybaba M, Lopez D. Case-control study of phyto-oestrogens and breast cancer. *Lancet* 1997;350:990-994.

Jenkins DJ, Kendall CW, Garsetti M, et al. Effect of soy protein foods on low-density lipoprotein oxidation and ex vivo sex hormone receptor activity—a controlled crossover trial. *Metabolism* 2000;49:537-543.

Jenkins DJ, Kendall CW, Vidgen E, et al. Effect of soy-based breakfast cereal on blood lipids and oxidized low-density lipoprotein. *Metabolism* 2000;49:1496-1500.

Kreijkamp-Kaspers S, Kok L, Grobbee DE, et al. Effect of soy protein containing isoflavones on cognitive function, bone mineral density, and plasma lipids in postmenopausal women. *JAMA* 2004;292:65-74.

Kritz-Silverstein D, Von Mühlen D, Barrett-Connor E, Bressel MA. Isoflavones and cognitive function in older women: the Soy and Postmenopausal Health In Aging (SOPHIA) Study. *Menopause* 2003;10:196-202.

Kuiper GG, Lemmen JG, Carlsson B, et al. Interaction of estrogenic chemicals and phytoestrogens with estrogen receptor beta. *Endocrinology* 1998;139:4252-4263.

Lichtenstein AH, Jalbert SM, Adlercreutz H, et al. Lipoprotein response to diets high in soy or animal protein with and without isoflavones in moderately hypercholesterolemic subjects. *Arterioscler Thromb Vasc Biol* 2002;22:1852-1858.

Manonai J, Songchitsomboon S, Chanda K, Hong JH, Komindr S. The effect of a soy-rich diet on urogenital atrophy: a randomized, cross-over trial. *Maturitas* 2006;54:135-140.

Marini H, Minutoli L, Polito F, et al. Effects of phytoestrogen genistein on bone metabolism in osteopenic postmenopausal women: a randomized trial. *Ann Intern Med* 2007;146:839-847.

Martin PM, Horwitz KB, Ryan DS, McGuire WL. Phytoestrogen interaction with estrogen receptors in human breast cells. *Endocrinology* 1978;103:1860-1867.

Mei J, Yeung SS, Kung AW. High dietary phytoestrogen intake is associated with higher bone mineral density in postmenopausal but not premenopausal women. *J Clin Endocrinol Metab* 2001;86:5217-5221.

Merz-Demlow BE, Duncan AM, Wangen KE, et al. Soy isoflavones improve plasma lipids in normocholesterolemic, premenopausal women. *Am J Clin Nutr* 2000;71:1462-1469.

Nelson HD, Vesco KK, Haney E, et al. Nonhormonal therapies for menopausal hot flashes: systematic review and meta-analysis. *JAMA* 2006;295:2057-2071.

Nestel PJ, Yamashita T, Sasahara T, et al. Soy isoflavones improve systemic arterial compliance but not plasma lipids in menopausal and perimenopausal women. *Arterioscler Thromb Vasc Biol* 1997;17:3392-3398.

Newton KM, Reed SD, LaCroix AZ, Grothaus LC, Ehrlich K, Guiltinan J. Treatment of vasomotor symptoms of menopause with black cohosh, multibotanicals, soy, hormone therapy, or placebo. *Ann Intern Med* 2006;145:869-879.

Nikander E, Rutanen EN, Nieminen P, Wahlstrom T, Ylikorkala O, Tiitinen A. Lack of effect of isoflavonoids on the vagina and endometrium in postmenopausal women. *Fertil Steril* 2005;83:137-142.

The North American Menopause Society. The role of isoflavones in menopausal health: consensus opinion of The North American Menopause Society. *Menopause* 2000;7:215-229.

Pepine CJ, von Mering GO, Kerensky RA, et al, for the WISE Study Group. Phytoestrogens and coronary macrovascular function in women with suspected myocardial ischemia: a report from the Women's Ischemia Syndrome Evaluation (WISE) Study. *J Womens Health* 2007;16:481-488.

Sacks FM, Lichtenstein A, Van Horn L, Harris W, Kris-Etherton P, Winston M. Soy protein, isoflavones and cardiovascular health: an American Heart Association Science Advisory for professionals from the Nutrition Committee. *Circulation* 2006;113:1034-1044.

Samman S, Lyons Wall PM, Chan GS, Smith SJ, Petocz P. The effect of supplementation with isoflavones on plasma lipids and oxidisability of low density lipoprotein in premenopausal women. *Atherosclerosis* 1999;147:277-283.

Schabath MB, Hernandez LM, Wu X, Pillow PC, Spitz MR. Dietary phytoestrogens and lung cancer risk. *JAMA* 2005;294:1493-1504.

Secreto G, Chiechi LM, Amadori A, et al. Soy isoflavones and melatonin for the relief of climacteric symptoms: a multicenter, double-blind, randomized study. *Maturitas* 2004;47:11-20.

Simons LA, von Konigsmark M, Simons J, Celermajer DS. Phytoestrogens do not influence lipoprotein levels or endothelial function in healthy, postmenopausal women. *Am J Cardiol* 2000;85:1297-1301.

St. Germain A, Peterson CT, Robinson JG, Alekel DL. Isoflavone-rich or isoflavone-poor soy protein does not reduce menopausal symptoms during 24 weeks of treatment. *Menopause* 2001;1:17-26.

Tikkanen MJ, Wahala K, Ojala S, Vihma V, Adlercreutz H. Effect of soybean phytoestrogen intake on low density lipoprotein oxidation resistance. *Proc Natl Acad Sci USA* 1998;95:3106-3110.

Unfer V, Casini ML, Costabile L, Mignosa M, Gerli S, Di Renzo GC. Endometrial effects of long-term treatment with phytoestrogens: a randomized, double-blind, placebo-controlled study. *Fertil Steril* 2004;82:145-148.

USDA-Iowa State University Database on the Isoflavone Content of Foods. 2007. Available at: http://www.ars.usda.gov/SP2UserFiles/Place/12354500/Data/isoflav/isoflav1-4.pdf. Accessed August 24, 2007.

van der Schouw YT, Pijpe A, Lebrun CE, et al. Higher usual dietary intake of phytoestrogens is associated with lower aortic stiffness in postmenopausal women. *Arterioscler Thromb Vasc Biol* 2002;22:1316-1322.

Wangen KE, Duncan AM, Xu X, Kurzer MS. Soy isoflavones improve plasma lipids in normocholesterolemic and mildly hypercholesterolemic postmenopausal women. *Am J Clin Nutr* 2001;73:225-231.

Welty FK, Lee KS, Lew NS, Zhou J-R. Effect of soy nuts on blood pressure and lipid levels in hypertensive, prehypertensive, and normotensive postmenopausal women. *Arch Intern Med* 2007;167:1060-1067.

Wiseman H, O'Reilly JD, Adlercreutz H, et al. Isoflavone phytoestrogens consumed in soy decrease F(2)-isoprostane concentrations and increase resistance of low-density lipoprotein to oxidation in humans. *Am J Clin Nutr* 2000;72:395-400.

Wood CE, Register TC, Franke AA, Anthony MS, Cline JM. Dietary soy isoflavones inhibit estrogen effects in the postmenopausal breast. *Cancer Res* 2006;66:1241-1249.

Herbs

Amato P, Christophe S, Mellon PL. Estrogenic activity of herbs commonly used as remedies for menopausal symptoms. *Menopause* 2002;9:145-150.

Anghelescu IG, Kohnen R, Szegedi A, Klement S, Kieser M. Comparison of *Hypericum* extract WS 5570 and paroxetine in ongoing treatment after recovery from an episode of moderate to severe depression: results from a randomized multicenter study. *Pharmacopsychiatry* 2006;39:213-219.

Avorn J, Monane M, Gurwitz JH, Glynn RJ, Choodnovskiy I, Lipsitz LA. Reduction of bacteriuria and pyuria after ingestion of cranberry juice. *JAMA* 1994;271:751-754.

Bailey DT, Dalton C, Joseph Daugherty F, Tempesta MS. Can a concentrated cranberry extract prevent urinary tract infections in women? A pilot study. *Phytomedicine* 2007;14:237-241.

Bal Dit Sollier C, Caplain H, Drouet L. No alteration in platelet function or coagulation induced by Egb761 in a controlled study. *Clin Lab Haematol* 2003;25:251-253.

Bent S, Padula A, Moore D, Patterson M, Mehling W. Valerian for sleep: a systematic review and meta-analysis. *Am J Med* 2006;119:1005-1012.

Bergmann J, Luft B, Boehmann S, Runnebaum B, Gerhard I. The efficacy of complex medication Phyto-Hypophyson L in female, hormone-related sterility. A randomized, placebo-controlled clinical double-blind study [in German]. *Forsch Komplementarmed Klass Naturheilkd* 2000;7:190-199.

Birks J, Grimley EV. Ginkgo biloba for cognitive impairment and dementia (Cochrane review). *Cochrane Database Syst Rev* 2007;2:CD003120.

Blumenthal M, Goldberg A, Brinckmann J, eds. *Herbal Medicine: Expanded Commission E Monographs*. Newton, MA: Integrative Medicine Communications, 2000.

Cagnacci A, Arangino S, Renzi A, Zanni AL, Malmusi S, Volpe A. Kava-kava administration reduces anxiety in perimenopausal women. *Maturitas* 2003;44:103-109.

Chenoy R, Hussain S, Tayob Y, et al. Effect of oral gamolenic acid from evening primrose oil on menopausal flushing. *BMJ* 1994;308:501-503.

Daniele C, Thompson Coon J, Pittler MH, Ernst E. Vitex agnus castus: a systematic review of adverse events. *Drug Sac* 2005;28:319-332.

David E, Morris D. Medicinal uses of licorice through the millennia: the good and plenty of it. *Mol Cell Endocrinol* 1991;78:1-6.

Duker E-M, Kopanski L, Jarry H, Wuttke W. Effects of extracts from *Cimicifuga racemosa* on gonadotropin release in menopausal women and ovariectomized rats. *Planta Med* 1991;57:420-424.

Fava M, Alpert J, Nierenberg AA, et al. A double-blind, randomized trial of St John's wort, fluoxetine, and placebo in major depressive disorder. *J Clin Psychopharmacol* 2005;25:441-447.

Fugh-Berman A. Herbs, phytoestrogens, and other CAM therapies. In: Lobo RA, ed. *Treatment of the Postmenopausal Woman: Basic and Clinical Aspects*, 3rd ed. San Diego, CA: Academic Press, 2007:684-690.

Gastpar M, Singer A, Zeller K. Comparative efficacy and safety of a once-daily dosage of hypericum extract STW3-VI and citalopram in patients with moderate depression: a double-blind, randomized, multicentre, placebo-controlled study. *Pharmacopsychiatry* 2006;39:66-75.

Geller SE, Studee L. Botanical and dietary supplements for mood and anxiety in menopausal women. *Menopause* 2006;14:541-549.

Hirata JD, Swiersz LM, Zell B, Small R, Ettinger B. Does dong quai have estrogenic effects in postmenopausal women? A double-blind, placebo-controlled trial. *Fertil Steril* 1997;68:981-986.

Hopkins MP, Androff L, Benninghoff AS. Ginseng face cream and unexplained vaginal bleeding. *Am J Obstet Gynecol* 1988;159:1121-1122.

Hudson T. *Women's Encyclopedia of Natural Medicine*. Los Angeles, CA: Keats Publishing, 1999.

Huntley AL, Ernst E. A systematic review of herbal medicinal products for the treatment of menopausal symptoms. *Menopause* 2003;10:465-476.

Hypericum Depression Trial Study Group. Effect of *Hypericum perforatum* (St John's wort) in major depressive disorder: a randomized controlled trial. *JAMA* 2002;287:1807-1814.

Israel D, Youngkin E. Herbal therapies for perimenopausal and menopausal complaints. *Pharmacotherapy* 1997;17:970-984.

Jacobson JS, Troxel AB, Evans J, et al. Randomized trial of black cohosh for the treatment of hot flashes among women with a history of breast cancer. *J Clin Oncol* 2001;19:2739-2745.

Jiang X, Williams KM, Liauw WS, et al. Effect of ginkgo and ginger on the pharmacokinetics and pharmacodynamics of warfarin in healthy subjects. *Br J Clin Pharmacol* 2005;59:425-432.

Kim HL, Streltzer J, Goebert D. St. John's wort for depression: a meta-analysis of well-defined clinical trials. *J Nerv Ment Dis* 1999;187:532-538.

Kontiokari T, Sundqvist K, Nuutinen M, Pokka T, Koskela M, Uhari M. Randomised trial of cranberry-lingonberry juice and Lactobacillus GG drink for the prevention of urinary tract infections in women. *BMJ* 2001;322:1571.

Kuhlmann J, Berger W, Podzuweit H, Schmidt U. The influence of valerian treatment on "reaction time, alertness and concentration" in volunteers. *Pharmacopsychiatry* 1999;32:235-241.

Lieberman S. A review of the effectiveness of *Cimicifuga racemosa* (black cohosh) for the symptoms of menopause. *J Womens Health* 1998;7:525-529.

Lindahl O, Lindwall L. Double blind study of a valerian preparation. *Pharmacol Biochem Behav* 1989;32:1065-1066.

Linde K, Mulrow CD, Berner M, Egger M. St John's wort for depression (Cochrane review). *Cochrane Database Syst Rev* 2005;2:CD000448.

Liske E. Therapeutic efficacy and safety of *Cimicifuga racemosa* for gynecologic disorders. *Adv Ther* 1998;15:45-53.

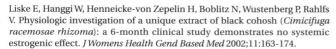

Liske E, Hanggi W, Henneicke-von Zepelin H, Boblitz N, Wustenberg P, Rahlfs V. Physiologic investigation of a unique extract of black cohosh (*Cimicifuga racemosae rhizoma*): a 6-month clinical study demonstrates no systemic estrogenic effect. *J Womens Health Gend Based Med* 2002;11:163-174.

Low Dog T, Powell KL, Weisman SM. Critical evaluation of the safety of *Cimicifuga racemosa* in menopause symptom relief. *Menopause* 2003;10:299-313.

Lucks BC. Vitex agnus castus essential oil and menopausal balance: a research update. *Complement Ther Nurs Midwifery* 2003;9:157-160.

Lucks BC, Sorensen J, Veal L. Vitexagnus-castus essential oil and menopausal balance: a self-care survey. *Complement Ther Nurs Midwifery* 2002;8:148-154.

Medical Economics. *Physician's Desk Reference (PDR) for Herbal Medicine*, 3rd ed. Montvale, NJ: Thomson Healthcare, 2004.

Nesselhut T, Scheillhase C, Dietrich R, Kuhn W. Studies on mammary carcinoma cells regarding the proliferative potential of herbal medications with estrogen-like effects. *Arch Gynecol Obstet* 1993;258:817-818.

Newall CA, Anderson LA, Phillipson JD, eds. *Herbal Medicines: A Guide for Health Care Professionals*. London, UK: Pharmaceutical Press, 1996.

Newton KM, Reed SD, LaCroix AZ, Grothaus LC, Ehrlich K, Guiltinan J. Treatment of vasomotor symptoms of menopause with black cohosh, multibotanicals, soy, hormone therapy, or placebo: a randomized trial. *Ann Intern Med* 2006;145:869-879.

Noe J. Angelic sinensis: a monograph. *J Naturopathic Med* 1997;7:66-72.

The North American Menopause Society. Treatment of menopause-associated vasomotor symptoms: position statement of The North American Menopause Society. *Menopause* 2004;11:11-33.

Osmers R, Friede M, Liske E, Schnitker J, Freudenstein J, Henneicke-von Zepelin H-H. Efficacy and safety of isopropanolic black cohosh extract for climacteric symptoms. *Obstet Gynecol* 2005;105:1074-1083.

Page RL 2nd, Lawrence JD. Potentiation of warfarin by dong quai. *Pharmacotherapy* 1999;19:870-876.

Raus K, Brucker C, Gorkow C, Wuttke W. First-time proof of endometrial safety of the special black cohosh extract (*Actaea* or *Cimicifuga racemosa* extract) CR BNO 1055. *Menopause* 2006;13:678-691.

Robbers JE, Tyler VE, eds. *Tyler's Herbs of Choice: The Therapeutic Use of Phytomedicinals*, 2nd ed. Binghamton, NY: Haworth Herbal Press, 1999.

Rotblatt M, Ziment I, eds. *Evidence-Based Herbal Medicine*. Philadelphia, PA: Haney & Belfus, 2002.

Schellenberg R. Treatment for the premenstrual syndrome with agnus castus fruit extract: prospective, randomised, placebo controlled study. *BMJ* 2001;322:134-137.

Seidl MM, Stewart DE. Alternative treatments for menopausal symptoms: qualitative study of women's experiences. *Can Fam Physician* 1998;44:1271-1276.

Seidl MM, Stewart DE. Alternative treatments for menopausal symptoms: systematic review of scientific and lay literature. *Can Fam Physician* 1998;44:1299-1308.

Shelton RC, Keller MB, Gelenberg A, et al. Effectiveness of St. John's wort in major depression. *JAMA* 2001;285:1978-1986.

Solomon PR, Adams F, Silver A, Zimmer J, DeVeaux R. Ginkgo for memory enhancement: a randomized controlled trial. *JAMA* 2002; 288:835-840.

Sprangler L, Newton KM, Grothaus LC, et al. The effects of black cohosh on lipids, fibrinogen, glucose and insulin. *Maturitas* 2007;57:195-204.

Szegedi A, Kohnen R, Dienel A, Kieser M. Acute treatment of moderate to severe depression with hypericum extract WS 5570 (St John's wort): randomized controlled double blind non-inferiority trial versus paroxetine. *BMJ* 2005;330:503.

Uebelhack R, Blohmer JU, Graubaum HJ, Busch R, Gruenwald J, Wernecke KD. Black cohosh and St. John's wort for climacteric complaints. *Obstet Gynecol* 2006;107:247-255.

Vogler BK, Pittler MH, Ernst E. The efficacy of ginseng: a systematic review of randomised clinical trials. *Eur J Clin Pharmacol* 1999;55:567-575.

Wiklund IK, Mattsson LA, Lindgren R, Limoni C, for the Swedish Alternative Medicine Group. Effects of a standardized ginseng extract on quality of life and physiological parameters in symptomatic postmenopausal women: a double-blind, placebo-controlled trial. *Int J Clin Pharmacol Res* 1999;19:89-99.

World Health Organization (WHO). *Rhizoma cimicifugae racemosae. WHO Monographs on Selected Medicinal Plants*. Geneva, Switzerland: WHO Publications, 2002.

Yuan CS, Wei G, Dey L, et al. Brief communication: American ginseng reduces warfarin's effect in healthy patients: a randomized, controlled trial. *Ann Intern Med* 2004;141:23-27.

Zava DT, Dollbaum CM, Blen M. Estrogen and progestin bioactivity of foods, herbs, and spices. *Proc Soc Exp Biol Med* 1998;217:369-378.

Zhu M, Chan KW, Ng LS, Chang Q, Chang S, Li RC. Possible influences of ginseng on the pharmacokinetics and pharmacodynamics of warfarin in rats. *J Pharm Pharmacol* 1999;51:175-180.

Zierau O, Bodinet C, Kolba S, Wulf M, Vollmer G. Antiestrogenic activities of Cimicifuga racemosa extracts. *J Steroid Biochem Mol Biol* 2002;80:125-130.

Notes

This section of the textbook addresses various issues to consider when counseling women about health issues related to menopause. Managing patients should involve addressing their concerns based on scientific evidence while also being respectful and considering their individual priorities.

Social and cultural aspects of care

Health status and health outcomes are determined by many factors in addition to the physical factors. They include education, income, social status, housing, employment, health services, community support, spirituality, personal health practices, and the physical environment.

Differences between middle-class Caucasian women and women of other social and cultural backgrounds have implications for the way they experience menopause and for their future health and well-being. Risk factors, morbidity and mortality patterns, and access to health care differ among these groups. However, there are few data on these differences as they relate to menopause, because much of the current body of health information is based on Caucasian, relatively healthy, middle-class women.

United States. From the 2000 census, there were approximately 40 million postmenopausal women in the United States. This includes more than 3.5 million African-American, 1 to 2 million Hispanic, and 1 million Asian women. In 2000, almost 10% of the US population was foreign born. Nearly 15% are estimated to speak a foreign language at home. Millions of American-born residents follow the traditions and beliefs of other cultures. The census also reported that about one in three US residents was multiethnic, multiracial, or multicultural; by mid-century, about 47% of the population will be nonwhite. Thus, it is likely that most practitioners in the United States will care for women of many races and cultures.

In the United States, rates of diabetes mellitus (DM), hypertension, and obesity are much higher among African-American, Hispanic-American, and American-Indian women than among Caucasian-American women. African-American women are reported to have a 50% higher prevalence of hypertension, and it develops at an earlier age. When treated for hypertension, African-American women have significantly greater risk reductions in fatal and nonfatal cardiovascular events and in all-cause mortality.

Osteoporosis rates are higher among Caucasian-American women than African Americans. This is most likely because of higher bone mineral densities (BMDs) in African-American women associated with fewer hip fractures (5.6% vs 15.3% for Caucasian Americans). African-American and Asian-American women have higher rates of lactose intolerance than do Caucasian-American women. African-American women have lower rates of endometrial cancer

(1.5% vs 2.6%) and breast cancer (7.3% vs 10.2%), although each of these cancers is more likely to be fatal.

Many immigrant groups present special challenges with disease risks different from those in the United States.

Canada. Canadian healthcare professionals face similar social and cultural challenges in meeting the needs of an increasingly diverse population. Currently, the growth rate of the immigrant population is approximately three times that of the Canadian-born population. Sources of immigration to Canada have also shifted recently. There are increasing numbers of immigrants from Asia, Central and South America, the Middle East, and Africa. Although there is a lack of ethnos-specific national data, some analyses suggest that recent immigrant women report better health and are less likely to engage in risky health behaviors, such as smoking and regular alcohol consumption, than Canadian-born women. Unfortunately, immigrant women are more likely to report poor health and higher morbidity than Canadian-born women over time.

Canadian Aboriginal women represent about 3% of the total population of Canadian women. However, they face multiple health burdens, including poor health status, poverty, violence, and substance abuse. Health practices of Aboriginal women are very different from those of the general Canadian female population. They are twice as likely to smoke and to have alcohol dependence. They are at higher risk for chronic diseases (eg, cardiovascular disease [CVD], DM, arthritis, cervical cancer, human immuno-deficiency virus [HIV], and acquired immune deficiency syndrome [AIDS]) and have higher death rates for heart disease and stroke. Their life expectancy is 5 years lower than the national average for Canadian women.

The Canadian Women's Health Surveillance Report identified other vulnerable groups. Single mothers were more likely than partnered women to be poor and to experience higher rates of distress, personal and chronic stress, violence, and emotional abuse. Incarcerated women were at higher risk of exposure to HIV/AIDS, antibiotic-resistant tuberculosis, hepatitis C infections, and sexually transmitted infections. Rural women had significantly higher rates of mortality than urban women.

Ethnicity and menopause. With respect to menopause, variations exist across racial and ethnic groups in the frequency and severity of menopause-related symptoms, and attitudes toward menopause, use of menopausal hormone therapy (HT), and the healthcare system.

The Study of Women's Health Across the Nation (SWAN) is a 10-year longitudinal trial of several ethnic groups of US women—including African Americans, Caucasian Americans, Chinese Americans, Japanese Americans, and Hispanic Americans—designed to examine group differences with respect to the transition to menopause.

In general, women's attitudes toward menopause were neutral to positive. Among the groups, African-American women were significantly more positive in attitude than other groups. The least positive groups were the less acculturated Chinese-American and Japanese-American women. The results also suggest that factors other than those directly associated with menopause status, including socioeconomics, smoking, and other demographic factors, had a substantial effect on attitudes toward menopause.

Other US surveys have also found similar attitudinal differences regarding menopause. These studies have shown that African-American, Japanese-American, and Chinese-American women report significantly fewer symptoms associated with menopause than Caucasian-American women. However, African-American women report more vasomotor symptoms than Caucasian-American women, although they do not find them as bothersome. Both Japanese-American and Chinese-American women have shown more negative attitudes toward menopause than Caucasian-American women, despite their report of fewer symptoms.

Multiple studies, with a variety of ethnic groups, suggest that assumptions cannot be made about the menopause experience of women from different ethnic communities living in Western countries. A study compared the experience of menopause and quality of life in a migrated Asian population living in the United Kingdom with a matched sample of Caucasian women in the same area and a sample of Asian women with a similar socioeconomic background living in Delhi, India. The women in India reported fewer hot flashes (32%) than the UK Asian (75%) and Caucasian (61%) groups. Both the UK Asian and Caucasian groups reported similar menopause experiences.

While some variability in menopause symptom severity can be attributed to differences in definitions, measurements, and analysis, some key comparative studies provide strong evidence that this variability is real, and it is possible to delineate the factors that account for it. Some of these factors are biological. For example, in populations in which many women experience surgical menopause, symptom frequency is higher than among those who experience natural menopause. Similarly, where more women smoke or the incidence of obesity is high, symptom frequency will be higher than in populations where these characteristics are rare.

It is also clear, however, that social factors play a significant role in explaining the experience of particular symptoms and the meaning attached to menopause as a phase of life. Such factors include socioeconomic status, definitions of women's position across the life cycle, prevalent ideas about body functioning, and norms related to femininity and aging. In addition, the healthcare industry has an important influence on the attitudes of women and clinicians.

Whether menopause is accepted as a natural phase of life or considered to be a medical condition requiring treatment will depend on many factors, including the extent to which therapies are available and accessible to the population and on clinicians' enthusiasm in recommending them. Different cultural beliefs and preferences for traditional treatments such as herbal remedies also affect acceptance of the menopause transition.

The risk and benefits of HT have mainly been evaluated in multicenter clinical trials enrolling predominantly Caucasian women.

Treatment regimens differ among sociocultural groups. In a 1996 study, African-American women treated menopause symptoms predominantly with nonprescription treatments (55% prefer diet, vitamins, exercise, or herbal remedies over HT). Knowledge deficits among African-American women, especially among low-income women, were identified regarding menopause and symptom management. The 1998 Commonwealth Fund Study found that HT use was most prevalent among well-educated, white, non-Hispanic women living in the midwestern United States who have partners and middle- to upper-range incomes.

Cross-cultural counseling. Studies among African-American women suggest that practitioners are not providing adequate information regarding menopause. Only 14% of African-American women identified their healthcare provider as the primary source of information on menopause; 60% identified their family and friends as the primary source, with literature second at 20%. In contrast, most Caucasian-American women (67%) rely on literature as their primary source, with their healthcare provider second at 17%.

The research on menopause experiences of women in other cultures illustrates the need to learn about women's cultural beliefs and the various complementary and alternative therapies that women use. Educational material that addresses those issues can be made available. These materials must be culturally sensitive and even translated, when appropriate.

Effective counseling requires that the clinician be aware of any cultural beliefs that can affect a woman's view of menopause and various treatment options. However, it is a mistake to stereotype women of foreign descent—they do not all observe the same traditions or exhibit the same cultural traits. As always, delivery of health care must respect each woman as a unique individual (see Table 1).

Multiple factors can increase diseases during menopause and beyond, but there are also barriers that lead to disparities in disease prevalence, such as income level, health insurance status, cultural values, transportation, and race or ethnicity. Many barriers can be overcome with advances in techniques to enhance patient and clinician education.

Table 1. Suggestions for cross-cultural counseling

- Encourage the woman to discuss her concerns. Ask why she thinks she has the symptoms and what her family and friends say about the symptoms.

- Ask her if she is using alternative or folk remedies or if she is consulting with others, such as healers. It is important to know all the medications or treatments she is using before a treatment plan can be prescribed.

- Do not disparage her current practices. Be willing to compromise to devise a plan acceptable to her.

- In some cultures, healing and religion are inextricably linked. A medical treatment plan may need to be designed to complement her other treatments to ensure continuance. Consider a plan that will treat the woman medically and traditionally.

- Have social workers experienced with a particular culture and interpreters available for consultation. Avoid using family members as interpreters. Face the woman when speaking, not an interpreter. A telephone-interpreter service is another option.

- Consider the role of the woman's family. They can help her follow instructions, as well as monitor therapy and keep records.

- If she does not speak English or is unfamiliar with Western medicine, set aside more time for counseling.

- Be aware that conversing in English does not necessarily mean that the woman can read English or her native language. One in five US adults is functionally illiterate. If illiteracy is suspected, have visual instructions that illustrate when to take the medication, such as a clock face or depictions of sunrise.

- Clarify the limitations of Western medicine. If the woman has symptoms that may not respond to therapy, make it clear to her.

- Explain in advance what you are going to be doing during a physical examination. Some women may not understand why you are examining parts of their body other than those affected.

- Keep in mind differences between populations and the differences within populations. Major differences in social class, economic status, and background exist within all ethnic groups.

Lesbian health

Up to 5% of women have their primary emotional and sexual relationships with other women. Lesbian (gay, homosexual) women live in all communities and represent a diverse group in race, ethnicity, education, age, and sexual practice. They may be celibate or sexually active with women, men, or both. Lesbians cannot be described as a group. However, some counseling guidelines can be offered.

Many healthcare providers assume that all women they are caring for are heterosexual. For the lesbian to receive appropriate health care, her sexual orientation and lifestyle must be known and understood by her healthcare provider. Often, providers do not ask this question. In a Canadian survey of nearly 500 lesbians about healthcare experiences, only 24% had been asked by a provider about their sexual orientation; this low proportion has remained the same over the last 25 years.

Women respond well to language free of heterosexual assumptions (eg, rather than asking "What method of birth control do you use," first ask, "Are you in need of birth control?"). In addition, it is important not to assume that the sexual relations of a lesbian are exclusively with other women.

The fear of sharing information with a clinician about sexual orientation and lifestyle keeps some lesbians from seeking health care as frequently as desirable or at all. In a survey conducted in the 1980s, lesbians (N = 1,921) were asked about their experiences with healthcare practitioners. Responses included many accounts of insensitivity and heterosexism and even homophobia. Fortunately, tolerance for diversity in sexual orientation has improved since that time, but problems remain. Lesbians in the United States are reported to see their healthcare providers less frequently than do other US women. In Canada, frequency is reported to be approximately equal to that of other Canadian women.

Although it is unknown whether lesbian women experience higher rates of certain chronic diseases that affect women at midlife and beyond (eg, certain cancers, cardiovascular disease), the higher incidence of relevant lifestyle risk factors suggest that this may be the case. The Women's Health Initiative (WHI), which includes the largest number of midlife and older women to identify themselves as lesbians in the medical literature (n = 500 over age 50), has found that the incidence of risk factors, such as alcohol consumption, smoking, and overweight, is higher in lesbian women. Recent population-based surveys confirm higher rates of smoking, alcohol use, and overweight/obesity among lesbians than among heterosexual women.

Lesbians underestimate their risk of developing cancer, particularly cervical cancer, perhaps from the infrequency of their heterosexual intercourse (although most lesbians have had heterosexual intercourse at some point in their lives). One large survey shows a lower rate of Pap smears in lesbians and bisexuals than in heterosexual women. Abnormal Pap smears and cervical cancer have been found even among lifelong lesbians. Pap smears are an important part of the appropriate evaluation of a lesbian woman's health.

Lesbians may be at a higher risk of breast cancer and they may have higher rates of cancer mortality, perhaps because they are less likely to be screened with mammograms and breast examinations. Because lesbian women are less likely to become pregnant, they may have a higher risk of certain diseases associated with nulliparity and low or no use of oral contraceptives such as ovarian cancer. In addition, high-risk lifestyle factors, such as obesity, smoking, and alcohol consumption, may increase cancer risk. Unfortunately, many lesbians do not think they need an annual gynecologic examination because they are not currently engaging in sexual relations with men. The WHI, a large trial of postmenopausal women, showed no difference in the rate of breast cancer among the lesbian and bisexual participants compared with heterosexual women. Low numbers do not permit a definitive answer.

Lesbians and their partners are at risk of contracting sexually transmitted infections (STIs). Many types of STIs, including *Trichomonas* infections, can be passed between female partners through skin-to-skin contact and through unsafe use of sex toys. Neither gonorrheal nor chlamydial infections have ever been reported in a woman who has had sex only with women, but the rate of bacterial vaginosis appears to be higher among lesbians. Viral infections (eg, herpes, human papillomavirus) can be transmitted from woman to woman, although some uncertainty exists with regard to HIV. Current thinking is that some women are at high risk of HIV and AIDS, but that risk is related to intravenous drug abuse and their heterosexual/bisexual practices.

It is important to screen for STIs, as indicated, and to encourage safer sex practices. There is evidence that lesbians who engage in high-risk behaviors are less likely than heterosexual women to limit risk by practicing safer sex. For tips on how lesbian and bisexual women can avoid STIs, see Section E, page 156.

Clinicians are advised to be alert to the possibility of current or previous physical/sexual abuse. It is estimated that approximately 38% of lesbians have had childhood sexual abuse. An estimated 40% report sexual assault, similar to women in the general population. Intimate-partner violence, while less common in lesbian relationships than in heterosexual ones, does occur and is less likely to be reported.

Lesbians seem to be at higher risk of generalized anxiety disorder and mood disorders, and are more likely to have had more than one lifetime psychiatric diagnosis. Lesbians are also targets for antigay verbal abuse, threats, violence, and discrimination. In one study, the excess of psychiatric diagnoses was associated with experiences of discrimination.

General counseling suggestions for lesbian women are found in Table 2.

Clinicians are encouraged to examine biases regarding sexual orientation. If they or their staff are uncomfortable when obtaining an in-depth sexual history and providing

---

Table 2. Suggestions when counseling lesbian women

- Use a questionnaire that includes a question about sexual orientation. One survey found that 97% of lesbians and gays revealed their sexual orientation through this procedure. Suggested questions may include:
  — Are you in a relationship?
  — Are you sexually active?
  — Do you have a partner or partners?
  — Is your partner a man or a woman?
  — Have you ever been sexually active with a man, woman, or both?
- Instill trust that the information will be treated with respect and confidentiality.
- Use language free of heterosexual assumptions until sexual orientation is known.
- Don't assume that sexual relations are exclusively with other women.
- Respect the role of the lesbian's partner in her life and health-related decisions, treating her as a spouse.
  — Instead of asking for the spouse's name, ask, "Who would you like to have involved in the discussion of your treatment/surgery?"
  — Give her partner complete access if she is hospitalized; if needed, suggest obtaining a durable power of attorney or healthcare power of attorney.
  — Be aware of insurance issues, especially when the partner is the only one working and the employer does not recognize the patient as a family member.

---

clinical care for lesbian women, referral is advised to other providers who provide a nonjudgmental attitude.

Lifestyle and behavior modification

Lifestyle. The menopause transition is an appropriate time for a comprehensive review of a woman's overall health, for assessment of risk factors for disease, and for counseling about options for health promotion and disease prevention. Many postmenopausal women are active participants in their health care. According to one survey, approximately 75% of postmenopausal women report making some type of health-related lifestyle change at menopause/midlife.

According to the US Preventive Services Task Force and the Canadian Task Force on Preventive Health Care, improved control of behavioral risk factors—such as use of tobacco, alcohol, and other drugs, lack of exercise, and poor nutrition—could prevent one half of all premature deaths, one third of all cases of acute disability, and nearly all cases of chronic disability. The economic consequences place a tremendous burden on society, in terms of lost productivity and increased demands on health and social services.

Although smoking may be the single greatest preventable cause of illness and premature death, clinicians also need to stress the importance of other factors to overall health (see Table 3).

Table 3. Lifestyle counseling issues for peri- and postmenopausal women

Substance use
- Tobacco cessation
- Alcohol/drug safety (eg, avoid use while driving, swimming, boating)
- Alcohol/drug abuse

Diet and exercise
- Limit fat and cholesterol intake
- Maintain caloric balance
- Consume a diet based on whole grains, fruits, vegetables, water
- Ensure adequate vitamin and mineral intake, especially calcium
- Emphasize importance of regular physical activity

Injury prevention
- Wear lap/shoulder belts in the car
- Institute fall prevention methods
- Wear appropriate helmet and other safety equipment when riding motorcycle, bicycle, or all-terrain vehicle
- Have adequate number of smoke and carbon monoxide detectors
- Ensure safe storage or removal of firearms
- Set water heater thermostat between 120°F (49°C) and 130°F (54°C) or lower
- Train household members to deliver CPR

Sexual behavior
- Institute prevention of STIs:
- Avoid high-risk sexual behavior
- Use condoms and/or female barrier
- Prevent unintended pregnancies with appropriate contraception

Dental health
- Stress importance of regular dental visits
- Floss and brush with fluoride toothpaste daily

Source: US Preventive Services Task Force 1996, 2006.

Behavior modification. Risky health behaviors are the leading cause of preventable morbidity and mortality. Individuals who are socially and economically disadvantaged, including those in low-income ethnic or racial minority groups, demonstrate the highest prevalence of these behaviors.

Behavior modification may reduce morbidity and mortality and improve quality of life across diverse populations. Counseling that results in behavior modification and improved lifestyle practices may prove to be more valuable for improving overall health than screening for diseases.

However, current rates of behavioral counseling by primary care practitioners fall far below target levels. Time and reimbursement are always issues. There is also a lack of scientific evidence that supports counseling recommendations. Evidence supporting the effectiveness of behavioral counseling by primary care practitioners is only beginning to appear in the literature. The following six health risk patterns have been identified as appropriate targets for behavior modification counseling:

- Dietary patterns
- Physical inactivity
- Cigarette smoking
- Risky sexual practices
- Problem drinking (addictive behaviors related to alcohol and/or street drugs are excluded)
- Accidental injury

Counseling to promote behavior change often requires more than giving brief advice. Effective interventions usually involve behavioral counseling techniques, multiple contacts, and use of other resources. Adjuncts to counseling include interventions by other healthcare team members (eg, nurses, health educators, pharmacists) and the use of other communication strategies (eg, telephone-, video-, or computer-assisted learning, self-help guides, handouts, or mailings). Certain situations will require referral to a structured counseling program that uses a longer time frame and a range of behavior modification methods.

Healthcare practitioners can play an important role in motivating and facilitating behavior change. They often have repeated contacts with women over many years, which provide continuity of care and contribute to a relationship of trust between the provider and patient. Studies have shown that patients expect primary care practitioners to provide preventive health information and recommendations and that these practitioners value their role in health promotion and disease prevention. Preliminary studies suggest that advice from one's healthcare provider based on personal health status is a strong motivator for health-promoting behavior.

Four categories of behavioral theories have contributed to the understanding of behavior change and compliance with counseling recommendations. These include communication, rational belief, a self-regulative system, and social learning models. Each has a slightly different perspective about risky health behaviors, but all refer to similar components: illness cognition, risk perception, motivation to change, acquisition of coping strategies, and appraisal of results. Most counseling strategies use a combination of components from complementary theories to form a theoretical framework.

Behavioral counseling strategies address complex behaviors that are part of daily living. They vary in intensity and scope according to the individual, and they require repeated action by both the provider and the recipient to achieve health improvement. Effective counseling interventions are goal-oriented and patient-centered, and require active participation from the provider and the patient.

The delivery of preventive health services, such as behavioral counseling, is often hindered by numerous barriers. These include a need to focus on more urgent medical issues, lack of resources (eg, time, training, reimbursement, support), and low demand. The existence of barriers reinforces the need for a consistent approach for behavioral counseling interventions. These interventions help to address barriers, improve patient access, and increase treatment effectiveness.

The Canadian Task Force on Preventive Health Care and the US Preventive Services Task Force have adopted a construct for behavioral counseling interventions called the "Five A's," chosen because it was found to have the highest degree of empirical support for each of its elements and because of its use in existing literature (see Table 4).

Table 4. The "Five A's" for clinical counseling

- **Assess.** Ask about and assess behavioral health risk(s) and factors affecting choice of goals and methods of behavior change.

- **Advise.** Give clear, specific, and personalized behavior change advice, including information about personal health harms and benefits.

- **Agree.** Collaboratively select appropriate treatment goals and methods based on the patient's interest in and willingness to change the behavior.

- **Assist.** Using behavior change techniques (self-help and/or counseling), aid the woman in achieving agreed-upon goals by acquiring the skills, confidence, and social/environmental strategies for behavior change, supplemented with adjunctive medical treatments when appropriate (eg, pharmacotherapy for tobacco dependence, contraceptive drugs/devices).

- **Arrange.** Schedule follow-up contacts (in person and by telephone) to provide ongoing assistance/support and to adjust the treatment plan as needed, including referral to more intensive or specialized treatment.

Source: Whitlock *Am J Prev Med* 2002.

Appreciating the effect of behavioral counseling strategies requires a population-based perspective. Individually, the brief, counseling interventions feasible in primary care settings may have only a modest impact on behavior change. However, this translates into significant health benefits when systematically delivered to a large population. Behavioral counseling strategies in the primary care setting are an important means of addressing risky health behaviors that are major contributors to preventable morbidity and mortality in North America.

Substance abuse. There are three major categories of substance abuse: legal drugs (such as nicotine and alcohol), illegal drugs (such as marijuana and cocaine), and prescription drugs (including benzodiazepines, opiates, and psychostimulants).

The lifetime incidence of alcoholism among North American women is approximately 10%. The lifetime incidence of illegal drug dependence among women is 5% to 6%. Rates of illegal drug and alcohol use are lower in women than in men; the rate of nicotine dependence is nearly equal to that in men.

Legal drugs.

- *Smoking.* Cigarette smoking is the leading preventable cause of premature death, disease, and disability. Smoking-related diseases are responsible for more than 178,000 deaths annually in women in the United States and 16,000 deaths per year in Canadian women. About one of every five US women aged 18 years and older smokes.

The three leading smoking-related causes of death in women are lung cancer, heart disease, and chronic lung disease. A total of 99% of all lung cancer deaths in women smokers are attributable to smoking. Lung cancer deaths among women have increased by more than 600% since 1950, and in 1987 lung cancer surpassed breast cancer as the leading cause of cancer-related deaths in women. Women must also avoid environmental (ie, secondhand) smoke—approximately 3,000 lung cancer deaths occur each year in US nonsmokers as a result of exposure to secondhand smoke.

Lung cancer risk among former smokers has been shown to decrease with increasing duration of smoking abstinence. However, the time that needs to pass before the risk of former smokers reaches that of never-smokers is less clear. The Iowa Women's Health Study, a large prospective cohort study of women aged 55 to 69 years, found that former smokers had an elevated lung cancer risk up to 30 years after smoking cessation. Smoking low tar or light cigarettes does not seem to reduce health risks of tobacco use.

Women who smoke have an increased risk for other cancers, including cancers of the oral cavity, pharynx, larynx, esophagus, pancreas, kidney, bladder, and uterine cervix. Use of snuff and tobacco also causes cancers of the oral cavity, esophagus, and larynx. Women who smoke double their risk for developing coronary heart disease (CHD) and increase by more than 10-fold their likelihood of dying from chronic obstructive pulmonary disease.

Smoking may double the risk for Alzheimer's disease. Postmenopausal women have lower BMD and higher risk of fracture, and may be at higher risk of developing rheumatoid arthritis and cataracts. The list of risks of smoking for reproductive-age women is longer. (See also Section E on Cancers and Cardiovascular disease.)

Smokers tend to reach menopause up to 2 years earlier than nonsmokers, placing smokers at increased risk for diseases associated with lower levels of endogenous estrogen. On the contrary, altered plasma levels of estradiol and estrone have not been associated with smoking in pre- or postmenopausal women. Among postmenopausal women who take oral HT, smokers have lower serum estrone and estradiol levels than nonsmokers.

The Nurses' Health Study (NHS) found that among current smokers, a younger age at natural menopause was associated with a higher risk of CHD. However, among those who did not smoke or who were past smokers, CHD risk was not affected. These same observations may also be true for women after induced menopause.

This same study also found that after women stopped smoking, one third of the excess risk of CHD was eliminated within 2 years. After 10 to 14 years, the excess risks for total mortality, as well as that for both CHD and total cancer mortality, approached that of women who never smoked.

Smoking during adolescence and early adulthood may impede the achievement of optimal peak bone mass. Smoking is also associated with more rapid bone loss in women and higher fracture rates. In the NHS, hip fracture risk increased linearly with greater cigarette consumption. Risk declined after quitting, but the benefit was not observed until 10 years after cessation. In this study, the increase in risk among current smokers and the decline in risk after smoking cessation were, in part, accounted for by differences in body weight. The mechanisms by which smoking might affect bone mass are not known, although some evidence suggests that some component of cigarette smoke interferes with estrogen metabolism.

Smoking cigarettes, as well as use of snuff and chewing tobacco, jeopardizes dental health for several reasons. It has a direct influence on gingival tissues caused by the heat and chemical constituents of tobacco smoke. It has antiestrogenic effects and contributes to the development of osteoporosis (which in turn might result in tooth loss). Smoking may also increase the likelihood of infection and periodontitis by inhibiting tissue oxygen levels, limiting gingival blood supply, and impairing antibacterial immune response.

Women who smoke cigarettes generally experience more hot flashes than nonsmokers, and the risk increases with the amount smoked. Anecdotal observations suggest that stopping smoking may lower the hot flash risk, but no study has specifically tested the effects of smoking cessation on the severity and rate of hot flashes. Although definitions of smoking status are not uniform, in the Iowa Women's Health Study, smoking status was classified as current (smoked ≥100 cigarettes in lifetime and currently smoking), former (smoked ≥100 cigarettes in lifetime and currently not smoking), and never (smoked <100 cigarettes in lifetime and currently not smoking). Former smokers were further classified according to years of smoking abstinence and pack-years of smoking (pack-years is defined as total years of smoking multiplied by cigarette packs smoked per day).

Smoking cessation is the most effective strategy for smokers to enhance the quality and duration of their lives. Nearly all smokers acknowledge that tobacco use is harmful to their health, but they underestimate the magnitude of their risk. The nicotine in tobacco is as addictive as heroin or cocaine. Tobacco use delivers nicotine to the brain rapidly and effectively, causing a rapid onset and maintenance of addiction. This results in both a physiologic and psychological dependence on tobacco, which explains the continued use of tobacco products in spite of the known health risks. Regardless of the health risks, many women are better motivated to quit smoking by understanding the contribution that this habit makes on facial wrinkles.

On average, women gain about 5 pounds after quitting, an amount that can be controlled through diet and exercise.

Smoking cessation is not a single event but a process that involves a change in lifestyle, personal values, social groups, perceptions, and coping skills.

Approximately one third of smokers try to stop smoking each year, but only 20% of them seek help. Those who do are more successful; less than 10% who try to stop on their own are successful over the long term. Several attempts are usually required before a smoker truly quits.

The most important step in addressing tobacco dependence is screening for tobacco use and offering minimal smoking cessation interventions (lasting 1-3 min) to all smokers, at every opportunity. Prominently displaying "quit smoking" posters and ensuring cessation materials are easily accessible deliver a strong message to clients that cessation assistance is available. Labeling of each client's chart with smoking status reminds healthcare providers to consistently integrate smoking cessation into their care. Progress can also be made by assessing each smoker's readiness to quit and helping her move closer to the stage of quitting.

Intensive intervention is appropriate for all smokers willing to participate and includes smoking history, motivation to quit, identification of high-risk situations and help with problem solving strategies for those situations. Proactive telephone counseling, group counseling, and individual counseling are all effective smoking cessation interventions.

Healthcare providers can offer a variety of prescription smoking cessation aids. The use of pharmacologic therapy approximately doubles the long-term abstinence rates over those produced by placebo. Government-approved, first-line medications for smoking cessation include slow-release bupropion (Zyban) and nicotine replacement therapy (NRT). NRT is available in gum, transdermal patch, and vapor inhaler in the United States and Canada. Other NRT options (eg, nasal spray, sublingual tablets, and lozenges) currently available in the United States (but not Canada) have been demonstrated to be effective and are recommended as first-line therapies. Varenicline (Chantix), a selective nicotinic-receptor agonist, was government approved in the United States in 2006. In a recent study, varenicline and slow-release bupropion were found to be superior to placebo in promoting abstinence from smoking during 7 weeks of active treatment, and varenicline (1 mg, twice daily) was most effective for smoking abstinence during 1 year.

Nonpharmacologic interventions to assist with smoking cessation include self-help books and materials, individual counseling, hypnosis, group programs, and mutual aid and self-help group support. A combination of behavior modification techniques and prescription drug therapy appears to be the most successful approach. Due to the high rate of relapse in the first 3 months after quitting, a greater emphasis on follow-up care and training in relapse prevention may improve long-term quit rates.

- *Alcohol.* Drinking alcohol has been associated with benefits and risks, depending on the quantity consumed. In peri- and postmenopausal women, the effect of alcohol on endogenous estrogen levels is unclear. Although some studies have suggested that alcohol consumption may lower estrogen levels, one study in postmenopausal women using HT found that acute alcohol consumption was associated with significant, sustained elevations in circulating estradiol, up to levels 300% higher than those used clinically.

Moderate alcohol consumption seems to lower the risk of hip fractures in women aged 65 years and older, possibly because moderate consumption increases endogenous estradiol concentrations and calcitonin excretion, which may inhibit bone resorption. In the NHS, women who consumed 75 g/week or more of alcohol had significantly higher BMD at the lumbar spine than nondrinkers, although alcohol intakes of less than 75 g/week were also

of benefit. This positive association was observed among current users and never-users of HT. However, alcohol consumption was not associated with a higher femoral BMD.

Women are more affected by alcohol than men because of many factors, including less water in their bodies to dilute the alcohol, fewer enzymes to digest the alcohol, and hormonal differences that may affect absorption. Death rates from alcohol abuse are 50% to 100% higher for women than they are for men.

Both women and men who drink have a higher risk of cancer. Women who consume one or two drinks daily may be at increased risk for breast cancer. The mechanism of this effect is not known, but the association may be related to carcinogenic actions of alcohol or its metabolites, or to alcohol-induced changes in levels of hormones, such as estrogen. (See also Section E on Cancers.)

Alcoholic beverages can also cause cancers of the oral cavity, esophagus, and larynx. The combined use of tobacco and alcohol leads to a greatly increased risk of oral and esophageal cancers. The effect of tobacco and alcohol combined is greater than the sum of their individual effects.

Compared with men, women who drink experience greater damage to the liver and a higher risk of stroke. Higher levels of alcohol use—defined as more than seven drinks per week (one drink equals 12 oz beer, 4 oz wine, or 1 oz liquor) or more than 3 per occasion—may increase certain cardiovascular risks, such as hypertension, stroke, and coronary artery disease. Heavy alcohol consumption has also been shown to increase the risk of falls and hip fractures. Excessive alcohol consumption may have detrimental effects on bones, the liver, and other body systems. Heavy drinkers who stop may have unpleasant withdrawal symptoms.

For more about how to evaluate alcohol abuse, see Section F, page 185.

Illegal drugs. Identification of women with alcohol or illegal drug dependence requires a careful history. It is important to be knowledgeable and willing to make inquiries regarding illegal drug (eg, marijuana, cocaine) use, as well as to evaluate for common comorbid issues, such as anxiety and depression. However, responses may vary from candid honesty to complete misrepresentation. Specific questions such as "how much" and "how often" might yield more honest responses than yes or no questions.

Prescription drugs. Peri- and postmenopausal women are more likely to abuse prescription medications if they have another identified chemical dependency, such as alcohol and/or nicotine. Some women obtain prescriptions for medications from several clinicians, none of whom is aware of prescriptions from the others. Often there is a history of repeated refill requests for reasons such as "lost prescription" or the alleged use of the prescription by family members or friends.

Women who are abusing mood-altering drugs may have many physical concerns consistent with menopause symptoms. These include mood changes, vasomotor instability, and insomnia. A primary psychiatric problem, such as a depressive or anxiety disorder, may also be part of the clinical picture.

To detect problematic drug use, it is helpful to look for preoccupation with a particular drug in conjunction with an entire lifestyle that appears centered around drug procurement and use. Assessment of adverse consequences of continued drug abuse (eg, physical, psychological, spiritual, social) is advised. Many women tend to minimize or deny their extent of abuse or adverse consequences. Such women typically lack insight into the problems created by their drug use. They may be quite unaware of the impact of their addiction on family members, friends, and business associates.

Address concern about use of alcohol or other drugs (including prescription medications) in an immediate and direct fashion. Beginning with a statement such as "I'm concerned about you" can be very effective. If uncomfortable dealing with these types of issues, a quick and easy referral to a more appropriate professional is also recommended here. This could include a physician or counselor who is experienced in dealing with addictive disorders. It is possible that detoxification may be required.

Physical activity. Regular physical activity can help prevent CVD, obesity, DM, and cancer, and maintain musculoskeletal strength and mental well-being. Other benefits may include a positive effect on vasomotor symptoms and better, more restorative sleep.

Current guidelines suggest 30 minutes of moderate exercise daily equivalent to brisk walking (which can be intermittent). For adults attempting to lose weight or maintain weight loss, at least 60 minutes of physical activity is recommended most days of the week. When performed regularly, activities such as brisk walking, running, aerobics, dancing, tennis, and strength training provide numerous health benefits.

Despite these recommendations, more than one third of US women aged 45 years and older participate in no leisure-time physical activity. Less than 20% participate in regular, sustained physical activity of at least 30 minutes five or more times per week. Reports in Canada are similar—only 15% of Canadian women aged 40 to 54 years are sufficiently active. Another 54% report regular participation in physical activity; 18% are occasionally active and 23% are inactive. The percentage of those physically inactive increases as Canadian women age; 72% of women over age 70 are inactive.

Guidance regarding which type(s) and level of physical activity are appropriate, and encouragement to work exercise into their routine for the rest of their lives is required. Brief interventions by healthcare providers can be effective in increasing physical activity in the short term. For exercise to be sustained a year later, follow-up sessions at 3- to 6-month intervals are required after the initial discussion. It is also helpful to provide written information about the benefits of regular activity and local opportunities available.

The three basic exercise types are:

- *Strength training* (eg, resistance exercises, weight-bearing exercises). This type of exercise, using free weights or weight machines, provides muscle resistance. Early in life, strength training promotes higher bone mass; later in life, it can have a modest impact on slowing bone loss. Older women in particular need these exercises to build strength, thereby improving balance to prevent falls.
- *Aerobic.* The cardiovascular and respiratory systems benefit from aerobic exercises, including brisk walking, jogging, rowing, and cycling. Low-impact aerobics are easier on the joints than high-impact aerobics and thus may be a better choice for women at midlife and beyond.
- *Flexibility.* Exercises such as yoga and stretching help maintain flexibility and reduce stiffness with aging. Improving flexibility and balance can also decrease the risk of fractures caused by falls.

Current activity level, physical condition, preferences, and personal circumstances are key determinants of the exercise prescription. For example, if a woman has been sedentary, advice can include starting slowly and progressing gradually. She should be screened for CVD before starting a regimen. Regimens can begin with strength exercises that engage all muscle groups, to be performed three times per week on alternate days for a minimum of 10 to 12 weeks, then reduced to two times per week with aerobic exercise added to the program.

Evidence also suggests that a *written* prescription for exercise to outline physical activity goals will be helpful and that follow-up at appropriate intervals may be more important than the length of each session. Finding ways to make exercise a permanent part of daily life will help ensure a healthier future. One way is to suggest partnering with a friend for regular walks or other physical activities.

Stress. Although menopause has not been shown to raise stress levels, women at midlife may face many new stressors. Stress negatively affects quality of life, produces various unpleasant symptoms, and may aggravate some medical conditions, including CVD.

Mind-body medicine, one of the most common types of complementary and alternative medicine, focuses on the interactions among the brain, mind, body, and behavior as well as the ways in which emotional, mental, social, spiritual, and behavioral factors can directly affect health. It typically includes intervention strategies thought to promote health. In 2002, more than 52% of the adult US population reported use of mind-body interventions, including prayer. (See Section I for more about complementary and alternative medicine.)

Research evidence suggests that:

- Mind-body therapies, such as combinations of stress management, coping skill training, cognitive-behavioral interventions, and relaxation therapy, may be appropriate adjunct treatments for coronary artery disease and pain-related disorders, such as arthritis.

- Multimodal mind-body approaches, such as cognitive-behavioral therapy, combined with an educational component, may be effective adjuncts for the management of chronic conditions.

- Presurgical use of mind-body therapies, such as imagery, hypnosis, and relaxation, may reduce pain and improve recovery time following surgery.

Research supports the benefit of paced respiration, a form of cognitive-behavioral technique, in reducing hot flashes when performed as a hot flash begins. In three randomized, prospective clinical trials, paced respiration significantly lowered hot flash frequency by approximately 50% more than the controls, a significant difference. Paced respiration involves taking slow, deep, abdominal breaths in through the nose and releasing them out through the mouth at the beginning of a hot flash.

Although not evaluated in controlled clinical trials, some women report fewer hot flashes when they engage in activities to enhance relaxation, such as meditation, yoga, massage, or even just a leisurely bath. Mind-body approaches appear to have positive effects on psychological functioning and quality of life, carry minimal risk, and are easily taught. Future research may lead to insights that will enhance their effectiveness and techniques for tailoring to meet individual needs.

Encourage women to recognize their own life stressors, to find stress-relieving strategies that work for them, and to take time to relax every day. (See also Section I on Complementary and alternative medicine.)

Nutrition. A healthy diet is an essential component of a healthy lifestyle and is associated with reduced risk for obesity, type 2 DM, hypertension, CVD, osteoporosis, some types of cancer, and other diseases.

Dietary guidelines developed in the United States and Canada recommend that nutrient needs be met primarily through a diet that is high in grain products, vegetables, and fruits, and low in saturated fats and cholesterol. This provides an array of nutrients and other compounds that have a beneficial effect on health. In some instances, fortified foods and dietary supplements may be useful sources of nutrients that would be consumed in less than recommended amounts. However, dietary supplements cannot replace a healthy diet.

Examples of eating patterns that exemplify dietary guidelines are the USDA Dietary Guidelines, the Dietary Approaches to Stop Hypertension (DASH) Eating Plan, and Canada's Food Guide. These eating patterns are designed so most individuals can integrate dietary recommendations into a healthy way to eat and are constructed across a range of calorie levels to meet the needs of various age and gender groups. Although originally developed to study the effects of an eating pattern on the prevention and treatment of hypertension, DASH is one example of a balanced eating plan consistent with the 2005 *Dietary Guidelines for Americans* and the 2006 diet recommendations of the American Heart Association. (See also Section E on Concomitant conditions.)

The recommended calorie intake will differ for individuals based on age, gender, and activity level. The recommended nutrient intake can be met without consuming the day's full calorie allotment if nutrient-dense foods are consumed. This allows flexibility with the remaining calories (also called discretionary calorie allowance) to consume some foods and beverages that may contain added fats, added sugars, and alcohol.

It is also important to incorporate the food preferences of different racial/ethnic groups, vegetarians, religious food requirements, and health-related food restrictions when planning diets and developing educational programs and materials. The *Dietary Guidelines for Americans*, Canada's Food Guide, and the DASH Eating Plan accommodate a range of food preferences and cuisines.

Many excellent tools are available to supplement the information given by the healthcare provider, including written information and interactive Web sites (www.smallstep.gov from the Department of Health and Human Services; and the Dieticians of Canada's www.eattracker.ca). Controlling portions can be achieved by using a smaller plate or a premeasured portion-control plate. Women with special considerations or medical conditions are best referred to a dietitian for specific dietary advice.

Of special significance to the population of peri- and postmenopausal women are strategies to prevent CVD, which is the leading killer of North Americans. The following are general diet and lifestyle recommendations from the AHA in 2006, which, if rigorously applied with other lifestyle recommendations, will significantly decrease the risk for CVD and noncardiac disease as well. For individuals who are at high risk of CVD, the recommendations may have to be intensified.

Maintain a healthy body weight. To avoid weight gain, adults must achieve energy balance (caloric intake = energy expenditure). Knowledge about the caloric content of foods and beverages per portion consumed may increase control of portion size and calorie intake. The macronutrient composition of a diet (the amount of fat, carbohydrate, and protein) has little effect on energy balance unless manipulation of those macronutrients influences total energy intake.

Consume a diet rich in vegetables and fruit. Increasing intake of vegetables and fruits meet micronutrient, macronutrient, and fiber requirements without adding substantially to overall energy consumption. Deeply colored vegetables and fruits (eg, spinach, carrots, peaches, berries) tend to be higher in micronutrients than others (eg, potatoes, corn). Compared with whole fruit, fruit juice has less fiber content and need not be emphasized.

Choose whole-grain, high-fiber foods. These products have been associated with increased diet quality and decreased risk of CVD and some cancers. At least one half of grain intake needs to come from whole grains, which include wild rice, barley, quinoa, millet, and wheat berries.

Consume fish, especially oily fish, at least twice a week. Eating two servings (approximately 8 oz) per week of fish that is high in omega-3 polyunsaturated fatty acids (eg, salmon) is associated with a decreased risk of sudden death and death from coronary artery disease in adults. Contamination of some fish (especially large, predatory fish such as shark, swordfish, king mackerel, or tilefish) with mercury and other organic compounds is of concern, especially in children and pregnant women. For middle-aged and older men and postmenopausal women, the benefits of fish consumption far outweigh the potential risks when the amounts eaten are within the recommendations established by the United States Food and Drug Administration and Environmental Protection Agency. Potential exposure to some contaminants can be reduced by removing the skin and surface fat from fish before cooking, and by eating smaller fish.

Limit intake of saturated and trans fat and cholesterol. The AHA recommends intakes of less than 7% of energy as saturated fat, less than 1% trans fat, and less than 300 mg of cholesterol per day. Strategies to reduce saturated fat and cholesterol usually involve replacement of animal fats with unsaturated (polyunsaturated and monounsaturated) fats and selection of lower-fat versions of foods, such as replacing full-fat dairy products with nonfat or low-fat versions. Replacing meats with vegetable alternatives and/or fish is another option. Reduction of trans-fatty acids usually requires substitution of partially hydrogenated fats with liquid vegetable oils, with the exception of tropical oils. Some margarines or butter products contain plant sterols useful in lowering cholesterol.

Minimize intake of beverages and foods with added sugars and caffeine. The primary reasons for this recommendation are to lower total caloric intake and promote nutrient adequacy. Evidence suggests that calories consumed as liquids have less satiety than those from solid foods. This may, in turn, negatively affect attempts to maintain a healthy body weight.

Caffeine-containing drinks (coffee, tea, colas, soft drinks) can have a negative effect on health (eg, trigger hot flashes, contribute to insomnia, increase dehydration). Since women are often unaware of the effects of caffeine or its sources, discuss their intake.

Choose and prepare foods with little or no salt. Reduced sodium intake can prevent hypertension, act as an adjunct to antihypertensive medication, and facilitate hypertension control. Because of the currently high-sodium food supply and high levels of sodium consumption, an interim recommendation for sodium intake has been set at 2.3 g/day (100 mmol/d). An optimal sodium intake is 1.5 g/day (65 mmol/d), which may not be easily achievable at present.

Consume alcohol in moderation. Alcohol can be addictive, and high intake has been associated with serious health and social consequences. The AHA recommends that alcohol consumption be limited to no more than two drinks per day for men and one drink per day for women, and ideally consumed with meals.

Follow the AHA 2006 diet and lifestyle recommendations when eating food prepared outside of the home. Foods prepared outside of the home or "take-away" foods tend to come in large portions and have high-energy density. They are often also high in saturated fat, trans fat, cholesterol, added sugars, and sodium, and low in fiber and micronutrients. There is an association between frequency of "fast food" consumption and total energy intake, weight gain, and insulin resistance. Individuals must be vigilant and make wise choices when eating food prepared outside of the home.

Weight. Efforts to manage weight in peri- and postmenopausal women are essential. The advice to eat a healthy diet, increase physical activity, and avoid further weight gain is appropriate for almost all women at or above a healthy weight. For those who are overweight or obese, weight loss is indicated. Both weight gain and loss involve the complex interaction of numerous physical, social, and emotional factors, making it difficult for people to change their eating habits and lifestyle.

Physical activity can help balance caloric intake with energy expenditure. Both physical activity and controlled caloric intake are necessary to achieve or maintain a healthy body weight.

No single diet or eating regimen is right for all women. Women seeking to shed weight can be encouraged to set realistic goals achieved through long-term lifestyle change. Place emphasis on changing eating habits rather than relying on diets, especially faddish diets. Support can be obtained from family members, coworkers, and friends. Various organization and support groups (eg, Weight Watchers, Overeaters Anonymous) offer help with dieting, although no one program has been proven superior.

With exercise, muscle mass often increases, while fat often decreases—and muscle mass weighs more than fat. When counseling regarding weight management, women will benefit from knowing that, as they build muscle mass, body measurements may be a more accurate reflection of success than weight.

At some point almost all dieters reach a plateau—they stop losing weight, and tend to get discouraged and backslide. Furthermore, a 2007 review by Mann et al of 31 of the most rigorous diet studies that contained a year of follow-up data found that dieters initially lost 5% to 10% of weight during the first 6 months, but most regained the weight—plus more—within 4 to 5 years. Since participants self-reported their last weight, the success rate is probably even worse. "Weight cycling" (repeatedly losing and gaining weight) is linked to adverse health effects (eg, CVD, DM), although the cause is unknown. Thus, some experts are advocating that "dieting" should not be recommended. Instead, eating in moderation, coupled with regular exercise, may be the key to sustained weight management.

Having too low a weight is also of concern. Premenopausal women who eat sparingly, overdiet, or overexercise can become so thin that they become amenorrheic. So long as their body fat remains low, this temporary low-estrogen state increases the risk of osteoporosis later in life. Specifically, women who weigh less than 127 pounds (57.7 kg) have an increased risk of osteoporosis.

For more detailed information about weight management, see Section C, page 68.

Abuse of women. Abuse of women is a significant public health concern. Types of abuse include threatened or actual physical, sexual, financial, emotional, or psychological abuse by partners or acquaintances. Abuse of women crosses all boundaries, including cultural, ethnic, lifestyle, educational, and socioeconomic. Especially vulnerable groups include single mothers, lesbians, women with mental health issues, women with disabilities, and elderly women.

Abuse of women has profound and enduring physical and emotional health consequences. Abused women have a significantly higher prevalence of the following physical and mental health problems: injury, gastrointestinal problems (especially chronic irritable bowel syndrome), chronic pain (head, neck, fibromyalgia), gynecologic problems (especially pelvic pain, urinary tract infections, STIs), and mental health problems (especially depression, anxiety, and low self-esteem). Assessment for abuse is especially important in women presenting with these symptoms.

Healthcare providers are challenged to routinely assess for abuse in ways that minimize barriers to disclosure and enhance the development of an effective plan of care based on each woman's abuse experience. Exploring the question of physical violence with women may occur less frequently than is recommended, possibly because clinicians feel they have nothing to offer the woman or that uncovering violence may necessitate complicated and time-consuming intervention strategies.

NAMS, and several other organizations, including the American Medical Association, the American College of Obstetricians and Gynecologists, the Society of Obstetricians and Gynaecologists of Canada, and the Registered Nurses' Association of Ontario (RNAO), recommend that healthcare providers look for signs and symptoms of abuse. Routine universal screening for abuse should be part of all evaluations.

Detecting abuse can be difficult because women are often reluctant to disclose their experience. An environment of openness, safety, and trust may help to facilitate disclosure. Displaying posters and print materials about domestic violence in public and private areas (such as the washroom) of the office gives women the opportunity to read the information without being seen and can educate them about options for responding to domestic violence. Many women are not aware of community outreach groups, safe shelters, or the full range of their services or how to contact them.

To facilitate disclosure, healthcare professionals must know how to ask the question and how to respond. Validated tools may be used or individuals may develop their own style of questioning as part of a health history. Include the following points:

- Explain that all women are being asked about abuse because it is so prevalent in society and is related to significant health consequences.

- Inform women they can expect to be screened each time a health history is taken.

- Conduct interviews in private—with no friends, relatives, or caregivers present.

- Use a flexible approach tailored to each individual using direct and nonjudgmental language that is culturally and linguistically appropriate.

- Before screening, inform the woman of any reporting requirements or other limits to provider/patient confidentiality.

- Give a clear message that violence is unacceptable.

Table 5 provides suggestions for direct questions.

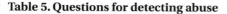

Table 5. Questions for detecting abuse

- Have you ever been emotionally or physically abused by your partner or someone important to you?

- Within the last year, have you been pushed or shoved, hit, slapped, kicked, or otherwise physically hurt by someone?

- Do you (or did you ever) feel controlled or isolated by your partner?

- Within the past year, has anyone forced you to have sexual activities?

- Are you afraid of your partner or anyone else?

- Do you feel you are in danger? Is it safe to go home?

- Has any of this happened to you in a previous relationship?

If a woman discloses abuse, the appropriate response is to:

- Acknowledge the abuse.
- Validate the woman's experience.
- Assess her immediate health needs and treat accordingly.
- Assess her immediate safety.
- Explore her options.
- Have a contact list of violence against women services available.
- Refer her to the appropriate services at the woman's consent.
- Document the interaction.

If a woman responds negatively to abuse but the practitioner suspects otherwise, it is appropriate to:

- Discuss what has been observed and explain continued concern about her health and safety.
- Offer educational information about the health effects and prevalence of abuse.
- Highlight referral services.
- Document the woman's responses.

In other situations where there is no disclosure, the practitioner is encouraged to share general information about the abuse and document the woman's response.

The RNAO has developed a comprehensive best-practice guideline called *Women Abuse: Screening, Identification and Initial Response*. Although created as a guide for nurses, the guideline provides comprehensive information appropriate for any healthcare professional to develop the knowledge and skills necessary to screen and respond appropriately and effectively. Identifying abuse and referral to specialized services, if the woman wishes, is the central process to follow in the guideline. Supporting the abused woman's choice is critical so as not to continue the experience of coercion and control.

Before initiating screening, the practitioner needs to inform the woman of the scope and limitations of confidentiality. In most US states and Canadian provinces, confidentiality cannot be guaranteed in cases of suspected child abuse or neglect, if there is a possibility of the woman harming herself or others, or when documents are subpoenaed by the courts.

Documentation must be comprehensive and legible, and accurately reflect screening practice. In the record, include a safety check, direct quotations of what the woman describes, direct observations made by the practitioner, and referrals that were made and/or information given. Again, women need to be aware, prior to screening, that the interaction will be documented and will become part of her health record that can be accessed at a later date if the woman wishes. Disclosure of any health information to any individual or organization outside of the healthcare team requires the woman's consent, except in cases described above.

Treatment counseling

When counseling a woman regarding treatment at menopause or beyond, the goal is to fully inform her about options and encourage her to take an active part in the decision-making process. Women who have more confidence in their ability to participate and who experience fewer barriers to participating are more likely to take an active role in the healthcare encounter and, in turn, are more satisfied with the decisions made.

Women who have no bothersome symptoms still need to understand the changes in risk profile at the time of menopause and the options that are available for risk reduction.

The woman's priorities for treatment and her concerns are key. The clinician can provide accurate and current information about the treatment options and help her examine the options and trade-offs in light of the outcome that is most important to her. The clinician can at this time reinforce the fact that menopause is a natural event, not a disease.

Some women may experience menopause-associated symptoms that interfere with their daily life. These women may be uncertain about what is happening to their bodies and need to understand the hormonal changes involved at menopause. Many changes may be related to aging, not menopause. Clinicians must be sensitive to individual concerns, recognizing that each woman is distinctively different in her response to menopause. Culture may influence communication style. Skills and sensitivity in communicating with women from different cultural backgrounds are essential.

Many women use alternative therapies, including herbal preparations, for symptom relief or for disease prevention. Because they are understood to be "natural," women may not think of these preparations as medicines. It is important for the clinician to assess all therapeutic strategies, including herbal preparations, when taking the history and conducting the physical examination. Clinicians need current information on alternative therapies and to alert women to those that have been shown to be effective or not effective through clinical trials and those for which there are no data. Women need to be informed about the lack of standardization among products, and they also need to know that side effects and interactions must be a consideration with so-called natural preparations as well as standard medications.

The decision for a woman to use hormones depends on many individual factors: her biological and psychological response to menopause/aging, tolerance for various symptoms, risk profile for disease in later years, contraindications to therapy, and feelings about medications. Clinicians can reinforce the concept of uniqueness and help women to become informed about the options available to them to achieve the outcomes they desire.

In the 1997 NAMS-Gallup Poll, a woman's decision to commence HT was more often made on the basis of physical symptom relief rather than prevention of disease. In a study of a nationally representative sample of women in the Commonwealth Fund 1998 Survey of Women's Health (N = 884), the two most common reasons for initiating HT were following a doctor's or other provider's recommendation (57%) and seeking relief of menopause symptoms (36%).

The WHI, which studied one type of oral HT in postmenopausal women, found surprising adverse health events from HT users. Awareness of these results differed among populations of US women. A survey of predominantly Caucasian women found 93% of the women were aware of the findings, and 56% had attempted to stop HT. In a smaller survey of Hispanic-American and African-American women, 74% had heard about the results, and almost all of them (87%) attempted to discontinue HT.

Results from the WHI trial have had an impact on women's use of HT. A study of women aged 50 to 69 years in a large health maintenance organization found that 56% of HT users tried to discontinue therapy during the 6 to 8 months after publication of the WHI results, although most women were not well informed regarding the results of the trial. A 2006 report on US prescribing patterns for HT between 2001 and 2003 showed a dramatic drop in prescriptions after publication of the WHI data—from 26.5 million to 16.9 million—with the rate of decline highest among the greatest number of users, women aged 50 years and over. This was the first decline in HT use after nearly two decades of increased numbers of prescriptions. Another study showed that in the months that followed, an estimated 40% reinitiated therapy.

Clinicians have a responsibility to ensure that women's decisions are informed and based on current information, including the risks and benefits of HT. In a telephone survey of 156 women in a managed care population, merely asking each woman a simple question regarding her level of knowledge was an effective clinical tool for identifying women who needed additional education about HT and menopause. Race, income, and discussion with a provider but not educational status were related to knowledge about HT.

A study evaluating 421 African-American and Caucasian-American women aged 50 to 54 years revealed that HT awareness was strongly influenced by race, educational level, and perception of "being in" or "having completed" menopause. Increased HT use among educated women may have resulted partly from increased awareness of HT. In this study, African-American women had a lower likelihood of HT awareness, even with adjustment for educational level. The study concluded that African-American women may view menopause and menopause-related symptoms differently than Caucasian-American women, considering it a natural process that does not require treatment.

Few studies have addressed the prevalence of HT counseling among US women. The 1994 National Health Interview Survey showed that among women aged 50 to 54 years, approximately 62% reported having received counseling regarding HT.

The 1998 NAMS survey (Part II) showed that 75.4% of 749 US women aged 50 to 65 years reported they had received HT counseling from healthcare providers. Women of low socioeconomic status and those who did not have a primary care provider were least likely to have received counseling. No differences were observed in prevalence of counseling between women in managed care settings and those with other types of health insurance.

In a 2000 survey of 1,800 Canadian women aged 45 to 64 years, 96% felt comfortable discussing menopause with their physician, and 70% felt that their physician provided adequate information about HT. However, 25% had not discussed HT mainly because they did not have menopause symptoms and a discussion was not necessary.

Improving medication continuance. *Continuance* is defined as using a medication regimen for the period of time and at the dosage needed to achieve the desired effect. It defines behavior beyond the initial decision to take a medication, referring to the daily decisions required to sustain medication-taking over time. The words *adherence* and *compliance* are often used interchangeably with *continuance*, although *compliance*, *comply*, and *compliant* are viewed by some women as paternalistic words referring to yielding or obedience rather than following a mutual decision. The important consideration is that the medication regimen is mutually agreed upon by the patient and provider. Such a process leads to the woman taking the medication to achieve her own goals.

Although medication continuance can refer to any medication taken over a period of time, much of the discussion for women at menopause centers on HT. In the Massachusetts Women's Health Study of 2,500 women aged 45 to 55 years given prescriptions for HT, 30% never filled the prescription, 20% stopped within 9 months, and 10% used HT only intermittently. In a 2006 retrospective chart analysis, 1,000 postmenopausal women who had received prescriptions for HT in 2002 to 2003 were tracked for continuance. Of those, 12% remained on HT in 2004 (a decline from 16% over 15 mo). Reasons for continuance included severity of menopausal symptoms, patient preference, and osteoporosis and osteopenia.

In a study of 449 women in a Massachusetts managed care health plan, the experience of certain side effects, such as irregular uterine bleeding, edema, and abdominal cramps/pelvic pain, was significantly associated with HT discontinuation. During the first few months of using HT, women were at greatest risk for discontinuing therapy because of side effects.

There is some evidence that continuance is greater with transdermal than with oral estrogen therapy (ET). Continuance is also greater with oral ET than with oral estrogen plus progestogen therapy (EPT) when the two hormones are taken separately. In one study, 30% of women stopped using progestogen and continued taking estrogen alone. A recent study involving longitudinal analysis of pharmacy claims data was conducted among 7,120 women who were new users of six EPT regimens. Higher rates of treatment continuation were seen with newer continuous-combined EPT regimens that caused fewer adverse effects, particularly uterine bleeding.

Most studies show that older women are more likely to discontinue HT than younger women. In one study, the relative risk of discontinuation was determined to be 1.1 for every 5 years of age. Older women appear to be particularly intolerant of uterine bleeding. In one study, 52% of those older than 65 years discontinued HT because of bleeding compared with 29% of those 55 years and younger.

The convenience of a regimen is also a factor in continuance. Continuance is correlated not with the number of drugs prescribed, but with the number of dosing times per day of all therapies. The fewer the number of doses, the greater the rate of continuance. The cost of therapy has not been linked conclusively to continuance.

In many cases, the reverse of the factors related to discontinuance can increase continuance. Women who feel better using HT are more likely to continue the regimen. Continuance has been shown to be higher in women whose symptoms were reduced after using HT. The absence of a uterus also enhances continuance, as uterine bleeding is eliminated. When the woman is asymptomatic, continuation is more problematic. When symptoms are severe, continuation is improved. For example, following

bilateral oophorectomy, women typically have severe symptoms, leading to improved HT continuance.

The current recommendation of using HT primarily for symptom relief supports the premise that continuance is more than ever a subjective decision that women must make for themselves. Good communication with their clinicians regarding the therapeutic potential of HT is essential.

With the conflicting data in the literature, many women feel inadequately informed about the risks and benefits of HT, and this can lead to inaccurate expectations and uncertainty. However, with guidance from an informed healthcare provider, women can address these issues by learning about the risks of HT and building realistic expectations of the therapy. Through discussion of therapeutic options and goals for using HT, and assessment of what is important to them, women can be fully informed to participate in the HT decision. Discussions are best supplemented with written information to take home.

Table 6 presents recommendations made by NAMS in its consensus opinion about HT continuance that are applicable to most medications.

Table 6. Counseling recommendations to improve continuance

- Involve the woman in the decision-making process, and recognize that decision making involves daily decisions.
- Share the decision making between the woman and her healthcare provider to optimize treatment planning and subsequent continuance.
- Explain the benefits and risks with clarity, personalizing information by translating population data to the personal risk profile.
- Determine the woman's preferences early in the decision-making process and use these preferences to modify a regimen to improve continuance.
- Provide educational information in words that the woman can understand.
- Help the woman systematize medication taking.
- Ensure adequate follow-up.
- Set the expectation that it may be necessary to try more than one regimen.

Source: The North American Menopause Society *Menopause* 1998.

In general, communication is key to the mutual decision making that enhances continuance with therapy. Let the communication lead to an understanding by the provider of the woman's goals, preferences, and concerns as well as to an understanding by the woman of the trade-offs of the therapy, potential side effects, and therapeutic outcomes. It is essential that the woman understand that it may take time to achieve the right therapeutic option, regimen, or dose. Women are most likely to discontinue medication at the time of initiating treatment, when changing treatment, or after a long period of treatment when a change occurs in their life. The key is to maintain communication channels so that if she chooses to discontinue she make contact with the clinician and discuss and possibly revise the regimen to achieve the clinical goal.

A number of barriers to counseling regarding continuance have been identified. These include a lack of available information concerning the risks and benefits (eg, lack of clinical trial data or conflicting data).

Decreased length of office visits is a trend in managed care, which may limit available clinician time for meeting educational and psychosocial needs. Creative approaches to education, including group support sessions, nurse counseling, printed material, suggested Web sites, and decision supports are additional resources for counseling. NAMS provides many educational materials that give assistance.

Some clinicians are unfamiliar with the variety of therapeutic regimens and how to use them if the initial one is unacceptable. Clinicians must continuously be informed about emerging data regarding medications, including complementary and alternative medicine therapies, to address specific therapeutic goals. NAMS offers a wide variety of provider educational materials and activities.

It is important to recognize that most data related to continuance are based on studies involving middle-class Caucasian women who live in the United States. Cultural experiences, education, and economics can affect women's health decisions. When caring for women of diverse cultural/ ethnic, educational, and/or economic backgrounds, it is vital to listen sensitively to the woman's preferences, goals, and perceptions. Written information may be particularly useful for diverse populations. (See also cross-cultural counseling on page 278.)

In summary, factors that increase the probability of continuance for the length of time to meet treatment goals include assessing the woman's goal in considering medication and ensuring active participation of the woman in the decision-making process. Continuance rates are greater when women have participated in the decision-making process and feel their expectations have been met, when the practitioner listens and respects their concerns, and when adequate information has been provided regarding their condition and therapeutic progress. Delivering instructions verbally and in writing reinforces continuance counseling.

Importance of listening and building trust

When providing health care for women at menopause and beyond, clinicians have many counseling responsibilities (see Table 7).

Listening and building trust are primary avenues toward fulfilling clinicians' counseling responsibilities. Actively listening to each woman's account of her menopause experience is significant to identify individual health beliefs, to motivate a change in behavior and level of commitment, to determine the best management approach, and to build trust in the therapeutic relationship.

Table 7. Clinician responsibilities
• Develop satisfactory clinical relationships through communication and listening.
• Provide all the information necessary for an informed decision.
• Provide unbiased, factual, and comprehensive information on the risks and benefits of any therapeutic initiative.
• Elicit and include the woman's preferences in any recommendations.
• Periodically evaluate treatment continuance and adjust the regimen as needed.
• Regardless of treatment continuance, the clinician still has ethical and legal responsibility. To fulfill this responsibility, the clinician must understand the woman's comprehension of the instructions and capacity to follow the instructions.

When counseling, consider the following suggestions:

• Put the woman at ease by ensuring as much privacy as possible during the interview. Use a concerned, friendly demeanor. Avoid taking phone calls.

• Maintain eye contact. This assures the woman that she is being heard and enables the provider to observe her expression. Don't look at your watch, glance toward the hallway, or interrupt the woman in midsentence. (Beware of cultural issues around eye contact, such as with American Indian women.)

• Encourage the woman to speak spontaneously through open-ended questions or reflective statements, and allow adequate time for her to respond. Listen carefully to the answer. Some research indicates that women who are heard first and have their emotions acknowledged are more likely to understand the information discussed.

• Avoid judgmental statements and questions, which may put the woman on the defensive and break down the lines of communication. Refrain from making social criticisms or allowing personal feelings of dislike or disapproval to interfere.

• Ask specific questions to clarify the woman's statements. Avoid closed-ended (ie, yes/no) questions, such as, "Do you understand the instructions?" Those types of questions do not elicit much information.

• Consider each woman as an individual. Don't assume that every woman will be influenced by the same information or motivators.

- Be aware of body language, both the woman's and your own.
- Ensure that the woman has personal control over her selection of treatment. Providing her with enough information for her to make an informed decision can help build a trusting relationship.
- Be sensitive to conversations about menopause, which may be viewed negatively by some women. Consider forming menopause discussion groups and forums for women to articulate their feelings about menopause with other women facing the same situation.
- Supplement verbal counseling with written instructions and take-home reading materials that can reinforce the message and allow the woman more time to absorb the information.
- Short words and sentences are easier to understand and facilitate learning. Avoid jargon and medical abbreviations that may be misunderstood.
- When explaining material, allow time for questions. Give reasons for important instructions.
- Be aware of (and avoid) perfunctory listening. This kind of listening is half-hearted and indifferent, and it does not convey the message of understanding that is necessary for a woman to feel as if she has been heard.
- Engage the woman in the treatment decision. Avoid counseling as if there were only one "right way." Shared decision making empowers the woman to take an active role in her health care. It may also reduce the risk of litigation if something goes wrong.
- Involve each woman in monitoring for adverse drug reactions and interactions. Knowing what to expect can enhance feelings of control over treatment and avoid potentially dangerous side effects.
- Schedule follow-up contacts either by phone or office visit. A woman who might not contact the provider with a question may be more apt to share her concerns if contacted by the office staff.
- Be attentive to financial factors associated with a treatment plan. A woman who will have difficulty paying for a medication is less likely to continue the treatment plan.
- Keep a list of available local and national resources.

A time of new beginnings

The menopause transition is a fact of life that will affect most women around the world. However, the physical and mental impact of this physiologic inevitability varies both within and across all cultures. There is no universal menopause experience. But, for all women, menopause can mark the beginning of an exciting new time of life.

Most postmenopausal women look back on the menopause experience as the beginning of many positive changes in their lives and, hopefully, their health. Yet in today's youth-obsessed society, a woman's perception of menopause can be influenced by many negative stereotypes—in the media, from friends, family, peers, and even healthcare professionals. Education and counseling can help dispel these myths and challenge outdated views.

In fact, a NAMS survey found that US women at midlife are divided in their opinions of menopause. Some considered it a medical condition requiring treatment, while others viewed it as a "natural transition that could be managed by natural means." Another survey found that women wanted more information about menopause, but that their major source of information was consumer magazines, not their healthcare providers. This survey also found that women have serious misunderstandings about their health risks after menopause.

Diversity in women, including social and cultural differences, can also apply to a woman's experience of menopause and her view of menopause treatments, as well as her overall health and well-being. Risk factors, patterns of disease and mortality, access to health care, economic status, existing medical therapies, and societal norms related to femininity and aging all differ across groups of women. There is very little research, however, on how these differences affect the experience of menopause. As discussed earlier, menopause research has focused mostly on middle-class Caucasian-American women. Although different populations are now being studied, considerable information is needed before many aspects of menopause are better understood.

As women experience the physical, emotional, and social changes of approaching menopause, each woman faces an opportunity to identify her own strategies for wellness. In fact, reaching menopause, whether natural or induced, is an ideal time to begin or reinforce a health promotion program that will provide benefits throughout the rest of the woman's life.

Each woman is the expert on her own body, and she benefits most if she is well informed. The primary message for a woman at this stage of life is that she can enjoy good health into old age provided she makes informed, responsible choices. The Mission of NAMS is to help in this process. Research continues—information keeps changing. The NAMS Web site (www.menopause.org) can be counted on as a reliable source of current information. ●

Suggested reading

Social and cultural aspects of care

Avis NE, Stellato R, Crawford S, et al. Is there a menopausal syndrome? Menopausal status and symptoms across racial/ethnic groups. *Soc Sci Med* 2001;52:345-356.

Bohannon AD. Osteoporosis and African American women. *J Womens Health* 1999;8:609-615.

Canadian Institute for Health Information. *Women's Health Surveillance Report: A Multi-dimensional Look at the Health of Canadian Women*. Ottawa, ON, Canada: Canadian Institute for Health Information, 2003.

Deeks AA. Psychological aspects of menopause management. *Best Pract Res Clin Endocrinol Metab* 2003;17:17-31.

Gold EB, Sternfeld B, Kelsey JL, et al. Relation of demographic and lifestyle factors to symptoms in a multi-racial/ethnic population of women 40-55 years of age. *Am J Epidemiol* 2000;152:463-473.

Gupta P, Sturdee DW, Hunter MS. Mid-aged health in women from the Indian subcontinent (MAHWIS): general health and the experience of menopause in women. *Climacteric* 2006;9:13-22.

Helenius IM, Korenstein D, Halm EA. Changing use of hormone therapy among minority women since the Women's Health Initiative. *Menopause* 2007;14:216-222.

Hunter M, Rendall M. Bio-psycho-socio-cultural perspectives on menopause. *Best Pract Res Clin Obstet Gynaecol* 2007;21:261-274.

MacLaren A, Woods NF. Midlife women making hormone therapy decisions. *Womens Health Issues* 2001;11:216-230.

Obermeyer CM. Cross-cultural perspectives on menopause. *Menopause* 2000;7:184-192.

Ramirez de Arellano A. Latino women: health status and access to health care. In: Falik M, Scott Collins K, eds. *Women's Health: The Commonwealth Fund Survey*. Baltimore, MD: Johns Hopkins University Press, 1996:123-144.

Sharps PW, Phillips J, Oguntimalide L, Sailing J, Yun S. Knowledge, attitudes, perceptions and practices of African-American women toward menopausal health. *J Natl Black Nurses Assoc* 2003;14:9-15.

Sommer B, Avis N, Meyer P, et al. Attitudes toward menopause and aging across ethnic/racial groups [erratum in: *Psychosom Med* 2000;62:96]. *Psychosom Med* 1999;61:868-875.

Statistics Canada, National Population Health Survey 1994-1995 and 2002-2003. Ottawa, ON, Canada: Statistics Canada, 1995-2003. Catalogue no. 82-F0001XCB; record no. 5003.

Utian W, Boggs P. The North American Menopause Society 1998 menopause survey. Part I: Postmenopausal women's perceptions about menopause and midlife. *Menopause* 1999;6:122-128.

Woods NF, Mitchell ES. Anticipating menopause: observations from the Seattle Midlife Women's Health Study. *Menopause* 1999;6:167-173.

Lesbian health

Bailey JV, Kavanagh J, Owen C, et al. Lesbians and cervical screening. *Br J Gen Pract* 2000;50:481-482.

Bonvicini KA, Perlin MJ. The same but different: clinician-patient communication with gay and lesbian patients. *Patient Educ Couns* 2003;51:115-122.

Case P, Austin SB, Hunter DJ, et al. Sexual orientation, health risk factors, and physical functioning in the Nurses' Health Study II. *J Womens Health* 2004;13:1033-1047.

Chu SY, Buehler JW, Fleming PL, et al. Epidemiology of reported cases of AIDS in lesbians, United States 1980-89. *Am J Public Health* 1990;80:1380-1381.

Christilaw JE, Davis V, Edwards C, et al. Society of Obstetricians and Gynaecologists of Canada clinical practice guidelines: lesbian health guidelines. *J SOGC* 2000;22:202-205.

Cochran SD, Mays VM, Bowen D, et al. Cancer-related risk indicators and preventive screening behaviors among lesbians and bisexual women. *Am J Public Health* 2001;91:591-597.

Cochran SD, Mays VM, Sullivan JG. Prevalence of mental disorders, psychological distress, and mental health services use among lesbian, gay, and bisexual adults in the United States. *J Consult Clin Psychol* 2003;71:53-61.

Diamant AL, Wold C. Sexual orientation and variation in physical and mental health status among women. *J Womens Health* 2003;12:41-49.

Dibble SL, Roberts SA, Nussey B. Comparing breast cancer risk between lesbians and their heterosexual sisters. *Womens Health Issues* 2004:14:60-68.

Dibble SL, Roberts SA, Robertson PA, Paul SM. Risk factors for ovarian cancer: lesbian and heterosexual women. *Oncol Nurs Forum* 2002;29:E1-E7.

Fethers K, Marks C, Mindel A, Estcourt CS. Sexually transmitted infections and risk behaviours in women who have sex with women. *Sex Transm Infect* 2000;76:345-349.

Gilman SE, Cochran SD, Mays VM, Hughes M, Ostrow D, Kessler RC. Risk of psychiatric disorders among individuals reporting same-sex sexual partners in the National Comorbidity Survey. *Am J Public Health* 2001;91:933-939.

Grushkin EP, Hart S, Gordon N, Ackerson L. Patterns of cigarette smoking and alcohol use among lesbians and bisexual women enrolled in a large health maintenance organization. *Am J Public Health* 2001;91:976-979.

Koh AS. Use of preventive health behaviors by lesbian, bisexual, and heterosexual women: questionnaire survey. *West J Med* 2000;172:379-384.

Marrazzo JM, Coffey P, Elliott MN. Sexual practices, risk perception and knowledge of sexually transmitted disease risk among lesbian and bisexual women. *Perspect Sex Reprod Health* 2005;37:6-12.

Marrazzo JM, Stine K. Reproductive health history of lesbians: implications for care. *Am J Obstet Gynecol* 2004;190:1298-1304.

Mays VM, Cochran SD. Mental health correlates of perceived discrimination among lesbian, gay, and bisexual adults in the United States. *Am J Public Health* 2001;91:1869-1876.

Price JH, Easton AN, Telljohann SK, Wallace PB. Perceptions of cervical cancer and Pap smear screening behavior by women's sexual orientation. *J Community Health* 1996;21:89-105.

Roberts SJ. Health care recommendations for lesbian women. *J Obstet Gynecol Neonatal Nurs* 2006;35:583-591.

Sandfort TG, de Graaf R, Bijl RV, Schnabel P. Same-sex sexual behavior and psychiatric disorders: findings from the Netherlands Mental Health Survey and Incidence Study (NEMESIS). *Arch Gen Psychiatry* 2001;58:85-91.

Skinner WF, Otis MD. Drug and alcohol use among lesbian and gay people in a southern US sample: epidemiological, comparative, and methodological findings from the Trilogy Project. *J Homosex* 1996;30:59-92.

Steele LS, Tinmouth JM, Lu A. Regular health care use by lesbians: a path analysis of predictive factors. *Fam Pract* 2006;23:631-636.

Valanis BG, Bowen DJ, Bassford T, Whitlock E, Charney P, Carter RA. Sexual orientation and health: comparisons in the Women's Health Initiative sample. *Arch Fam Med* 2000;9:843-853.

Lifestyle and behavior modification

Elford RW, MacMillan HL, Wathen CN, for the Canadian Task Force on Preventive Health Care. Counseling for risky health habits: a conceptual framework for primary care practitioners. Available at: http://www.ctfphc.org/Full_Text/Counseling_TR.htm. Accessed June 19, 2007.

Merzel C, D'Afflitti J. Reconsidering community-based health promotion: promise, performance, and potential. *Am J Public Health* 2003;93:557-574.

Minkler M, Schauffler H, Clements-Nolle K. Health promotion for older Americans in the 21st century. *Am J Health Promot* 2000;14:371-379.

Smedley BD, Syme SL, for the Committee on Capitalizing on Social Science and Behavioral Research to Improve the Public's Health. Promoting health: intervention strategies from social and behavioral research. *Am J Health Promot* 2001;15:149-166.

US Preventive Services Task Force. *Guide to Clinical Preventive Services*. 2005. Washington, DC: US Department of Health and Human Services, 2005.

Warren MP, Artacho CA, Hagey AR. Role of exercise and nutrition. In: Lobo RA, ed. *Treatment of the Postmenopausal Woman: Basic and Clinical Aspects*, 3rd ed. San Diego, CA: Academic Press, 2007:655-682.

Whitlock EP, Orleans CT, Pender N, Allan J. Evaluating primary care behavioral counseling interventions: an evidence-based approach. *Am J Prev Med* 2002;22:267-284.

Substance abuse

Centers for Disease Control and Prevention. Cigarette smoking among adults—United States, 2004. Available at: http://www.cdc.gov/mmwr/preview/mmwrhtml/mm5444a2.htm. Accessed June 19, 2007.

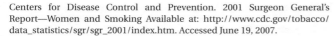

Centers for Disease Control and Prevention. 2001 Surgeon General's Report—Women and Smoking Available at: http://www.cdc.gov/tobacco/data_statistics/sgr/sgr_2001/index.htm. Accessed June 19, 2007.

Di Castelnuovo AD, Costanzo S, Bagnardi V, Donati MB, Iacoviello L, Gaetano G. Alcohol dosing and total mortality in men and women: an updated meta-analysis of 34 prospective studies. *Arch Intern Med* 2006;166:2437-2445.

Fiellin DA, Reid MC, O'Connor PG. Outpatient management of patients with alcohol problems. *Ann Intern Med* 2000;133:815-827.

Nides M, Oncken C, Gonzales D, et al. Smoking cessation with varenicline, a selective alpha4beta2 nicotinic receptor partial agonist: results from a 7-week, randomized, placebo- and bupropion-controlled trial with 1-year follow-up. *Arch Intern Med* 2006;166:1561-1568.

Novotny TE, Giovino GE. Tobacco use. In: Brownson RC, Remington PL, Davis JR, eds. *Chronic Disease Epidemiology and Control*, 2nd ed. Washington, DC: American Public Health Association, 1998:117-148.

Registered Nurses' Association of Ontario. *Integrating Smoking Cessation into Daily Nursing Practice*. Revised. Toronto, ON, Canada: Registered Nurses' Association of Ontario, 2007.

Single E, Robson L, Xie X, Rehm J. The economic costs of alcohol, tobacco and illicit drugs in Canada, 1992. *Addiction* 1998;93:991-1006.

Sorocco KH, Ferrell SW. Alcohol use among older adults. *J Gen Psychol* 2006;133:453-467.

US Department of Health and Human Services. *Report on Carcinogens*, 11th ed. Washington, DC: US Department of Health and Human Services, Public Health Service, National Toxicology Program, 2005.

Ustun B, Compton W, Mager D, et al. WHO Study on the reliability and validity of the alcohol and drug use disorder instruments: overview of methods and results [erratum in: *Drug Alcohol Depend* 1998;50:185-186]. *Drug Alcohol Depend* 1997;47:161-169.

Winger G, Woods JH, Hofmann FG, eds. *A Handbook on Drug and Alcohol Abuse: The Biomedical Aspects*, 4th ed. New York: Oxford University Press, 2004.

Zhang SM, Lee IM, Manson JE, Cook NR, Willett WC, Buring JE. Alcohol consumption and breast cancer risk in the Women's Health Study. *Am J Epidemiol* 2007;165:667-676.

Physical activity

American Heart Association Nutrition Committee, Lichtenstein A, Appel L, Brands M, et al. Diet and lifestyle recommendations revision 2006: a scientific statement from the American Heart Association Nutrition Committee. *Circulation* 2006;114:82-96.

Brockie J. Exercise for women in the early postmenopausal years. *J Br Menopause Soc* 2006;12:126-127.

McPherson R, Frohlich J, Fodor G, Genest J, for the Canadian Cardiovascular Society. Canadian Cardiovascular Society position statement—Recommendations for the diagnosis and treatment of dyslipidemia and prevention of cardiovascular disease [Erratum in: *Can J Cardiol* 2006;22:1077]. *Can J Cardiol* 2006;22:913-927.

National Institute for Health and Clinical Excellence (NICE). Four commonly used methods to increase physical activity: brief interventions in primary care, exercise referral schemes, pedometers and community based exercise programs for walking and cycling. 2006. Available at: http://www.nice.org.uk/page.aspx?o=PHI002&c=publichealth. Accessed June 19, 2007.

Taylor-Piliae RE, Haskell WL, Froelicher ES. Hemodynamic responses to a community-based Tai Chi exercise intervention in ethnic Chinese adults with cardiovascular disease risk factors. *Eur J Cardiovasc Nurs* 2006;5:165-174.

Stress

Barnes P, Powell-Griner E, McFann K, Nahin R. CDC Advance Data Report #343. Complementary and alternative medicine use among adults: United States, 2002. Available at: http://nccam.nih.gov/news/camstats.htm. Accessed June 19, 2007.

Hunter M, Rendall M. Bio-psycho-socio-cultural perspectives on menopause. *Best Pract Res Clin Obstet Gynaecol* 2007;21:261-274.

National Center for Complementary and Alternative Medicine. Mind-body medicine: An overview. Available at: http://nccam.nih.gov/health/backgrounds/mindbody.htm. Accessed June 19, 2007.

Weight and nutrition

American Heart Association Nutrition Committee, Lichtenstein AH, Appel LJ, Brands M, et al. Diet and lifestyle recommendations revision 2006: a scientific statement from the American Heart Association Nutrition Committee. *Circulation* 2006;114:82-96.

Appel LJ, Brands MW, Daniels SR, Karanja N, Elmer PJ, Sacks FM, for the American Heart Association. Dietary approaches to prevent and treat hypertension: a scientific statement from the American Heart Association. *Hypertension* 2006;47:296-308.

Buse J, Ginsberg HN, Bakris GL, et al, for the American Heart Association, American Diabetes Association. Primary prevention of cardiovascular disease in people with diabetes mellitus: a scientific statement from the American Heart Association and the American Diabetes Association. *Circulation* 2007;115:114-126.

Calle EE, Rodriguez C, Walker-Thurmond K, Thun MJ. Overweight, obesity, and mortality from cancer in a prospectively studied cohort of US adults. *N Engl J Med* 2003;348:1625-1638.

Dansinger ML, Gleason JA, Griffith JL, Selker HP, Schaefer EJ. Comparison of the Atkins, Ornish, Weight Watchers, and Zone diets for weight loss and heart disease risk reduction. *JAMA* 2005;293:43-53.

Drewnowski A, Warren-Mears VA. Does aging change nutrition requirements? *J Nutr Health Aging* 2001;5:70-74.

Gardner CD, Kiazand A, Alhassan S, et al. Comparison of the Atkins, Zone, Ornish, and LEARN diets for change in weight and related risk factors among overweight premenopausal women. The A to Z Weight Loss Study: a randomized trial. *JAMA* 2007;297:969-977.

Godfrey JR. Toward optimal health: Robert Kushner, M.D., offers a practical approach to assessment of overweight patients. *J Womens Health* 2006;15:991-995.

Health Canada. Eating well with Canada's food guide. 2007. Available at: http://www.hc-sc.gc.ca/fn-an/food-guide-aliment/index_e.html. Accessed September 6, 2007.

Kris-Etherton P, Eckel RH, Howard BV, St. Jeor S, Bazzarre TL, for the Nutrition Committee, Population Science Committee, and Clinical Science Committee of the American Heart Association. AHA science advisory: Lyon Diet Heart Study. Benefits of a Mediterranean-style diet. National Cholesterol Education Program/American Heart Association step I dietary pattern on cardiovascular disease. *Circulation* 2001;103:1823-1825.

Mann T, Tomiyama AJ, Westling E, Lew AM. Samuels B, Chatman J. Medicare's search for effective obesity treatments: diets are not the answer. *Am Psychol* 2007;62:220-233.

National Heart, Lung, and Blood Institute. Your guide to lowering your blood pressure with DASH. 1998; rev. 2006. Available at: http://www.nhlbi.nih.gov/health/public/heart/hbp/dash/new_dash.pdf. Accessed June 19, 2007.

National Women's Health Report. Women and obesity. *National Women's Health Report* 2006;28:1-4.

Obarzanek E, Sacks FM, Vollmer WM, et al, for the DASH Research Group. Effects on blood lipids of a blood pressure-lowering diet: the Dietary Approaches to Stop Hypertension (DASH) Trial. *Am J Clin Nutr* 2001;74:80-89.

Park HS, Lee KU. Postmenopausal women lose less visceral adipose tissue during a weight reduction program. *Menopause* 2003;10:222-227.

Ponnampalam EN, Mann NJ, Sinclair AJ. Effect of feeding systems on omega-3 fatty acids, conjugated linoleic acid and trans fatty acids in Australian beef cuts: potential impact on human health. *Asian Pac J Clin Nutr* 2006;15:21-29.

Sacks FM, Svetkey LP, Vollmer WM, et al, for the DASH-Sodium Collaborative Research Group. Effects on blood pressure of reduced dietary sodium and the Dietary Approaches to Stop Hypertension (DASH) diet. *N Engl J Med* 2001;344:3-10.

Snelling AM, Crespo CJ, Schaeffer M, Smith S, Walbourn L. Modifiable and nonmodifiable factors associated with osteoporosis in postmenopausal women: results from the Third National Health and Nutrition Examination Survey, 1988-1994. *J Womens Health Gend Based Med* 2001;10:57-65

Svetkey LP, Sacks FM, Obarzanek E, et al, for the DASH-Sodium Collaborative Research Group. The DASH Diet, Sodium Intake and Blood Pressure Trial (DASH-sodium): rationale and design. *J Am Diet Assoc* 1999;99(Suppl 8):96S-104S.

US Department of Health and Human Services, Office of Disease Prevention and Health Promotion Program. *Healthy People 2010.* Washington, DC: US Department of Health and Human Services, 2002. Available at: www.health. gov/healthypeople. Accessed July 2, 2007.

US Department of Health and Human Services and US Dept. of Agriculture. *Dietary Guidelines for Americans, 2005,* 6th ed. Washington, DC: US Government Printing Office, 2005. Available at: http://www.healthierus.gov/ dietaryguidelines. Accessed June 19, 2007.

US Preventive Services Task Force. Screening for obesity in adults: recommendations and rationale. *Ann Intern Med* 2003;139:930-932.

Abuse of women

Family Violence Prevention Fund. National Consensus Guidelines on Identifying and Responding to Domestic Violence Victimization in Health Care Settings. 2002. Available at http://endabuse.org/programs/healthcare/ files/Consensus.pdf. Accessed June 20, 2007.

Halpern KLR, Perciaccante VJ, Hayes C, et al. A protocol to diagnose intimate partner violence in the emergency department. *J Trauma* 2006;60:1101-1105.

Kahn A, Plummer D, Hussain R, Minichiello V. Sexual risk assessment in general practice: evidence from a New South Wales survey. *Sex Health* 2007;4:1-8.

MacMillan HL, Wathen CN, Jamieson E, et al. Approaches to screening for intimate partner violence in health care settings: a randomized trial. *JAMA* 2006;296:530-536.

Moracco KE, Runyan CW, Bowling JM, Earp JA. Women's experiences with violence: a national study. *Womens Health Issues* 2007;17:3-12.

Registered Nurses' Association of Ontario. Woman abuse: Screening, identification and initial response. Toronto, ON, Canada: Registered Nurses' Association of Ontario, 2005.

Treatment counseling

Akkuzu G, Eroğlu K. The effect of education and counseling services on compliance to therapy of women taking hormone therapy for the first time. *Menopause* 2005;12:763-773.

Anderson LA, Caplan LS, Buist DS, et al. Perceived barriers and recommendations concerning hormone replacement therapy counseling among primary care providers. *Menopause* 1999;6:161-166.

Berman RS, Epstein RS, Lydick EG. Risk factors associated with women's compliance with estrogen replacement therapy. *J Womens Health* 1997;6:219-226.

Burg MA, Fraser K, Gui S, et al, for the Florida Behavioral Health Research Consortium. Treatment of menopausal symptoms in family medicine settings following the Women's Health Initiative. *J Am Board Fam Med* 2006;19:122-131.

Cano A. Compliance to hormone replacement therapy in menopausal women controlled in a third level academic centre. *Maturitas* 1995;20:91-99.

Castelo-Branco C, Peralta S, Ferrer J, et al. The dilemma of menopause and hormone replacement—challenge for women and health-care providers: knowledge of menopause and hormone therapy in Spanish menopausal women. *Climacteric* 2006;9:380-387.

Connelly MT, Rusinak D, Livingston W, Raeke L, Inui T. Patient knowledge about hormone replacement therapy: implications for treatment. *Menopause* 2000;7:266-272.

Coulter A. Patient-centered decision making: empowering women to make informed choices. *Womens Health Issues* 2001;11:325-330.

Ettinger B, Grady D, Tosteson AN, Pressman A, Macer JL. Effect of the Women's Health Initiative on women's decisions to discontinue postmenopausal hormone therapy. *Obstet Gynecol* 2003;102:1225-1232.

Ettinger B, Woods NF, Barrett-Connor E, Pressman A. The North American Menopause Society 1998 Menopause Survey: Part II. Counseling about hormone replacement therapy: association with socioeconomic status and access to medical care. *Menopause* 2000;7:143-148.

Faulkner DL, Young C, Hutchins D, et al. Patient noncompliance with hormone replacement therapy: a nationwide estimate using a large prescription claims database. *Menopause* 1998;5:226-229.

Hersh AL, Stefanick ML, Stafford RS. National use of postmenopausal hormone therapy: annual trends and response to recent evidence. *JAMA* 2004;291:47-53.

Hing E, Brett KM. Changes in US prescribing patterns of menopause hormone therapy, 2001-2003. *Obstet Gynecol* 2006;108:33-40.

Jacobs Institute of Women's Health Expert Panel on Menopause Counseling. *Guidelines for Counseling Women on the Management of Menopause.* Washington, DC: Jacobs Institute of Women's Health, 2000.

Kaufert P, Boggs PP, Ettinger B, Woods NF, Utian WH. Women and menopause: beliefs, attitudes, and behaviors: The North American Menopause Society 1997 menopause survey. *Menopause* 1998;5:197-202.

Kroll J, Rothert M, Davidson WS, et al. Predictors of participation in health care at menopause. *Health Commun* 2000;12:339-360.

MacLaren A, Woods NF. Midlife women making hormone therapy decisions. *Womens Health Issues* 2001;11:216-230.

Motheral BR, Fairman KA. Patient education programs and continuance with estrogen replacement therapy: evaluation of the Women's Health Exchange. *Menopause* 1998;5:35-42.

Ness J, Aronow WS. Prevalence and causes of persistent use of hormone replacement therapy among postmenopausal women: a follow-up study. *Am J Ther* 2006;13:109-112.

The North American Menopause Society. Achieving long-term continuance of menopausal ET/EPT: consensus opinion of The North American Menopause Society. *Menopause* 1998;5:69-76.

Reynolds RF, Obermeyer CM, Walker AM, Guilbert D. Side effects and sociobehavioral factors associated with the discontinuation of hormone therapy in a Massachusetts health maintenance organization. *Menopause* 2001;8:189-199.

Reynolds RF, Walker AM, Obermeyer CM, Rahman O, Guilbert D. Discontinuation of postmenopausal hormone therapy in a Massachusetts HMO. *J Clin Epidemiol* 2001;54:1056-1064.

Sharps PW, Phillips J, Oguntamalide L, Saling J, Yun S. Knowledge, attitudes, perceptions and practices of African-American women toward menopausal health. *J Natl Black Nurses Assoc* 2003;14:9-15.

Simon JA, Wysocki S, Brandman MS, Axelsen K. A comparison of therapy continuation rates of different hormone replacement agents: a 9 month retrospective, longitudinal analysis of pharmacy claims among new users. *Menopause* 2003;10:37-44.

Utian WH, Boggs PP. The North American Menopause Society 1998 Menopause Survey. Part I: postmenopausal women's perceptions about menopause and midlife. *Menopause* 1999;6:122-128.

White VE, Bennett L, Raffin S, Emmett K, Coleman MJ. Use of unopposed estrogen in women with uteri: prevalence, clinical implications, and economic consequences. *Menopause* 2000;7:123-128.

Zhang P, Tho G, Anderson LA. Prevalence of and factors associated with hormone replacement therapy counseling: results from the 1994 National Health Interview Survey. *Am J Public Health* 1999;89:1575-1577.

Importance of listening and building trust

Anderson LA, Caplan LS, Buist DS, et al. Perceived barriers and recommendations concerning hormone replacement therapy counseling among primary care providers. *Menopause* 1999;6:161-166.

Boggs PP. Telling isn't teaching: tips for optimal clinician-patient communication. *Menopause Management* 1998;7:13-21.

Jacobs Institute of Women's Health, Expert Panel on Menopause Counseling. *Guidelines for Counseling Women on the Management of Menopause.* Washington, DC: Jacobs Institute of Women's Health, 2000.

Kaufert P, Boggs PP, Ettinger B, Woods NF, Utian WH. Women and menopause: beliefs, attitudes, and behaviors: The North American Menopause Society 1997 menopause survey. *Menopause* 1998;5:197-202.

Nichols MP. *The Lost Art of Listening.* New York: Guildford Press, 1995.

Utian WH, Boggs PP. The North American Menopause Society 1998 menopause survey. Part I: Postmenopausal women's perceptions about menopause and midlife. *Menopause* 1999;6:122-128.

Woods NF. Midlife women health care patterns and choices. In: Falik M, Collins K, eds. *Women's Health: The Commonwealth Fund Survey.* Baltimore, MD: Johns Hopkins Press, 1996:145-174.

Anemia, iron deficiency, 34, 247–248
Angeliq, 210t
Angina, 71, 195
Angiotensin II receptor blockers (ARBs), 133, 135, 137
Angiotensin-converting enzyme (ACE), 72
Angiotensin-converting enzyme (ACE) inhibitors, 135, 137
Anovulation, 22
Anovulatory bleeding, 31
Antacids, 39–40
Antiandrogens
    for androgenic alopecia, 77
    for hirsutism, 78
Antibiotics, for pyometra, 34
Anticholinergic medications, 63t, 64, 65t
Anticoagulants, 243, 250, 263–264, 264t
Anticonvulsants. See also specific drugs
    for epilepsy, 160–161
    interaction with hormonal contraceptives, 32, 160–161
    for migraine prophylaxis, 44
    osteoporosis induced by, 161
    for vulvodynia, 56
Antidepressants. See also specific drugs and classes
    for depression, 49, 51
    estrogen potentiation of, 50
    for hot flashes, 39
        combined with gabapentin, 40
    for migraine prophylaxis, 44
    for premenstrual dysphoric disorder, 49
    prophylaxis for tension-type headache, 44
    for vulvodynia, 56
Antiepileptic drugs. See Anticonvulsants
Antihypertensive therapy, 133
    for diabetic patients, 137
    for glaucoma, 79
Anti-Müllerian hormone (AMH), 21
Antioxidants
    cognitive function and, 243
    in prevention of cardiovascular disease or cancer, 131, 243–244
Antithrombin III, 72
Antithyroid drugs, 160
Anxiety, 47–48, 280
Apo-imipramine, for urge incontinence, 63t
Appetite suppressants, 70
AR (attributable risk/absolute risk), 16
Arava (leflunomide), for rheumatoid arthritis, 81
ARBs (angiotensin II receptor blockers), 133, 135, 137
Aricept (donepezil), for Alzheimer's disease, 46
Aromatase inhibitors
    endometrial cancer and, 147
    to reduce breast cancer risk, 146
    vaginal effects of, 52
Arrhythmias, 71, 72
Arthralgia, 81–82
Arthritis, 80–81
    osteoarthritis, 80–81
    rheumatoid, 81
Ascorbic acid, 240
    cardiovascular disease and, 131
    food sources of, 240
    recommended intake of, 238t, 240
    supplementation of, 240
    toxicity of, 240
Aspirin
    gastrointestinal bleeding induced by, 132
    for migraine, 44

for prevention of cardiovascular events, 132
    in diabetic patients, 137
    to reduce colorectal cancer risk, 154
    for tension-type headache, 44
Assisted reproductive technologies, 29, 30, 108
Asthma, 161
Astroglide, 252
ATA (American Thyroid Association), 159, 160
Atherosclerosis. See also Coronary heart disease
    diabetes mellitus and, 133
    hypercholesterolemia and, 132
    testing for, 195
Atkins diet, 262
ATP III (Expert Panel on Detection, Evaluation, and Treatment of High Blood Cholesterol in Adults), 129, 130, 130t, 131, 133, 195
Attitudes about menopause and aging, 9–10, 278, 293
Attributable risk (AR), 16
AUB. See Abnormal uterine bleeding
Audiometric testing, 80
Auditory examination, 189
Australian Therapeutic Goods Authority, 268
AutoCyte Prep, for cervical cancer screening, 150
Autoimmune disorders, premature menopause and, 106
Avage (tazarotene), for photoaging, 75
Aygestin, 213t
Ayurvedic medicine, 260

B

Back pain, 117–118
    due to osteoporotic vertebral fracture, 117
        management of, 128
Bacterial vaginosis (BV), 156–157, 196, 280
Bacteriuria, asymptomatic, 66
Bannayan-Riley-Ruvalcaba syndrome, 144
Bariatric surgery, 70–71
Barium enema, 154, 154t, 190
Barrier contraceptive methods, 30
Bartholin's gland cyst, 53, 56
Bartholin's gland infection, 52, 53
Basal cell carcinoma, 155–156
Bazedoxifene, 125
BCDDP (Breast Cancer Detection Demonstration Project), 141, 151
Beaver Dam Eye Study, 79
Beck Depression Inventory, 50
Behavioral counseling, 281–282
Behavioral therapies
    for sleep disturbances, 41–42
    for urinary incontinence, 63t
Bellergal (phenobarbital, ergotamine tartrate, and belladonna alkaloids), for hot flashes, 40
Benzodiazepines, for sleep disturbances, 42
Beta-blockers
    for cardiovascular disease, 135
    for hypertension, 133
    for migraine prophylaxis, 44
Beta-carotene, 131, 244
BHT (bioidentical hormone therapy), 217–218
Biochanin A, 264
Biofeedback, 261
    for tension-type headache, 44
    for vulvodynia, 56
Bioidentical hormone therapy (BHT), 217–218
Bisexual women, 156
Bisphosphonates, for osteoporosis, 119, 120–125, 120t
    adverse effects of, 123–124

FSH. *See* Follicle-stimulating hormone

G
Gabapentin (Neurontin), 161
  adverse effects of, 39, 40
  for hot flashes, 39–40, 161
    combined with antidepressants, 40
  interaction with antacids, 39–40
  for vulvodynia, 56
GAIT (Glucosamine/chondroitin Arthritis Intervention Trial), 252
Galactosemia, 103
Galantamine (Razadyne; Reminyl), for Alzheimer's disease, 46
Gallbladder disease, 136, 161–162, 187
Gardasil (human papillomavirus vaccine), 139, 150–151
Garlic, 264
Gastrointestinal effects
  of S-adenosyl methionine, 252
  of antidepressants, 39
  aspirin-induced bleeding, 132
  of bisphosphonates, 123–124
  of black cohosh, 268
  of calcium supplements, 247
  of chemotherapy agents, 108
  of clonidine, 40
  of estrogen-progestin oral contraceptives, 39
  of menopausal hormone therapy, 219
Genetic factors/disorders
  age at menopause and, 19, 19t
  bone loss due to, 117t
  bone mineral density and, 114
  breast cancer risk and, 140, 143, 144, 146
  colorectal cancer and, 153
  metabolic syndrome and, 129
  ovarian cancer risk and, 140, 151
  premature ovarian failure and, 103
Genistein, 264
Genital herpes, 157, 196
Genital warts, 53, 56–57
German chamomile, 43
Gestational carriers, 29
Gestodene, 213
GFR (glomerular filtration rate), in diabetes, 137
Ginger, 264
Gingivitis, 73
Ginkgo biloba, 46, 264, 269
Ginseng, 38, 264, 269–270
Glaucoma, 79
Glomerular filtration rate (GFR), in diabetes, 137
Glucocorticoids, 24, 116
Glucosamine, 81, 251–252
Glucosamine/chondroitin Arthritis Intervention Trial (GAIT), 252
Glucose dysregulation, 129
Glucose screening, 136–137, 195
Glycated hemoglobin (HbA1C) level, 134, 136, 138
Glycitein, 264
GnRH. *See* Gonadotropin-releasing hormone
GOG (Gynecologic Oncology Group), 147
Goiter, 160
Gonadotropin-releasing hormone (GnRH), 23–24
Gonadotropin-releasing hormone (GnRH) agonists
  for abnormal uterine bleeding, 34
  for chronic pelvic pain, 68
  temporary amenorrhea induced by, 103
Gonorrhea, 157, 196
GPR30, 25

Graves' disease, 159–160
Greene Climacteric Scale, 183, 184
Gynecologic Cancer Foundation, 151, 152
Gynecologic history, 183
Gynecologic Oncology Group (GOG), 147

H
Hair changes, 76–78
  androgenic alopecia and hair thinning, 76–77
  chemotherapy-induced hair loss, 108
  hirsutism, 76, 77–78
HbA1C (glycated hemoglobin) level, 134, 136, 138
HBV (hepatitis B virus) infection, 82, 157, 196
HBV (hepatitis B virus) vaccine, 139, 157
hCG (human chorionic gonadotropin), 24
HDL-C. *See* High-density lipoprotein cholesterol
Headache, 43–45
  causes of, 43–44
    role of hormones, 43–44
  cluster, 43, 45
  drug-induced
    antidepressant withdrawal, 39
    clonidine patch, 40
    estrogen-progestin oral contraceptives, 39
    menopausal hormone therapy, 219t, 220t
  management of, 44–45
  migraine, 43, 44–45
  serious conditions indicated by, 43
  tension-type, 43, 44
Headache diary, 43
Healing touch, 262
Health Canada, 135, 238, 268
Health Outcomes and Reduced Incidence with Zoledronic Acid Once Yearly (HORIZON) Pivotal Fracture Trial, 123
Health status, 9, 183
Hearing impairment, 80, 189
Heart and Estrogen/progestin Replacement Study (HERS), 134, 135, 138, 161, 217, 220, 221
Heart disease. *See* Cardiovascular disease
Heart Outcomes Prevention Evaluation (HOPE), 243
Heart Protection Study Collaborative Group, 243–244
Heart rate, during hot flashes, 35, 72
Height, 186
  loss of, 117, 118, 186
  measurement of, 186
Hemangiomas, 155
Hematometra, 32, 34
Hematuria, 189
Hepatitis B virus (HBV) infection, 82, 157, 196
Hepatitis B virus (HBV) vaccine, 139, 157
Her Option, 35
Herbal therapies, 237, 262–264, 267–272. *See also specific herbs*
  administration of, 263
  adverse effects of, 263, 267
  counseling about use of, 289–290
  for depression, 49
  drug interactions with, 263–264
  history of, 263
  for hot flashes, 38
  regulation of, 263, 267
  safety and efficacy of, 263, 267
  for sleep disturbances, 43
  in Traditional Chinese Medicine, 38, 259–260
  for weight reduction, 70
Hereditary nonpolyposis colorectal cancer (HNPCC), 151, 153

Notes

Designated activity:
Menopause Practice: A Clinician's Guide, 3rd Edition

The North American Menopause Society (NAMS) is accredited by the Accreditation Council for Continuing Medical Education (ACCME) to provide continuing medical education for physicians. NAMS designates this educational activity for a maximum of 25 *AMA PRA Category 1 Credits*™. Physicians should only claim credit commensurate with the extent of their participation in the activity.

To receive CME credit, please read this textbook, then answer the following questions on the Answer Sheet found on page 334. No administrative fee is required. Credit can be awarded only if returned to NAMS before the expiration date of October 31, 2009 (see page 3 for more).

Section A

1. Which of the following types of studies is <u>not</u> considered an experimental study?
   ___ A. randomized controlled trial
   ___ B. case-control study
   ___ C. crossover trial

2. Which of the following statements is correct?
   ___ A. An exposure's relative risk of less than 2.0 suggests that it lowers risk.
   ___ B. If a study is statistically significant, it will be clinically significant.
   ___ C. Absolute risk provides a measure of an exposure's public health impact.

3. Which of the following statements is correct?
   ___ A. The average age of natural menopause in the Western world is 50 years.
   ___ B. Early menopause is defined by NAMS as menopause reached at or under age 45.
   ___ C. Premature menopause is defined by NAMS as menopause reached under age 40.

Section B

4. Which of the following factors is <u>not</u> associated with influencing age of natural menopause?
   ___ A. lifetime history of major depression
   ___ B. epilepsy
   ___ C. type 2 diabetes mellitus

5. Which of the following factors is associated with delaying natural menopause?
   ___ A. prior use of oral contraceptives
   ___ B. nulliparity
   ___ C. alcohol consumption

6. Which of the following statements is true?
   ___ A. During the menstrual cycle, inhibin B levels are low for most of the follicular phase, then rise in midcycle, subsequently falling and then rising again to reach the highest levels during the luteal phase.
   ___ B. Most follicular loss results from ovulation.
   ___ C. During the menopause transition, progesterone is often lower than in normal-cycling women, even during ovulatory cycles.

7. Classic endocrine findings during postmenopause include which of the following?
   ___ A. levels of FSH greater than levels of LH
   ___ B. estradiol becomes the predominant circulating estrogen
   ___ C. increased levels of progesterone

8. Which of the following statements is <u>not</u> true?
   ___ A. Smoking is associated with decreased adrenal androgens.
   ___ B. Cortisol and ACTH levels rise with increasing age.
   ___ C. Progesterone receptor-β dominates the breast.

Section C

9. Which of the following statements is true?
   ___ A. Fertility declines significantly in women around age 35 to 38.
   ___ B. Maternal age of 45 is associated with a 25% increased risk for spontaneous miscarriage.
   ___ C. Tubal ligation has a failure rate of about 15 per 1,000.

10. The definition of metrorrhagia is:
   ___ A. uterine bleeding that occurs every 21 days or less.
   ___ B. frequent uterine bleeding that occurs between periods.
   ___ C. prolonged or excessive uterine bleeding.

11. Which of the following conditions is associated with menorrhagia?
____ A. hypothyroidism
____ B. hyperthyroidism
____ C. hyperprolactinemia

12. Which of the following herbal therapies does NAMS not recommend for hot flash relief?
____ A. black cohosh
____ B. evening primrose oil
____ C. isoflavones

13. Which of the following is among the most common causes of vulvar pruritis?
____ A. lichen sclerosus
____ B. vulvodynia
____ C. lichen planus

14. Which of the following statements is true about androgen production in women?
____ A. Bilateral oophorectomy decreases circulating levels of testosterone by 75%.
____ B. Androgen depletion is seen with Addison's disease.
____ C. High androgen concentration occurs in women with advanced cancer.

15. Which of the following statements is true about oral health after menopause?
____ A. For each 1% per year decrease in whole-body BMD, the risk for tooth loss almost doubles.
____ B. Hormone receptors are found in basal and spinous layers of the epithelium and connective tissue of the gingiva.
____ C. Burning mouth syndrome is localized to the tongue and/or lips.

16. Which of the following statements is true about hair loss?
____ A. In women, thinning of the hair begins between the ages of 12 and 40 years.
____ B. Alopecia occurs more often in men than women.
____ C. Finasteride is effective in treating hair loss in women.

Section D

17. Which of the following is not a known cause of premature ovarian failure?
____ A. mumps parotitis
____ B. uterine artery embolization for uterine fibroids
____ C. smoking

18. Among the following tests, which is not routinely recommended for women with premature ovarian failure?
____ A. progestogen-withdrawal challenge test
____ B. FSH, LH, and estradiol measurements on at least two occasions
____ C. karyotype when under age 40 and have short stature

19. Which of the following types of menopause is associated with more intense menopause symptoms?
____ A. premature spontaneous menopause
____ B. high-dose pelvic radiation–induced menopause
____ C. chemotherapy-induced menopause

20. Which of the following cancer treatments is most likely to result in subsequent resumption of fertility in a 42-year-old premenopausal woman?
____ A. chemotherapy with an alkylating agent
____ B. radiation therapy for cervical cancer
____ C. radiation therapy for Hodgkin's disease

Section E

21. Which of the following T-scores defines osteoporosis, according to World Health Organization criteria?
____ A. below or equal to –2.5
____ B. below or equal to –1.5
____ C. between –2.0 and –2.5

22. NAMS recommends measuring BMD in which of the following populations?
____ A. postmenopausal women >55 years with medical causes of bone loss
____ B. postmenopausal women ≥65 years
____ C. postmenopausal women ≥65 years with one additional risk factor

23. Which of the following systolic blood pressure levels (in mm Hg) is classified by the JNC 7 guidelines as prehypertension?
____ A. 115-120
____ B. 140-159
____ C. 120-139

24. Which of the following statements is true?
____ A. The American Heart Association encourages limiting alcohol consumption to no more than two drinks per day.
____ B. Light to moderate use of alcohol lowers cardiovascular mortality among women over age 50.
____ C. Over five drinks per week may increase risk of hypertension.

25. Which of the following is a potential risk factor for breast cancer?
    ____ A. history of breast cancer in a father
    ____ B. having the first child after age 25
    ____ C. menarche below age 15

26. Which of the following is associated with a reduction in breast density?
    ____ A. increasing age
    ____ B. use of estrogen therapy
    ____ C. use of estrogen-progestogen therapy

27. Which of the following cancer risks is not increased with smoking?
    ____ A. colorectal cancer
    ____ B. cervical cancer
    ____ C. endometrial cancer

Section F

28. Which of the following is not a validated instrument for measuring health-related quality of life in peri- and postmenopausal women?
    ____ A. Kupperman Index
    ____ B. Greene Climacteric Scale
    ____ C. Short Form-36 Health Survey

29. Which of the following hormonal evaluations does NAMS recommend for perimenopausal women?
    ____ A. salivary estrogen
    ____ B. inhibin B
    ____ C. thyroid-stimulating hormone

30. According to the National Institutes of Health, which of the following BMI values (in kg/m^2) is classified as "normal weight" for women?
    ____ A. 24.0
    ____ B. 25.5
    ____ C. 26.5

31. Which of the following is not recommended by NAMS for all women over age 40?
    ____ A. yearly clinical breast examination
    ____ B. annual pelvic examination regardless of whether the woman is sexually active
    ____ C. fecal occult blood test with stool sample obtained in office

Section G

32. Which of the following is the most common side effect of transdermal estrogen therapy?
    ____ A. irritation at the patch application site
    ____ B. headaches
    ____ C. mood swings

33. When comparing the incidence of endometrial hyperplasia with use of various estrogen progestogen (EPT) regimens, which of the following is true?
    ____ A. Cyclic EPT regimens provide more protection than continuous-combined regimens.
    ____ B. Progestins provide more endometrial protection than progesterone.
    ____ C. Continuous EPT regimens provide protection similar to cyclic regimens.

34. What is the brand name of the only oral intermittent-combined regimen of estrogen-progestin approved by the FDA?
    ____ A. Angeliq
    ____ B. Prefest
    ____ C. Estalis

35. What is the most biologically active human estrogen?
    ____ A. estradiol
    ____ B. estrone
    ____ C. estriol

36. Which of the following oral contraceptives is also FDA approved for the treatment of symptoms of premenstrual dysphoric disorder?
    ____ A. Seasonale
    ____ B. Yaz
    ____ C. Cyclessa

Section H

37. In the United States, dietary supplement marketers can make health claims without providing documentation for efficacy and safety for which of the following conditions?
    ____ A. hot flashes
    ____ B. osteoporosis
    ____ C. depression

38. Which of the following statements about vitamin D is not correct?
    ____ A. 2007 guidelines from the National Osteo-porosis Foundation recommend 800 to 1000 IU/day of vitamin D for adults age 50 and over.
    ____ B. Vitamin D_2 is more effective than vitamin D_3 for treating vitamin D deficiency.
    ____ C. Wearing a sunscreen with a sun protection factor of 8 or more blocks the skin's ability to produce vitamin D by 95%.

39. Absorbability of calcium in a supplement is most closely associated with which of the following?
    ____ A. formulation of supplement
    ____ B. type of calcium salt
    ____ C. taking less than 400 mg at one time

40. Which of the following supplements is contraindicated for a woman with seafood allergies?

    ____ A. SAM-e

    ____ B. glucosamine

    ____ C. coenzyme Q10

Section I

41. Which of the following treatments has <u>not</u> been approved by the FDA for at least one health indication?

    ____ A. acupuncture

    ____ B. soy protein

    ____ C. black cohosh

42. Good evidence supports that soy and soy isoflavones:

    ____ A. are not safe for breast cancer survivors.

    ____ B. provide benefits in the prevention of post-menopausal bone loss.

    ____ C. may have small benefits in the treatment of vasomotor symptoms in the short term.

43. Which of the following herbs has been shown to increase the anticoagulant effect of warfarin?

    ____ A. ginkgo

    ____ B. ginseng

    ____ C. vitex

Section J

44. Research has found that after women stopped smoking, which of the following occurred?

    ____ A. One third of the excess risk for CHD was eliminated within 1 year.

    ____ B. After 5 years, the excess risk for CHD approached that of women who never smoked.

    ____ C. After 10-14 years, the excess risk for total mortality approached that of women who never smoked.

45. Studies have found that women who smoke cigarettes:

    ____ A. have an increased risk of periodontitis.

    ____ B. experience more hot flashes than non-smokers, but this risk does not increase with the amount smoked.

    ____ C. experience fewer hot flashes when they stop smoking.

Menopause Practice: A Clinician's Guide, 3rd Edition
Answer Sheet

Please circle the correct answers:

1.	A	B	C	13.	A	B	C	24.	A	B	C	35.	A	B	C
2.	A	B	C	14.	A	B	C	25.	A	B	C	36.	A	B	C
3.	A	B	C	15.	A	B	C	26.	A	B	C	37.	A	B	C
4.	A	B	C	16.	A	B	C	27.	A	B	C	38.	A	B	C
5.	A	B	C	17.	A	B	C	28.	A	B	C	39.	A	B	C
6.	A	B	C	18.	A	B	C	29.	A	B	C	40.	A	B	C
7.	A	B	C	19.	A	B	C	30.	A	B	C	41.	A	B	C
8.	A	B	C	20.	A	B	C	31.	A	B	C	42.	A	B	C
9.	A	B	C	21.	A	B	C	32.	A	B	C	43.	A	B	C
10.	A	B	C	22.	A	B	C	33.	A	B	C	44.	A	B	C
11.	A	B	C	23.	A	B	C	34.	A	B	C	45.	A	B	C
12.	A	B	C												

Post-Test Evaluation

Your evaluation of this CME activity will help NAMS plan future educational offerings. Please answer the following questions by circling your response:

A. Were the stated learning objectives met?   Yes   No

B. Was the topic of this activity relevant and valuable to your practice?   Yes   No

C. Will this activity lead you to modify your clinical practice?   Yes   No

D. Was this activity fair, balanced, and free of commercial bias?   Yes   No

To Apply for CME Credit

To receive credit for this activity, this page must be completed, then faxed or postmarked by the activity's expiration date of October 31, 2009. There is no administrative charge. Mail or fax a copy of this completed form to:

The North American Menopause Society
Post Office Box 94527
Cleveland, OH 44101, USA
Fax: 440/442-2660

Keep a copy for your file. Each participant will receive a confidential report of his/her results along with the correct answer to each question. A certificate of credit will be sent to those who successfully complete the examination.

Name (please print) _____

Address _____

City_____

State/Province_____ Zip/Country Code_____ Country_____

Telephone_____ Fax _____ E-Mail _____